Medical Disorders
in Obstetric Practice

Medical Disorders in Obstetric Practice

EDITED BY

Michael de Swiet

MD FRCP
Consultant Physician, Queen Charlotte's
Hospital for Women: Senior Lecturer,
Department of Paediatrics, Cardiothoracic
Institute, Brompton Hospital, London; and
Honorary Consultant Physician, University
College Hospital, London

Blackwell Scientific Publications

OXFORD LONDON EDINBURGH

BOSTON PALO ALTO MELBOURNE

© 1984 by Blackwell Scientific
Publications
Editorial offices:
Osney Mead, Oxford, OX2 0EL
8 John Street, London, WC1N 2ES
23 Ainslie Place, Edinburgh EH3 6AJ
52 Beacon Street, Boston
    Massachusetts 02108, USA
667 Lytton Avenue, Palo Alto
    California 94301, USA
107 Barry Street, Carlton
    Victoria 3053, Australia

First published 1984
Reprinted 1986

Set and printed by
The Alden Press Ltd, Oxford
and bound by William Clowes Ltd, Beccles

DISTRIBUTORS

USA
    Blackwell Mosby Book Distributors
    11830 Westline Industrial Drive
    St Louis, Missouri 63141

Canada
    The C. V. Mosby Company
    5240 Finch Avenue East,
    Scarborough, Ontario

Australia
    Blackwell Scientific Book Distributors
        (Australia) Pty Ltd
    107 Barry Street
    Carlton, Victoria 3053

British Library
Cataloguing in Publication Data

Medical disorders in obstetric practice.
    1. Pregnancy. Complications of
    I. De Swiet, M
    618.3   RG571

ISBN 0-632-00876-8

Contents

List of Contributors

RICHARD BEARD MD, FRCOG, Professor, Department of Obstetrics and Gynaecology, St Mary's Hospital Medical School, London.

VINTON CHADWICK MD, FRCP, Senior Lecturer & Honorary Physician, Royal Postgraduate Medical School, The Hammersmith Hospital, London.

JOHN DAVISON BSc, MD, MSc, MRCOG, Consultant Obstetrician, Medical Research Council Human Reproduction Group, Princess Mary Maternity Hospital, Newcastle upon Tyne.

MICHAEL DE SWIET MD, FRCP, Consultant Physician, Queen Charlotte's Hospital for Women, and Senior Lecturer, Cardiothroacic Institute, Brompton Hospital, London.

ELIZABETH FAGAN BSc, MBBS, MSc, MRCP, Lecturer, Honorary Senior Registrar, Liver Unit, King's College Hospital, London.

ANTHONY HOPKINS MD, FRCP, Physician-in-Charge, Department of Neurological Sciences, St Bartholomew's Hospital, London.

ROSALINDE HURLEY MD, FRCPath, Professor of Microbiology, Institute of Obstetrics and Gynaecology, Queen Charlotte's Maternity Hospital, London.

ELIZABETH LETSKY MB, BS, MRCPath, Consultant Haematologist, Queen Charlotte's Hospital for Women, London.

IAN RAMSAY MD, FRCP, MRCPE, Consultant Physician, Department of Endocrinology, North Middlesex Hospital, London.

CHRISTOPHER REDMAN MB, BChir, FRCP, Lecturer in Obstetric Medicine, Nuffield Department of Obstetrics and Gynaecology, The John Radcliffe Hospital, Oxford.

BARRY WALTERS FRACP, Senior Registrar in Obstetric Medicine, Institute of Obstetrics and Gynaecology, Queen Charlotte's Maternity Hospital, London.

Preface

This book has been produced to replace *Medical Disorders in Obstetric Practice* which was written by my predecessor, as Consultant Physician at Queen Charlotte's Maternity Hospital, Cyril Barnes. In many ways Cyril Barnes established the subspecialty of obstetric medicine in Great Britain. Some would argue that obstetric medicine is not a subspecialty at all; that the already established subspecialties, such as cardiology and haematology, embrace a sufficient body of knowledge to deal adequately with all medical complications of pregnancy. I disagree. The physiology of the pregnant woman is so altered, and the constraint of the welfare of the fetus is so important, that subspecialists who can oversee the two widely different fields of obstetrics and medicine are needed.

Barnes' text was a model of clarity, and a tribute to his considerable clinical experience. I hope that with this book, we have been able to continue in the tradition of my predecessor. In particular, I hope that the obstetrician who may not always have optimal medical support, will find practical answers to his medical problems here. In addition, this is now a multi-author book, and we have tried to include the latest advances in a very rapidly progressing subject.

M. de Swiet
Queen Charlotte's
Maternity Hospital,
London

Acknowledgements

I am most grateful to my co-authors for the hard work that they have freely given in writing their chapters. I would also like to thank my clinical colleagues at Queen Charlotte's Maternity Hospital for referring me patients and thus giving me the clinical experience that is so necessary to write and edit a book such as this. Many medical complications of pregnancy are not common; for the same reason, I therefore wish to thank other colleagues both in the United Kingdom and overseas, who have discussed the problems of their patients with me.

Much of the work involved in preparing this book was done while I was visiting professor at Queen Victoria Medical Centre, Monash University in Melbourne. I am deeply grateful to Professor William Walters and Professor Michael Adamson for inviting me to Monash and making this time available to me. In addition, Georgina Going, librarian at the Institute of Obstetrics and Gynaecology, Queen Charlotte's Maternity Hospital and the University and Hospital librarians at the Queen Victoria Medical Centre gave invaluable help. Jony Russell and his colleagues at Blackwell Scientific Publications have been quite exceptional in the assistance that they have given me.

The following colleagues kindly read various chapters of the book, and otherwise gave invaluable information: Dr John de Louvois, Dr Robert Dinwiddie, Professor Rosalinde Hurley, Professor Stephen Jeffcoate, Dr Barbara Morgan, Dr Bonnie Sibbald, Dr Michael Snaith and Dr Stephen Spiro. Finally, I would like to acknowledge the invaluable secretarial assistance of Susan Cowley, and the patient and understanding support of my wife and family.

1 Diseases of the Respiratory System

Michael de Swiet

Disorders of the lungs severe enough to cause respiratory failure are rare in pregnancy (Gaensler *et al* 1953) since the major causes, chronic bronchitis and emphysema, are more common in men or in women past their childbearing years. Nevertheless, respiratory failure may occur in bronchial asthma, in overwhelming infection and occasionally in connective tissue disorders. It may be the cause of death in postanaesthetic complications. Before considering these and other respiratory diseases in pregnancy, we should first review the physiological changes in the respiratory system that occur during pregnancy. For more detailed reviews of physiology see de Swiet (1980), Fishburne (1979) and Milne (1979).

Physiological adaptation to pregnancy

Oxygen consumption, PaO_2 and CO_2 production

During pregnancy oxygen consumption rises by about 45 ml/min (Alaily *et al* 1978, Gazioglu *et al* 1970). Since the oxygen consumption at rest is approximately 300 ml/min (Knuttgen and Emerson 1974, Emerson *et al* 1972, Pernoll *et al* 1975) the increase is about 18 per cent. About one-third of the increased oxygen consumption is necessary for the metabolism of the fetus and placenta. The remainder is supplied for the extra metabolism of the mother, in particular the extra oxygen consumption associated with the increased cardiac output and the extra work of increased secretion and reabsorption by the kidney (de Swiet 1980).

The majority of authors find little change in PaO_2 during pregnancy. The normal value is about 103 mmHg at the end of pregnancy (Templeton and Kelman 1976). Those authors such as Lucius (1970) that have found a PaO_2 reduced to 85 mmHg in pregnancy have usually not specified the position of their patients. Pao_2 may fall by up to 13 mmHg on changing from the sitting to the supine position (Ang *et al* 1969) probably due to a combination of haemodynamic alterations and changes in functional residual capacity and closing volume. These changes cause mismatching of ventilation and perfusion and subsequent hypoxaemia. Therefore arterial blood gas measurements should always be made in pregnancy in the sitting position if they are used for diagnostic purposes such as in suspected pulmonary embolism (p. 99).

The increase in oxygen consumption is associated with a corresponding increase in carbon dioxide output. Since the respiratory quotient increases from 0.76 before pregnancy to 0.83 in late pregnancy, the increase in CO_2 production is proportionately greater than the increase in oxygen uptake (Knuttgen and Emerson 1974, Emerson *et al* 1972). This effect is likely to be due to an increase in the proportion of carbohydrate to fat metabolised during pregnancy.

Tidal volume

The increase in oxygen consumption is associated with a marked increase in ventilation of up to 40 per cent in pregnancy. This increase in ventilation is achieved efficiently by increasing tidal volume from 500 to 700 ml (Cugell *et al* 1953) rather than by any increase in respiratory rate (Pernoll *et al* 1975) (Fig. 1.1). It occurs early in pregnancy (Milne *et al* 1977a). Effective alveolar ventilation is further increased by a reduction of 20 per cent in residual volume—the volume of air in the lungs that remains at the end of expiration and with which the incoming air is diluted (Alaily *et al* 1978) (Fig. 1.2).

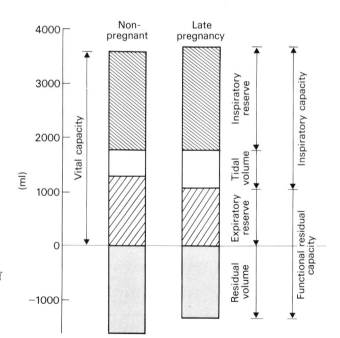

Fig. 1.1 Sub-divisions of lung volume and their alterations in pregnancy. (From Hytten and Chamberlain 1980.)

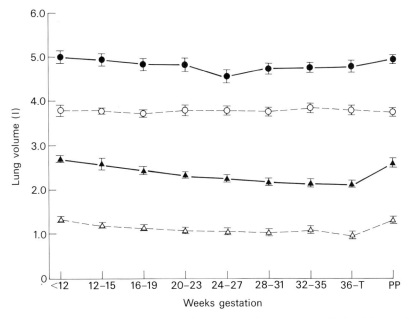

Fig. 1.2   Serial values of static lung volume during normal pregnancy and after delivery. (Values are mean ± SEM.) ● Total lung capacity; ○ vital capacity; ▲ functional residual capacity; △ residual volume.

Ventilatory equivalent, Paco₂ and pH

The increase in ventilation of 40 per cent compared to the increase in oxygen consumption of 20 per cent causes a considerable increase in ventilatory equivalent—the minute volume divided by oxygen consumption—which rises from 3.2 l/min/100 ml oxygen consumed to 4.0 l/min/100 ml oxygen consumed. Therefore, the $Paco_2$ falls in pregnancy from nonpregnant levels of 35–40 mmHg to about 30 mmHg (Eng *et al* 1975). Most authors (e.g. Milne 1979) find that $Paco_2$ falls early in pregnancy in parallel with the change in ventilation, but Lucius (1970) and Bouterline-Young and Bouterline-Young (1956) found a progressive fall in $Paco_2$. The fall in $Paco_2$ is even greater at altitude where the mother is hyperventilating further in an attempt to maintain the Pao_2 as high as possible. Hellegers *et al* (1959) found a $Paco_2$ of 28 mmHg at 4400 m and Sobrevilla *et al* (1971) recorded a $Paco_2$ of 24 mmHg at altitude.

The fall in $Paco_2$ is matched by an equivalent fall in plasma bicarbonate concentration and all the evidence suggests that arterial pH is not altered from the normal nonpregnant level of about 7.40.

The stimulus to hyperventilation

The increase in ventilation and associated fall in $Paco_2$ occurring in pregnancy, is due to progesterone (Döring and Loeschche 1947) which lowers the threshold of the respiratory centre to CO_2 (Willbrand *et al* 1959). In addition, during pregnancy, the sensitivity of the respiratory centre increases (Lyons and Antonio 1959) so that an increase in $Paco_2$ of 1 mmHg increases ventilation by 6 l/min in pregnancy, compared to 1.5 l/min in the nonpregnant state (Prowse and Gaensler 1965, Pernoll *et al* 1975, Eng *et al* 1975). It is also possible that progesterone acts as a primary stimulant to the respiratory centre independently of any change in CO_2 sensitivity or threshold (Skatrud *et al* 1978). Not only does progesterone stimulate ventilation, but it also increases the level of carbonic anhydrase B in the red cell (Schenker *et al* 1972, Paciorek and Spencer 1980). An increase in carbonic anhydrase will facilitate carbon dioxide transfer, and also tend to decrease $Paco_2$ independently of any change in ventilation. The respiratory stimulant effect of progesterone has been used in the treatment of respiratory failure and emphysema with varying success (Cullen *et al* 1959, Lyons and Huang 1968, Sutton *et al* 1975). A similar but smaller increase in ventilation is observed in the luteal phase of the menstrual cycle (England and Farhi 1976, Milne *et al* 1977b) and in patients taking some oral contraceptives (Milne 1979).

We have so far described the increase in oxygen consumption and the way in which this occurs in pregnancy, how the increase in ventilation is driven by progesterone and the effect of the increase in ventilation on blood gases. However, there are some other aspects of pulmonary physiology which must be considered concerning the woman's adaptation to pregnancy.

Vital capacity

The vital capacity, the maximum volume of gas that can be expired after a maximum inspiration, probably does not change in pregnancy (Figs 1.1 & 1.2). Some have found that it increases (Gazioglu *et al* 1970, Knuttgen and Emerson 1974), others have found that it decreases (Eng *et al* 1975, Rubin *et al* 1956); the majority have found no change (Cugell *et al* 1953, Sims *et al* 1976, Alaily and Carrol 1978, Milne 1979). Cugell *et al* (1953) found a transient fall in vital capacity in the puerperium. As the authors themselves noted, it is likely that this was due to maternal discomfort from, for example, episiotomy sutures preventing full cooperation.

Anatomical changes

The findings of no change in vital capacity with a reduction in residual volume are in keeping with the observed changes in the configuration of the chest during pregnancy. The level of the diaphragm rises by about 4 cm early in pregnancy even before it is under pressure from the enlarging uterus (Mobius 1961). This would account for the decrease in residual volume since the lungs would be relatively compressed at forced expiration.

Airways resistance

The work done in breathing may be partitioned into work done in overcoming the total airways resistance of the tracheobronchial tree—where the resistance of large airways (greater than 2 mm in diameter) is much more important than small airways function (Macklem and Mead 1967)—and work done in expanding the lungs and chest wall, the compliance.

Measurements of forced expiratory volume in one second (FEV_1) and peak expiratory flow rate are indirect measurements that depend on both airways resistance and lung compliance. Neither measurement is affected by pregnancy (Sims *et al* 1976), nor is airways conductance (Milne *et al* 1977a) nor lung compliance (Gee *et al* 1967).

Bevan *et al* (1974) and Garrard *et al* (1978) found an increased closing volume in pregnancy with closure beginning during normal tidal volume in half their subjects. This would suggest that the calibre of small airways less than 2 mm in diameter decreases in pregnancy to the point where some airways close during respiration. However, Craig and Toole (1975) and Baldwin *et al* (1977) found no change in the point of airways closure during normal pregnancy, and Farebrother and McHardy (1974) suggested that an increased closing volume was only a feature of complicated pregnancy. More work is necessary in this field. If some airways do close during tidal breathing, this would lead to impairment of ventilation perfusion ratio and a decreased efficiency of pulmonary gas exchange causing hypoxaemia.

Gas transfer (pulmonary diffusing capacity)

This factor is a measure of the ease with which carbon monoxide and therefore oxygen is transported across the pulmonary membrane. Earlier studies showed no change in transfer factor during pregnancy (Bedell and Adams 1962, Krumholtz *et al* 1964). However, more recently, Milne *et al* (1977c) showed a marked decrease in transfer factor early in pregnancy (Fig. 13). This could be related to the fall in haematocrit, but would be offset by the increase in cardiac output occurring early in pregnancy. A

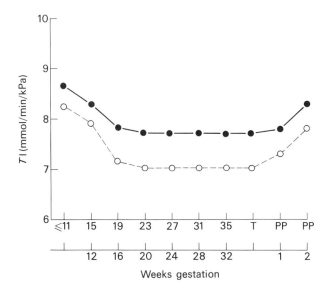

Fig. 1.3 Change in pulmonary transfer factor during normal pregnancy and after delivery (PP). ● Corrected for Hb and alveolar volume; ○ observed values. (After Milne 1976.)

reduction in transfer factor would be one effect acting against the increase in ventilation to improve the efficiency of gas exchange in pregnancy.

In summary, the mother more than compensates for the increased oxygen consumption required by her and the fetus with a marked increase in tidal volume, leading to a considerable reduction in $Paco_2$. This is driven by progesterone, and respiratory efficiency is augmented by the decrease in residual volume. These effects could be offset by an increase in closing volume and a decrease in transfer factor.

Breathlessness in pregnancy

Breathlessness is a subjective symptom and the degree to which patients are aware of the profound changes in ventilation occurring in pregnancy as breathlessness varies enormously between patients and in the same patient in different pregnancies.

The degree of breathlessness felt by women in pregnancy has been documented by Thomson and Cohen (1938), Cugell *et al* (1953) and Milne *et al* (1978). Milne found that about 50 per cent of women were aware of breathlessness before 20 weeks' gestation. The maximum incidence of breathlessness at rest occurred between 28 and 31 weeks' gestation. However, the symptom of breathlessness cannot in general be correlated with any single parameter of respiratory function. Therefore, the reason for the maximum incidence of dyspnoea at 28–31 weeks' gestation remains unknown.

It is clearly important for the clinician to be aware that dyspnoea is a normal feature of pregnancy and does not necessarily represent cardiorespiratory disease. In the absence of any other symptoms of cardiorespiratory disease, normal findings on examination and a normal chest X-ray should be sufficient to exclude any serious pathology in the majority of women with breathlessness in pregnancy. Measurement of arterial blood gases and transfer factor should be reserved for those who are markedly breathless with particular relevance to pulmonary embolus and the possibility of diffuse infiltrative lung conditions, such as idiopathic pulmonary fibrosis.

General comments on disorders of the respiratory system in pregnancy

Pregnancy stresses the respiratory system very little compared to its effect on the cardiovascular system. During pregnancy the minute ventilation increases by about 40 per cent from 7.5 l/min to 10.5 l/min and oxygen consumption increases by about 18 per cent from about 250 ml/min to 300 ml/min. Yet, in exercise, minute ventilation can increase to 80 l/min (Comroe *et al* 1962), a tenfold increase. Cardiac output also rises by approximately 40 per cent from 4.5 l/min to 6 l/min in pregnancy (p. 117), but in contrast, the maximum cardiac output achieved in exercise is probably no greater than 12 l/min, an increase of threefold. Thus, although cardiac output and minute ventilation both increase by an equal fraction in pregnancy, the increase in cardiac output represents a far greater proportion of the maximum that the body is capable of than does the increase in ventilation. Patients with respiratory disease are therefore less likely to deteriorate in pregnancy than those with cardiac disease since they have greater reserve.

Bronchial asthma

Asthma is a common condition affecting about 1 per cent of women in their childbearing years (Schaefer and Silverman 1961, Williams 1959). More recently, Hernandez *et al* (1980) reported that 1 per cent of 4529 pregnancies at Johns Hopkins Hospital were complicated by acute asthma; 0.15 per cent had severe attacks requiring hospitalization. It is therefore the commonest respiratory disorder complicating pregnancy. For other general reviews see Weinstein *et al* (1979), Hernandez *et al* (1980), Weinberger *et al* (1980), Turner *et al* (1980) and Fishburne (1979).

THE EFFECT OF PREGNANCY ON ASTHMA

Asthma is a very variable condition. Its severity depends on the patient's exposure to allergens, and the presence of respiratory infection, both also dependent on the season of the year. In addition, the patient's emotional state is important. If sufficient patients are studied to allow for these other influences, pregnancy has no consistent effect on asthma. For example, Hiddlestone (1964) found that pregnancy improved asthma, whereas Gordon *et al* (1970) and Schaefer and Silverman (1961) found that pregnancy was associated with a deterioration in bronchial asthma. Turner *et al* (1980) reviewed 1054 cases reported in nine different publications: 48 per cent showed no change in pregnancy, 29 per cent improved and 23 per cent deteriorated. Patients do not necessarily change in the same way during different pregnancies. Williams (1967) found that 37 per cent of 63 patients with asthma reacted differently in different pregnancies; this difference did not depend on the sex of the fetus (Williams 1967). When we followed measurements of FEV_1 serially through pregnancy in 27 patients with asthma, we were unable to find any consistent changes during pregnancy, or between pregnancy and the nonpregnant state (Sims *et al* 1976); this is in keeping with studies in nonasthmatic patients reviewed above.

If pregnancy does not cause any net change in airways resistance either in normal subjects or those with asthma, this is likely to be the sum of several factors acting in opposing directions. The bronchodilator influences are increased progesterone secretion, which may cause bronchodilatation by increasing beta adrenergic activity (Raz *et al* 1973), and increased free cortisol (Chapter 12); the bronchoconstrictor influences are the reduced residual volume (Briscoe and Dubois 1958), reduced $Paco_2$ (Newhouse *et al* 1964) and increased prostaglandin $F_{2\alpha}$ secretion (Hyman *et al* 1978). Prostaglandin $F_{2\alpha}$ should therefore not be used in obstetric practice (therapeutic abortion, induction of labour), particularly in asthmatic patients (Fishburne *et al* 1972a, 1972b, Hyman *et al* 1978, Kreisman *et al* 1975, Smith 1973). Prostaglandin E is used more widely and is the preferred prostaglandin for use in asthmatic patients, although there is controversy as to whether it may be bronchoconstrictor or bronchodilator (Smith 1973).

THE EFFECT OF ASTHMA ON PREGNANCY

Schatz (1975) found no excess risk to the fetus in 70 pregnancies of patients receiving corticosteroids for asthma, apart from a slight excess of prematurity; this risk was also noted by Bahna and Bjerkedal (1972). It has been suggested that perinatal mortality is doubled over 'normals' in patients with asthma in pregnancy, but this effect was largely confined to a black, presumably socially deprived population (Gordon *et al* 1970). We found no extra risk to the fetus if the mother suffered from asthma in pregnancy, although there was a tendency towards growth retardation, particularly amongst fetuses of mothers taking oral steroid therapy (Sims *et al* 1976). These patients were more severely affected by asthma, and may have been intermittently hypoxic. Templeton (1977) suggested that hypoxia was the cause of recurrent growth retardation that he noted in a patient with bronchiectasis. Alternatively, hyperventilation which may be associated with acute attacks of asthma, often causes hypocapnia, and this also has been related to fetal hypoxia (Wulf *et al* 1972, Moya *et al* 1965). Animal data would suggest that maternal respiratory alkalosis also causes fetal hypoxia (Motoyama *et al* 1967) and both respiratory alkalosis and hypocapnia may act via a reduction in maternal placental perfusion (Moya *et al* 1965, Motoyama *et al* 1966). In summary there may be a slight increased risk to the fetus of the mother with asthma, but this effect is very small, and should not be exaggerated when counselling individual patients.

MANAGEMENT OF ASTHMA IN PREGNANCY

The diagnosis of bronchial asthma is made on the basis of the history of recurrent episodes of wheeze and breathlessness, often associated with trigger factors such as exposure to allergens (dust, pollen), infection or psychological factors. An arbitrary definition is a variation in peak expiratory flow rate or FEV_1 by more than 20 per cent, either spontaneously or as a result of treatment. Some patients may present with a history of cough only. Patients with attacks only at night or on exercise may have a primary cardiac cause rather than bronchial asthma, but these usually have other signs of heart disease, or cardiomegaly on the chest radiograph. It is now possible to purchase inexpensive peak expiratory flow meters. Patients can use these at home to record their peak flows throughout the day on diary cards. In patients with asthma these records often show characteristic dips in peak flow at night or during the early morning.

In addition pulmonary embolus may also rarely present as bronchospasm (Windebank 1973) and this should be remembered as a possibility in patients who have their first attack of 'asthma' in pregnancy (Gurewich *et al* 1965) (Chapter 4).

GENERAL MEASURES

Asthma is by definition a variable condition which inevitably affects the patient's emotions. Also emotional upsets to which patients are particularly susceptible in pregnancy adversely affect asthma. It is therefore particularly important for the patient to develop a good relationship with an obstetrician and a physician whom she can trust.

Barbiturates and other sedative drugs should not be used because of the risk of respiratory depression; even diazepam is unsafe. The anxiety is much better treated by relief of symptoms with effective therapy. If the patient has any evidence of chest infection, as indicated by purulent sputum, this should be treated with an appropriate antibiotic (*see* below). However, eosinophilia may cause yellow sputum which looks purulent. Chest infection is probably overdiagnosed as a cause of exacerbation of asthma and such exacerbation should always be managed with an increase in bronchodilator therapy. In addition, it should be remembered that expectorants containing iodine should not be used in pregnancy, because the iodine may block thyroxine synthesis in the fetus making it hypothyroid or giving it a goitre (Carswell *et al* 1970, Galina *et al* 1962). Since iodine is preferentially excreted in breast milk (Varheer 1974), mothers who are breast feeding should also not use iodine-containing expectorants or cough medicine.

Those clinicians who use desensitisation in the treatment of asthma have not found any problems particular to pregnancy (Metzger *et al* 1978), although the risk of desensitisation (i.e. anaphylaxis) remains.

The use of bronchodilator drugs is considered below. However, a reasonable strategy in the patient presenting with asthma for the first time in pregnancy would be to use a selective beta β_2 sympathomimetic inhaler such as salbutamol or terbutaline for the acute attack. If this is being used more than twice a day, the inhaled β_2 sympathomimetic should be taken regularly, two puffs four times per day. If this regime does not give adequate control, a short course of regular disodium chromoglycate (Intal) inhalations could be used, but this treatment is only occasionally effective. My own preference would be to add regular betamethasone inhalations, two puffs, four times per day. Oral slow release aminophylline can also be used at this stage. If the patient is still no better, a short course of oral prednisone should be given, starting at 60 mg/day, reducing the dose rapidly, and aiming to stop oral steroids completely within ten days. Oral beta sympathomimetics are often used, but they tend to cause tremor and anxiety, and they are not usually helpful.

If there is any difficulty in controlling asthma that patient should be admitted to hospital, particularly in pregnancy. Status asthmaticus is difficult to define and has been renamed acute severe asthma, but deteriorating asthma which fails to respond promptly to regular medication is a life-threatening condition (MacDonald *et al* 1976) which has been shown to be particularly dangerous in pregnancy (Gordon *et al* 1970). It is likely that this is because the condition is managed initially by those with an obstetric orientation. It is notoriously easy to underestimate the severity of attacks of asthma (MacDonald *et al* 1976). Therefore all patients with acute severe asthma in pregnancy should be managed in cooperation with a physician interested in respiratory disease, preferably in an intensive care unit. Ominous signs are a heart rate greater than 100–120/min, respiratory rate greater than 30/min, pulsus paradoxus of more than 18–20 mmHg, and peak expiratory flow of less than 120 l/min in addition to dyspnoea, accessory muscle use and wheeze (Fischl *et al* 1981).

The patient should be monitored with regular measurements of peak flow rate and blood gases. If this is done, there is no need for controlled oxygen therapy, and the patient can have oxygen, 10 l/min, given via an M C mask. Because of the maternal risk, the patient should be managed as if she were not pregnant, giving optimal therapy for the respiratory condition. However, as outlined below, treatment with steroids, beta sympathomimetics or theophyllines is unlikely to affect the fetus in any case. The only drug that should not be used is tetracycline (p. 18), but fortunately there are other, better, broad spectrum antibiotics available. Despite this, antibiotics should only be given if there is clear evidence of infection.

Ventilation is rarely necessary but should the patient require it, either because of exhaustion or rising $Paco_2$, it is clear that maternal Pao_2 should be maintained as near physiological levels as possible; indeed, this is the usual purpose of ventilation. As noted previously, Wulf *et al* (1972) showed that as maternal Po_2 fell from 91 to 47 mmHg, fetal umbilical vein Po_2 fell from 32 to 27 mmHg. However, hypocapnia ($Pco_2 < 17$) and alkalosis (pH < 7.6) should also be avoided, since these are associated with reduced fetal oxygenation, probably due to impaired placental transport (Moya *et al* 1965, Turner *et al* 1980, Wulf *et al* 1972).

Beta-sympathomimetic drugs (isoprenaline, salbutamol, terbutaline, fenoterol)

A beta sympathomimetic inhaler is the first drug to use in treating patients who have occasional attacks of bronchospasm. It may be used prophylactically if the patient is particularly at risk, for example, from exercise-induced asthma. Although most of the beta sympathomimetics such as salbutamol, terbutaline and fenoterol that are used for the treatment of asthma are relatively selective, stimulating β_2 rather than β_1 receptors, the dosage given is still limited by cardiac side-effects of tachycardia and irregularities of heart rhythm. In addition, patients may notice tremor and a feeling of anxiety or apprehension. These effects are more marked with non-selective beta sympathomimetic drugs such as isoprenaline, which should not be used. There is little to choose between one selective beta sympathomimetic drug and another. My own preference is to use salbutamol, which has been widely studied in pregnant and nonpregnant patients.

There is considerable experience of the use of beta sympathomimetic agents in pregnancy, not only for the treatment of asthma, but also for premature labour (Lewis *et al* 1980). There is no evidence of teratogenicity and ephedrine in particular has been shown to be safe (Heinonen *et al* 1977). However, in the case of adrenaline when given in the first four months of pregnancy (Heinonen *et al* 1977) there was a small nonspecific increased risk of teratogenicity (minor eye and ear abnormalities) found by the Perinatal Collaborative Project; but it is possible that the acute condition for which adrenaline was given, rather than the drug itself, was the cause of the malformations.

The most worrying side-effects in pregnancy are pulmonary oedema and metabolic acidosis (de Swiet and Fidler 1981). Although it is possible to demonstrate metabolic (Lunell *et al* 1978, Wager *et al* 1981) and cardiovascular (Lunell *et al* 1978) side-effects after oral salbutamol, these serious complications are unlikely with normal therapy, providing the manufacturer's instructions are complied with. High dose intravenous therapy is much more likely to cause side-effects in patients receiving beta sympathomimetics for premature labour, rather than in the treatment of asthma where intravenous sympathomimetic drugs have only been used in the treatment of acute severe asthma and where more patients receive inhaled beta sympathomimetics.

Oral beta sympathomimetic therapy will cause hyperglycaemia in pregnant patients with diabetes (Wager *et al* 1981). Since control of blood glucose is so important in diabetic pregnancy (Chapter 10), patients who have impaired glucose tolerance and develop asthma should either not be given oral beta sympathomimetics or should have their blood glucose controlled particularly carefully.

Because beta sympathomimetics are used in the treatment of premature labour, their use for asthma might be expected to delay the onset or impede the progress of normal labour. The fact that this does not occur (Sims *et al* 1976) is perhaps not surprising in view of doubts about their efficacy in premature labour (Hemminki and Starfield 1978).

Theophyllines

Aminophylline has been widely used and is safe in pregnancy (Greenberger and Patterson 1978). It is available as a soluble preparation, a slow-release preparation, or as rectal suppositories in varying dosages. The oral dose is up to 10 mg/kg/day. The slow-release preparation acts for up to twelve hours and should therefore be used in preference to suppositories for the control of nocturnal and early morning asthma (Alkader and Cole 1978). Theophylline is also available as an elixir which is rapidly absorbed, giving therapeutic blood levels at 15 minutes (Fixley *et al* 1977). Optimal treatment, particularly in acute severe asthma is achieved by maintaining blood levels between 5 and 20 μg/ml (Weinstein *et al* 1979, Abramowicz 1978). The recommended infusion rate to achieve this in nonpregnant subjects is 0.7 mg/kg/hour for the first twelve hours after a 6 mg/kg bolus, followed by 0.5 mg/kg/hour thereafter. Since theophylline pharmacokinetics do not change during pregnancy (Sutton *et al* 1978) this regime is also recommended for the pregnant state (Marx and Fraser 1981) but may need to be modified according to the theophylline blood level. Amniophylline may cause nausea and also causes tachyarrhythmias, especially when given intravenously. The bolus dose should therefore be given slowly. Because aminophylline is also a pulmonary vasodilator, the patient should be receiving oxygen during intravenous administration to avoid hypoxaemia.

Aminophylline is assumed to cross the placenta (Weinstein *et al* 1979) and is excreted in breast milk in small quantities (Yurchak and Jusko 1976) but this has not been shown to cause any long-term harm in the fetus (Nelson and Forfar 1971). The safety of theophyllines in pregnancy is also suggested by a recent study in which aminophylline was given to women at risk of premature delivery. Therapy was associated with a decrease in the incidence of neonatal respiratory distress syndrome and perinatal mortality. There were no adverse side-effects (Hadgjigeogiou *et al* 1979). However, there are case reports (Arwood *et al* 1979), Yeh and Pildes 1977) of three newborn infants who showed theophylline toxicity (jitteriness, tachycardia, opisthotonos) after the mother had been given theophylline or aminophylline in late pregnancy. There were no long-term sequelae in any of these infants.

Disodium chromoglycate

Disodium chromoglycate is inhaled from a 'Spinhaler' or conventional aerosols but the aerosols only deliver a small dose. It is used as a prophylactic to prevent the occurrence of asthma attacks. It appears to be safe for the fetus (Dykes 1974, Weinstein *et al* 1979). Since the drug is taken by inhalation, the quantity entering the blood stream (8 per cent) is very small (Dykes 1974) and so little is transferred to the fetus. It occasionally causes bronchospasm at the time of inhalation and this can be avoided by using a combination preparation of disodium chromoglycate and isoprenaline.

Anticholinergic drugs, such as atropine or more recently ipratropium bromide given by aerosol, are also used in the prophylaxis of asthma (Van Arsdel and Paul 1977). Atropine has not been associated with any increased risk of teratogenesis (Heinonen *et al* 1977), and fetal tachycardia is the only likely side-effect.

Steroids

If patients cannot be managed with β_2-adrenergic stimulants, inhaled steroids, theophylline preparations, disodium chromoglycate or anticholinergic drugs, an oral corticosteroid preparation should be used. The patient who is having repeated severe attacks of asthma should receive steroids relatively early, before all other forms of treatment have been tried. An alternate day, oral steroid regime appears to lessen the side-effects of glucocorticoid therapy, although this has not been confirmed in pregnancy (Abramowicz 1975).

There is considerable debate concerning the use of steroids in pregnancy. Inhaled steroid therapy, e.g. beclomethasone, represents a considerable advance, since it permits the reduction or omission of oral therapy with prednisone. Inhaled beclomethasone acts locally on the bronchi, and is not absorbed if less than 1 mg (20 puffs becotide) is inhaled (Harris 1975). It has been used widely in pregnancy (Morrow Brown and Storey 1975). The side-effects which occur with long-term use are monilial infections of the upper respiratory and gastrointestinal tracts, but these are not a specific risk of pregnancy and are only a problem in 5 per cent of users. If patients are changed from chronic oral to inhaled steroid therapy, the dosage of oral steroid therapy should be reduced very slowly—no more rapidly than 1 mg reduction of prednisone per day every four weeks, if the dosage of prednisone is less than 10 mg/day. More rapid reduction has been associated with Addisonian collapse, a flare up of other atopic manifestations such as allergic rhinitis, or just lethargy and nonspecific malaise.

If patients require oral corticosteroid therapy for asthma, this should not be withheld because they are pregnant. Corticosteroids are said to cause cleft palate (Francis and Smellie 1964) but this risk appears to be confined to the rabbit (Fainstall 1954). Schatz *et al* (1975) did not find any excess of congenital malformations in 70 pregnancies complicated by asthma, treated with corticosteroids (average daily dose of prednisone, 8 mg) and this has been confirmed in other clinical studies (Bongiovanni and McPadden 1960, Heinonen *et al* 1977, Synder and Synder 1978) and reviewed by Turner *et al* (1980).

Steroid therapy will depress maternal adrenal activity. This can lead to a reduction in the maternal secretion and urinary secretion of oestriol if the dose is more than 30 mg of prednisone a day (Driscoll 1969, Morrison and Kilpatrick 1969, Wallace and Michie 1966). This effect, which is important if oestriol levels are used as an index of fetal wellbeing, may occur at dosages below 30 mg prednisone per day, but this has not been documented.

There is always concern that the hypothalamo-pituitary adrenal axis of the fetus may be suppressed by maternal steroid therapy (Warrell and Taylor 1968); this would make the infant liable to collapse in the neonatal period. In practice this does not occur, perhaps because little prednisone crosses the placenta. The maternal:fetal concentration of prednisone is 10:1 (Beitins *et al* 1972), in comparison to hydrocortisone 6:1, and betamethasone 3:1 (Ballard *et al* 1975). Also, the fetoplacental unit is relatively lacking in the enzymes to convert prednisone to its active metabolite, prednisolone (Ballard *et al* 1975), and placental 11 beta-ol-dehydrogenase is very efficient, deactivating 87 per cent of an injected dose of prednisone (Levitz *et al* 1978).

The management of labour

It is unusual for labour to be complicated by attacks of asthma. Perhaps this is because of an even greater secretion of glucocorticoids from the adrenal cortex (Jolivet *et al* 1974) and possibly also catecholamines from the adrenal medulla. Increased prostaglandin secretion during labour may also cause bronchodilation. For attacks of asthma which do occur in labour, conventional treatment with inhaled beta sympathomimetics should be used first, with earlier resource to parenteral steroid therapy if the patient does not improve rapidly. Because of the risk of maternal suppression of the hypothalamo-pituitary adrenal axis, it is conventional to give hydrocortisone 100 mg i.m. 6 hourly, to cover the period of labour, if she has taken continuous steroid therapy for more than two weeks in the previous year; Addisonian collapse in labour is very rare.

Anaesthesia and analgesia

Epidural anaesthesia is preferable to general anaesthesia (Marx 1974) because of the risk of atelectasis and subsequent chest infection. If a general anaesthetic cannot be avoided, halothane should be used because of its bronchodilating properties. Nebulised salbutamol can be given pre- and post-operatively. Opiates such as pethidine are best avoided because they cause bronchoconstriction, and respiratory depression; but these remain relative rather than absolute contraindications, and it would not be correct to deny a patient with asthma any effective analgesia at all if epidural anaesthesia was not available.

Breast feeding

Breast feeding should be encouraged. There is some, though conflicting, evidence that women with asthma in particular should breast feed because it may confer protection from food allergy in atopic individuals (Jellife and Jellife 1977). Turner *et al* (1980) have reviewed the secretion of drugs used in the treatment of asthma in breast milk. None of these drugs, including steroids, is likely to be secreted in sufficient quantities to harm the neonate, except tetracycline and iodides. In general, patients with asthma should therefore breast feed their infants.

Genetic counselling

The overall risk of any child having asthma is about 4 per cent. If one parent has asthma, the risk that the child will have asthma increases to 8–16 per cent, depending on whether the parent is also atopic. If both parents have asthma, and are also atopic, the risk may be as high as 30 per cent (Sibbald 1981).

In conclusion, asthma is a common condition affecting many women who are pregnant. It is not usually a problem in pregnancy, either to the mother or the fetus. The major difficulties lie in realising that the majority of drugs used in the treatment of pregnancy do not harm the fetus, and in maintaining the treatment of a potentially life-threatening illness despite the mother's pregnancy.

Tuberculosis

Pulmonary tuberculosis is now a rare complication of pregnancy in the general population of the UK, although some subgroups such as the Gujurati Indians have an incidence that is up to 100 times greater than the national figure. At Queen Charlotte's Hospital we see one case every 2–3 years, delivering approximately 4000 patients per year. For this reason we and others (Glass *et al* 1960, Bonebrake *et al* 1978, Mattox 1973) do not routinely perform chest X-rays in pregnancy, despite contrary recommendations (Sulavik 1975). In our population routine chest radiographs are not worth the financial cost, or the very minimal extra risk to the fetus of irradiating the mother. Nevertheless, there should be no hesitation in performing chest X-rays if there is any clinical indication.

Before antituberculous drugs were available, the results of pregnancy complicated by tuberculosis were poor for both mother and fetus (Cohen *et al* 1952); there was a particular tendency for patients to deteriorate in the puerperium (Hedvall 1953, Barnes 1974). However, Selikoff and Dormann (1965) reported that pregnancy did not affect the 15–30 per cent of patients with untreated active tuberculosis, who deteriorated in the first 30 months after diagnosis. More recently, de March (1975) was unable to find any deleterious effect of pregnancy in 100 patients with tuberculosis who had been pregnant, compared with 108 patients with pulmonary tuberculosis who had not been pregnant. Schaefer *et al* (1975) found that progression of pulmonary tuberculosis occurred in less than 1 per cent of patients managed during pregnancy at the New York Lying-In Hospital, between 1957 and 1972. There is also no conclusive evidence that the outcome of pregnancy is adversely affected by tuberculosis (Schaefer *et al* 1975, Selikoff and Dormann, 1965). However, Bjerkedal *et al* (1975) did notice an increased risk of abortion to 20 per 1000 patients with tuberculosis compared to two per 1000 controls. But 2/1000 is a very low incidence of abortion for the controls and this data should therefore be questioned. There is certainly no longer any justification for therapeutic abortion in maternal tuberculosis either for the sake of maternal health or because the fetus would otherwise be at such risk. Tuberculosis only very rarely affects the fetus by transplacental passage (Kapllan *et al* 1980) but, if the mother has open tuberculosis, the neonate is at risk.

In pregnancy, pulmonary tuberculosis may present because of symptoms—cough, purulent sputum, haemoptysis, fever, weight loss, chest pain (tuberculous pleural effusion)—or as an incidental finding when a chest X-ray is taken for a different reason. The diagnosis is based on the chest X-ray appearance and sputum culture and examination for acid-fast bacilli. Occasionally the diagnosis may be made by examination of the pleural effusion, pleural biopsy, liver biopsy or by bone marrow aspiration. The Mantoux test will become positive within 4–12 weeks after the initial infection. Despite previous suggestions (Finn *et al* 1972), Mantoux status is not affected by pregnancy itself (Present and Comstock 1975).

The problem in managing a pregnant patient with tuberculosis is not her potential respiratory impairment, but the possible effects on the fetus of the chemotherapeutic drugs used. This subject has recently been extensively reviewed by Snider *et al* (1980). Overall, their findings were very encouraging, since 94 per cent of all pregnancies terminated with the delivery of apparently normal infants, and only 3 per cent of the infants exposed in utero were classified as having birth defects (Snider *et al* 1980).

The drugs for which there is considerable information are ethambutal, isoniazid, streptomycin and rifampicin. In addition, it is believed that ethionamide is teratogenic (Potworoska *et al* 1966).

Ethambutol has replaced para-amino salicylic acid (PAS) as a 'front-line' anti-tuberculous drug, because it is so much easier for the patient to take. Although it may cause retrobulbar neuritis in adults in high doses (Citron 1969), there is no evidence from abortion specimens (Lewitt *et al* 1974) or the neonate (Brobowitz 1974) that the fetus is affected. Snider *et al* (1980) found only 14 infants or fetuses with abnormalities in 655 pregnancies treated with ethambutol, and none had optic nerve abnormalities. This drug must therefore be considered safe in pregnancy.

The same is true of isoniazid. There have been 16 abnormal fetuses reported in a total of 1480 pregnancies (Snider *et al* 1980). This abnormality rate is lower than the normal hospital population. Monnet *et al* (1967) noted that 4 of the 5 abnormal fetuses in their series of 125 patients treated with isoniazid, had CNS abnormalities. Since isoniazid is known to cause peripheral neuritis, this is the potential difficulty in the use of isoniazid in pregnancy, but it must be emphasised that this high incidence of CNS abnormalities was only seen in one group of patients, all of whom had also received ethionamide (Monnet *et al* 1967). In addition, the Collaborative Drug Project (Heinonen *et al* 1977) found a small (twice excess) nonspecific increase of congenital abnormalities in patients taking isoniazid. Because of the possible higher requirement of pyridoxine in pregnancy, all patients taking isoniazid in pregnancy should also take pyridoxine 20 mg/day to reduce the risk of peripheral neuritis (Brummer 1972).

The real problems concern the use of streptomycin and rifampicin. Although at one time it was considered that streptomycin was relatively innocuous in pregnancy (Conway and Birt 1965), this cannot be the current opinion. Conway and Birt (1965) found no disabled children from 17 patients in whom the mother had been treated with streptomycin in pregnancy, but eight children had abnormal caloric tests and/or abnormal audiograms. Severe hearing loss was reported by Robinson and Cambon (1964). Snider *et al* (1980) found 34 cases of eighth nerve damage amongst the reports of 206 patients treated with streptomycin. This incidence of over 10 per cent appears excessive. Furthermore, the risk of eighth nerve damage will persist after the period of organogenesis, throughout gestation.

Although Scheinhorn and Angelillo (1977) initially suggested that rifampicin did not affect the fetus, Snider *et al* (1980) also found reports of 14 abnormal fetuses amongst 442 patients treated with rifampicin. The malformations were variable and severe. Nine of these cases have been reported in detail by the manufacturers (Steen and Stainton Ellis 1977).

In summary, the patient presenting with tuberculosis in the first trimester of pregnancy, should be treated with isoniazid and ethambutol in standard dosage unless the tuberculosis is very widespread or deteriorating. After organogenesis is complete at 16 weeks' gestation, it should be safe to use rifampicin. It may be necessary to admit the patient to establish the diagnosis, in which case she should be in a single room rather than have strict barrier nursing. The patient should also be in a single room when she is admitted for labour. However, now that antituberculous therapy is so effective, the majority of treatment can be given as an outpatient. Nine months' treatment with isoniazid and rifampicin is considered sufficient for pulmonary tuberculosis.

If the patient's organism is sensitive to isoniazid, the new-born infant should be given isoniazid and isoniazid-resistant BCG to prevent infection from the mother and allow the infant to acquire immunity, respectively (Gaisford and Griffiths 1961). Without these measures the risk of the child developing active disease may be as high as 50 per cent (Kendig 1969). If the organism is isoniazid resistant and the mother is considered infectious, the neonate will have to be separated until the child has become Mantoux positive.

Sarcoidosis and erythema nodosum

Although sarcoid is commonest in women aged 20–40 years, pulmonary sarcoid is rarely reported as a complication of pregnancy—perhaps 0.05 per cent of all pregnancies are affected by the condition (Grossman and Littner 1976). However, there have been less than five cases reported where there was any marked symptomatic impairment in respiratory function (Grossman and Littner 1976, Reisfield *et al* 1969) and only two maternal deaths (Krupp 1957), one of which may have been due to pre-eclampsia (Given and DiBenedetto 1963). This combination may have been significant, since pre-eclamptic toxaemia is associated with an increase in pulmonary vascular resistance (*see* p. 138). Nevertheless, specialist referral centres have experience of large numbers of patients with sarcoid in pregnancy (James 1970). The consensus of opinion is that sarcoidosis, if it changes, improves in pregnancy, perhaps due to the increase in free as well as total cortisol (p. 138); however, there is a tendency for the condition to relapse in the puerperium (Weinberger *et al* 1980, O'Leary 1962, Fried 1964, Scadding 1961), and also to appear in the puerperium (Fried 1964). Nevertheless, the relapse is unlikely to be serious and should not be a contraindication to pregnancy, except in the rare patient who is severely affected. Apart from the pulmonary complications of sarcoid, patients may very rarely have life-threatening heart, renal and neurological disease.

The usual presentation is with symmetrical bilateral hilar lymphadenopathy and mediastinal lymphadenopathy found on chest X-ray, either by chance or in a patient with pyrexia or erythema nodosum. The patient may also have cervical lymphadenopathy. The differential diagnoses include lymphoma such as Hodgkin's disease (Case and Benaroya 1980) and tuberculosis. In tuberculosis and Hodgkin's disease the hilar lymphadenopathy is usually not symmetrical and tuberculosis is usually associated with parenchymal lung lesions in the acute attack in women of this age. The Kveim test is positive in the majority of women with sarcoid presenting with bilateral lymphadenopathy. If there is any doubt the patient should have fibreoptic bronchoscopy with transbronchial aspiration. If this is negative, mediastinotomy, mediastinoscopy or liver biopsy may be necessary to prove or disprove the diagnosis.

More advanced sarcoid is associated with diffuse lung infiltration, when the patient is more likely to be breathless and will frequently have a reduced transfer factor. Those patients that are symptomatic can be given alternate-day steroid therapy (*see* p. 12), particularly if there is evidence of deteriorating pulmonary function. Since hilar lymphadenopathy may be absent, the differential diagnosis of this condition is wide, ranging from hypersensitivity to drugs to connective tissue diseases and organic dust diseases. Lymphangiomyomatosis, proliferation of lymphatic vessels, is a very rare cause of diffuse pulmonary infiltration that can occur in pregnancy but one that is specific to women in their childbearing years (McCarty *et al* 1980). In the absence of any clinical clues, transbronchial, fibreoptic lung biopsy is usually the definitive investigation. The late manifestations of sarcoid include lung fibrosis and cor pulmonale due to hypoxaemia. Steroid therapy rarely helps at this stage.

No special management is necessary for the average case in pregnancy. Systemic steroids should not be withheld (*see* p. 12) if they are indicated for the pulmonary condition (O'Leary 1962). However, there is no evidence that steroid therapy influences the natural course of the disease. Sarcoid is not transmitted to the fetus (Barnes 1974), although sarcoid granulomata have been reported in the placenta in one patient (Keleman and Mandl 1969) but not in others (Reisfeld 1958). Since patients often take extra vitamins in pregnancy, they should be particularly warned not to take extra vitamin D, to which they may be very sensitive (James 1970).

ERYTHEMA NODOSUM

This topic is included here because erythema nodosum frequently complicates sarcoid and tuberculosis. However, it may also complicate other infections (streptococcal, pertussis, measles, coccidiomycosis), drug therapy (particularly sulphonamides) and inflammatory bowel disease. In many patients, the precipitating cause, if there is one, is not found. The rash consists of tender, pretibial red or purple nodules. New lesions appear while old ones are resolving, and each lesion lasts a few days to a few weeks. The whole illness may last several months, and be accompanied by fever and arthralgia.

Erythema nodosum occurs not infrequently in pregnancy. We see about one case per 1000 maternities at Queen Charlotte's Maternity Hospital. If the patient has none of the clinical conditions outlined above, a normal chest X-ray and a blood count that is normal for pregnancy, she may be reassured that the condition is most unlikely to have any sequelae and that her pregnancy will not be affected.

Salvatore and Lynch (1980) reported 21 cases occurring in pregnancy, or in patients taking oral contraceptives. Since they could find no cause for ten of these, they believed that pregnancy or oestrogen therapy could be precipitating factors. This remains unproven, since erythema nodosum occurs most frequently in women during their childbearing years.

Other respiratory tract infections

UPPER RESPIRATORY TRACT

At least half of the infections of the upper respiratory tract are viral and due to adeno-, rhino- and para-influenza viruses. In addition, acute bronchitis may be bacterial in origin due to organisms such as *Haemophilus influenzae.* Viral upper respiratory tract infections require no specific treatment. The condition is self-limiting and the patient improves with symptomatic therapy—analgesics and antipyretics (e.g. paracetamol) and bed rest. A high fluid intake is encouraged. If the patient has purulent sputum, a sample should be sent for culture and appropriate antibiotic therapy should be started. For acute bronchitis this should be broad spectrum therapy with ampicillin, amoxycillin or a cephalosporin. Erythromycin can be used in patients who are sensitive to penicillin. The safety of cotrimoxazole has not been established in pregnancy and tetracycline should definitely not be used because of the risks of abnormal bone formation and permanent discolouration of the child's teeth (Elder *et al* 1971). In addition, tetracycline therapy has been related to multiple congenital abnormalities (Corcoran and Castles 1977), and parenteral tetracycline has caused pancreatitis and fatal liver failure in pregnancy (Kunelis *et al* 1965). Treatment for bronchitis should also include steam inhalation to liquefy secretions, but iodine-containing expectorants should not be used because of the adverse effects of iodine on the fetus (p. 390). Bronchodilators to relieve bronchospasm may also be helpful (p. 10).

PNEUMONIA

This is associated with the clinical and radiological signs of lung consolidation. The patient presents with fever, cough, purulent sputum or chest pain. Patients frequently have a history of antecedent chest illness and the majority are smokers (Hopwood 1965). No cause for the infection can be found in up to 52 per cent of cases (White *et al* 1981). The majority are bacterial in origin, due to *Streptococcus pneumoniae* (the pneumococcus) but many other organisms may be involved, particularly in epidemics. Hospital-acquired infection may be with *Haemophilus influenzae*, haemolytic streptococcus, *Staph. aureus* or *Klebsiella pneumoniae* in the very debilitated. However, the influenza virus is an important cause of pneumonia during epidemics and mycoplasma may also cause pneumonia, although many causes previously thought to be due to mycoplasma may have been caused by *Legionella pneumophilus*. Therapy in the first instance should be with penicillin on the assumption that the patient has a *Strep. pneumoniae* infection. If the patient is sensitive to penicillin, she should receive erythromycin; this will also treat Legionnaire's disease and mycoplasma infection. If the patient is thought to have a hospital-acquired infection, she should also have a broad spectrum antibiotic (amoxycillin, cephalosporin, erythromycin) pending the results of sputum, blood culture and sensitivities, when further antibiotics may be necessary. Patients should also receive paracetamol as an antipyretic and may require tepid sponging and full nursing care is they are very sick.

Pneumonia used to have a bad reputation in pregnancy with many patients aborting and a 20 per cent maternal mortality (Oxorn 1955). Now that effective antibiotics are available, this is no longer so, except in the case of premature labour which remains a definite risk, presumably related to pyrexia (Oxorn 1955). In contrast, it is generally believed that viral pneumonia has a high mortality in pregnancy (Greenberg *et al* 1958); during influenza epidemics pneumonia may be responsible for half the cases of maternal mortality (Freeman and Barno 1959) and Griffith (1974) has reported a case of adult respiratory distress syndrome associated with influenza and pneumonia. However, such high maternal mortalities have not been reported recently, and the additional risk of influenza pneumonia due to pregnancy has probably been exaggerated (*Contemporary Obstetrics and Gynaecology* 1976).

Fungal lung infections are very rare in the United Kingdom. However, Harris (1966) has reviewed the clinical outcome in 50 cases of coccidioidomycosis from North America, 22 of which became disseminated in pregnancy with a maternal mortality of nearly 100 per cent if untreated with amphotericin B (Smale and Waechter 1974).

Cystic fibrosis

Cystic fibrosis is the commonest important genetic disorder in Caucasians with a gene frequency of 1 in 20 (*British Medical Journal* 1979). Since heterozygotes are asymptomatic, homozygous patients who suffer from the condition are relatively common. The incidence is about 1 in 2000 live births (*British Medical Journal* 1979). Recently the mortality has improved markedly, so that many more women are surviving to become pregnant. Even in 1974 there were 648 women in North America with cystic fibrosis over the age of 17 years (Cystic Fibrosis Foundation 1976) and it is predicted that there will be 4000 patients in this age group by 1985 (Corkey *et al* 1981). Over 70 per cent of children identified in the first year of life now survive beyond twelve years (Mearns 1974). This, in turn, is likely to increase the future genetic load in the community, and intensive efforts are being made to develop tests which will detect the heterozygote for preconceptual counselling and to establish the antenatal diagnosis of the homozygote for counselling concerning termination of pregnancy. The improvement of mortality has come from improved prophylactic bronchial toilet and widespread use of antibiotics, rather than any single therapeutic advance. In addition, pancreatic enzymes and vitamins are added to a high protein and low fat diet. Carbohydrates are given as sugar to increase calorie intake.

Case reports of cystic fibrosis in pregnancy have been published first by Siegel and Siegel (1960) and also by Grand *et al* (1966), Plotz *et al* (1967), Novy *et al* (1967), Rosenow and Lee (1968), Ayers (1970), Larsen (1972), Visser *et al* (1977), and Friedman *et al* (1979). Phelan (1981) reported the successful results of three pregnancies in 66 women aged more than 16 years, attending the Royal Children's Hospital, Melbourne. He comments that the low incidence of pregnancy is possibly due to fear of producing affected children, as well as possible infertility.

The most recent extensive review of cystic fibrosis in pregnancy was by Cohen *et al* (1980). A postal survey was performed of 119 centres in North America and reported the outcome in 129 patients delivered before 1975. Although 19 per cent of patients had therapeutic abortions, the incidence of spontaneous abortion (5 per cent) was not elevated. However, both the perinatal mortality (11 per cent) and the maternal mortality (12 per cent within 6 months of delivery) were considerably greater than in the rest of the population. Although the maternal mortality is alarming it was no greater than reported for patients with cystic fibrosis who were not pregnant (Cystic Fibrosis Foundation 1976, Warwick *et al* 1975). Corkey *et al* (1981) reported the outcome of eleven pregnancies in seven patients. Only one pregnancy required termination and these authors suggested that this prognosis is better when pancreatic function is maintained.

It has been reported that patients with cystic fibrosis show a decrease in residual volume as do normal women in pregnancy, but they are unable to maintain vital capacity. Although they increase oxygen uptake, they do not show the 'hyperventilation' associated with normal pregnancy (Novy *et al* 1967).

The judgement of individual physicians is likely to be coloured by their most recent experience of relatively few cases, and this would account for a wide diversity of clinical opinions regarding the advisability of pregnancy in patients with cystic fibrosis. Several indices have been suggested as a guide to the success of pregnancy, based on the presence or absence of emphysema, cor pulmonale and such abnormalities in respiratory function as vital capacity less than 50 per cent predicted for height (Schwachman and Kulczyki 1958, Taussig *et al* 1973, Larsen 1972). Although a vital capacity of less than 50 per cent than that predicted has been recommended as an indication for termination (Visser *et al* 1977), many patients with a vital capacity of less than this in cystic fibrosis and other conditions such as kyphoscoliosis, have a normal pregnancy. Since patients die because of uncontrollable recurrent chest infection and cor pulmonale (which is in turn related to hypoxaemia) it is suggested that these should be the parameters considered when counselling patients. If there is any doubt about the presence of hypoxaemia, the arterial blood gases should be measured. From the data of di Saint'Agnese and Davis (1979), it would appear that an arterial Po_2 of less than 60 mmHg, when the patient is free from infection and breathing air, is associated with an NIH score of less than 50. This is the score at which pulmonary hypertension is present (Siassi *et al* 1971). Pulmonary hypertension has a particularly poor outcome in pregnancy (*see* Chapter 5). In addition, if there is any doubt about the presence of pulmonary hypertension, the pulmonary artery pressure should be measured. When a flow-directed, Swan–Ganz catheter is used, X-ray screening may be unnecessary. If the pulmonary artery systolic pressure is less than 35 mmHg, the patient does not have cor pulmonale. This is a much more reliable measurement than inference from clinical signs, chest radiographs, or the electrocardiograph.

Physicians should also be aware that patients with cystic fibrosis may have liver disease (Psacharopoulos *et al* 1981) and diabetes mellitus (Plotz *et al* 1967). However, the reported incidence of cirrhosis varies between 0.5 per cent (Crozier 1974) and 90 per cent (Isenberg and L'Heureuse 1976) and this has not yet been reported to be a problem in pregnancy.

Apart from a high level of medical and obstetric care, there are no special measures which should be taken in the antenatal period. Because of the ototoxic and renal side-effects of the aminoglycosides reviewed above, these antibiotics should be avoided if possible in pregnancy, and the penicillins should be used instead. Nebulized gentamicin may represent a real advantage here. However, it is reassuring that there were no congenital abnormalities amongst the 129 cases reviewed by Cohen *et al* (1980) of whom 26 received aminoglycosides during pregnancy.

During labour, particular care should be taken concerning fluid and electrolyte balance. Patients with cystic fibrosis lose large quantities of sodium in sweat and may easily become hypovolaemic. However, they will also be very intolerant of overhydration, if there is any degree of cor pulmonale. Oxygen may be freely administered if the $Paco_2$ is not elevated. Because of the risk of postanaesthetic atelectasis, inhalation anaesthesia is better avoided and epidural or caudal anaesthesia substituted.

Whitelaw and Butterfield (1977) reported that the sodium content of breast milk from women with cystic fibrosis may be as high as 280 mmol/l, and suggested that this was a reason for these mothers not to breast feed. However, Alpert and Cormier (1983) have found normal electrolyte content in milk from mothers with cystic fibrosis, and believe that the electrolyte contents found by Whitelaw and Butterfield were abnormally high because the milk was expressed from a woman that was not lactating freely. Such expressed milk was demonstrated to have abnormally high electrolyte contents even if the mothers did not have cystic fibrosis. It would seem sensible to check the sodium content of breast milk from women with cystic fibrosis who are lactating, but it is unlikely that this will be a contraindication to breast feeding.

Chronic bronchitis, emphysema and bronchiectasis

Since these conditions are now rarely important in patients during childbearing years, there is little information on their outcome in pregnancy. Although Templeton (1977) has reported intrauterine growth retardation in a patient with bronchiectasis, this does not regularly occur (Howie and Milne 1978). If pregnancy does occur in patients with bronchiectasis, they can be severely debilitated and will need to be treated as high-risk patients with regular supervision and attention to postural drainage and physiotherapy. Chest infection, and airways obstruction should be managed as described earlier. As suggested by Lalli and Rafa (1981) a successful outcome to pregnancy may be limited by the presence of pulmonary hypertension and hypoxaemia (*see* above). In a single case report, emphysema due to α_1 antitrypsin deficiency did not affect the successful outcome of pregnancy (Giesler *et al* 1977).

Kyphoscoliosis

The reported incidence of kyphoscoliosis is 0.1–0.7 per cent of pregnancies (Kopenhager 1977) but much depends on the definition in mild cases. Kopenhager noted a marked increase in perinatal mortality to 102 per 1000, possibly due to maternal hypoxia. In Mendelson's series (1958) only one patient had a vital capacity of less than one litre, and she was in heart failure during labour. However, we have successfully delivered two patients with kyphoscoliosis who have vital capacities of less than one litre with no overt problems. As in cystic fibrosis, the limiting factors are hypoxaemia and pulmonary hypertension, rather than the results of any particular respiratory function tests. These patients are more likely to require Caesarean section, because of associated abnormalities of the bony pelvis. Notwithstanding the spinal deformities, epidural anaesthetic is preferable to general anaesthesia.

Adult respiratory distress syndrome, shock lung

This is the end point of several different types of obstetric disaster including inhalation of gastric contents during anaesthesia (*see* p. 25). In addition, it may occur with disseminated intravascular coagulation (DIC) in pre-eclampsia, eclampsia, abruptio placentae, dead fetus syndrome, and amniotic fluid embolism (*see* Chapter 3). The syndrome is also associated with hypovolaemic shock from postpartum haemorrhage with or without sepsis (Andersen *et al* 1980) and with severe anaphylaxis. It is also found with metastatic cancer or, in pregnancy, with hydatidiform mole (Orr *et al* 1980).

Changes in maternal physiology may be the reason for the apparent frequency of pregnancy as an underlying cause of adult respiratory distress in women. However, if this is so, it is not clear which is the critical function, or functions, that change. Alternatively, and more plausibly, it may be that other secondary causes, such as anaesthesia, shock from haemorrhage and DIC (p. 76) are more likely to be present in women in the pregnant than the nonpregnant state.

These patients are severely ill and should be managed in an intensive care unit. The clinical picture is of a patient who develops acute severe hypoxaemia, despite a high inspired oxygen concentration (Ashbaugh *et al* 1967), and shows diffuse infiltrates on the chest radiograph—where signs may take 24 hours to develop. It is assumed that the primary problem is in the lung, where compliance and permeability are reduced due to extravasation of liquid, rather than in the heart. However, it may be necessary to prove that there is not a primary cardiac abnormality by demonstrating a normal (less than 14 mmHg) pulmonary artery wedge pressure, i.e. a normal left ventricular end diastolic pressure using a flow-guided Swan–Ganz catheter (Keefer *et al* 1981). Such a catheter (if left in place) can be of great assistance for management, since it can provide measurements of pulmonary artery pressure and cardiac output by green dye or thermodilution. Peripheral oedema, elevated jugular venous pressure and cardiomegaly are unusual and suggest cardiac, rather than pulmonary, pathology.

The therapeutic options available are correction of the underlying cause, artificial ventilation, and medication with steroids, diuretics and antibiotics.

Correction of the underlying cause is usually limited to reversal of DIC with fresh frozen plasma (followed by delivery of the dead fetus if present) and treatment of infection. Andersen *et al* (1980) suggest ventilation, preferably with an inspired oxygen concentration of less than 60 per cent, maintaining an end expiratory pressure of 5–35 cmH_2O to try to keep the arterial Po_2 greater than 60 mmHg. The use of positive end expiratory pressure (PEEP) may help by thinning the layer of water in the alveolus and increasing alveolar area to improve gas exchange.

Fluid balance is crucial. If the patients are hypovolaemic, cardiac output and perfusion will decrease; hence infusion of albumen or blood (increasing oxygen carrying capacity) can be helpful, although there is a risk of further protein loss into the alveoli (*see* p. 79) for a further discussion of which fluid may be best in this situation). If they are hypervolaemic, there will be increased extravasation of fluid and increased preload, decreasing oxygenation and cardiac output. Diuretic therapy will then be necessary. The indication for manipulating blood volume and its effect, can be determined by repeated measurement of pulmonary artery wedge pressure and cardiac output, using the Swan–Ganz catheter. Corticosteroids may reverse excess capillary permeability (Wilson 1972), but they may also increase susceptibility to infection (Blaisdell and Schlobohm 1973).

Despite these measures, the mortality of adult respiratory distress syndrome is 50–60 per cent (Shanies 1977). Nevertheless, every effort should be made in treating these patients since those who survive recover well. It is hoped, though not proven, that early aggressive treatment will reduce the mortality from this condition (Andersen *et al* 1980).

Pneumothorax and pneumomediastinum

Both these conditions occur infrequently in pregnancy, but probably more commonly than in the nonpregnant state. They most commonly occur in susceptible individuals due to the expulsive efforts of labour (Spellacy and Prem 1963, Burgener and Solmes

1979), but pneumomediastinum in particular may occur at other times—for example in association with bronchial asthma (Hague 1980). Pneumothorax may occur in association with other chest conditions, such as emphysema or pulmonary tuberculosis. In pneumomediastinum, which is commoner in pregnancy than pneumothorax, a false passage is created between the airways and the mediastinal tissues. Air tracks through the mediastinum to the neck, and there may be widespread subcutaneous emphysema over the thorax or even the whole body. This produces a quite characteristic crackling sound and sensation on palpation, which does not occur in any other condition. In addition, there may be a crunching noise—Hamman's sign (Hamman 1945)—synchronous with the heart beat at the left sternal edge. In pneumothorax there is a false passage between the airways and the pleural cavity. Pneumothorax accompanies about one-third of the cases of pneumomediastinum that occur in pregnancy (Sulavik 1975) but may also occur independently. In both conditions, the patient complains of the sudden onset of chest pain and breathlessness and the diagnosis is confirmed by chest radiography. In tension pneumothorax the patient will become cyanosed and hypotensive due to the reduction in the venous return. A similar variant of pneumomediastinum—'malignant mediastinum' (Gray and Hanson 1966)—also occurs but is much rarer.

Pneumomediastinum normally clears spontaneously and the treatment is therefore usually conservative, with oxygen and analgesics. Malignant mediastinum requires urgent relief either by multiple incisions over the subcutaneous tissue where air is trapped (Gray and Hanson 1966) or by splitting the sternum. Pneumothorax should be drained via an underwater seal if the lung is more than 25 per cent collapsed. Tension pneumothorax requires immediate relief by a large-bore needle inserted through the chest wall overlying the pneumothorax. If pneumothorax or pneumomediastinum has occurred in pregnancy, elective forceps delivery should be performed to minimise the chance of recurrence, caused by raised intrapulmonary pressure due to maternal straining.

Anaesthetic considerations

The most recent confidential maternal mortality report, which examined all maternal deaths occurring in England and Wales in the years 1976–8, indicates that there were 14 deaths due to inhalation of stomach contents, out of a total of 227 maternal deaths (Department of Health & Social Security 1982). The management of adult respiratory distress syndrome has been discussed above. Further treatment of inhalation includes bronchoscopy for the patient who becomes acutely cyanotic following regurgitation of large particles of food which have obstructed major airways. It is also important to realise that pulmonary aspiration may occur without frank vomiting or regurgitation (Benson and Adriani 1954). The differential diagnosis of amniotic fluid embolism and aspiration is considered on pp. 83–4 and, in general, in Chapter 4.

Much of modern obstetric medical practice involves prevention of the complication of gastric aspiration. It is common practice to starve women during labour, but the stomach will continue to secrete fluid, even though in reduced quantities; also gastric emptying from meals taken before the onset of labour is much reduced. On the assumption that it is the acid component of gastric contents that is harmful, patients in labour are often given up to 30 ml of antacid (magnesium trisilicate mixture) every two hours to maintain the pH greater than 3.5 (Cohen 1979, Pedersen and Finster 1979). However, the confidential maternal mortality series indicate that the number of deaths from aspiration during 1973–5, when antacid administration was widespread, was no less than the number occurring in 1970–2, before antacids were generally used (Scott 1978). Furthermore, Bond *et al* (1979) have described pulmonary aspiration syndrome after inhalation of stomach contents of pH 6.4, in a patient who had been given regular antacid therapy with magnesium and aluminium hydroxide. This would suggest that the hydrogen ion concentration is not the only determinant of the pulmonary aspiration syndrome; either the antacid itself or other constituents of the gastric fluid must contribute. Perhaps 0.3 M sodium citrate solution is a safer antacid (Tatersall 1983). Alternative approaches are to use an H_2 antagonist such as cimetidine (Dundee *et al* 1981, McCaughey *et al* 1981) which decreases acid secretion, or metoclopramide therapy which increases gastric emptying (Howard and Sharp 1973). Large-scale comparative studies are necessary to determine which is the most effective.

In the patient who has respiratory impairment, general anaesthesia should be avoided because of the slight risk of intrapartum hypoxia, due to deteriorating ventilation perfusion imbalance, and the greater risk of postoperative atelectasis. Epidural, caudal or spinal anaesthetics are obvious substitutes.

References

Abramowicz M. (1975) Alternate-day corticosteroid therapy. *Medical Letters on Drugs and Therapeutics* **17**, 95.

Abramowicz M. (1978) Drugs for asthma. *Medical Letters on Drugs and Therapeutics* **20**, 69.

Alaily A.B. & Carrol K.B. (1978) Pulmonary ventilation in pregnancy. *British Journal of Obstetrics and Gynaecology* **85**, 518–24.

Alkader A.A. & Cole R.B. (1978) Effect of aminophylline on FEV_1 in patients with nocturnal asthma. *Thorax* **88**, 536–7.

Alpert S.E. & Cormier A.D. (1983) Normal electrolyte and protein content in milk from mothers with cystic fibrosis: An explanation for the initial report of elevated milk sodium concentration. *Journal of Pediatrics* **102**, 77–80.

Andersen H.F., Lynch J.P. & Johnson T.R.B. (1980) Adult respiratory distress syndrome in obstetrics and gynecology. *Obstetrics and Gynecology* **55**, 291–5.

Anderson, G.J., James G.B., Mathers N.P., Smith E.L. & Walker J. (1969) The maternal oxygen tension and acid base status during pregnancy. *American Journal of Obstetrics and Gynecology* **100**, 1–6.

Ang C.K., Tan T.H., Walters Wan & Wood C. (1969) Postural influence on maternal capillary oxygen and carbon dioxide tension. *British Medical Journal* **4**, 201.

Arwood L.L., Dasta J.F. & Friedman C. (1979) Placental transfer of theophylline: two case reports. *Pediatrics* **63**, 844–6.

Ashbaugh D.G., Bigelow D.B. & Petty T.L. (1967) Acute respiratory distress in adults. *Lancet* **2**, 319.

Ayers M.A. (1970) Pregnancy and cystic fibrosis of lungs and pancreas. A case report. *Ohio Medical Journal* **66**, 53–4.

Bahna S.L. & Bjerkedal T. (1972) The course and outcome of pregnancy in women with bronchial asthma. *Acta Allergologica* **27**, 397–400.

Baldwin G.R., Moorthi D.S., Whelton J.A. & MacDoneal K.F. (1977) New lung functions and pregnancy. *American Journal of Obstetrics and Gynecology* **127**, 235.

Ballard P.L., Granberg P. & Ballard R.A. (1975) Glucocorticoid levels in maternal and cord serum after prenatal beclomethasone therapy to prevent respiratory distress syndrome. *Journal of Clinical Investigation* **56**, 1548–54.

Barnes C.G. (1974) *Medical Disorders in Obstetric Practice.* Blackwell Scientific Publications, Oxford.

Bedell G.N. & Adams R.S. (1962) Pulmonary diffusing capacity during rest and exercise. A study of normal persons and persons with atrial septal defect, pregnancy and pulmonary disease. *Journal of Clinical Investigation* **41**, 1908.

Beitins R., Baynard F., Ances I.G., Kowarsk A. & Migeon C.J. (1972) The transplacental passage of prednisone and prednisolone in pregnancy near term. *Journal of Pediatrics* **81**, 936–45.

Benson W. & Adriani J. (1954) 'Silent' regurgitation and aspiration during anesthesia. *Anesthesiology* **15**, 644.

Bevan D.R., Holdcroft A., Loh L., MacGregor W.G., O'Sullivan J.C. & Sykes M.K. (1974) Closing volume and pregnancy. *British Medical Journal* **i**, 13–15.

Bjerkedal T., Bahna S.L. & Lehmann E.H. (1975) Cause and outcome of women with pulmonary tuberculosis. *Scandinavian Journal of Respiratory Disease* **56**, 245–50.

Blaisdell F.W. & Schlobohm R.M. (1973) The respiratory distress syndrome: A review. *Surgery* **74**, 251.

Bond V.K., Stoetling R.K. & Gupta C.D. (1979) Pulmonary aspiration syndrome after inhalation of gastric fluid containing antacids. *Anesthesiology* **51**, 452–3.

Bonebrake C.R., Noller K.L., Loehnen C.P., Muhm J.R. & Fish C.R. (1978) Routine chest roentography in pregnancy. *Journal of the American Medical Association* **240**, 2747–8.

Bongiovanni A.M. & McPadden A.J. (1960) Steroids during pregnancy and possible fetal consequences. *Fertility and Sterility* **11**, 181–6.

Bouterline-Young H. & Bouterline-Young E. (1956) Alveolar carbon dioxide levels in pregnant parturient and lactating subjects. *Journal of Obstetrics and Gynaecology of the British Empire* **63**, 509.

Briscoe W.A. & Dubois A.B. (1958) The relationship between airway resistance, airway conductance and lung volume in subjects of different age and body size. *Journal of Clinical Investigation* **37**, 1279.

British Medical Journal (1979) Editorial: Cystic fibrosis in Adults. *British Medical Journal* **2**, 626.

Brobowitz I.D. (1974) Ethambutol in Pregnancy. *Chest* **66**, 20–4.

Brummer D.L. (1972) Letter to the editor. *American Review of Respiratory Disease* **106**, 785.

Burgener L. & Solmes J.G. (1979) Spontaneous pneumothorax and pregnancy. *Canadian Medical Association Journal* **120**, 19.

Carswell F., Kerr M.M. & Hutchinson J.H. (1970) Congenital goitre and hypothyroidism produced by maternal ingestion of iodides. *Lancet* **1**, 1241.

Case B.W. & Benaroya S. (1980) Dyspnoea in a pregnant young woman. *Canadian Medical Association Journal* **122**, 890–6.

Citron K.M. (1969) Ethambutol: A review with special reference to ocular toxicity. *Tubercle* Suppl. **32**.

Cohen J.D., Patton E.A. & Badger T.L. (1952) The tuberculous mother. *American Review of Tuberculosis* **65**, 1–23.

Cohen L.F., Di Sant'Agnese P.A. & Friedlander J. (1980) Cystic fibrosis and pregnancy. A national survey. *Lancet* **2**, 842–4.

Cohen S.E. (1979) Aspiration syndromes in pregnancy. *Anesthesiology* **51**, 375–7.

Comroe J.J., Forster R.E., Dubois A.B., Briscoe W.A. & Carlsen E. (1962) *The Lung: Clinical Physiology and Pulmonary Function Tests.* Year Book Medical Publishers, Chicago.

Contemporary Obstetrics and Gynecology (1976) Editorial: Pregnant patients and swine flue vaccine. *Contemporary Obstetrics and Gynaecology* **8**, 74–5.

Conway N. & Birt B.D. (1965) Streptomycin in pregnancy: effect on fetal ear. *British Medical Journal* **2**, 260–3.

Corcoran K. & Castles J.M. (1977) Tetracycline for acne vulgaris and possible teratogenesis. *British Medical Journal* **2**, 807–8.

Corkey C.W.B., Newth C.J.L., Corey M. & Levison H. (1981) Pregnancy in cystic fibrosis: A better prognosis in patients with pancreatic function? *American Journal of Obstetrics and Gynecology* **140**, 737–42.

Craig D.R. & Toole M.A. (1975) Airway closure in pregnancy. *Canadian Anaesthetists Society Journal* **22**, 665.

Crozier M.D. (1974) Cystic fibrosis—a not-so-fatal disease. *Pediatric Clinics of North America* **21**, 935–7.

Cugell D.W., Frank N.R., Gaensler E.A. & Badger T.L. (1953) Pulmonary function in pregnancy. I. Serial observations in normal women. *American Review of Tuberculosis* **67**, 568–97.

Cullen J.H., Brum V.O. & Reid T.W.H. (1959) The respiratory effects of progesterone in severe pulmonary emphysema. *American Journal of Medicine* **27**, 551–7.

Cystic Fibrosis Foundation (1976) *1974 Report on Survival of Patients with Cystic Fibrosis.* Cystic Fibrosis Foundation, Rockville, Maryland, USA.

de March P. (1975) Tuberculosis and pregnancy. Five-to-ten-year review of 215 patients in their fertile age. *Chest* **68**, 800–4.

Department of Health & Social Security (1982) *Report on confidential enquiries into maternal deaths in England and Wales 1976–1978.* HMSO, London.

de Swiet M. (1980) The respiratory system. In Hytten F. and Chamberlain G. (eds) *Clinical Physiology in Obstetrics.* Blackwell Scientific Publications, Oxford.

de Swiet M. & Fidler J. (1981) Heart disease in pregnancy: Some controversies. *Journal of the Royal College of Physicians* **15**, 183–6.

di Saint Agnese P.A. & Davis P.B. (1979) Cystic fibrosis in adults. *American Journal of Medicine* **66**, 121–32.

Döring G.K. & Loeschche H.H. (1947) Atmung und Saure—Basengleichgewicht in der Schwangershaft. *Pflügers Archiv für die gesamte Physiologie des Menschen und der Tierre* **249**, 437.

Driscoll A.M. (1969) Urinary oestriol excretion in pregnant patients given large doses of Prednisone. *British Medical Journal* **1**, 556–7.

Dundee J.W., Moore J., Johnston J.P. & McCaughey W. (1981) Cimetidine and obstetric anaesthesia. *Lancet* **2**, 252.

Dykes M.H.M. (1974) Evaluation of an anti asthmatic agent cromolyn sodium (Aarare, Intal). *Journal of the American Medical Association* **227**, 1061–2.

Elder H.A., Santamarine B.A.G., Smith S. & Kass E.H. (1971) The national history of asymptomatic bacteriuria during pregnancy: The effect of tetracycline on the clinical course and outcome of pregnancy. *American Journal of Obstetrics and Gynecology* **111**, 441–62.

Emerson K., Saxena B.N. & Poindexter E.L. (1972) Caloric cost of normal pregnancy. *Obstetrics and Gynaecology* **40**, 786–94.

Eng M., Butler J. & Bonich J.J. (1975) Respiratory function in pregnant obese women. *American Journal of Obstetrics and Gynecology* **123**, 241.

England S.J. & Fahri L.E. (1976) Fluctuations in alveolar CO_2 and in base excess during the menstrual cycle. *Respiration Physiology* **26**, 157.

Fainstall T. (1954) Cortisone-induced congenital cleft palate in rabbits. *Endocrinology* **55**, 520–4.

Farebrother M.J.B. & McHardy G.J.R. (1974) Closing volume and pregnancy. *British Medical Journal* **1**, 454.

Finn R., St. Hill C.A., Govan A.J., Ralfs I.G., Gurney F.J. & Denye V. (1972) Immunological responses in pregnancy and survival of fetal homograft. *British Medical Journal* **3**, 150–2.

Fischl M.A., Pitchenik A. & Gardner L.B. (1981) An index predicting relapse and need for hospitalization in patients with acute bronchial asthma. *New England Journal of Medicine* **305**, 783–9.

Fishburne J.I. (1979) Physiology and diseases of the respiratory system in pregnancy. A review. *Journal of Reproductive Medicine* **22**, 177–89.

Fishburne J.I., Brenner W.E., Braaksma J.T. & Hendricks C.H. (1972a) Bronchospasm complicating intravenous prostaglandin F_{2a} for therapeutic abortion. *Obstetrics and Gynecology* **39**, 892–6.

Fishburne J., Brenner W.E., Braaksma J.T., Staurovsky L.G., Mueller R.A., Hoffer J.L. & Hendricks C.H. (1972b) Cardiovascular and respiratory responses to intravenous infusion of prostaglandin F_{2a} in the pregnant woman. *American Journal of Obstetrics and Gynecology* **114**, 765–72.

Fixley M., Shen D.D. & Azarnoff D.L. (1977) Theophylline bioavailability. A comparison of the oral absorption of a Theophylline Elixir and two combination theophylline tablets to intravenous aminophylline. *American Review of Respiratory Disease* **115**, 955–62.

Francis H.H. & Smellie J. (1964) General diseases in pregnancy. *British Medical Journal* **1**, 887–90.

Freeman D.W. & Barno A. (1959) Deaths from Asian influenza associated with pregnancy. *American Journal of Obstetrics and Gynecology* **78**, 1172–5.

Fried K.H. (1964) Sarcoidosis and pregnancy. *Acta Medica Scandinavica* **176**, Suppl 425, 218–21.

Friedman A.J., Haseltine F.P. & Berkowitz R.L. (1979) Pregnancy in a patient with cystic fibrosis and idiopathis thrombocytopenic purpura. *Obstetrics and Gynecology* **55**, 511–14.

Gaensler E.A., Patton W.E. & Verstraeten J.M. (1953) Pulmonary functions in pregnancy: III. Serial observations in patients with pulmonary insufficiency. *American Review of Tuberculosis* **67**, 779–97.

Gaisford W. & Griffiths M.I. (1961) A freeze-dried vaccine from isioniazid-resistant BCG. *British Medical Journal* **1**, 1500–1.

Galina M.P., Avnet N.L. & Einhorn A. (1962) Iodides during pregnancy: Apparent cause of fetal death. *New England Journal of Medicine* **267**, 1124.

Garrard C.G., Littler W.A.W. & Redman C.W.G. (1978) Closing volume during normal pregnancy. *Thorax* **33**, 484.

Gazioglu K., Kaltreider N.L., Rosen M. & Yu P.N. (1970) Pulmonary function during pregnancy in normal women and in patients with cardiopulmonary disease. *Thorax* **25**, 445–50.

Gee J.B.L., Packer B.S., Millen J.E. & Robin E.D. (1967) Pulmonary mechanics during pregnancy. *Journal of Clinical Investigation* **46**, 945–52.

Giesler C.F., Buehler J.H. & Depp, R. (1977) Alpha-antitrypsin deficiency: severe obstructive lung disease and pregnancy. *Obstetrics and Gynecology* **49**, 31–4.

Given F.R. & DiBenedetto R.L. (1963) Sarcoidosis and pregnancy. *Obstetrics and Gynecology* **22**, 355–9.

Glass D.D., Ginsburgh F.W. & Boucot K.K. (1960) Screening procedures for pulmonary disease in prenatal patients. *American Review of Respiratory Disease* **82**, 689.

Gordon M., Niswander K.R., Berendes H. & Kantor A.G. (1970) Fetal morbidity following potentially anoxigenic obstetric conditions. VII. Bronchial asthma. *American Journal of Obstetrics and Gynecology* **106**, 421–9.

Grand R.J., Talamo R.C., Di Saint Agnese P.A. & Schwartz R.H. (1966) Pregnancy in cystic fibrosis of the pancreas. *Journal of the American Medical Association* **195**, 993–1000.

Gray J.M. & Hanson G.C. (1966) Mediastinal emphysema: Aetiology, diagnosis and treatment. *Thorax* 325–31.

Greenberg M., Jacobziner H., Pakter J. & Weisel B.A.G. (1958) Maternal mortality in the epidemic of Asian influenza New York City 1957. *American Journal of Obstetrics and Gynecology* **76**, 897–902.

Greenberger P. & Patterson R. (1978) Safety of therapy for allergic symptoms during pregnancy. *Annals of Internal Medicine* **89**, 234–7.

Griffith E.R. (1974) Viral pneumonia in pregnancy: Report of a case complicated by disseminated intravascular coagulation and acute renal failure. *American Journal of Obstetrics and Gynecology* **120**, 201–2.

Grossman II J.H. & Littner M.D. (1976) Severe sarcoidosis in pregnancy. *Obstetrics and Gynecology* **50** (Suppl.), 81–4S.

Gurewich V., Sasahara A.A. & Stein M. (1965) In Sasahara A.A. & Stein M. (eds) *Pulmonary Embolic Disease*, p. 162. Grune & Stratton, New York.

Hadjigeogiou E., Kitsiou S., Psaroudakis A., Segos C., Nicolopoulos D. & Kaskarelis D. (1979) Antepartum aminophylline treatment for prevention of respiratory distress syndrome in premature infants. *American Journal of Obstetrics and Gynecology* **135**, 257–60.

Hague W.M. (1980) Mediastinal and subcutaneous emphysema in a pregnant asthmatic. *British Journal of Obstetrics and Gynaecology* **87**, 440–3.

Hamman L. (1945) Mediastinal emphysema. *Journal of the American Medical Association* **128**, 1.

Harris D.M. (1975) Some properties of beclomethasone diproprionate and related steroids in man. *Postgraduate Medical Journal* (Suppl. 4) **51**, 20–5.

Harris R.E. (1966) Coccidiodomycosis complicating pregnancy. Report of three cases and review of the literature. *Obstetrics and Gynecology* **28**, 401–5.

Hedvall E. (1953) Pregnancy and tuberculosis. *Acta Medica Scandinavica (Supplement)* **147**, *Supplement 286*, 1–101.

Heinonen O.P., Slone D. & Shapiro S. (1977) *Birth Defects and Drugs in Pregnancy*. Publishing Sciences Group Inc., Littleton, Mass.

Hellegers A., Metcalfe J., Huckabee W., Meschia G., Prystowsky H. & Barron D. (1959) The alveolar Pco_2 and Po_2 in pregnant and non-pregnant women at altitude. *Journal of Clinical Investigation* **38**, 1010.

Hemminki E. & Starfield B. (1978) Prevention and treatment of premature labour by drugs: Review of clinical trials. *British Journal of Obstetrics and Gynaecology* **85**, 411–17.

Hernandez E., Angel C.S. & Johnson J.W.C. (1980) Asthma in pregnancy: Current concepts. *Obstetrics and Gynecology* **55**, 739–43.

Hiddlestone H.J.H. (1964) Bronchial asthma and pregnancy. *New Zealand Medical Journal* **63**, 521–3.

Hopwood H.G. (1965) Pneumonia in pregnancy. *Obstetrics and Gynecology* **25**, 875.

Howard F.A. & Sharp D.S. (1973) Effect of metoclopramide on gastric emptying during labour. *British Medical Journal* **1**, 446–8.

Howie A.D. & Milne J.A. (1978) Pregnancy in patients with bronchiectasis. *British Journal of Obstetrics and Gynaecology* **85**, 197–200.

Hyman A.L., Spannha K.E.E.W. & Kadowitz Q.J. (1978) Prostaglandins and the lung: State of the art. *American Review of Respiratory Disease* **117**, 111–36.

Isenberg J.N. & L'Heureuse D.R. (1976) Clinical observation on the biliary system in cystic fibrosis. *American Journal of Gastroenterology* **65**, 134–9.

James D.G. (1970) Sarcoidosis. *Disease-A-Month* **1**, 43.

Jellife D.B. & Jelliffe E.F.P. (1977) 'Breast is Best': Modern meanings. *New England Journal of Medicine* **297**, 912–15.

Jolivet A., Blanchier H., Gantray J.P. & Dhem N. (1974) Blood cortisol variations during late pregnancy and labour. *American Journal of Obstetrics and Gynecology* **119**, 775–83.

Kapllan C., Benirschke K. & Tarzy B. (1980) Placental tuberculosis in early and late pregnancy. *American Journal of Obstetrics and Gynecology* **137**, 858–60.

Keefer J.R., Strauss R.G., Civetta J.M. & Burke T. (1981) Non-cardiogenic pulmonary edema and invasive cardiovascular monitoring. *Obstetrics and Gynecology* **58**, 46–51.

Keleman J.T. & Mandl L. (1969) Sarcoidose in der placenta. *Zentralblatt fur Allgemeine Pathologie und Pathologische Anatomie* **112**, 18.

Kendig E.L. (1969) The place of BCG vaccine in the management of infants born of tuberculous mothers. *New England Journal of Medicine* **281**, 520–3.

Knuttgen H.G. & Emerson K. (1974) Physiological response to pregnancy at rest and during exercise. *Journal of Applied Physiology* **36**, 549.

Kopenhager T. (1977) A review of 50 pregnant patients with kyphoscoliosis. *British Journal of Obstetrics and Gynaecology* **84**, 585.

Kreisman H., Van De Wiel N. & Mitchell C.A. (1975) Respiratory function during prostaglandin-induced labour. *American Review of Respiratory Diseases* **111**, 564–6.

Krumholz R.A., Echt C.R. & Ross J.C. (1964) Pulmonary diffusing capacity, capillary blood volume, lung volumes and mechanics of ventilation in early and late pregnancey. *Journal of Laboratory and Clinical Medicine* **63**, 648.

Krupp P.J. (1957) Maternal mortality at Charity Hospital. *American Journal of Obstetrics and Gynecology* **73**, 248.

Kunelis C.T., Peters J.L. & Edmondson H.A. (1965) Fatty liver of pregnancy and its relationship to tetracycline therapy. *American Journal of Medicine* **38**, 359–77.

Lalli C.M. & Raju L. (1981) Pregnancy and chronic obstructive pulmonary disease. *Chest* **80**, 759–61.

Larsen J.W. (1972) Cystic fibrosis and pregnancy. *Obstetrics and Gynecology* **39**, 880–3.

Levitz M., Jansen V. & Dancis J. (1978) The transfer and metabolism of corticosteroids in the perfused human placenta. *American Journal of Obstetrics and Gynecology* **132**, 363–6.

Lewis P.J., de Swiet M., Boylan P. & Bulpitt C.J. (1980) How obstetricians in the United Kingdom manage preterm labour. *British Journal of Obstetrics and Gynaecology* **87**, 574–7.

Lewitt T., Neibel L., Terracina S. & Karman S. (1974) Ethambutol in pregnancy: Observations on embryogenesis. *Chest* **66**, 25–6.

Lucius H., Gahlenbeck H., Kleine H.O., Fabel H. & Bartels H. (1970) Respiratory functions, buffer system and electrolyte concentrations of blood during human pregnancy. *Respiration Physiology* **9**, 311.

Lunell N.O., Wager J., Fredholm B.B. & Person B. (1978) Metabolic effects of oral salbutamol in late pregnancy. *European Journal of Clinical Pharmacology* **14**, 95–9.

Lyons H.A. & Antonio R. (1959) The sensitivity of the respiratory centre in pregnancy and after the administration of progesterone. *Transactions of the Association of American Physicians* **72**, 173.

Lyons H.A. & Huang C.T. (1968) Therapeutic use of progesterone in alveolar hypoventilation associated with obesity. *American Journal of Medicine* **44**, 881–8.

McCarty K.S., Mossler J.A., McLelland R. & Seiker H.O. (1980) Pulmonary lymphangiomyomatosis responsive to progesterone. *New England Journal of Medicine* **303**, 1461–5.

McCaughey W., Howe J.P., Moore J. & Dundee J.W. (1981) Cimetidine in elective Caesarian section: effect on gastric acidity. *Anaesthesia* **36**, 167–72.

MacDonald J.B., MacDonald E.T., Seaton A. & Williams D.A. (1976) Asthma deaths in Cardiff 1963–1974: 53 deaths in hospital. *British Medical Journal* **2**, 721–3.

Maklem P.T. & Mead J. (1967) Resistance of central and peripheral airways measured by a retrograde catheter. *Journal of Applied Physiology* **22**, 395.

Marx G.F. (1974) Obstetric anesthesia in the presence of medical complications. *Clinics in Obstetrics and Gynecology* **17**, 165–81.

Marx C.M. & Fraser D.G. (1981) Treatment of asthma in pregnancy. *Obstetrics and Gynecology* **57**, 766–7.

Mattox J.H. (1973) The value of a routine prenatal chest X-ray. *Obstetrics and Gynecology* **41**, 243–5.

Mearns M.R. (1974) Cystic fibrosis. *British Journal of Hospital Medicine* **12**, 497–506.

Mendelson C.L. (1958) Pregnancy and kyphoscoliotic heart disease. *American Journal of Obstetrics and Gynecology* **56**, 457.

Metzger W.J., Turner E. & Patterson R. (1978) The safety of immunotherapy during pregnancy. *Journal of Allergy and Clinical Immunology* **61**, 268–72.

Milne J.A. (1979) The respiratory response to pregnancy. *Postgraduate Medical Journal* **55**, 318–24.

Milne J.A., Howie A.D. & Pack A.I. (1978) Dyspnoea during normal pregnancy. *British Journal of Obstetrics and Gynaecology* **84**, 448.

Milne J.A., Mills R.J., Howie A.D. & Pack A.I. (1977a) Large airways function during normal pregnancy. *British Journal of Obstetrics and Gynaecology* **84**, 448–51.

Milne J.A., Pack A.I. & Coutts J.R.T. (1977b) Gas exchange and acid base status during ovulatory cycles and those regulated by oral contraceptives. *Journal of Endocrinology* **75**, 17P.

Milne J.A., Pack A.I. & Coutts J.R.T. (1977c) Maternal gas exchange and acid base status during normal pregnancy. *Scottish Medical Journal* **22**, 108.

Möbius W.V. (1961) Abrung and Schwangershaft. *Munchener medizinische Wokenschrift* **103**, 1389.

Monnet P., Kalb J.C. & Pujol M. (1967) De l'influence nocive de l'isoniazide sur le produit de conception. *Lyon Medical* **218**, 431–55.

Morrison J. & Kilpatrick N. (1969) Low urinary oestriol excretion in pregnancy associated with oral prednisone therapy. *Journal of Obstetrics and Gynecology of the British Commonwealth* **76**, 719–20.

Morrow Brown H. & Storey G. (1975) Treatment of allergy of the respiratory tract with beclomethasone dipropionate steroid aerosol. *Postgraduate Medical Journal* (Suppl. 4) **51**, 59–94.

Motoyama E.K., Rivard G., Acheson F. & Cook C.D. (1966) Adverse effect of maternal hyperventilation on the fetus. *Lancet* **1**, 286–8.

Motoyama E.K., Rivard G., Acheson F. & Cook C.D. (1967) The effect of changes in maternal pH and Pco_2 on the Po_2 of fetal lambs. *Anesthesiology* **28**, 891–903.

Moya F., Morishima H.O., Shnider S.M. & James L.S. (1965) Influence of maternal hyperventilation on the new born infant. *American Journal of Obstetrics and Gynecology* **91**, 76–84.

Nelson M.M. & Forfar J.O. (1971) Associations between drugs administered during pregnancy and congenital abnormalities of the fetus. *British Medical Journal* **1**, 523–7.

Newhouse M.T., Becklaile M.R., Macklem P.T. & McGregor M. (1964) Effect of alterations in end-tidal CO_2 on flow resistance. *Journal of Applied Physiology* **19**, 745.

Novy M.J., Tyler J.M., Scwachman H., Easterday C.L. & Reid D.E. (1967) Cystic fibrosis and pregnancy. *Obstetrics and Gynecology* **30**, 530–6.

Old J.M., Ward R.H.T., Petrou M., Karagözlu F., Modell B. & Weatherall D.J. (1982) First-trimester fetal diagnosis for haemoglobinopathies: three cases. *Lancet* **2**, 1913–16.

O'Leary J.A. (1962) Ten year study of sarcoidosis and pregnancy. *American Journal of Obstetrics and Gynecology* **84**, 462.

Orr J.W., Austin J.M., Hatch K.D., Shingleton H.M., Younger L.B. & Boots L.R. (1980) Acute pulmonary edema associated with molar pregnancy: A high-risk factor for development of persistent trophoblastic disease. *American Journal of Obstetrics and Gynecology* **136**, 412–14.

Oxorn H. (1955) The changing aspects of pneumonia complicating pregnancy. *Obstetrics and Gynecology* **70**, 1057.

Paciorek J. & Spencer N. (1980) An association between plasma progesterone and erythrocyte carbonic anhydrase 1 concentration in women. *Clinical Science* **58**, 161–4.

Pedersen H. & Finster M. (1979) Anesthetic risk in the pregnant surgical patient. *Anesthesiology* **51**, 439–51.

Pernoll M.L., Metcalfe J., Kovach P.A., Wachter R. & Dunham M.J. (1975) Ventilation during rest and exercise in pregnancy and postpartum. *Respiration Physiology* **25**, 295.

Phelan P.D. (1981) Cystic fibrosis and pregnancy. *Medical Journal of Australia* **1**, 58.

Plotz E.J., Patterson P.R. & Streit J.H. (1967) Pregnancy in a patient with cystic fibrosis (mucoviscidosis) and diabetes mellitus. *American Journal of Obstetrics and Gynecology* **98**, 1105–10.

Potworoska M., Sianoẓeka E. & Szufladowicz R. (1966) Ethionamide treatment and pregnancy. *Polish Medical Journal* **5**, 1152–8.

Present P.A. & Comstock G.W. (1975) Tubercular sensitivity in pregnancy. *American Review of Respiratory Disease* **112**, 413–16.

Prowse C.M. & Gaensler E.A. (1965) Respiratory and acid base changes during pregnancy. *Anesthesiology* **26**, 381.

Psacharopoulos H.T., Howard E.R., Portmann B., Mowatt A.P. & Williams R. (1981) Hepatic complications of cystic fibrosis. *Lancet* **2**, 78–80.

Raz S., Zeigler M. & Caine M. (1973) The effect of progesterone on the adrenergic receptors of the urethra. *British Journal of Urology* **45**, 131.

Reisfeld D.R. (1958) Boeck's sarcoid and pregnancy. *American Journal of Obstetrics and Gynecology* **75**, 795–801.

Reisfield D.R., Yahia C. & Laurenz G.A. (1969) Pregnancy and cardiorespiratory failure in Boeck's sarcoid. *Surgery, Gynecology and Obstetrics* **109**, 412–16.

Robinson G.C. & Cambon K.G. (1964) Hearing loss in infants of tuberculous mothers treated with streptomycin during pregnancy. *New England Journal of Medicine* **271**, 949–51.

Rosenow E.C. & Lee R.A.C. (1968) Cystic fibrosis and pregnancy. *Journal of American Medical Association* **203**, 227–9.

Rubin A., Russo N. & Goucher D. (1956) The effect of pregnancy upon pulmonary function in normal women. *American Journal of Obstetrics and Gynecology* **72**, 963.

Salvatore M.A. & Lynch P.J. (1980) Erythema nodosum, estrogens, and pregnancy. *Archives of Dermatology* **116**, 557–8.

Scadding J.G. (1961) Prognosis of intrathoracic sarcoidosis in England: A review of 136 cases after five years' observation. *British Medical Journal* **2**, 1165–72.

Schaefer G. & Silverman F. (1961) Pregnancy complicated by asthma. *American Journal of Obstetrics and Gynecology* **82**, 182–9.

Schaefer G., Zervoudakis I.A., Fuchs F.F. & David S. (1975) Pregnancy and pulmonary tuberculosis. *Obstetrics and Gynecology* **46**, 706–15.

Schatz M., Patterson R. & Zeitz S. (1975) Corticosteroid therapy for the pregnant asthmatic patient. *Journal of the American Medical Association* **233**, 804–7.

Scheinhorn D.J. & Angelillo V.A. (1977) Antituberculous therapy in pregnancy: risks to the fetus. *Western Journal of Medicine* **127**, 195–8.

Schenker J.G., Ben-Yoseph Y. & Shapira E. (1972) Erythrocyte carbonic anhydrase B levels during pregnancy and use of oral contraceptives. *Obstetrics and Gynecology* **39**, 237–40.

Schwachman H. & Kulczyki L.L. (1958) Longterm study of one hundred and five patients with cystic fibrosis. *American Journal of Diseases of Children* **96**, 6–15.

Scott D.B. (1978) Mendelson's syndrome. *British Journal of Anaesthesia* **50**, 81–2.

Selikoff I.J. & Dormann H.L. (1965) Management of tuberculosis. In *Medical, Surgical and Gynecologic Complications of Pregnancy*, 2nd Ed., p. 111. The Williams & Wilkins Co., Baltimore.

Shanies H.M. (1977) Non-cardiogenic pulmonary oedema. *Medical Clinics of North America* **61**, 1319.

Siassi B., Moss A.J. & Dooley R.R. (1971) Clinical recognition of cor pulmonale in cystic fibrosis. *Journal of Pediatrics* **78**, 794.

Sibbald B. (1981) A family study approach to the genetic basis of asthma. University of London Ph.D. thesis.

Siegel B. & Siegel S. (1960) Pregnancy and delivery in a patient with cystic fibrosis of the pancreas. *Obstetrics and Gynecology* **16**, 438–40.

Sims C.D., Chamberlain G.V.P. & de Swiet M. (1976) Lung function tests in bronchial asthma during and after pregnancy. *British Journal of Obstetrics and Gynaecology* **88**, 434–7.

Skatrud J.B., Dempsey J.A. & Kaiser D.G. (1978) Ventilatory response to medroxy-progesterone acetate in normal subjects: time course and mechanism. *Journal of Applied Physiology: Respiration Environmental and Exercise Physiology* **44**, 939–44.

Smale L.E. & Waechter K.G. (1974) Dissemination of coccidiomycosis. *American Journal of Obstetrics and Gynecology* **107**, 356–61.

Smith A.P. (1973) The effects of intravenous infusion of graded doses of prostaglandins $F_{2\alpha}$ and E_2 on lung resistance in patients undergoing termination of pregnancy. *Clinical Science* **44**, 17–25.

Snider D.E., Layde P.M., Johnson M.W. & Lyle H.A. (1980) Treatment of tuberculosis during pregnancy. *American Review of Respiratory Diseases* **122**, 65–78.

Sobrevilla L.A., Cassinelli M.T., Carcelen A. & Malaga J.W. (1971) Human fetal and maternal oxygen tension and acid-base status during delivery at high altitude. *American Journal of Obstetrics and Gynaecology* **111**, 1111.

Spellacy W.N. & Prem K.A. (1963) Subcutaneous emphysema and pregnancy: Report of three cases. *Obstetrics and Gynecology* **22**, 521–3.

Steen J.S.M. & Stainton-Ellis D.M. (1977) Rifampicin in pregnancy. *Lancet* **2**, 604–5.

Sulavik S.B. (1975) Pulmonary disease. In Burrow G.N. and Ferris T.F. (eds) *Medical Complications During Pregnanacy*, p. 549. W. B. Saunders, Philadelphia.

Sutton F.D. Jr., Zwillich C.W., Creag H.C.E., Pierson D.J. & Weil J.V. (1975) Progesterone for outpatient treatment of Pickwickian syndrome. *Annals of Internal Medicine* **83**, 476–9.

Sutton P.L., Koup J.R. & Rose B.S. (1978) The pharmokinetics of theophylline in pregnancy. *Journal of Allergy and Chemical Immunology* **61**, 174.

Synder R.D. & Synder D.L. (1978) Corticosteroids for asthma during pregnancy. *Annals of Allergy* **41**, 340–1.

Tatersall M.P. (1983) Prescribing drugs in pregnancy. *British Journal of Hospital Medicine* **29**, 382.

Taussig L.M., Kattwinkel J., Freidwald W.T. & di Sant'Agnese P.A. (1973) A new prognostic score and clinical evaluation system for cystic fibrosis. *Journal of Pediatrics* **82**, 380–90.

Templeton A. (1977) Intrauterine growth retardation associated with hypoxia due to bronchiectasis. *British Journal of Obstetrics and Gynaecology* **84**, 389–90.

Templeton A. & Kelman G.P. (1976) Maternal blood gases (PAO_2—P_aO_2) physiological shunt and V_D/V_T in normal pregnancy. *British Journal of Anaesthesia* **48**, 1001–4.

Thomson K.J. & Cohen M.E. (1938) Studies on the circulation in pregnancy. II: Vital capacity observations in normal pregnant women. *Surgery, Gynecology and Obstetrics* **66**, 591.

Turner E.S., Greenberger P.A. & Patterson R. (1980) Management of the pregnant asthmatic patient. *Annals of Internal Medicine* **6**, 905–18.

Van Arsdel P.P.J. & Paul G.H. (1977) Drug therapy in the management of asthma. *Annals of Internal Medicine* **87**, 68–74.

Varheer H. (1974) Drug excretion in breast milk. *Postgraduate Medicine* **56**, 97–104.

Visser G.H.A., Huisjes H.J., ten Kate L.P., Smit Sibinga C.T. & Wiers P.W.J. (1977) Pregnancy in cystic fibrosis: Report of a case, complicated by hemophilia A, and review of the literature. *European Journal of Obstetrics, Gynecology and Reproductive Biology* **7**, 109–15.

Wager J., Fredholm B.B., Lunell N-O. & Persson B. (1981) Metabolic and circulatory effects of oral salbutamol in the third trimester of pregnancy in diabetic and non-diabetic women. *British Journal of Obstetrics and Gynaecology* **88**, 352–61.

Wallace S.J. & Michie E.A. (1966) A follow-up study of infants born to mothers with low oestriol excretion during pregnancy. *Lancet* **2**, 560–3.

Warrell D.W. & Taylor R. (1968) Outcome for the fetus of mother receiving prednisolone during pregnancy. *Lancet* **1**, 117–18.

Warwick W.J., Progue R.E., Gerber H.M. & Nesbitt C.J. (1975) Survival patterns in cystic fibrosis. *Journal of Chronic Diseases* **28**, 609–22.

Weinberger S.E., Weiss S.T., Cohen W.R., Weiss J.W. & Johnson T.S. (1980) Pregnancy and the lung. *American Review of Respiratory Disease* **121**, 559–81.

Weinstein A.M., Dubin B.D., Podleski W.K., Spector S.L. & Farr R.S. (1979) Asthma and pregnancy. *Journal of the American Medical Association* **241**, 1161–5.

White R.J., Blainey A.D., Harrison K.J. & Clarke S.K.R. (1981) Causes of pneumonia presenting to a district general hospital. *Thorax* **36**, 566–70.

Whitelaw A. & Butterfield A. (1977) High breast milk sodium in cystic fibrosis. *Lancet* **2**, 1288.

Wilbrand U., Porath Ch., Matthaes P. & Jaster R. (1959) Der einfluss der Ovarialsteroide auf die Funktion des Atemzentrums. *Archiv für Gynäkologie* **191**, 507.

Williams D.A. (1959) Definition, prevalence, predisposing and contributory factors. In Jamar J.M. (ed.) *International Textbook of Allergy*, pp. 90–100. Blackwell Scientific Publications, Oxford.

Williams D.A. (1967) Asthma and pregnancy. *Acta Allergolica* **22**, 311–23.

Wilson J.W. (1972) Treatment or prevention of pulmonary cellular damage with pharmacological doses of corticosteroids. *Surgery, Gynecology and Obstetrics* **134**, 675.

Windebank W.J., Boyd G. & Moran F. (1973) Pulmonary thromboembolism presenting as asthma. *British Medical Journal* **1**, 90.

Wulf K.H., Kunzel S. & Lehman V. (1972) Clinical aspects of placental gas exchange. In Longo L.D. and Bartels H. (eds) *Respiratory gas exchange and blood flow in the placenta*. US Department of Health, Education & Welfare, Bethesda, Maryland, USA.

Yeh T.F. & Pildes R.S. (1977) Transplacental aminophylline toxicity in a neonate. *Lancet* **1**, 910.

Yurchak A.M. & Jusko W.J. (1976) Theophylline secretion in breast milk. *Pediatrics* **75**, 518–20.

2 Blood Volume, Haematinics, Anaemia

Elizabeth Letsky

Blood volume

Although the 'plethora' of pregnancy was recognised early in the nineteenth century and German work as far back as 1854 showed a rise of blood volume in pregnant laboratory animals, the evidence for plethora in pregnant women rested primarily on the demonstration of reduced concentration of solids and cells in the blood until the early twentieth century (Miller *et al* 1915). The best estimate of total blood volume is obtained when plasma volume and red cell mass are measured simultaneously; however, the majority of published reports of blood volume in pregnancy are based on either measured plasma volume or total red cell mass, the fraction not directly estimated being calculated from body haematocrit.

PLASMA VOLUME

The measurement of plasma volume in pregnancy has a long history which was comprehensively reviewed by Hytten and Leitch (1971). Plasma volume rises progressively throughout pregnancy, with a tendency to plateau in the last eight weeks (Pirani *et al* 1973). The terminal fall in plasma volume described by almost all investigators previously, occurs only when measurements are made in the supine position. The underestimation in the supine position is due to the bulky uterus obstructing venous return from the lower limbs resulting in incomplete mixing of dye (Chesley and Duffus 1971)—a similar condition to the reduction in cardiac output seen in patients in the supine position (Chapter 5).

There is little doubt that the amount of increase in plasma volume is correlated with obstetric outcome and the birthweight of the baby (Hytten and Leitch 1971, Pirani *et al* 1973). Since second and subsequent pregnancies tend to be more successful than the first, with bigger babies, a larger plasma volume increase in multigravidae would be expected; however, the evidence for this is not entirely satisfactory (Hytten and Leitch 1971).

Women with multiple pregnancy have proportionately higher increments of plasma volume. The plasma volume at term was found to be approximately 1940 ml above control in eight women with twins and 2400 ml above control in two women with triplets (Rovinsky and Jaffin 1965). One woman with a quadruplet pregnancy had raised her plasma volume by 2400 ml above her non-pregnant value by 34 weeks (Fullerton *et al* 1965).

In contrast, women with poorly growing fetuses (particularly multigravidae with a history of poor reproductive performance) have a correspondingly poor plasma response (Gibson 1973).

In summary, healthy women in a normal first pregnancy increase their plasma volume from a nonpregnant level of almost 2600 ml by about 1250 ml. Most of the rise takes place before 32–34 weeks' gestation; thereafter there is relatively little change. In subsequent pregnancies, the increase is greater. The increase is related to the size of the fetus and there are particularly large increases in association with multiple pregnancy.

RED CELL MASS

The red cell 'mass' is a confusing term which expresses the total volume of red cells in the circulation. The more logical alternative of red cell volume cannot be used because of its specific meaning in haematology of the volume of a single erythrocyte.

There is less published information on red cell mass than plasma volume and the results are more variable. There is still disagreement as to how much the red cell mass increases in normal pregnancy. The extent of the increase is considerably influenced by iron medication which will cause the red cell mass to rise in apparently healthy women even if they have no clinical evidence of iron deficiency.

The literature is summarised by Hytten and Leitch (1971). If one accepts a figure of about 1400 ml for the volume of red cells in the average healthy woman before pregnancy, then the rise in pregnancy for women not given iron supplements is about 240 ml (18%) and for those given iron 400 ml (30 per cent). The red cell mass increases steadily between the end of the first trimester and term. As with plasma volume, the extent of the increase is related to the size of the conceptus, particularly large increases being seen in association with multiple pregnancy (Rovinsky and Jaffin 1965; Fullerton *et al* 1965).

The red cell mass falls immediately at delivery as a result of blood loss (de Leeuw *et al* 1968). Nonpregnant blood volumes are reached around three weeks after delivery (Chesley 1972).

TOTAL HAEMOGLOBIN

The haemoglobin concentration, haemotocrit, and red cell count, fall during pregnancy because the expansion of the plasma volume is greater than that of the red cell mass. Paradoxically there is a rise in total circulating haemoglobin directly related to the increase in red cell mass. This in turn is dependent partly on the iron status of the individual. Published evidence for the rise in total haemoglobin is unsatisfactory and is confused by the varying iron status of the women studied. It is impossible to give physiological limits for the expected rise in total haemoglobin until better figures are available, and controversies resolved.

The lowest normal haemoglobin in the healthy adult *nonpregnant* woman living at sea level is defined as 12.0 g/dl (World Health Organisation 1972). In most published studies the mean minimum in pregnancy is between 11 and 12 g/dl. The lowest haemoglobin observed in a carefully studied iron supplemented group was 10.44 g/dl (de Leeuw *et al* 1966). The mean minimum acceptable to the World Health Organisation is 11.0 g/dl (World Health Organisation 1972).

IRON METABOLISM

In pregnancy the demand for iron is increased to meet the needs of the expanding red cell mass and requirements of the developing fetus and placenta. By far the greatest single demand for iron is that for the expansion of the red cell mass. The fetus derives its iron from the maternal serum by active transport across the placenta mainly in the last four weeks of pregnancy (Fletcher and Suter 1969). The total requirement for iron is of the order of 700–1400 mg. Overall the requirement is 4 mg per day, but this rises to 6.6 mg per day in the last few weeks of pregnancy. This can be met only by mobilising iron stores in addition to achieving maximum absorption of dietary iron, because a normal mixed diet supplies about 14 mg of iron each day of which only 1–2 mg (5–15%) is absorbed.

Iron absorption is increased when there is erythroid hyperplasia—rapid iron turnover—and a high concentration of unsaturated transferrin, all of which are part of the physiological response in the healthy pregnant woman. There is evidence that absorption of dietary iron is enhanced in the latter half of pregnancy (Apte and Iyengar 1970; Hytten and Leitch 1971), but this would still not provide enough iron for the needs of pregnancy and the puerperium for a woman on a normal mixed diet.

IRON ABSORPTION

There are at least two distinct pathways for iron absorption: one for inorganic iron and one for iron attached to haem. The availability of food iron is quite variable. In most foods inorganic iron is in the 'ferric' form and has to be converted to the ferrous form before absorption can take place. In foods derived from grain, iron often forms a stable complex with phytates and only small amounts can be converted to a soluble form. The iron in eggs is poorly absorbed because of binding with phosphates present in the yolk. Milk, particularly cows' milk, is poor in iron content. Tea inhibits the absorption of iron. The traditional Scotsman's breakfast of porridge and eggs washed down with milky tea is rich in protein but provides very little, if any, absorbable iron!

The intestinal mucosal control of iron absorption is complex and incompletely understood; however, in general, absorption is enhanced in times of increased need and deficiency. Haem iron derived from the haemoglobin and myoglobin of animal origin is more effectively absorbed than non-haem iron. Factors interfering with or promoting the absorption of inorganic iron have no effect on the absorption of haem iron. This puts vegetarians at a disadvantage in terms of iron sufficiency. The amount of iron absorbed will depend very much on the extent of the iron stores, the content of the diet and whether or not iron supplements are given. It was found, in a carefully controlled study in Sweden (Svanberg 1975), that absorption rates differed markedly between those pregnant women receiving 100 mg ferrous iron supplements daily and those receiving a placebo. Iron absorption increased steadily throughout pregnancy in the placebo group. In the supplemented group there was no increase between the 12th and 24th week of gestation and thereafter the increase was only 60 per cent of the placebo group. After delivery the mean absorption in the placebo group was markedly higher. These differences can be explained by the difference in storage iron between the two groups (Svanberg 1975).

The commonest haematological problem in pregnancy is anaemia resulting from iron deficiency. The bulk of iron in the body is contained in the haemoglobin of the circulating red cells. Since many women enter pregnancy with depleted stores, it is not surprising that iron deficiency in pregnancy and the puerperium is so common when, in addition to the demands of the fetus and blood loss at delivery, the absolute red cell mass increases by approximately 25 per cent.

Over the years there have been many studies which have proved without doubt that iron supplements prevent the development of anaemia (Lund 1951; Magee and Milligan 1951; Gatenby 1956; Stott 1960; Morgan 1961; Chanarin *et al*; 1965, Chisholm 1966) and that even in women on a good diet who are not apparently anaemic at booking, the mean haemoglobin level can be raised by oral iron therapy throughout pregnancy. The difference in favour of those so treated is most marked at term when the need for adequate haemoglobin is maximal (Morgan 1961; de Leeuw *et al* 1966; Fenton *et al* 1977).

Diagnosis of iron deficiency

HAEMOGLOBIN

A reduction in concentration of circulating haemoglobin is a relatively late develop-ment in iron deficiency. This is preceded by a depletion of iron stores and then a reduction in serum iron before there is any detectable change in haemoglobin level. However, measurement of haemoglobin is the simplest, non-invasive practical test at our disposal and is the one investigation on which further action is usually taken.

The changes in blood volume and haemodilution are so variable that the normal range of haemoglobin concentration in healthy pregnancy at 30 weeks' gestation in women who have received parenteral iron is from 10.0 to 14.5 g/dl. However, haemoglobin values of less than 10.5 g/dl in the second and third trimesters are probably abnormal and require further investigation.

RED CELL INDICES

The appearance of red cells on a stained film is a relatively insensitive gauge of iron status in pregnancy. Most hospital laboratories now possess electronic counters which perform accurate red cell counts. The size of the red cell (MCV), its haemoglobin content (MCH), and haemoglobin concentration (MCHC) can be calculated from the red cell count (RBC), haemoglobin concentration and packed cell volume (PCV). A better guide to the diagnosis of iron deficiency in pregnancy is the examination of these red cell indices (Table 2.1, p. 52).

The ealiest effect of iron deficiency on the erythrocyte is a reduction in cell size (MCV) and with the dramatic changes in red cell mass and plasma volume of pregnancy this appears to be the most sensitive indicator of underlying iron deficiency. Hypochromia and a fall in MCHC only appear with more severe degrees of iron depletion.

Of course some women enter pregnancy with already established anaemia due to iron deficiency or with grossly depleted iron stores and they will quickly develop florid anaemia with reduced MCV, MCH and MCHC. These do not present any problems in diagnosis. It is those women who enter pregnancy in precarious iron balance with a normal haemoglobin who present the most difficult diagnostic problems.

SERUM IRON AND TOTAL IRON BINDING CAPACITY (TIBC)

In health, the serum iron of adult nonpregnant women lies between 13 and 27 μmol/l. It shows marked individual diurnal variation and fluctuates even from hour to hour. The total iron binding capacity in the nonpregnant state lies in the range 45–72 μmol/l. It is raised in association with iron deficiency and found to be low in chronic inflammatory states. In the non-anaemic individual the TIBC is approximately one-third saturated with iron.

Most workers report a fall in the serum iron and percentage saturation of the TIBC in pregnancy; the fall in serum iron can largely be prevented by iron supplements. Serum iron even in combination with TIBC is not a reliable indication of iron stores because it fluctuates so widely and is also affected by recent ingestion of iron and other factors (such as infection not directly involved with iron metabolism). With these considerable reservations a serum iron of less than 12 μmol/l and a TIBC saturation of less than 15% indicate deficiency of iron during pregnancy.

FERRITIN

Ferritin, a high-molecular-weight glycoprotein thought previously to be a totally intracellular iron storage compound, circulates in the plasma of healthy adults in amounts in the range of 15–300 μg/l (Jacobs *et al* 1972). It is stable, not affected by recent ingestion of iron, and appears to reflect the iron stores accurately and quantitatively—particularly in the lower range associated with iron deficiency which is so important in pregnancy. A study of serum ferritin during the course of pregnancy in 154 women has been carried out in Cardiff (Fenton *et al* 1977a). The patients were divided randomly into roughly equal groups, one of which received oral iron supplements. Although there was a rapid decrease in iron stores during early pregnancy in all women studied, the stores (as assessed by serum ferritin levels) were prevented from reaching iron deficient levels during the latter half of pregnancy in the supplemented group. This pattern has been demonstrated previously in an examination of the stainable iron in bone marrow at term (de Leeuw *et al* 1966). Interestingly, the concentration of ferritin in the cord blood was substantially greater than the maternal level at term in all cases but the babies born to iron-deficient mothers had significantly decreased cord ferritin levels compared to the others.

This trend was apparent in the data of another study of maternal and infant iron stores (Rios *et al* 1975), although the authors interpreted their data without reference to this trend. There is a reduction in the iron accumulated by the fetuses of mothers with depleted iron stores and this may have an important bearing on the iron stores of the child during the first year of life.

Serum ferritin is estimated by a sensitive immunoradiometric assay. Not all hospital laboratories can offer this service and if the Supraregional Assay Service is used there is a delay in obtaining results. Recently a number of commercial kits have become available which will facilitate the test being done in individual hospitals, but they are still rather expensive. Even if there is a delay in obtaining the result, it is valuable to have an accurate assessment of iron stores before therapy is started.

MARROW IRON

The most rapid and reliable method of assessing iron stores in pregnancy is by examination of an appropriately stained preparation of a bone marrow sample. If properly performed, marrow aspiration need not result in any major discomfort—in skilful hands the procedure takes no more than ten minutes. The iliac crest (anterior or posterior) should always be used as the aspiration site in preference to the sternum, for the benefit and comfort of the patient. In the absence of iron supplementation there is no detectable stainable iron in over 80 per cent of women at term (de Leeuw *et al* 1966). A block of incorporation of iron into haemoglobin occurs in the course of chronic inflammation particularly of the urinary tract even if iron stores are replete. This problem will be revealed by examination of the marrow aspirate stained for iron.

Management of iron deficiency

In the UK the management of iron deficiency in pregnancy has largely become one of prevention by daily oral supplements. Oral supplementation of 60–80 mg elemental iron per day from early pregnancy maintains the haemoglobin in the recognised normal range for pregnancy but does not maintain or restore the iron stores (Fleming *et al* (1974a, de Leeuw *et al* 1966). The World Health Organisation (1972) recommends that supplements of 30–60 mg per day be given to those pregnant women who have normal iron stores and 120–240 mg to those women with none. Whether all pregnant women need iron is controversial and is discussed below, but if it is accepted that iron is necessary, a bewildering number of preparations of varying expense are available for use. In those women to whom additional iron cannot be given by the oral route either because of non-compliance or because of unacceptable side-effects, intramuscular injection of 1000 mg iron more than ensures iron sufficiency for that pregnancy. The injections are painful and can be skin staining but there is no extra risk of incurring malignancy at the injection site in man as Richmond (1959) reported in rats.

There is no haematological benefit in giving parenteral as opposed to oral iron, but the failure rate of some women to take oral preparations is high and the sole advantage is that the physician can be sure they have received adequate supplementation.

The side-effects of oral administration of iron have been shown to be related to the quantity administered (Hallberg *et al* 1966): if the daily dose is reduced to 100 mg they are rare with any preparation. Although some women do have gastric symptoms the most common complaint is constipation which is usually easily overcome by simple measures. Slow-release preparations, which are generally more expensive, are said to be relatively free of side-effects. This is only because much of the iron is not released at all, is unabsorbed and excreted unchanged. This means that double doses may have to be given to cover requirements, thereby further increasing expense. The majority of women tolerate the cheaper preparations with no significant side-effects and in the interests of economy these should be tried first.

All the preparations used routinely in pregnancy are now combined with an appropriate dose of folic acid (*see* below). Prophylaxis therefore depends partly on good antenatal care, but ultimately on regular attendance at the antenatal clinic and cooperation in taking the prescribed medication.

The management of iron deficiency anaemia diagnosed late in pregnancy presents a particular challenge to the obstetrician because a satisfactory response has to be obtained in a limited space of time. Parental iron is invaluable in the management of this condition, particularly if it is diagnosed late. Iron sorbitol citrate can be given as a series of intramuscular injections but it is associated with toxic reactions such as headache, nausea and vomiting if given simultaneously with oral iron (Scott 1963).

Iron dextran is an extensively used preparation and may be administered as a series of intramuscular injections or by total dose infusion. Rare anaphylactic reactions do occur in the case of intravenous infusion, but usually during the period when the first few millilitres are being given (Clay *et al* 1965). For this reason infusion should always be started slowly and the patient watched carefully for the first few minutes. This preparation does not appear to be associated with toxicity if given simultaneously with oral iron (Scott 1962).

In the absence of any other abnormality an increase in haemoglobin concentration of 1 g/dl per week can be reasonably expected with adequate treatment of iron, whether oral or parenteral. If there is not time to achieve a reasonable haemoglobin concentration before delivery, blood transfusion is indicated.

THE CASE FOR PROPHYLACTIC IRON THERAPY

There is still considerable controversy about whether the fall in haemoglobin concentration which occurs in healthy women during pregnancy is an indication of iron deficiency and whether raising the haemoglobin with iron confers any benefit (Anon 1978). Many authors are not able to accept that the physiological requirements for iron in pregnancy are considerably higher than the usual intake of most healthy women with apparently good diets in industrialised countries. The arguments about policy among nutritionists wishing to prevent iron deficiency are complicated by the varying problems of applying strategies in countries with differing standards of living. Paradoxically the greatest experience in prevention comes from those countries where iron deficiency is least common and least severe (Jacobs and Worwood 1982).

There is no doubt that in the poorly developed countries the incidence of anaemia and iron deficiency is high and many women enter pregnancy who are either anaemic or who have grossly depleted iron stores. A small but careful study of anaemia in pregnancy from Nigeria (Ogunbode *et al* 1979) showed that once the major problems of malaria and the haemoglobinopathies were partially solved by giving antimalarials and folic acid routinely throughout pregnancy, iron deficiency was also present in many of the patients with pregnancy anaemia. The conclusion was that the deficiency was primarily due to poor iron content in the diet and routine iron supplementation was recommended. Another larger controlled trial from the Phillippines (Kuizon *et al* 1979) showed clearly that those women with normal haemoglobins given iron throughout pregnancy maintained their haemoglobin; anaemic women on a larger dose of iron raised their haemogloins if compared to those taking placebo or ascorbic acid alone.

One of the earliest large studies in the UK came from Manchester (Magee and Milligan 1951). Over 2000 women were studied during pregnancy. In those not taking iron a progressive drop in the haemoglobin was observed—the lowest level being reached at 32 weeks' gestation—but it took more than a year after delivery before the prepregnancy haemoglobin level was re-achieved. Those women who took iron had consistently higher haemoglobins and the effects persisted into the postnatal period—prepregnancy haemoglobin levels being much more rapidly re-achieved. However, the majority of the women, whether taking iron or not, were perfectly healthy and had no complaints. This raises the question of whether a haemoglobin level raised by iron therapy is in itself an advantage. There was no advantage in terms of subjective health conferred by iron treatment in another double-blind study (Paintin *et al* 1966) in Aberdeen.

'In general there is no convincing evidence that the normal pregnant woman is at an advantage if she takes extra iron' (Hytten and Leitch 1971). The fact that the fall of haemoglobin concentration in normal multigravidae has been found to be greater than in primigravidae has been interpreted as indirect evidence of depletion of iron concentration by repeated pregnancy; however, multigravidae have a greater rise of plasma volume than primigravidae and therefore a correspondingly lower haemoglobin is to be expected. All these findings emphasise the important principle that 'normality' in pregnancy cannot be judged by reference to nonpregnant standards. Curiously enough a fall in haemoglobin concentration due to haemodilution seems to cause anxiety; however, a satisfactory level of haemoglobin concentration may indicate an unsatisfactory increase of plasma volume. Moreover the human female is not alone in depleting the concentration of her circulating red cell mass during pregnancy: this phenomenon is observed in other mammalian species as different as the dog, elephant and monkey.

Hemminki and Starfield (1978) have recently reviewed controlled clinical trials of iron administration during pregnancy in developed western countries. Seventeen trials were found which fulfilled their stated criteria. As a result of their analysis they concluded that there was no beneficial effect in terms of birthweight, length of gestation, maternal and infant morbidity and mortality in those woman receiving iron compared with controls. They maintain that while age, economic status and poor nutrition affect the outcome, pregnancy anaemia is not related and is simply associated with other risk factors. They did not take into account the withdrawal of anaemic patients from the trials they reviewed. Their analysis may be correct but anaemia remains a potential danger in pregnancy especially in the face of haemorrhage. The majority of women who do not receive iron supplements have no stores at all at the end of pregnancy (Fenton *et al* 1977, de Leeuw *et al* 1966). Also offspring of non-anaemic women who have not received supplements have less iron stores than those of iron replete women (Fenton *et al* 1977). An analysis of factors leading to a 20 per cent reduction in iron deficiency in Swedish women of childbearing age in the ten year period 1965–75 attributed this to greater prescribing of iron tablets (10%) and fortification of food (7–8 per cent); oral contraception also played a part (2–3 per cent) (Hallberg *et al* 1979).

The crucial information needed to decide the interpretation of the physiological anaemia of pregnancy is whether or not the average young woman has a sufficiency of storage iron. Svanberg (1975) comments that the absence of iron stores in women of fertile age is not physiological and that the increased iron demand during pregnancy cannot be met by increased absorption. The conclusion is that, even with maximum iron content in the diet, the immediate demands of pregnancy cannot be covered by an increased absorption from the diet. From the evidence that is available it would appear that a high proportion of women in reproductive years do lack storage iron (Fenton *et al* 1977, de Leeuw *et al* 1966).

The reasons may be different in different populations. Over thousands of years man has changed his way of living and eating, from a society based on hunting and fishing to the present one with a lower intake of iron, meat and fish. Recent dietary changes in industrialised countries have made it difficult for women to build up iron stores so that iron balance can be maintained in pregnancy. There is no epidemiological evidence of reduced iron stores in normal women in the reproductive years, mainly because the only rapid safe method available in the recent past was examination of a suitably stained bone marrow specimen. This is cumbersome, semiquantitative and unjustifiable in a healthy young woman. Now that a relatively simple noninvasive method of assessing iron stores is available by estimation of serum ferritin levels, perhaps this epidemiological evidence can be obtained.

Meanwhile, with the evidence that is available, I feel it is safer, more practical and, in the long-term, less expensive in terms of investigation, hospital admission and treatment, to give all women iron supplements throughout pregnancy, especially as this appears to do no harm (Kullander and Källen 1976).

Folic acid

FOLATE METABOLISM

Folic acid and iron are particularly important in nutrition during pregnancy. At a cellular level folic acid is reduced first to dehydrofolic acid (DHF) and then to tetrahydrofolic acid (THF) which forms the pivot of cellular folate metabolism since it is fundamental (through linkage with L-carbon fragments) both to cell growth and cell division. The more active a tissue is in reproduction and growth, the more dependent it will be on the efficient turnover and supply of folate co-enzymes. Bone marrow and epithelial linings are therefore particularly at risk.

Requirements for folate are increased in pregnancy to meet the needs of the fetus, the placenta, uterine hypertrophy and the expanded maternal red cell mass. The placenta transports folate actively to the fetus even in the face of maternal deficiency, but maternal folate metabolism is altered early in pregnancy like many other maternal functions, before fetal demands act directly.

PLASMA FOLATE

With the exception of haemoglobin concentration and plasma iron, folic acid must be one of the most studied substances in maternal blood, but there are comparatively few serial data available. It is generally agreed, however, that plasma folate levels fall as pregnancy advances so that at term they are about half the nonpregnant values (Ball and Giles 1964; Chanarin 1979; Fleming *et al* 1974b; Landon 1975). Plasma clearance of folate by the kidneys is more than doubled by as early as the eighth week of gestation (Fleming 1972, Landon and Hytten 1971). It has been suggested that urinary loss may be a major factor in the fall of serum folate. Although the glomerular filtration rate is raised (Chapter 7), the marked contrast between the comparatively unchanging plasma levels and the wide variation in urinary loss suggests a change in tubular reabsorption, rather than some alteration in folate metabolism. It is unlikely that this is a major drain on maternal resources and it cannot play more than a marginal role (Landon 1975).

There have been conflicting reports about the part intestinal malabsorption may play in the aetiology of folate deficiency of pregnancy. Traditionally absorption has been assessed from plasma levels following an oral load. Earlier reports of decreased absorption (Chanarin *et al* 1959) were probably due to the underestimation of the rapid clearance of folate following an oral dose. Placenta and maternal tissues contribute from an early stage probably under the influence of oestrogens, as oral contraceptives also increase plasma clearance of folate (Stephens *et al* 1972). There is no change in absorption of either folate monoglutamates or polyglutamates in healthy pregnancy (Landon and Hytten 1972; McLean *et al* 1970). There is invariably a wide scatter of results. The incidence of abnormally low serum folates in late pregnancy varies with the population studied and presumably reflects the local nutritional standards.

Substantial day to day variation of plasma folate is possible and postprandial increases have been noted. This variability limits the diagnostic value of plasma folate estimations when occasional samples taken at a casual antenatal clinic visit are considered.

It could be argued that the changes noted in pregnancy are positively advantageous. There is no logical reason why reduced plasma levels of nutrients such as folate should indicate deficiency, while others such as glucose and amino acids are disregarded. The reduced levels may aid conservation in the face of a raised glomerular filtration rate. It is possible that the placenta may be able to compete more effectively with maternal tissues for folate supplies at lower maternal plasma levels and compensate for its relatively small receptive area (Landon 1975).

RED CELL FOLATE

The estimation of red cell folate may provide more useful information than plasma folate as it does not reflect the daily and other short-term variations of plasma folate. It is thought to give a better indication of overall body tissue levels, but the turnover of red blood cells is slow and there will be a delay before significant reductions in the folate concentrations of the red cells, due to folate deficiency, are evident.

A number of investigations of erythrocyte folate in pregnancy have shown a slight downward trend even though, as would be expected, the fall is not so marked as that noted for plasma (Avery and Ledger 1970, Chanarin *et al* 1968). There is evidence that patients who have a low red cell folate at the beginning of pregnancy develop megaloblastic anaemia in the third trimester (Chanarin *et al* 1968).

EXCRETION OF FORMIMINOGLUTAMIC ACID (FIGLU)

A loading dose of histidine leads to increased FIGLU excretion in the urine when there is folate deficiency. As a test for folate deficiency in pregnancy it no longer has much to recommend it, primarily because the metabolism of histidine is altered (Chanarin 1979) and this results in increased FIGLU excretion in normal early pregnancy (Stone *et al* 1967).

FOLIC ACID POSTPARTUM

In the six weeks following delivery there is a tendency for all indices of folate metabolism to return to nonpregnant values. However, should any deficiency of folate have developed and remained untreated in pregnancy, it may present clinically for the first time in the puerperium and its consequences may be detected for many months after delivery. Lactation provides an added folate stress. A folate content of 5 μg per 100 ml of human milk and a yield of 500 ml daily implies a loss of 25 μg folate daily in breast milk. In the Bantu, megaloblastic anaemia appears frequently in the year following pregnancy in association with lactation. Dietary folate intake is poor and it has been shown that folate deficiency becomes more apparent, as demonstrated by using FIGLU excretion, as lactation continues (Shapiro *et al* 1965). Red cell folate levels in lactating mothers are significantly lower than those of their infants during the first year of life (Chanarin 1979). In the UK, as early as 1919, Osler described the severe anaemias of pregnancy which had a high colour index and a striking incidence in the postpartum period.

INTERPRETATION OF INVESTIGATIONS

The value of these various investigations in predicting megaloblastic anaemia and assessing subclinical folate deficiency has been the subject of numerous reports. Using these various tests it appears that folate 'deficiency' in pregnancy is not always accompanied by significant haematological change (Shapiro *et al* 1965; Stone *et al* 1967).

Even in the absence of any significant haematological changes in the peripheral blood megaloblastic haemopoiesis should be suspected when the expected response to adequate iron therapy is not achieved. Evidence of megaloblastic haemopoiesis may become apparent only after iron therapy even though the rise in haemoglobin concentration appears adequate. No help can be expected from the use of tests of folate status. 'Abnormal' results are obtained with most of the tests but these are not significantly different from results in healthy pregnant women. The decline of serum folic acid levels from a mean of 6.0 μg/l in the nonpregnant to 3.4 μg/l at term should be viewed only as the physiological consequence of maternal tissue uptake, urinary loss and placental transfer—not of evidence of folate deficiency. The delay in fall of red cell folate makes this too impractical a test for folate deficiency in pregnancy. Therefore the diagnosis of folate deficiency in pregnancy has to be made ultimately on morphological grounds; this usually involves examination of a suitably prepared marrow aspirate.

Megaloblastic anaemia

FOLIC ACID DEFICIENCY

The cause of megaloblastic anaemia in pregnancy is nearly always folate deficiency. Vitamin B12 is only very rarely implicated (see below). A survey of reports from the UK over the past two decades suggest an incidence ranging from 0.2 to 5.0%, but a considerably greater number of women have megaloblastic changes in their marrow which are not suspected on examination of the peripheral blood only (Lowenstein *et al* 1966; Chanarin 1979). The incidence of megaloblastic anaemia in other parts of the world is considerably greater and is thought to reflect the nutritional standards of the population. Several workers have pointed to the poor socioeconomic status of their patients as the major aetiological factor contributing to the anaemia (Coyle and Geoghegan 1962, Chanarin 1979), which may be further exacerbated by seasonal changes in the availability of stable foodstuffs. Food folates are only partially available and the amount of folate supplied in the diet is difficult to quantify. In the UK, analysis of daily folate intake in foodstuffs showed a range of 129–300 μg (Chanarin 1975). The folate content of 24 hour food collections in various studies in Sweden and Canada proved to be about 200 μg, with a range as large as 70–600 μg (Chanarin 1979).

Foods that are very rich in folate include broccoli, spinach and brussel sprouts, but up to 90% of their folate content is lost within the first few minutes, by boiling or steaming, and they are unlikely to be eaten raw. Asparagus, avocados, and mushrooms also have a fairly high folate content but are expensive. Natural folates are protected from oxidation and degradation by the presence of reducing substances such as ascorbate. The results of analysis of folate content of food will give very low results if ascorbate is not added to the assay system—as occurred in the very earliest studies (Chanarin 1979). Having established the content of folate in food, there is only indirect evidence about its absorption. Monoglutamates are almost completely absorbed. Polyglutamates from different sources are variably available, but in general are less well absorbed, so that total folate intake should be combined with information about the source of food folate to give a realistic appraisal of the available folate content. In general, dietary intake is likely to be greater, rather than smaller, during pregnancy but obviously in certain areas of the world malnutrition is an essential aetiological factor in determining folate status.

The effects of dietary inadequacy may be further amplified by frequent childbirth and multiple pregnancy. An incidence of 1 in 11 in twin pregnancies compared with the expected incidence of 1 in 80 was noted in one survey of over 1000 patients (Chanarin 1979).

The normal dietary folate intake is inadequate to prevent megaloblastic changes in the bone marrow in approximately 25% of pregnant women. The fall in serum and red cell folate could be a physiological phenomenon in pregnancy but the incidence of megaloblastic change in the bone marrow is reduced only when the blood folate levels are maintained in a steady state by adequate oral supplements. There is much controversy about the requirement for folate, particularly during pregnancy. World

Health Organisation recommendations for daily folate intake are as high as 800 μg in the antenatal period, 600 μg during lactation, and 400 μg in the nonpregnant adult (WHO 1972). There is an increased need of about 100 μg folic acid daily during pregnancy which, without supplements, must be found from natural folates in the diet (Chanarin 1979). The WHO recommended intakes clearly overestimate the needs. The daily amount of folate that has been given prophylactically in pregnancy varies from 30 μg to 500 μg and even to pharmacological doses of 5–15 mg (Chanarin 1979). 30 μg daily was found to be too small to influence folate status appreciably (Chanarin *et al* 1965) but supplements of 100 μg or more all reduced the frequency of megaloblastic changes in the marrow and eliminated megaloblastic anaemia as a clinical entity (Chanarin 1979).

In order to meet the folate needs of those women with a dietary intake well below average, the daily supplement during pregnancy should be about 200–300 μg daily—still very much below the WHO's Recommended Daily Intake. The case for giving prophylactic folate throughout pregnancy is strong (Giles 1966; Chanarin 1979), particularly in countries where overt megaloblastic anaemia is frequent.

The main point at issue over recent years, however, is whether the apparently intrinsic folate deficiency of pregnancy can predispose the mother to a wide variety of other obstetric abnormalities and complications, in particular abortion, fetal deformity, prematurity and antepartum haemorrhage (Chanarin 1979, Coyle and Geoghegan 1962, Gatenby and Lillie 1960, Rae and Robb 1970). The extensive literature would seem to be almost equally divided in its opinion, but there is virtually no evidence that the routine use of folic acid supplements during pregnancy has reduced the incidence of anything but megaloblastic anaemia (Fletcher *et al* 1971, Landon 1975) except in areas of malnutrition where an increase in birthweight has been noted (Baumslag *et al* 1970; Iyengar 1971). However, a more recent report (Smithells *et al* 1980) of a controlled trial of periconceptional vitamin supplementation suggests that this supplementation may prevent neural tube defects. The mothers in the supplemented group were given Pregnavite Forte F for at least 28 days before conception and continuing at least until the date of the second missed period.

Pregnavite Forte contains vitamins A, B, C, D and E, as well as calcium and iron. Folic acid is only one component of this multivitamin supplement, but such a simple solution to a devastating congenital problem obviously deserves further investigation.

Severe megaloblastic anaemia is now uncommon in the UK during pregnancy or the puerperium but may still be a problem. Two case histories of severe macrocytic anaemia presenting in the puerperium with pancytopenia were recently published (McCann *et al* 1980). In both cases leukaemia was considered because of the increase in promyelocytes in the bone marrow as well as florid megaloblastic change. Both responded completely to therapy with folic acid. A similar case was recently seen at Queen Charlotte's Maternity Hospital, transferred from another hospital late in pregnancy, having been treated with iron alone for anaemia.

The risk of adverse effects from folate in a pregnant woman also suffering from B12 deficiency is very small indeed (*see* below). Folic acid should never be given without supplemental iron. A wide variety of preparations supplying both iron and folate are available and, provided that the folate content is not less than 100 μg daily, all are satisfactory for prophylaxis in pregnancy.

Once megaloblastic haemopoiesis is established treatment of folic acid deficiency becomes more difficult, presumably due to megaloblastic changes in the gastrointestinal tract resulting in impaired absorption. There are a small number of patients (Giles 1966) who fail to respond to parenteral folate therapy and who only recover after delivery. It is far better to intervene before these difficulties arise and give routine prophylaxis throughout pregnancy.

ANTICONVULSANT DRUGS AND PREGNANCY

The additional demand for folate during pregnancy leads to a rapid fall in red cell folate and to a high incidence of megaloblastic anaemia in those women taking anticonvulsant drugs for control of epilepsy. This is not surprising because non-pregnant individuals on anticonvulsants tend to become folate deficient (Chanarin 1979).

The risk of interfering with the control of epilepsy by the regular administration of iron–folate preparations during pregnancy and the precipitation of status epilepticus (Strauss and Bernstein 1974) has been overestimated. Anticonvulsant therapy during pregnancy is associated with an increased incidence of congenital abnormality (Hill *et al* 1974) and prematurity and low birthweight (Bjerkedal and Bahna 1973). Therefore folate supplements should be given to all epileptic women taking anticonvulsants in pregnancy (*see* p. 463). In addition, neonates born to women taking anticonvulsant drugs may have low prothrombin times and are at risk of bleeding. This risk appears to be preventable by giving the mothers vitamin K, 20 mg daily for two weeks before delivery (Deblay *et al* 1982).

VITAMIN B12 DEFICIENCY

Muscle, red cell and serum vitamin B12 concentrations fall during pregnancy (Ball and Giles 1964; Chanarin 1979; Edelstein and Metz 1969; Temperley *et al* 1968). Non-pregnant serum levels of 205–1025 μg/l fall to 20–510 μg/l at term, with low levels in multiple pregnancy (Temperley *et al* 1968). Women who smoke tend to have lower serum B12 levels (McGarry and Andrews 1972), which may account for the positive correlation between birthweight and serum levels in nondeficient mothers.

Vitamin B12 absorption is unaltered in pregnancy (Chanarin 1979, Cooper 1973). It is probable that tissue uptake is increased by the action of oestrogens as oral contraceptives also cause a fall in serum vitamin B12 (Briggs and Briggs 1972). Cord blood serum vitamin B12 is higher than that of maternal blood. The fall in serum vitamin B12 in the mother is related to preferential transfer of absorbed B12 to the fetus at the expense of maintaining the maternal serum concentration (Chanarin 1979), but the placenta does not transfer vitamin B12 with the same efficiency as it does folate. Low serum vitamin B12 levels in early pregnancy in vegetarian Hindus do not fall further while their infants often have subnormal concentrations (Roberts *et al* 1973). The vitamin B12 binding capacity of plasma increases in pregnancy analogous to the rise in iron binding capacity. The rise is confined to the liver-derived transcobalamin II concerned with transport rather than the leucocyte-derived transcobalamin I which is raised in other myeloproliferative conditions (Fleming 1975).

Pregnancy does not make a great impact on maternal vitamin B12 stores. Adult stores are of the order of 3000 μg or more and vitamin B12 stores in the newborn infant are about 50 μg (Chanarin 1979, Roberts *et al* 1973).

Addisonian pernicious anaemia does not usually occur during the reproductive years. Vitamin B12 deficiency is associated with infertility and pregnancy is likely only if the deficiency is remedied (Jackson *et al* 1967). However, severe vitamin B12 deficiency may be present without morphological changes in haemopoietic and other tissues. Pregnancy in such patients may be followed by death in utero or may proceed uneventfully (Chanarin 1979). Vitamin B12 deficiency in pregnancy may be associated with chronic tropical sprue. The megaloblastic anaemia which develops is due to longstanding vitamin B12 deficiency and superadded folate deficiency; the cord vitamin B12 levels remain above the maternal levels in these cases, but the concentration in the breast milk follows the maternal serum levels (Chanarin 1979).

The recommended intake of vitamin B12 is 2.0 μg per day in the nonpregnant and 3.0 μg per day during pregnancy (World Health Organisation 1972). This will be met by almost any diet which contains animal products, however deficient in other essential substances. Strict vegans who will not eat any animal-derived substances may have a deficient intake of vitamin B12 and their diet should be supplemented during pregnancy.

Haemoglobinopathies

Following the influx of immigrants from all parts of the world, obstetricians in the UK frequently encounter women with genetic defects of haemoglobin that are seldom seen in the indiginous population. It is important to recognise the specific defects early in pregnancy for the following reasons.

1   The clinical effects may complicate obstetric management and appropriate precautions can be taken.
2   It is now possible to offer prenatal diagnosis to those women carrying a fetus at risk of a serious defect of haemoglobin synthesis or structure at a time when termination of pregnancy is feasible (Alter 1981).

The haemoglobinopathies are inherited defects of haemoglobin, resulting from impaired globin synthesis (thalassaemia syndromes) or from structural abnormality of globin (haemoglobin variants). Only some of these anomalies are of practical importance, so particular emphasis will be placed on those where adverse effects may be aggravated during the stress of pregnancy. A proper appreciation of these defects requires some understanding of the structure of normal haemoglobin.

The haemoglobin molecule consists of four globin chains each of which is associated with a haem complex. There are three normal haemoglobins in man—HbA, HbA$_2$ and HbF—each of which contains two pairs of polypeptide globin chains. The synthesis and structure of the four globin chains alpha, beta, gamma and delta are under separate control (Fig. 2.1). The adult levels shown in Fig. 2.1 are those achieved by six months of age. It is obvious that only those conditions affecting the synthesis or structure of HbA ($\alpha_2 \beta_2$) which should comprise over 95% of the total circulating haemoglobin in the adult, will be of significance for the mother during pregnancy. Alpha chain production is under the control of four genes, two inherited from each parent, and as can be seen the alpha chains are common to all three haemoglobins. Beta chain production, on the other hand, is under the control of only two genes—one inherited from each parent.

The thalassaemia syndromes

The thalassaemia syndromes are the commonest genetic disorders of the blood and constitute a vast public health problem in many parts of the world. The basic defect is a reduced rate of globin chain synthesis resulting in red cells being formed with an inadequate haemoglobin content. The syndromes are divided into two main groups, the alpha and the beta thalassaemias depending on whether the alpha or the beta globin chain synthesis of adult haemoglobin (HbA $\alpha_2 \beta_2$) is depressed.

ALPHA THALASSAEMIA

Normal individuals have four functional alpha globin genes. Alpha thalassaemia, unlike beta thalassaemia, is often, but not always, a gene deletion defect. There are two forms of alpha thalassaemia trait, the result of inheriting two or three normal alpha genes instead of the usual four. They are called α_1 and α_2 thalassaemia (Fig. 2.2). Hb H disease is an intermediate form of alpha thalassaemia in which there is only one functional alpha gene and is the name given to the unstable haemoglobin formed by tetramers of the beta chain (β_4), when there is a relative lack of alpha chains. Alpha thalassaemia major in which there are no functional alpha genes (both parents having transmitted α_1 thalassaemia) is incompatible with life and pregnancy ends usually prematurely in a hydrops which will only survive a matter of hours if born alive. This is a common condition in South-East Asia. The name Hb Barts was given to tetramers of

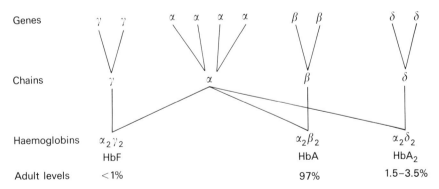

Fig. 2.1 Genetic control of globin synthesis. The adult levels shown are those reached by six months of age.

the gamma chain of fetal haemoglobin (HbF $\alpha_2 \gamma_2$). The tetramer (γ_4) forms in utero when no alpha chains are made and was first identified in a Chinese baby born at St Bartholomew's Hospital, London.

MANAGEMENT OF ALPHA THALASSAEMIA

During pregnancy, with its stress on the haemopoietic system, carriers of alpha thalassaemia, particularly those with α_1 thalassaemia (two deleted genes) may become very anaemic. They can be identified for further tests at booking, by finding abnormal red cell indices (Table 2.1). They have smaller red cells (MCV) and a reduced individual cell content of haemoglobin (MCH), although the mean cell haemoglobin concentration (MCHC) is usually within the normal range (Table 2.1). These changes are often minimal in α_2 thalassaemia (one deleted gene) (Fig. 2.2) but this condition is not so important as α_1 thalassaemia in terms of genetic counselling and prenatal diagnosis. The diagnosis can only be confirmed by globin chain synthesis studies or, in the case of gene deletion, by DNA analysis of nucleated cells. There is no abnormal haemoglobin made or excess or lack of one or other of the normal haemoglobins. These individuals need iron and folate oral supplements throughout the antenatal period. Sometimes intramuscular folic acid is helpful but parenteral iron should *never* be given (*see* below). If the haemoglobin is not thought to be adequate for delivery at term, transfusion is indicated (*see* p. 42).

Patients with HbH disease have a chronic haemolytic anaemia and have 5–30% HbF in their peripheral blood which can be identified on haemoglobin electrophoresis. They have a normal life expectancy but require daily oral folate supplements to cover the demands of increased marrow turnover. During pregnancy it is recommended to give 5.0 mg folate daily to women with HbH disease. They will transmit either α_1 or α_2 thalassaemia to their offspring.

Table 2.1   Red cell indices in iron deficiency and thalassaemia. In thalassaemia, unlike iron deficiency, there is a disproportionate decrease in MCV and MCH compared with the MCHC, which can be in the normal range.

	Normal range	Iron deficiency	Thalassaemia
$\dfrac{PCV}{RBC} = MCV$	75–99 fl	Decrease	Large decrease
$\dfrac{Hb}{RBC} = MCH$	27–31 pg	Decrease	Large decrease
$\dfrac{Hb}{PCV} = MCHC$	32–36 g/dl	Decrease	No change

PCV Packed cell volume, RBC Red cell count, Hb Haemoglobin, MCV mean corpuscular value, MCH mean corpuscular haemoglobin, MCHC mean corpuscular haemoglobin concentration.

Pregnancy with an alpha thalassaemia hydrops is associated with severe, sometimes life-threatening, pre-eclampsia in the mother (cf. severe rhesus haemolytic disease). Vaginal deliveries are associated with obstetric complication, due to the large fetus and very bulky placenta. If routine screening of the parents (*see* below) indicates that the mother is at risk of carrying such a child—both parents having α_1 thalassaemia—she should be referred for prenatal diagnosis (*see* below).

BETA THALASSAEMIA

Thalassaemia major, homozygous thalassaemia resulting from the inheritance of a defective beta globin gene from each parent was the first identified form of the thalassaemia syndromes. It was described in the 1920s by Cooley, a physician in practice in the United States. The first few cases were found in the children of Greek and Italian immigrants. The name thalassaemia was derived from the Greek '*thalassa*' meaning the sea, or in the classical sense the Mediterannean, because it was thought to be confined to individuals of Mediterannean origin; however, we know now that the distribution is virtually world-wide, although the defect is concentrated in a broad band which does include the Mediterannean and the Middle and Far East. It does not constitute a major health problem in the UK, but there are a fair number of heterozygotes, particularly in the immigrant Cypriot and Asian populations. The child of parents who are both carriers of beta thalassaemia has a 1 in 4 chance of inheriting thalassaemia major. The carrier rate in the UK is thought to be around 1 in 10 000 compared with 1 in 7 in Cyprus. There are between 300 and 400 patients with thalassaemia major in the UK today, most of them concentrated round the Greater London area, but world-wide there are over 100 000 babies born each year with the condition.

Before the days of regular transfusion, a child born with homozygous beta thalassaemia would die in the first few years of life from anaemia, congestive cardiac failure and intercurrent infection. Now that regular transfusion is routine where blood is freely available, survival is prolonged into the teens and early twenties. The management problem becomes one of iron overload derived mainly from the transfused red cells. This results in hepatic and endocrine disfunction and, most important of all, myocardial damage—the cause of death being cardiac failure in the vast majority of cases. Puberty is delayed or incomplete. Successful pregnancy in a truly transfusion-dependent thalassaemic girl is very rare (Goldfarb *et al* 1982). It remains to be seen how effective recently instituted intensive iron chelation programmes will be.

MANAGEMENT OF BETA THALASSAEMIA

Sometimes survival is possible without regular transfusion in thalassaemia major but this usually results in severe bone deformities due to massive expansion of marrow tissue, the site of largely ineffective erythropoiesis. Although iron loading still occurs from excessive gastrointestinal absorption, stimulated by the accelerated marrow turnover, it is much slower than in those who are transfused and pregnancy may occur in this situation. Extra daily folate supplements should be given but iron in any form is contraindicated. The anaemia should be treated by transfusion during the antenatal period.

Perhaps the commonest problem associated with haemoglobinopathies and pregnancy in the UK today is the anaemia developing in the antenatal period in women who have thalassaemia minor, heterozygous beta thalassaemia. They can be identified for further examination of the booking blood by finding, as in alpha thalassaemia, low MCV and MCH together with a normal MCHC (Table 2.1). The level of haemoglobin at booking may be normal or slightly below the normal range. The diagnosis will be confirmed by finding a raised concentration of HbA_2 ($\alpha_2 \delta_2$) with or without a raised HbF ($\alpha_2 \gamma_2$), excess alpha chain combining with delta and gamma chains because of the relative lack of beta chains (Fig. 2.2).

The women with beta thalassaemia minor require the usual *oral* iron and folate supplements in the antenatal period. Oral iron for a limited period will not result in significant iron loading, even in the presence of replete iron stores, but parenteral iron should *never* be given. In our experience at Queen Charlotte's Maternity Hospital many women with thalassaemia minor enter pregnancy with depleted iron stores as do many women with normal haemoglobin synthesis. Iron deficiency has also been shown in women in the UK with thalassaemia minor in a study of serum ferritin levels (Hussein *et al* 1975). If the anaemia does not respond to oral iron, and intramuscular folic acid has been tried, transfusion is indicated to achieve an adequate haemoglobin for delivery at term.

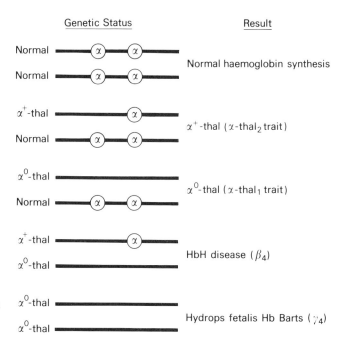

Fig. 2.2   Normal alpha gene status and the various forms of alpha thalassaemia resulting from gene deletion.

Haemoglobin variants

Over 250 structural variants of the globin chains of normal human haemoglobins (Fig 2.3) have been described but the most important by far, both numerically and clinically, is sickle cell haemoglobin (HbS). This is a variant of the beta globin chain where there is one amino acid substitution at the sixth position, a glutamine replacing a valine residue. HbS has the unique physical property that, despite being a soluble protein in its oxygenated form, in its reduced state the molecules become stacked on one another, forming tactoids, which distort the red cell to the characteristic shape which gives the haemoglobin its name. Because of their rigid structure these sickled cells tend to block small blood vessels. The sickling phenomenon occurs particularly in conditions of lowered oxygen tension but may also be favoured by acidosis or dehydration and cooling which cause stasis in small blood vessels.

SICKLE CELL SYNDROMES

The sickling disorders include the heterozygous state for sickle cell haemoglobin, sickle cell trait (HbAS), homozygous sickle cell disease (HbSS), compound heterozygotes for Hb variants, the most important of which is sickle cell/HbC disease (HbSC), and sickle cell thalassaemia. Although these disorders are most commonly seen in black people of African Origin, they can be seen in Saudi Arabian, Indian and even white Mediteraneans.

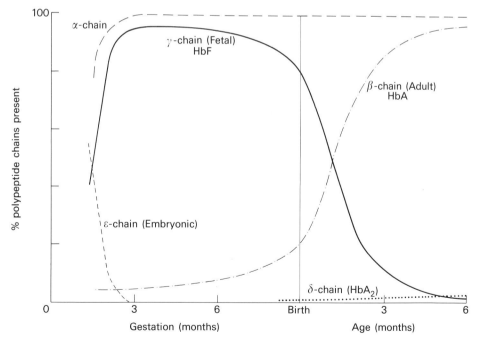

Fig. 2.3   The developmental changes in human haemoglobin chains. (After Huehns *et al* 1964.)

The characteristic feature of homozygous sickle cell anaemia (HbSS) is the occurrence of periods of health punctuated by periods of crisis. Between 3 and 6 months of age, when normal HbA production usually becomes predominant, a chronic haemolytic anaemia develops—the haemoglobin level being between 6 g/dl and 9 g/dl. Even if the haemoglobin is in the lower part of the range, symptoms due to anaemia are surprisingly few because of the low affinity of HbS for oxygen; oxygen delivery to the tissues being facilitated. The acute episodes due to intravascular sickling are of far greater practical importance since they cause vascular occlusion resulting in tissue infarction. The affected part is painful and the clinical manifestations are extremely variable, depending on the site at which sickling takes place. Sickling crises are often precipitated by infection and may be exacerbated by any accompanying dehydration. The majority of deaths are due to massive sickling following an acute infection. Prognosis depends greatly on environment: in Africa, a large proportion of children with this disorder die within the first five years and probably less than 10% reach adulthood. In the West Indies, however, where prompt treatment and prophylaxis of infection is more easily available, many women with sickle cell disease need management during pregnancy. Thomas *et al* (1982), reviewing 241 mortalities from homozygous sickle cell disease in the West Indies, found that ten were associated with pregnancy and often due to pulmonary embolus (Chapter 4) which has been reported with heterozygotes (van Dinh *et al* 1982). Renal complications are a constant finding; there is a progressive inability to concentrate the urine and haematuria is common. Both these defects result from sickling in the renal medullary circulation. Inability to concentrate the urine adequetely makes pregnant women unduly prone to dehydration during labour.

Sickle cell haemoglobin C disease (HbSC) is a milder variant of HbSS with normal or near normal levels of haemoglobin. One of the dangers of this condition is that, owing to its mildness, neither the woman nor her obstetrician may be aware of its presence. These women are at risk of massive, sometimes fatal, sickling crises during pregnancy and particularly in the puerperium. It is therefore vital that the abnormality is detected so that the appropriate precautions can be taken.

Clinical manifestations of the doubly heterozygous condition, sickle cell thalassaemia, are usually indistinguishable from HbSS although those who make detectable amounts of HbA are usually less severely affected but still at risk from sickling crises during pregnancy.

Sickle cell trait (HbAS) results in no detectable abnormality under normal circumstances although it is easily diagnosed by specific investigations including haemoglobin electrophoresis (*see* below). Affected subjects are not anaemic even under the additional stress of pregnancy, unless there are additional complications and sickling crises occur only in situations of extreme anoxia.

MANAGEMENT OF SICKLE CELL SYNDROMES

At present there is no effective long-term method of reducing the liability of red cells to sickle *in vivo*. Once a crisis is established, there is no evidence that alkalis, hyperbaric oxygen, vasodilators, plasma expanders, urea or anticoagulants are of any value. Where beneficial effects have been reported they can usually be attributed to the meticulous care and supportive therapy received by the patient, rather than to the specific measures themselves. Adequate fluid administration alone probably accounts for the benefit. However, Huehns *et al* (1981) have recently suggested that fresh frozen plasma as an adjunct to rehydration can relieve pain, reduce the amount of analgesia required and shorten the duration of admission in painful sickling crises. Further evaluation of this relatively simple approach is indicated.

Women with sickle cell disease present special problems in pregnancy (Tuck 1982). Fetal loss is high, presumably due to sickling infarcts in the placental circulation. Abortion, premature labour and other complications are more common than in women with normal haemoglobin. Although many women with sickle cell disease have no complications, the outcome in any individual case is always in doubt. The only consistently successful way of reducing the incidence of complications is by regular blood transfusion at approximately six week intervals, to maintain the proportion of HbA at 60–70% of the total (Huehns 1982). Between 3 and 4 units of blood should be given at each transfusion. This regime has two effects: it dilutes the circulating sickle haemoglobin and, by raising the haemoglobin, reduces the stimulus to the bone marrow and therefore the amount of sickle haemoglobin produced.

Sickle cells have a shorter life than normal red cells and so the effect of each successive transfusion is more beneficial. If this regime has been instituted a general anaesthetic may be given with safety and sickling crises in the course of normal labour are much less likely.

Some authors recommend elective Caesarean section at 36 weeks, preceded by partial exchange transfusion, because it gives more overall control of the situation. A transfusion of 3–4 units is given and a week later a further transfusion of a similar amount; the first transfusion raises the haemoglobin and suppresses the output of sickle cells by the bone marrow; the second further dilutes the circulating sickle cells. The aim is to achieve more than 60% circulating HbA.

If the disorder presents late in pregnancy and there is more urgency because, for instance, the woman is profoundly anaemic or is suffering a crisis, exchange transfusion can be used.

The following suggested exchange transfusion regime for patients with sickle cell disease, has been used with success in a large number of patients (Brozovic, personal communication).

Exchange transfusion in patients with sickle cell disease

1   Ensure free-flowing infusion in one arm. At least 1 litre of fluid (dextrose, saline, FFP) is required before the exchange is started.
2   Have cross-matched blood ready. (Preferably whole blood. Do not pack.)
3   Venesect 1 pint from the other arm. Often a 50–100 cm^3 syringe must be used.
4   Give 1 pint of blood.

5 Venesect another pint. If this is still very difficult and slow, venesection can be carried out at the same time as transfusion.

6 Exchange 1 blood volume; estimate proportion of A to S. If S less than 40% and Hb less than 8 g it is usually safe to 'top up' to approximately 13–14 g/dl.

7 It is often impossible to exchange more than 2 units on the first day. Venesection usually becomes easier after 2–3 units of exchange.

8 Do not give diuretics. Keep fluid balance chart, watch blood pressure, pulse, note any headache, drowsiness (CNS sludging), shortness of breath, etc.

9 Maintain the usual 3 litres of fluid/m^2/24 hours during exchange.

10 Give penicillin because of the probability of splenic infarction and possibility of overwhelming pneumococcal infection. Treat other infections as indicated.

It is obvious from the complexity of the above regime, that it would be far better to prevent the emergency situation during pregnancy; however, even after preparation with regular transfusion, tissue anoxia, acidosis and dehydration should be avoided because they would make the patient's own remaining sickle cells more likely to sickle. Tourniquets should not be used. To minimise pulmonary infection, prophylactic antibiotics are desirable to cover all anaesthetics.

No special preparation with blood transfusion is required in pregnancy for women with sickle cell trait (HbAS). However, as in patients with HbSS, it is essential that anoxia and dehydration are avoided during anaesthesia and labour, particularly in the immediate postdelivery period. In fact the majority of unexpected deaths associated with HbS have occurred in patients with sickle cell trait in the immediate postoperative or postpartum period.

Detection of HbS

Any test designed to screen for the presence of HbS should detect not only sickle cell disease but also distinguish HbSC, HbS thalassaemia and sickle cell trait. The classic sickling test in which the red cell is suspended in a reducing agent is difficult to interpret and may occasionally give false-negative results. Furthermore it is time consuming and its usefulness is limited when diagnosis is urgent. A proprietary product (Sickledex) is available that overcomes these drawbacks; it detects HbS by precipitation of de-oxygenated HbS. It is rapid, reliable and does not give false negatives. Definitive diagnosis of the particular sickle cell syndrome involved requires haemoglobin electrophoresis and sometimes, in the case of sickle cell/thalassaemia, family studies.

Screening for haemoglobinopathy

Selection for screening in a busy antenatal clinic may be more time consuming than it is worth and, to be efficient, should involve detailed documentation of a woman's heritage before excluding her from testing. For this reason, and because of the remote possibility of missing such a defect in the nonimmigrant population, general screening for haemoglobinopathies is carried out routinely on every woman's blood during pregnancy at Queen Charlotte's Maternity Hospital, which serves a cosmopolitan population. This involves examination of red cell indices (Table 2.1), haemoglobin electrophoresis and, where indicated, quantitation of HbA_2 and HbF on every sample of blood taken at booking. If a haemoglobin variant or thalassaemia is found, the husband is requested to attend so that his blood can also be examined. By this means we are able to assess the chances of a serious haemoglobin defect in the baby early in pregnancy and to advice the parents of the potential hazard and offer them prenatal diagnosis if they so desire.

Prenatal diagnosis of haemoglobinopathy

Until the mid-1970s the prenatal diagnosis of thalassaemia major and of sickle cell disease (also a β globin chain defect) was thought to be a relatively unrealistic goal, first because information concerning β chain synthesis in the first and second trimesters of human pregnancy was lacking, and secondly because it was believed that any techniques necessary for acquisition of fetal blood would prove prohibitively dangerous with respect to maintenance of the pregnancy.

Much is owed to Huehns and his colleagues at University College Hospital, who showed that adult haemoglobin (HbA $\alpha_2\beta_2$) could be detected in the red cells of the fetus as early as 8–10 weeks' gestation (Huehns *et al* 1964) (Fig. 2.3). If the haemoglobin is labelled with a radioactive amino acid and then globin chain separation effected by use of carboxymethyl cellulose urea chromatography (Clegg *et al* 1966), the amount of β chain synthesis can be quantitated and compared to γ chain derived from fetal haemoglobin (HbF $\alpha_2\gamma_2$) (Wood and Weatherall 1973). The $\beta:\gamma$ ratio was determined for fetuses with normal haemoglobin at various gestations on abortuses where termination was being carried out for nonhaematological reasons (Alter 1979). The next stage was to find the $\beta:\gamma$ ratios on fetuses of Cypriot women in London, where offspring were at risk for thalassaemia and the women had already opted for a termination. The normal $\beta:\gamma$ ratio at 18 weeks' gestation is about 0.11. It was found that those fetuses who had thalassaemia minor had $\beta:\gamma$ ratios at or above 0.045, and those with thalassaemia major had ratios of 0.025 or below (Chang *et al* 1975).

The diagnosis of sickle cell disease is much simpler, and does not require quantitation of β globin chain synthesis because structural differences give the haemoglobin different electrophoretic properties.

Two methods for obtaining fetal blood have been tried. The first and simplest approach is that of placental aspiration, pioneered in the UK by Fairweather at University College Hospital: the placenta is located by ultrasound, a 20 gauge needle is placed in the fetal surface of the placenta and a small sample (less than 0.1 ml) is aspirated with or without ultrasound guidance. There is bleeding into the amniotic fluid immediately following withdrawal of the needle and a sample of the blood-stained amniotic fluid often contains a high percentage of fetal cells. The second approach, developed at Yale (Hobbins and Mahoney 1974) involves the modification of fetoscopy to equip a small fibreoptic fetoscope with an aspirating needle such that a fetal vein on the surface of the placenta can be identified.

The fetal blood sampling is performed at 18–20 weeks' gestation when the placenta is sufficiently thick and the vessels large enough to provide a specimen enriched in fetal blood. By both methods of placental aspiration a mixture of fetal and maternal blood may be obtained. A Coulter particle size analyser can be used in the operating room to determine rapidly the relative proportion of the large fetal erythrocytes and small maternal red cells. The obstetrician can stop as soon as an adequate sample is taken.

Pure fetal blood samples are not required for the diagnosis of haemoglobinopathies. In the absence of maternal reticulocytosis as little as 10 μl of fetal cells would suffice even in the presence of as much as 80 per cent maternal cell contamination. The reason for this is that fetal red cells synthesise globin chains at a much higher rate than do mature adult red cells. It is also possible to concentrate fetal red cells in a mixture of maternal and fetal cells because of antigenic and biochemical differences between them (Kan *et al* 1974, Boyer *et al* 1976).

What are the risks of the procedure? The most important by far is fetal loss. This may be due to fetal exsanguination (which is associated more commonly with placental aspiration) or may be secondary to premature labour (which is more frequent when the fetoscope is used). Sometimes amniotic fluid leak follows the investigation, usually when the fetoscope is used, but does not necessarily herald premature labour and the pregnancy may continue to term with no ill effect (Alter 1979).

Studies of fetal blood from cases at risk for haemoglobinopathies began in 1974 in collaborative studies between Boston Children's Hospital and University College Hospital in London (Alter *et al* 1976) and in San Francisco (Kan *et al* 1977). Nearly 2000 cases have now been studied in approximately 15 centres round the world (Alter 1981), including University College Hospital and King's College Hospital, London. Ninety per cent were at risk for thalassaemia and the others for sickle cell disorders. It is of interest that most of the prenatal tests have been performed for thalassaemia, although sickle cell disease is more common in the United States where prenatal diagnosis using fetal blood analysis started. However, sickle cell disease has variable severity while thalassaemia is more often fatal in children. Current treatment for thalassaemia is cumbersome, expensive and difficult. Thus the decision regarding abortion of affected fetuses is easier.

The overall fetal loss rate is now 5 per cent, much less than the 12–15 per cent loss rate of earlier studies (Alter 1979). There have been 1 per cent incorrect diagnoses due primarily to the grey area in the $\beta:\gamma$ ratio between the heterozygote and β^+ homozygote, resulting in terminations of pregnancies in which the fetus proved to have thalassaemia minor or allowing pregnancies with thalassaemia major to go to term.

It is obvious that if fetal blood sampling could be avoided the risks of prenatal diagnosis would be considerably less.

Examination of the DNA of amniocentesis fibroblasts can be used in those conditions where there is a gene deletion, such as in some forms of alpha thalassaemia (Kan *et al* 1976) as it occurs in the Far East (Fig. 2.2) and delta/beta thalassaemia (Orkin *et al* 1978).

It may be asked why prenatal diagnosis for alpha thalassaemia should be attempted when the major form of the disease is incompatible with life, and HbH disease probably does not adversely affect life expectancy. One reason is that pregnancy with an alpha thalassaemia hydrops is associated with severe, sometimes life-threatening, pre-eclampsia in the mother. Also, vaginal deliveries are associated with obstetric complications due to the large fetus and very bulky placenta while the mothers are usually of Oriental origin and so are small in stature. The advantages in terminating such a pregnancy in the second trimester are obvious.

Discovery of polymorphisms in human DNA sequences linked to the sickle cell gene has made it possible to use restriction endonuclease gene mapping for the prenatal diagnosis of some cases of sickle cell disease (Kan and Dozy 1978). It was found that the β gene in normal individuals was in a 7.6 kilobase piece of DNA if the enzyme HpaI was used. Many patients, particularly those of West African origin with sickle cell disease, had a 13.0 kilobase piece instead and this information has been used to study DNA from amniotic fluid fibroblasts in fetuses at risk. Further advances and possible discoveries of similar linkages with the β gene may allow the diagnosis of beta thalassaemia by DNA analysis of amniotic fluid cells. Such a linkage has been found recently in cases of beta thalassaemia occuring in Sardinia (Kan *et al* 1980).

However, although amniocentesis is safer than fetal blood sampling, sufficiently large samples for analysis are not obtained any earlier with this procedure. This means that termination of an affected pregnancy may be delayed until late in the second trimester—a particularly unpleasant and depressing experience for the mother.

Details of a new technique have recently been published which may make prenatal diagnosis a possibility in the first trimester (Williamson *et al* 1981). Samples of trophoblast were obtained by transcervical aspiration before elective abortion in 8–14 week pregnancies. DNA was extracted from chorionic villi and sufficient was obtained to perform restriction endonuclease mapping (Old *et al* 1982). The potential advantages of DNA analysis may be utilised in this way in the future for prenatal diagnosis not only of the haemoglobinopathies but other conditions such as cystic fibrosis, where there is no means of detecting the carrier state (Anon 1981). However, the realisation of this technique does not only depend on the ability to analyse DNA variations in the laboratory. The method of obtaining chorionic villi must be proved to be safe, with risks of fetal loss and morbidity no greater than with current procedures. It also demands early diagnosis of pregnancy and family DNA studies as soon as it is recognised that a couple are at risk.

Meanwhile the procedure of the fetal blood sampling remains the method used in most cases of beta thalassaemia and some cases of sickle cell disease.

Miscellaneous anaemias

Many forms of anaemia, in particular the anaemia of renal failure, are made worse by pregnancy. However, supportive and prophylactic therapy for the various medical conditions concerned is improving and maternal risks for the most part have been reduced, as have the risks to the fetus. Each case has to be considered individually; there are no general rules that can be applied in terms of management.

APLASTIC ANAEMIA

There have been sporadic case reports of refractory hypoplastic anaemia, sometimes recurrent, developing in pregnancy and appearing to be related in some way to the pregnancy (Taylor *et al* 1968). Occasionally pregnancy occurs when chronic acquired aplastic anaemia is present as an underlying disease. It has been generally considered that in both these situations pregnancy exacerbates the marrow depression, results in rapid deterioration, and should be terminated. It is true that many cases do remit spontaneously after termination (Evans 1968), but there is no record of excessive haemorrhage at delivery in spite of profound thrombocytopenia. Supportive measures in this situation are improving and pregnancy should be maintained as long as the health of the mother is not seriously impaired (Lewis 1974).

AUTOIMMUNE HAEMOLYTIC ANAEMIA AND SYSTEMIC LUPUS ERYTHEMATOSUS

The rare combination of autoimmune haemolytic anaemia (AIHA) and pregnancy carries great risks to both the woman herself and the fetus. Very careful antenatal supervision and adjustment to steroid therapy is required (Chaplin *et al* 1973).

Pregnancy may result in exacerbations of systemic lupus erythematosus (SLE), although up to 50 per cent of women with this condition are reported to improve during pregnancy especially in the third trimester (Dubois 1966). (*See also* Chapter 8.)

Haemolytic anaemia, leukopenia and thrombocytopenia (*see* p. 86) have all been observed in infants of women with active disease, presumably due to IgG antibody involved in the disease process crossing the placenta. There have been a number of reports in which women have been treated with steroids and other immune suppressives throughout pregnancy for a variety of conditions including ITP, DLE, AIHA and some forms of malignancy. Possible effects of azothioprine are considered in Chapter 7 and of steroids in Chapter 1. The problems of their use are essentially the same as those outside pregnancy but more frequent monitoring and adjustment are required due to the rapidly changing blood volume and changes in the circulating hormones during the antenatal and postnatal periods.

LEUKAEMIA

One in 1000 pregnancies is complicated by malignant disease (Rothman *et al* 1973). The incidence of leukaemia in pregnancy should not exceed 1 in 75 000 pregnancies, but the information used to calculate this incidence is obtained from cases recorded in the literature—a method with serious limitations. Although peak incidence years for cancer do not coincide with the peak reproductive years, leukaemia was reported in 1969 as the second most common cause of death from malignant disease in females aged 15–34 in the USA (Vital Statistics of the United States 1969). Several hundred cases of leukaemia in association with pregnancy have now been reported; most papers give an account of a specific case or cases and include a review of the published literature (e.g. Ewing and Whittaker 1973; Gokal *et al* 1976; Nicholson 1968) and some include management considerations (e.g. McLain 1974).

Adult leukaemia is almost invariably fatal and one of the reasons why acute leukaemia is seen so rarely in association with pregnancy is that, without the aggressive treatment with cytotoxic drugs instituted in the last decade, the disease is characterised by rapid deterioration and death within weeks of diagnosis.

There is no objective evidence that pregnancy has a deleterious effect on leukaemia (McLain 1974; Ewing and Whittaker 1973). Survival times in pregnant women with leukaemia do not differ statistically from those of nonpregnant women. The application of modern treatment can result in remission of the disease that is sometimes repeated, and more affected women may now have the opportunity to conceive or to survive until the fetus is viable.

The diagnosis during pregnancy is made most frequently in the second and third trimesters although the disease may have been present earlier. This is because the early symptoms are nonspecific, the most common being fatigue, which is often attributed by the woman and her obstetrician to the pregnancy itself. This emphasises the importance of carrying out proper investigations, including bone marrow examination, of unexplained anaemia in pregnancy.

The occurrence of pregnancy in a woman suffering from or developing acute leukaemia creates special clinical problems which fall into two main groups—those arising from the disease process and those arising from its treatment. There are increased risks of infection, haemorrhage and abortion arising from the disease process itself. Fetal loss occurs in approximately 14.0 per cent of women with chronic myeloid leukaemia and 33 per cent of women with acute leukaemia. Haemorrhage may result from thrombocytopenia due to bone marrow infiltration or from a consumptive coagulopathy which is a particularly common problem in acute myelomonocytic leukaemia. The powerful cytotoxic drugs which are often used to achieve remission in acute adult leukaemia include cytosine arabinoside, rubidomycin and thioguanine. Such agents have been shown to be toxic to fetal tissue in experimental animals. Malformations have occurred after treatment with cytotoxic drugs in the first trimester (Nicholson 1968). Methotrexate, a folic acid antagonist, is the most teratogenic drug known to man. Its administration early in pregnancy always results in either abortion or congenital malformation. Other published data have indicated that cytotoxic drugs can be given with safety in the second and third trimesters (Nicholson 1968, Gokal *et al* 1976).

It has been suggested (Gokal *et al* 1976) that a pregnant leukaemic woman should be treated with aggressive chemotherapy until a remission is achieved. The risk of a malformed fetus in a woman so treated in the first trimester is high and termination should be considered once she is in remission and this can be performed with safety. Termination of pregnancy when therapy is started in the second or third trimester has to be carried out on moral and medicosocial grounds, as the fetus is likely to develop normally. Examination of chromosomes of fetal amniotic fluid cells and of fetal hair under the scanning electron microscope may provide evidence of fetal damage in those cases where treatment is started early in the second trimester (Gokal *et al* 1976).

Not one case of leukaemia has been reported in the newborn infant of a mother suffering from the disease, but long-term follow-up should be carried out on the offspring of mothers treated with cytotoxic drugs for late development of neoplasm and possible adverse drug effects, such as rubidomycin-induced cardiotoxicity.

Splenic irradiation alone with careful shielding of the uterus has been used with success to manage chronic myeloid leukaemia during pregnancy (McLain 1974, Richards and Spiers 1974), though the late carcinogenic effects of a fetus exposed to irradiation in utero have to be borne in mind. Treatment with drugs such as Busulfan, Thioguanine, or 6 mercaptopurine should be reserved until the third trimester or, if possible, until after safe delivery of the infant.

References

Alter B.P. (1979) Prenatal diagnosis of haemoglobinopathies and other haematologic diseases. *Journal of Pediatrics* **95**, 501–13.

Alter B.P. (1981) Prenatal diagnosis of haemoglobinopathies: A status report. *Lancet* **ii**, 1152–5.

Alter B.P., Modell C.B., Fairweather D., Hobbins J.C., Mahoney M.J., Frigoletto F.D., Sherman A.S. & Nathan D.G. (1976) Prenatal diagnosis of haemoglobinopathy: A review of 15 cases. *New England Journal of Medicine* **295**, 1437–43.

Anon (1978) Do all pregnant women need iron? *British Medical Journal* **ii**, 1317.

Anon (1981) Antenatal diagnosis of haemoglobin disorders. *Lancet* **ii**, 1147–8.

Apte S.V. & Iyengar L. (1970) Absorption of dietary iron in pregnancy. *American Journal of Clinical Nutrition* **23**, 73–7.

Avery B. & Ledger W.J. (1970) Folic acid metabolism in well nourished pregnant women. *Obstetrics and Gynecology* **35**, 616–24.

Ball E.W. & Giles C. (1964) Folic acid and vitamin B_{12} levels in pregnancy and their relation to megaloblastic anaemia. *Journal of Clinical Pathology* **17**, 165–74.

Baumslag N., Edelstein T. & Metz J. (1970) Reduction of incidence of prematurity by folic acid supplementation in pregnancy. *British Medical Journal* **1**, 16–17.

Bjerkedal T. & Bahna S.L. (1973) The course and outcome of pregnancy in women with epilepsy. *Acta Obstetrica et Gynaecologica Scandinavica Supplement* **52**, 245–8.

Boyer S.H., Noyes A.N. & Boyer M.L. (1976) Enrichment of erythrocytes of fetal origin from adult-fetal blood mixtures via selective haemolysis of adult blood cells: an aid to antenatal diagnosis of haemoglobinopathies. *Blood*, **47**, 883–97.

Briggs M. & Briggs M. (1972) Endocrine effect on serum Vitamin B_{12}. *Lancet* **ii**, 1037.

Brozovic M. (1981) Exchange transfusion in sickle cell crisis. *Personal communication.*

Chanarin I. (1975) The folate content of foodstuffs and the availability of different folate analogues for absorption. In *Getting the Most out of Food*, p. 41. Van den Bergh and Jurgens Ltd., London.

Chanarin I. (1979) Megaloblastic anaemia of pregnancy. In *The Megaloblastic Anaemias*, 2nd edn. Blackwell Scientific Publications, Oxford.

Chanarin I., MacGibbon B.M., O'Sullivan W.J. & Mollin D.L. (1959) Folic acid deficiency in pregnancy; the pathogenesis of megaloblastic anaemia of pregnancy. *Lancet* **ii**, 634–9.

Chanarin I., Rothman D. & Berry V. (1965) Iron deficiency and its relation to folic acid status in pregnancy: Results of a clinical trial. *British Medical Journal* **i**, 480–5.

Chanarin I., Rothman D., Ward A. & Perry J. (1968) Folate status and requirement in pregnancy. *British Medical Journal* **ii**, 390–4.

Chang H., Modell C.B., Alter B.P., Dickinson M.J., Frigoletto F.D., Huehns E.R. & Nathan D.G.

(1975) Expression of the β thalassaemia gene in the first trimester fetus. *Proceedings of the National Academy of Sciences, U.S.A.* **72**, 3633–7.

Chaplin H., Cohen R., Bloomberg G., Kaplan H.J., Moore J.A. & Dorner I. (1973) Pregnancy and idiopathic auto-immune haemolytic anaemia. A prospective study during 6 months gestation and 3 months post-partum. *British Journal of Haematology* **24**, 219–29.

Chesley L.C. (1972) Plasma and red cell volumes during pregnancy. *American Journal of Obstetrics and Gynecology* **112**, 440–50.

Chesley L.C. & Duffus G.M. (1971) Posture and apparent plasma volume in late pregnancy. *Journal of Obstetrics and Gynaecology of the British Commonwealth* **78**, 406–12.

Chisholm, J. (1966) A controlled clinical trial of prophylactic folic acid and iron in pregnancy. *Journal of Obstetrics and Gynaecology of the British Commonwealth* **73**, 191–6.

Clay B., Rosenberg B., Sampson N. & Samuels S.I. (1965) Reactions to total dose intravenous infusion of iron dextran (imferon). *British Medical Journal* **i**, 29–31.

Clegg J.B., Naughton M.A. & Weatherall D.J. (1966) Abnormal human haemoglobins: Separation and characterisation of the γ and β chains by chromatography and the determination of two new variants Hb. Chesapeake and Hb.J (Bangkok). *Journal of Molecular Biology* **19**, 91–108.

Cooper B.A. (1973) Folate and Vitamin B_{12} in pregnancy. *Clinics in Haematology* **2**, 461–76.

Coyle C. & Geoghegan F. (1962) The problem of anaemia in a Dublin maternity hospital. *Proceedings of the Royal Society of Medicine* **55**, 764–6.

Deblay M.F., Vert P., Andre M. & Marchal F. (1982) Transplacental vitamin K prevents haemorrhagic disease of infant of epileptic mother. *Lancet* **1**, 1247.

Dubois E.L. (1966) *Lupus Erythematosus.* McGraw Hill, New York.

Edelstein T. & Metz J. (1969) The correlation between Vitamin B_{12} concentration in serum and muscle in late pregnancy. *Journal of Obstetrics and Gynaecology of the British Commonwealth* **76**, 545–48.

Evans I.L. (1968) Aplastic anaemia in pregnancy remitting after abortion. *British Medical Journal* **3**, 166–7.

Ewing P.A. & Whittaker J.A. (1973) Acute leukaemia in pregnancy. *Obstetrics and Gynecology* **42**, 245–51.

Fenton V., Cavill I. & Fisher J. (1977) Iron stores in pregnancy. *British Journal of Haematology* **37**, 145–9.

Fleming A.F. (1972) Urinary excretion of folate in pregnancy. *Journal of Obstetrics and Gynaecology of the British Commonwealth* **79**, 916–20.

Fleming A.F. (1975) Haematological changes in pregnancy. *Clinics in Obstetrics and Gynaecology* **2**, 269–83.

Fleming A.F., Martin J.D., Hähnel R. & Westlake A.J. (1974a). Effects of iron and folic acid antenatal supplements on maternal haematology and fetal well-being. *Medical Journal of Australia* **ii**, 429–36.

Fleming A.F., Martin J.D. & Stenhouse N.S. (1974b). Pregnancy anaemia, iron and folate deficiency in Western Australia. *Medical Journal of Australia* **ii**, 479–84.

Fletcher J., Gurr A., Fellingham F.R., Pranker T.A.J., Brant H.A. & Menzies D.N. (1971) The value of folic acid supplements in pregnancy. *Journal of Obstetrics and Gynaecology of the British Commonwealth* **75**, 781–5.

Fletcher J. & Suter P.E.N. (1969) The transport of iron by the human placenta. *Clinical Science* **36**, 209–20.

Fullerton W.T., Hytten F.E., Klopper A.E. & McKay E. (1965) A case of quadruplet pregnancy. *Journal of Obstetrics and Gynaecology of the British Commonwealth* **72**, 791–6.

Gatenby, P.B.B. (1956) The anaemias of pregnancy in Dublin. *Proceedings of the Nutrition Society* **15**, 115–19.

Gatenby P.B.B. & Little E.W. (1960) Clinical analysis of 100 cases of severe megaloblastic anaemia of pregnancy. *British Medical Journal* **ii**, 1111–14.

Gibson H.M. (1973) Plasma volume and glomerular filtration rate in pregnancy and their relation to differences in fetal growth. *Journal of Obstetrics and Gynaecology of the British Commonwealth* **80**, 1067–74.

Giles C. (1966) An account of 335 cases of megaloblastic anaemia of pregnancy and the puerperium. *Journal of Clinical Pathology* **19**, 1–11.

Gokal R., Durrant J., Baum J.D. & Bennett M.J. (1976) Successful pregnancy in acute monocytic leukaemia. *British Journal of Cancer* **34**, 299–302.

Goldfarb A.W., Hochner-Celnikier D., Beller U., Menashe M., Dagan I. & Palti Z. (1982) A successful pregnancy in transfusion dependent homozygous β-thalassaemia: a case report. *International Journal of Gynaecology and Obstetrics* **20**, 319–22.

Hallberg L., Bengtsson C., Garby L., Lennartsson J., Rossander L. & Tibblin E. (1979) An analysis of factors leading to a reduction in iron deficiency in Swedish women. *Bulletin of the World Health Organisation* **57**, 947–54.

Hallberg I., Ryttinger L. & Sölvell L. (1966) Side effects of oral iron therapy. *Acta Medica Scandinavica Supplement* **459**, 3–10.

Hegde U.M., Bowes A., Powell D.K. & Joyner M.V. (1981) Detection of platelet bound and serum antibodies in thrombocytopenia by enzyme linked assay. *Vox Sanguinis* **41**, 306–12.

Hemminki E. & Starfield B. (1978) Routine administration of iron and vitamins during pregnancy: Review of controlled clinical trials. *British Journal of Obstetrics and Gynaecology* **85**, 404–10.

Hill R.M., Verniaud W.M., Horning M.G., McCulley L.B. & Morgan N.F. (1974) Infants exposed in utero to anti-epileptic drugs. *American Journal of Diseases in Childhood* **127**, 645–53.

Hobbins J.C. & Mahoney M.J. (1974) In utero diagnosis of haemoglobinopathies: Techniques for obtaining fetal blood. *New England Journal of Medicine* **290**, 1065–7.

Holmberg L., Bjorn C., Cordesius E., Kristofferson A.L., Ljung R., Löfberg L., Strömberg P. & Nilsson I.M. (1980) Prenatal diagnosis of haemophilia β by an immunoradiometric assay of Factor IX. *Blood* **56**, 397–401.

Homer L.W., Lindsten J., Blömbalk M., Hagenfeldt L., Cordesius E., Strömberg P. & Gustavii B. (1979) Prenatal evaluation of fetus at risk for severe Von Willebrand's Disease. *Lancet* **ii**, 191–2.

Huehns E.R. (1982) The structure and function of haemoglobin: Clinical disorders due to abnormal haemoglobin structure. In (eds) Hardisty R.M. and Weatherall D.J. *Blood and its Disorders* p. 364. 2nd edn. Blackwell Scientific Publications, Oxford.

Huehns E.R., Dance N., Beaven G.H., Hecht F. & Motulsky A.G. (1964) Human embryonic haemoglobins. Cold Spring Harbor Symposium. *Quantitative Biology* **29**, 327–31.

Huehns E.R., Davies S.C. & Brozovic M. (1981) Fresh frozen plasma for vaso-occlusive crises in sickle cell disease. *Lancet* **i**, 1310–11.

Hussein S.S., Hoffbrand A.V., Laulicht M., Attock B. & Letsky E.A. (1975) Serum ferritin levels in beta thalassaemia trait. *British Medical Journal* **2**, 920.

Hytten F.E. & Leitch I. (1971) The volume and compositon of the blood. In *The Physiology of Human Pregnancy*, 2nd edn, pp. 1–68. Blackwell Scientific Publications, Oxford.

Iyengar L. (1971) Folic acid requirements of Indian pregnant women. *American Journal of Obstetrics and Gynecology* **111**, 13–16.

Jackson I.M.D., Doig W.B. & McDonald G. (1967) Pernicious anaemia as a cause of infertility. *Lancet* **ii**, 1159.

Jacobs A., Miller F., Worwood M., Beamish M.R. & Wardrop C.A. (1972). Ferritin in serum of normal subjects and patients with iron deficiency and iron overload. *British Medical Journal* **4**, 206–8.

Jacobs A. & Worwood M. (1982) Iron metabolism, iron deficiency and iron overload. In Hardisty

R.M. and Weatherall D.J. (eds) *Blood and its Disorders*, 2nd ed. Blackwell Scientific Publications, Oxford.

Kan Y.W. & Dozy A.M. (1978) Antenatal diagnosis of sickle cell anaemia by DNA. Analysis of amniotic fluid cells. *Lancet* **2**, 810–12.

Kan Y.W., Golbus M.S. & Dozy A.M. (1976) Prenatal diagnosis of α thalassaemia: Clinical application of molecular hybridization. *New England Journal of Medicine* **295**, 1165–7.

Kan Y.W., Lee K.Y., Forbetta M., Angus A. & Cao A. (1980) Polymorphism of DNA sequence in β globin gene region. Application to prenatal diagnosis of β thalassaemia in Sardinia. *New England Journal of Medicine* **302**, 185–8.

Kan Y.W., Nathan D.G., Cividalli G. & Crookston M.C. (1974) Concentration of fetal red blood cells from a mixture of maternal and fetal blood anti-i serum: an aid to prenatal diagnosis of haemoglobinopathy. *Blood* **43**, 411–15.

Kan Y.W., Trecartin R.F., Golbus M.S. & Filly, R.A. (1977). Prenatal diagnosis of β thalassaemia and sickle cell anaemia. Experience with 24 cases. *Lancet* **i**, 269–71.

Kuizon M.D., Platon T.P., Ancheta L.P., Angeles J.C., Nunez C.B. & Macapinlac M.P. (1979) Iron supplementation among pregnant women. *South East Asian Journal of Tropical Medicine* **10**, 520–7.

Kullander S. & Källen, B. (1976) A prospective study of drugs and pregnancy. *Acta Obstetrica Gynecologica Scandinavica Supplement* **55**, 287–95.

Landon M.J. (1975) Folate metabolism in pregnancy. *Clinics in Obstetrics and Gynaecology* **2**, 413–30.

Landon M.J. & Hytten F.E. (1971) The excretion of folate in pregnancy. *Journal of Obstetrics and Gynaecology of the British Commonwealth* **78**, 769–75.

Landon M.J. & Hytten F.E. (1972) Plasma folate levels following an oral load of folic acid during pregnancy. *Journal of Obstetrics and Gynaecology of the British Commonwealth* **79**, 577–83.

Lazarchick J. & Hoyer L.W. (1978) Immunoradiometric measurement of the Factor VIII procoagulant antigen. *Journal of Clinical Investigation* **62**, 1048–52.

Leeuw N.K.M. de., Lowenstein L. & Hsieh Y.S. (1966) Iron deficiency and hydremia in normal pregnancy. *Medicine, Baltimore* **45**, 291–315.

Leeuw N.K.M. de., Lowenstein L., Tucker E.C. & Dayal S. (1968) Correlation of red cell loss at delivery with changes in red cell mass. *American Journal of Obstetrics and Gynecology* **100**, 1092–1101.

Lewis S.M. (1982) Aplastic anaemia in pregnancy. In Hardisty R.M. and Weatherall D.J. (eds). *Blood and its Disorders*, 2nd ed. Blackwell Scientific Publications, Oxford.

Lowenstein L., Brunton L. & Hsieh, Y.-S. (1966) Nutritional anemia and megaloblastosis in pregnancy. *Canadian Medical Association Journal*, **94**, 636–45.

Lund C.J. (1951) Studies on the iron deficiency anaemia of pregnancy including plasma volume, total hemoglobin, erythrocyte protoporphyrin in treated and untreated normal and anemic patients. *American Journal of Obstetrics and Gynecology* **62**, 947–61.

McCann S.R., Lawlor E., McGovern M. & Temperley I.J. (1980) Severe megaloblastic anaemia of pregnancy. *Journal of the Irish Medical Association* **73**, 197–8.

McGarry J.M. & Andrews J. (1972) Smoking in pregnancy and Vitamin B_{12} metabolism. *British Medical Journal* **ii**, 74–7.

MacKenzie I.Z., Sayers L., Bonnar J. *et al* (1975) Coagulation changes during second trimester abortion induced by intra-amniotic Prostaglandin E_2 and hypertonic solutions. *Lancet* **2**, 1066–9.

McLain C.R. (1974) Leukemia in pregnancy. *Clinical Obstetrics and Gynecology* **17**, No. 4. 185–94.

McLean F.W., Heine M.W., Held B. & Streiff R.R. (1970) Folic acid absorption in pregnancy: comparison of the pteroylpolyglutamate and pteroylmonoglutamate. *Blood* **36**, 628.

McMillan R. (1981) Chronic idiopathic thrombocytopenic purpura. *New England Journal of Medicine* **304**, 1135–47.

Magee H.E. & Milligan E.H.M. (1951) Haemoglobin levels before and after labour. *British Medical Journal* **ii**, 1307–10.

Marengo Rowe A.J., Murff, G., Leveson J.E. & Cook J. (1972) Haemophilia-like disease associated with pregnancy. *Obstetrics and Gynecology* **40**, 56.

Miller J.R., Keith N.M. & Rowntree L.G. (1915) Plasma and blood volume in pregnancy. *Journal of the American Medical Association* **65**, 779–82.

Morgan, E.H. (1961) Plasma iron and haemoglobin levels in pregnancy. The effect of oral iron. *Lancet* **i**, 9–12.

Nicholson H.O. (1968) Leukaemia and pregnancy. *Journal of Obstetrics and Gynaecology of the British Commonwealth* **75**, 517–20.

Ogunbode O., Akinyele I.O. & Hussain, M.A. (1979) Dietary iron intake of pregnant Nigerian women with anaemia. *International Journal of Gynaecology and Obstetrics* **17**, 290–3.

Old J.M., Ward R.H.T., Petrou M., Karagözlu F., Modell B. & Weatherall D.J. (1982) First-trimester fetal diagnosis for haemoglobinopathies: three cases. *Lancet* **2**, 1413–16.

Orkin S.H., Alter B.P., Altay C., Mahoney M.J., Lazarus H., Hobbins, J.C. & Nathan D.G. (1978) Application of endonulease mapping to the analysis and prenatal diagnosis of thalassaemias caused by globin gene deletion. *New England Journal of Medicine* **299**, 166.

Osler, W. (1919) Observations on the severe anaemias of pregnancy and the post-partum state. *British Medical Journal* **1**, 1–3.

Paintin D.B., Thomson, A.M. & Hytten F.E. (1966) Iron and the haemoglobin level in pregnancy. *Journal of Obstetrics and Gynaecology of the British Commonwealth* **73**, 181–90.

Pirani, B.B.K., Campbell D.M. & MacGillivray I. (1973) Plasma volume in normal first pregnancy. *Journal of Obstetrics and Gynaecology of the British Commonwealth* **80**, 884–7.

Rae P.G. & Robb P.M. (1970) Megaloblastic anaemia of pregnancy, a clinical and laboratory study with particular reference to the total and labile serum folate levels. *Journal of Clinical Pathology* **23**, 379–91.

Richards H.G. & Spiers A.S. (1974) Chronic granulocytic leukaemia in pregnancy. *Journal of Clinical Pathology* **27**, 927.

Richmond H.G. (1959) Induction of sarcoma in the rat by iron-dextran complex. *British Medical Journal* **1**, 947–9.

Rios E.R., Lipschitz, D.A., Cook J.D. & Smith N.J. (1975) Relationship of maternal and infant iron stores as assessed by determination of plasma ferritin. *Paediatrics* **55**, 694–9.

Roberts P.D., James H., Petrie A., Morgan J.O. & Hoffbrand A.V. (1973) Vitamin B_{12} status in pregnancy among immigrants to Britain. *British Medical Journal* **iii**, 67–72.

Rothman L.A., Cohen C.J. & Astarloa J. (1973) Placental and fetal involvement by maternal malignancy: A report of rectal carcinoma and review of the literature. *American Journal of Obstetrics and Gynecology* **116**, 1023–33.

Rovinsky J.J. & Jaffin H. (1965) Cardiovascular hemodynamics in pregnancy. I. Blood and plasma volumes in multiple pregnancy. *American Journal of Obstetrics and Gynecology* **93**, 1–13.

Scott, J.M. (1962) Toxicity of iron sorbitol citrate. *British Medical Journal* **2**, 480–1.

Scott J.M. (1963) Iron sorbitol citrate in pregnancy anaemia. *British Medical Journal* **2**, 354–7.

Shapiro J., Alberts H.W., Welch P. & Metz J. (1965) Folate and vitamin B_{12} deficiency associated with lactation. *British Journal of Haematology* **11**, 498–504.

Smithells R.W., Sheppard S., Schorah C.J., Seller M.J., Nevin N.C., Harris R., Read A.P. & Fielding D.W. (1980) Possible prevention of neural tube defects by periconceptional vitamin supplementation. *Lancet* **i**, 339–40.

Stephens H.E.M., Craft I., Peters T.J. & Hoffbrand A.V. (1972) Oral contraceptives and folate metabolism. *Clinical Science* **42**, 405–14.

Stone M.L., Luhby A.L., Feldman R., Gordon M. & Cooperman J.M. (1967) Folic acid metabolism in pregnancy. *American Journal of Obstetrics and Gynecology* **90**, 638–48.

Stott, G. (1960) Anaemia in Mauritius. *Bulletin of the World Health Organisation* **23**, 781–91.

Strauss R.G. & Bernstein R. (1974) Folic acid and dilantin antagonism in pregnancy. *Obstetrics and Gynecology* **44**, 345–8.

Svanberg, B. (1975) Absorption of iron in pregnancy. *Acta Obstetricia et Gynecologica Scandinavica Supplement* **48**, 7–108.

Taylor J.J., Studd J.W.W. & Green I.D. (1968) Primary refractory anaemia and pregnancy. *Journal of Obstetrics and Gynaecology of the British Commonwealth* **75**, 963–8.

Temperley I.J., Meehan M.J.M. & Gattenby P.B.B. (1968) Serum Vitamin B_{12} levels in pregnant women. *Journal of Obstetrics and Gynaecology of the British Commonwealth* **75**, 511–16.

Thomas A.N., Pattison C. & Serjeant G.R. (1982) Causes of death in sickle-cell disease in Jamaica. *British Medical Journal* **285**, 633–5.

Tuck S.M. (1982) Sickle cell disease and pregnancy. *British Journal of Hospital Medicine* **28**, 125–7.

Van Dinh T., Boor P.J. & Garza J.R. (1982) Massive pulmonary embolism following delivery of a patient with sickle cell trait. *American Journal of Obstetrics and Gynecology* **143**, 722–4.

Van Leeuwen E.F., Halmerhorst F.M., Engelfriet C.P. & Von Dem Borne A.E.G. Kr. (1981) Maternal autoimmune thrombocytopenia and the newborn. *British Medical Journal* **2**, **283**, 104.

Williamson R., Eskdale J., Coleman D.V., Niazi M., Loeffler F.E. & Modell, B.M. (1981) Direct gene analysis of chorionic villi: a possible technique for first trimester antenatal diagnosis of haemoglobinopathies. *Lancet* **ii**, 1125–7.

Wood W.G. & Weatherall D.J. (1973) Haemoglobin synthesis during human fetal development. *Nature* **244**, 162–5.

World Health Organisation (1972) Nutritional anaemias. *Technical Report Series*, No. **503**.

3 Haemostasis and Haemorrhage

Elizabeth Letsky

Haemostasis and pregnancy

Healthy haemostasis depends on normal vasculature, platelets, coagulation factors and fibrinolysis. These act together to confine the circulating blood to the vascular bed and arrest bleeding after trauma. Normal pregnancy is accompanied by dramatic changes in the coagulation and fibrinolytic systems where there is a marked increase in some of the coagulation factors, particularly fibrinogen. Fibrin is laid down in the uteroplacental vessel walls and fibrinolysis is suppressed. These changes, together with the increased blood volume, help to combat the hazard of haemorrhage at placental separation, but play only a secondary role to the unique process of myometrial contraction which reduces blood flow to the placental site. They also produce a vulnerable state for intravascular clotting, and a whole spectrum of disorders involving coagulation occur in complications of pregnancy, falling into two main groups— thromboembolism (*see* Chapter 4) and bleeding due to disseminated intravascular coagulation. To make more understandable the measures taken to deal with these obstetric emergencies, a short account follows of haemostasis during pregnancy and how it differs from that in the nonpregnant state.

VASCULAR INTEGRITY

It is not known how vascular integrity is normally maintained but it is clear that the platelets have a key role to play because conditions in which their number is depleted or their function is abnormal are characterised by widespread spontaneous capillary

70

haemorrhages. It is thought that the platelets in health are constantly sealing microdefects of the vasculature, with mini fibrin clots being formed and the unwanted fibrin being removed by a process of fibrinolysis. Generation of prostacyclin appears to be the physiological mechanism which protects the vessel wall from excess deposition of platelet aggregates, and explains the fact that contact of platelets with healthy vascular endothelium is not a stimulus for thrombus formation (Moncada and Vane 1979).

Prostacyclin (PGI_2) is an unstable prostaglandin first discovered in 1976. It is the principal prostanoid synthesised by blood vessels, a powerful vasodilator and potent inhibitor of platelet aggregation. Moncada and Vane (1979) have proposed that there is a balance between the production of prostacyclin by the vessel wall, and the production of the vasoconstrictor and powerful aggregating agent thromboxane by the platelet. Prostacyclin prevents aggregation at much lower concentrations than are needed to prevent adhesion, therefore vascular damage leads to platelet adhesion but not necessarily to aggregation and thrombus formation.

When the injury is minor, small platelet thrombi form and are washed away by the circulation as described above, but the extent of the injury is an important determinant of the size of the thrombus—and whether or not platelet aggregation is stimulated (*see* below). Prostacyclin synthetase is abundant in the intima and progressively decreases in concentration from the intima to the adventitia, whereas the pro-aggregating elements increase in concentration from the subendothelium to the adventitia. It follows that severe vessel damage or physical detachment of the endothelium will lead to the development of a large thrombus as opposed to simple platelet adherence.

There are several conditions in which the production of prostacyclin could be impaired, thereby upsetting the normal balance. Deficiency of prostacyclin production has been suggested in platelet consumption syndromes such as haemolytic uraemic syndrome and thrombotic thrombocytopenic purpura (Lewis 1982). Prostacyclin production has been shown to be reduced in fetal and placental tissue from pre-eclamptic pregnancies, and the current role of prostacyclin in pathogenesis of this disease and potential for treatment in hypertension of pregnancy is undergoing active investigation.

There have been several conflicting reports concerning the platelet count during pregnancy, the main problem being the definition of normal pregnancy. There is probably no significant change in uncomplicated, healthy pregnancy even towards term (Fenton *et al* 1977), but a decrease in the platelet count has been observed in pregnancies with fetal growth retardation, whether or not pre-eclampsia was implicated (Redman *et al* 1978). There is no evidence of changes in platelet function (Shaper *et al* 1968) or differences in platelet lifespan (Rakoczi *et al* 1979) between healthy nonpregnant and pregnant women; however, the lifespan is shortened significantly in pre-eclampsia.

ARREST OF AFTER TRAUMA BLEEDING

An essential function of the haemostatic system is a rapid reaction to injury which remains confined to the area of damage. This requires control mechanisms which will stimulate coagulation after trauma, and limit the extent of the response. The substances involved in the formation of the haemostatic plug normally circulate in an inert form, until activated at the site of injury, or by some factor released into the circulation which will trigger intravascular coagulation.

LOCAL RESPONSE

Platelets adhere to collagen on the injured basement membrane, which triggers a series of changes in the platelets themselves, including shape change and release of ADP and other substances. ADP release stimulates further aggregation of platelets, which triggers the coagulation cascade, and the action of thrombin leads to the formation of fibrin which converts the lone platelet plug into a firm, stable wound seal. The role of platelets is of less importance in injury involving large vessels, because platelet aggregates are of insufficient size and strength to breach the defect. The coagulation mechanism is of major importance here, together with vascular contraction.

COAGULATION SYSTEM

The end result of blood coagulation is the formation of an insoluble fibrin clot from the soluble precursor fibrinogen in the plasma. This involves a complex interaction of clotting factors, and a sequential activation of a series of proenzymes which has been termed the coagulation cascade (Fig. 3.1). When a blood vessel is injured, blood coagulation is initiated by activation of Factor XII by collagen (intrinsic mechanism) and activation of Factor VII by thromboplastin release (extrinsic mechanism) from the damaged tissues. Both the intrinsic and extrinsic mechanisms are activated by components of the vessel wall and both are required for normal haemostasis. Strict divisions between the two pathways do not exist and interactions between activated factors in both pathways have been shown. They share a common pathway following the activation of Factor X.

The intrinsic pathway (or contact system) proceeds spontaneously and is relatively slow, requiring 5–20 minutes for visible fibrin formation. All tissues contain a specific lipoprotein, thromboplastin (particularly concentrated in lung and brain), which markedly increases the rate at which blood clots. The placenta is also very rich in tissue factor, which will produce fibrin formation within twelve seconds; the acceleration of coagulation is brought about by bypassing the reactions involving the contact (intrinsic) system (*see* Fig. 3.1). Blood coagulation is strictly confined to the site of tissue injury in normal circumstances. Powerful control mechanisms must be at work to prevent dissemination of coagulation beyond the site of trauma.

The action of thrombin *in vivo* (particularly its absorption onto the locally formed fibrin) is controlled by a number of mechanisms, and the presence of a potent inhibitor, antithrombin III, an α_2 globulin, which destroys thrombin activity. Heparin, which potentiates the action of anti X^a, may be identical to antithrombin III (Biggs *et al* 1970). This is the rationale for the use of small-dose heparin as prophylaxis in patients at risk for thromboembolic phenomena postoperatively, in pregnancy and in the puerperium.

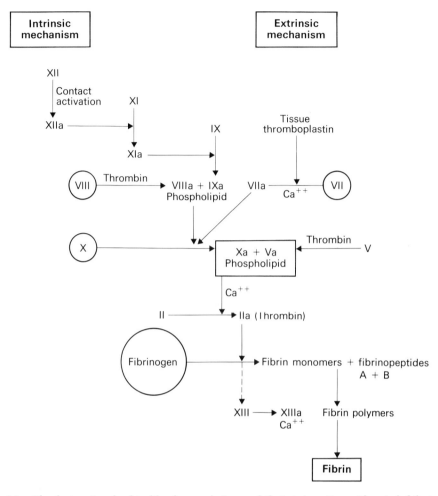

Fig. 3.1 The factors involved in blood coagulation and their interactions. The circled factors show significant increases in pregnancy.

Normal pregnancy is accompanied by major changes in the coagulation system, with increases in levels of Factors VII, VIII and X, and a particularly marked increase in the level of plasma fibrinogen (Bonnar 1981) (Fig. 3.1), which is probably the chief cause of the accelerated erythrocyte sedimentation rate observed during pregnancy. The effect of pregnancy on the coagulation factors can be detected from about the third month of gestation, and the amount of fibrinogen in late pregnancy is at least double that of the nonpregnant state (Bonnar 1981).

FIBRINOLYSIS

Fibrinolytic activity is an essential part of the dynamic, interacting haemostasis mechanism, and is dependent on plasminogen activator in the blood (Fig. 3.2). Fibrin

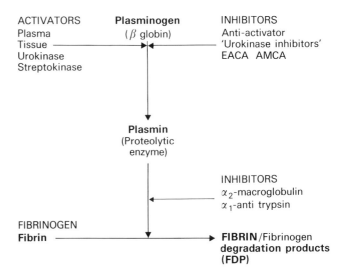

Fig. 3.2 Components of
the fibrinolytic system.

and fibrinogen are digested by plasmin, a proenzyme derived from an inactive plasma
precursor plasminogen.

Increased amounts of activator are found in the plasma after strenuous exercise,
emotional stress, surgical operations and other trauma. Tissue activator can be
extracted from most human organs with the exception of the placenta. Tissues
especially rich in activator include the uterus, ovaries, prostate, heart, lungs, thyroid,
adrenals and lymph nodes. Activity in tissues is concentrated mainly around blood
vessels, veins showing greater activity than arteries. Venous occlusion of the limbs will
stimulate fibrinolytic activity, a fact which should be remembered if tourniquets are
applied for any length of time before blood is drawn for measurement of fibrin
degradation products (FDP).

The inhibitors of fibrinolytic activity are of two types—anti-activators (anti-
plasminogens) and the antiplasmins. Inhibitors of plasminogen include epsilon amino
caproic acid (EACA) and tranexamic acid (AMCA). Aprotonin (Trasylol) is another
antiplasminogen which is commercially prepared from bovine lung.

Platelets, plasma and serum exert a strong inhibitory action on plasmin. Normally
plasma antiplasmin levels exceed levels of plasminogen and hence the levels of potential
plasmin; otherwise we would dissolve away our connecting cement! When fibrinogen
or fibrin is broken down by plasmin, fibrin degradation products are formed; these
comprise the high-molecular-weight slip products X and Y, and smaller fragments A, B,
C, D and E (Fig. 3.3). When a fibrin clot is formed, 70 per cent of fragment X is retained
in the clot, Y, D and E being retained to a somewhat lesser extent. Therefore serum, even
under normal circumstances, can contain small amounts of fragment X and larger
amounts of Y, D and E. All of these components have antigenic determinants in
common with fibrinogen and will be recognised by antifibrinogen antisera. It is
important to be aware of this when examining blood for the presence of FDPs as
confirmation of excess fibrinolytic activity (e.g. in disseminated intravascular coagula-

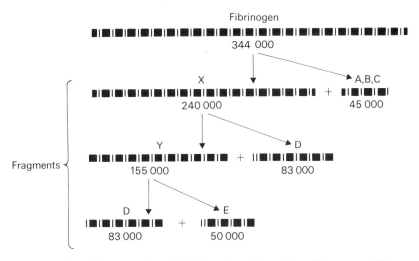

Fig. 3.3 Fibrin degradation products (FDPs) produced by action of plasma on fibrinogen. The molecular weights are shown.

tion). Blood should be taken by clean venepuncture and the tourniquet should not be left on too long (*see* above). The blood should be allowed to clot in the presence of an antifibrinolytic agent such as EACA to stop the process of fibrinolysis which would otherwise continue in vitro.

Plasma fibrinolytic activity is decreased during pregnancy, remains low during labour and delivery and returns to normal within one hour of delivery of the placenta (Bonnar *et al* 1970). The rapid return to normal of systemic fibrinolytic activity following delivery of the placenta and the fact that the placenta has been shown to contain inhibitors which block fibrinolysis, suggests that inhibition of fibrinolysis during pregnancy is mediated through the placenta.

SUMMARY OF CHANGES IN HAEMOSTASIS IN PREGNANCY

The changes in the coagulation system in normal pregnancy are consistent with a continuing low grade process of coagulant activity. Using electron microscopy, fibrin deposition can be demonstrated in the intervillous space of the placenta and in the walls of the spiral arteries supplying the placenta (Sheppard and Bonnar 1974). As pregnancy advances, the elastic lamina and smooth muscle of these spiral arteries are replaced by a matrix containing fibrin. This allows expansion of the lumen to accommodate an increasing blood flow and reduces the vascular resistance of the placenta. At placental separation during normal childbirth, a blood flow of 500–800 ml per minute has to be staunched within seconds, or serious haemorrhage will occur. Myometrial contraction plays a vital role in securing haemostasis by reducing the blood flow to the placental site. Rapid closure of the terminal part of the spiral artery will be further facilitated by the structural changes within the walls. The placental site is rapidly covered by a fibrin mesh following delivery. The increased levels of fibrinogen, and other coagulation factors, will be advantageous to meet the sudden demand for haemostatic components at placental separation.

Disseminated intravascular coagulation

The changes in the haemostatic system during pregnancy, and the local activation of the clotting system during parturition, carry with them risks, not only of thromboembolism (*see* Chapter 4), but of disseminated intravascular coagulation (DIC), consumption of clotting factors and of platelets leading to severe bleeding (particularly uterine and sometimes generalised). Despite the advances in obstetric care and highly developed blood transfusion services, haemorrhage still constitutes a major factor in maternal mortality and morbidity.

The first problem with DIC is its definition. It is never primary, but always secondary to some general stimulation of coagulation activity by release of procoagulant substances into the blood (Fig. 3.4). Hypothetical triggers of this process in pregnancy include the leaking of placental tissue fragments, amniotic fluid, incompatible red cells or bacterial products into the maternal circulation. There is a wide spectrum of manifestations of the process of DIC, ranging from a compensated state with no clinical manifestation but evidence of increased production and breakdown of coagulation factors, to the condition we all fear—massive uncontrollable haemorrhaging with very

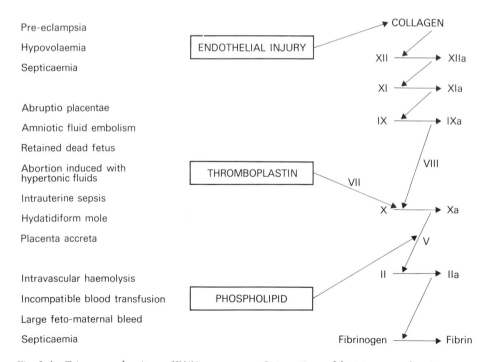

Fig. 3.4 Trigger mechanisms of DIC in pregnancy. Interactions of the trigger mechanisms occur in many of these obstetric complications.

low concentrations of plasma fibrinogen, pathological raised levels of fibrin degradation products and variable degrees of thrombocytopenia.

Fibrinolysis is stimulated by DIC, and the FDPs resulting from the process interfere with the formation of firm fibrin clots; a vicious circle is established which results in further disastrous bleeding. Obstetric conditions particularly associated with DIC include abruptio placentae, amniotic fluid embolism, septic abortion and intrauterine infection, retained dead fetus, hydatidiform mole, placenta accreta, pre-eclampsia and eclampsia, and prolonged shock from any cause (Fig. 3.4).

Haematological management

There have been many reports concerning both small series of patients and individual patients with coagulation failure during pregnancy. However, no significant controlled trials of the value of the many possible therapeutic measures have been carried out. This is mainly because no one person or unit is likely to see enough cases to randomise them into groups in which the number would achieve statistical significance. Also, the complex and variable nature of the conditions associated with DIC, which are often self-correcting or treated with a variety of measures, make it impossible to make an objective assessment of the published reports. What follows is an outline of the strategy to deal with haemorrhage in the obstetric patient, arrived at by friendly, though often heated, discussion of published reports and personal and collective experience at Queen Charlotte's Maternity Hospital.

The management of the bleeding obstetric patient is an acute and frightening problem. There is little time to think and there should be a routine, planned practice decided on by haematologist, physician, anaesthetist, obstetrician and nursing staff in any materinity unit, to deal with this situation whenever it arises. Good, reliable, continuing communication between the various clinicians and nursing, paramedical and laboratory staff is essential. As soon as there is any concern about a patient bleeding for any reason, approximately 15 ml of venous blood should be taken and stored in a set of bottles kept in an emergency pack, together with a set of laboratory request forms, previously made out, which only require the patient's name and identification number added to them. This blood can be taken at the time of setting up an intravenous infusion, if the patient does not already have one. It is essential that the blood should not be contaminated with even the smallest amount of heparin, or the results obtained will be meaningless and create even further panic! If heparin has been used to set up an intravenous infusion then the blood *must* be taken from another site. The venous line cannot be 'washed through' sufficiently to eliminate all heparin. The blood should be divided as follows:

1   2.5 ml into EDTA for full blood count with emphasis on Hb, PCV, and platelet count.
2   4.5 ml into citrate for coagulation screen.
3   2.0 ml into EACA for estimation of FDPs.
4   The rest, approximately 6.0 ml, into a plain tube for cross-matching.

Useful rapid screening tests for haemostatic failure include the platelet count, partial thromboplastin time, or accelerated whole blood clotting time (which tests intrinsic coagulation), prothrombin time (which tests extrinsic coagulation), the thrombin time and estimation of fibrinogen (*see* Fig. 3.1). Elevation of FDPs is not specific to DIC and only confirms the diagnosis. The estimation is carried out on a clotted specimen delivered into EACA which prevents further fibrinolysis taking place in vitro. Of the tests of coagulation, probably the thrombin time (an estimation of the thrombin-clottable fibrinogen in a citrated sample of plasma), is the most valuable, overall rapid screen of haemostatic competence of coagulation factors. The normal thrombin time is about 10–15 seconds, and the newly formed fibrin clot is firm and stable. In the most severe forms of DIC, there is no clottable fibrinogen in the sample, and no fibrin clot appears, even after 2–3 minutes. Indication of severe DIC is usually obtained by a prolonged thrombin time with a friable clot, which may dissolve on standing, due to fibrinolytic substances present in the plasma. A crude, but valuable rapid estimation of the fibrinogen level is obtained by performing the thrombin time test, using serial dilutions of the patient's plasma.

There is no point in the obstetrician, anaesthetist or nursing staff wasting time trying to perform bedside whole blood clotting tests. Whole blood clotting normally takes up to five minutes. The test must be performed in clean tubes in a 37°C water bath with suitable controls. The valuable hands at the bedside are of more use doing the things they are trained to do in this emergency situation, rather than wasting time performing a test which is time consuming, of little value or significance unless performed under strict control conditions, and will not contribute much, if anything, to management. The alerted laboratory worker will be able to provide significant results within half an hour, at the most, of receiving the specimen in the laboratory.

The tests referred to above are straightforward and should be available from any routine haematology laboratory. It is not necessary to have a sophisticated coagulation laboratory to perform these simple screening tests to confirm or refute a diagnosis of DIC. Once the blood has been sent off to the laboratory for investigation, place two units of fresh, frozen plasma in a 37°C water bath to thaw. Fresh frozen plasma does not have to be cross-matched or given to patients of the same group from which it was taken, although it is prefereable to use the same ABO and Rhesus group as the recipient if possible. While waiting for the plasma to thaw and for cross-matched blood, the circulating blood volume should be maintained with a plasma substitute. Treatment of severe haemorrhage must include prompt and adequate fluid replacement in order to avoid renal shutdown. If effective circulation is restored without too much delay, FDPs will be cleared from the blood mainly by the liver, which will further aid restoration of normal haemostasis. This is an aspect of management which is often insufficiently emphasised (Pritchard 1973).

PLASMA SUBSTITUTES

There is much controversy around which plasma substitute to use in any bleeding patient. The remarks which follow appertain to the supportive management of acute haemorrhage from the placental site, and should not be taken to apply to those situations in which hypovolaemia may be associated with severe hypoproteinaemia, such as occurs in septic peritonitis, burns and bowel infarction. The choice lies between simple crystalloids—Hartmann's solution or Ringer lactate, and artificial colloids—dextrans, hydroxyethyl starch, gelatin solution or the very expensive preparations of human albumin (albuminoids). If crystalloids are used, 2–3 times the volume of estimated blood loss should be administered because the crystalloid remains in the vascular compartment for a shorter time than do colloids.

Dextrans adversely affect platelet function, may cause pseudo-agglutination and interfere with interpretation of subsequent blood grouping and cross-matching tests. They are, therefore, contraindicated in the woman who is bleeding in pregnancy where there is a high chance of there being an associated, serious, haemostatic defect. Dextrans can also cause allergic anaphylactoid reactions. Albuminoids are thought to be associated less with anaphylactoid reactions, but they may be particularly harmful when transfused in the shocked patient by contributing to renal and pulmonary failure, adversely affecting cardiac function and further impairing haemostasis (Cash 1981).

Many studies have suggested that the best way to deal initially with hypovolaemic shock is by transfusing simple balanced salt solutions (crystalloid), followed by red cells and fresh frozen plasma (Carey *et al* 1970; Moss 1972; Virgilio *et al* 1979). More recent work (Hauser *et al* 1980) has challenged this approach, and suggests that albumin-containing solutions are superior to crystalloids for volume replacement in postoperative shocked patients with respiratory insufficiency (*see* Chapter 1). This aspect of the management of shocked patients with blood loss will remain controversial pending the results of further clinical trials. At Queen Charlotte's Maternity Hospital we use a derivative of bovine gelatin—polygeline (Haemaccel)—for immediate resuscitation. It has a shelf life of eight years, can be stored at room temperature, is iso-oncotic and does not interfere with platelet function or subsequent blood grouping or cross-matching. It is not associated with anaphylactoid reaction, and renal function is improved when it is administered in hypovolaemic shock.

The infusion of plasma substitutes, i.e. plasma protein, dextran, gelatin and starch solutions, may result in adverse reactions. Although the incidence of severe reactions is rare, they are diverse in nature, varying from allergic urticarial manifestation and mild fever to life-threatening anaphylactic reactions due to spasm of smooth muscle, with cardiac and respiratory arrest (Doenicke *et al* 1977). The anaphylactoid reaction accompanying infusion of dextrans are probably related to IgG and IgM antidextran antibodies which are found in high concentration in all patients with severe reactions.

Haemaccel is generally considered to be non-immunogenic, and therefore does not trigger the production of antibodies in man, even on repeated challenge. The reactions which occur, related to Haemaccel infusion, are thought to be due to histamine release (Lorenz *et al* 1976), the incidence and severity being proportional to the extent of histamine release. There have been very few reports of severe reactions with bronchospasm and circulatory collapse, but they do occur rarely and there has been one report of a fatality associated with Haemaccel administration (Freeman 1979). Nevertheless, whatever substitute is used, it should be considered as only temporary until suitable blood component therapy can be administered.

WHOLE BLOOD AND COMPONENT THERAPY

Whole 'fresh' blood is no longer generally available because there is insufficient time to complete hepatitis surface antigen and blood grouping tests before it is released from the Transfusion Centre. To release it earlier than the usual 18–24 hours would increase the risk of transmitting viral B hepatitis and of serologically incompatible transfusions. Syphilis, cytomegalovirus (CMV) and Epstein–Barr virus are examples of other microbes which may be transmitted in fresh blood. Their viability diminishes rapidly on storage at 4°C. These infections, particularly in immunosuppressed or pregnant patients, can be particularly hazardous. Apart from the hazards of giving whole blood less than 6–24 hours old, its use today represents a serious waste of vitally needed components required for patients with specific isolated deficiencies. The use of fresh frozen plasma followed by bank red cells provides all the components (apart from platelets) which are present in whole fresh blood and allows the plasma from the freshly donated unit to be used to make the much needed blood components.

PLASMA COMPONENT THERAPY

Fresh frozen plasma (FFP) contains all the coagulation factors present in plasma obtained from whole blood within six hours of donation. Frozen rapidly and stored at −30°C, the factors are well preserved for at least one year. Plasma stored at −20°C does degenerate, and should be used within six months of preparation. Freeze-dried plasma is prepared by pooling blood donations prior to dispensing and freezing; hence there is an increased risk of transmitting hepatitis. This product is also deficient in Factors V and VIII. Its advantage is that it can be stored in the dark, below 25°C, for up to eight years. It can be of value in providing colloid in the management of surgical or traumatic haemorrhage.

Concentrated fibrinogen should *not* be used in obstetric haemorrhage associated with DIC. The depletion of fibrinogen in these conditions is well known but undue importance is attributed to the lack of fibrinogen which is only part of a general consumptive coagulopathy. FFP provides abundant fibrinogen together with Factors V and VIII which are also depleted, and the coagulation inhibitor antithrombin III (*see* above). Concentrated fibrinogen prepared from pooled donations carries a great risk of subsequent hepatitis, and administration has been shown to result in a sharp fall in levels of antithrombin III, suggesting that the concentrates may aggravate intravascular coagulation (Bonnar 1981), thus adding 'fuel to the fire'.

Platelets, an essential haemostatic component, are not present in FFP and their functional activity rapidly deteriorates in stored blood. The platelet count reflects both the degree of intravascular coagulation and the amount of bank blood transfused. A patient with persistent bleeding and very low platelet count (less than 20×10^9/l) may require concentrated platelets although we have never yet had to give them to achieve haemostasis at Queen Charlotte's Maternity Hospital. Platelet concentrates are specially prepared at the Transfusion Centre in packs using 3–5 donations of blood, and have a shelf life of only 72 hours.

RED CELL TRANSFUSION

Cross-matched blood should be available within 40 minutes of the maternal specimen reaching the laboratory. If the woman has had all her antenatal care at the same hospital, her blood group will be known, and there is a good case for giving uncross-matched blood of her same group should the situation warrant it, provided that blood has been properly processed at the Transfusion Centre. If the blood group is unknown, uncross-matched group O, Rhesus-negative blood may be given if necessary. By the time that two units of Group O, Rhesus-negative blood have been given, laboratory screening tests of haemostatic function should be available. If these prove to be normal, but vaginal bleeding continues, the cause is nearly always trauma. It is imperative that the source of bleeding, often an unsuspected uterine or genital laceration, be located and treated. Prolonged hypovolaemic shock, or indeed shock from any cause, may also trigger off DIC and this may lead to haemostatic failure and further prolonged haemorrhage.

Whole blood that has been stored, even under optimal conditions, undergoes certain deleterious changes. The oxygen affinity of red cells, plasma K^+ and H^+, all increase. These changes are not significant until after four days of shelf life. Platelets deteriorate rapidly within the first 24 hours and after 72 hours they have lost all haemostatic function. The activity of the labile coagulation Factors V and particularly VIII fall within the first 24 hours of donation and, after six days' storage, micro-aggregates of platelets, white cells and fibrin form. If the blood loss is replaced only by stored bank blood, which is deficient in the labile clotting Factors V and VIII and platelets, the circulation will rapidly become depleted in these essential components of haemostasis even if the cause of haemorrhage is not initially DIC. It is advisable to transfuse one unit of fresh frozen plasma for every 4–6 units of bank red cells administered. It would seem sensible in any event, whatever the cause of bleeding, to replace the initial plasma substitute with two units of fresh frozen plasma once it has thawed, while waiting for compatible blood to be available. Finally, citrate used as an anticoagulant in transfused blood may complex calcium ions which are also necessary for haemostasis. Some centres recommend giving one ampoule (10 ml) of 10 per cent calcium gluconate slowly over ten minutes for every six units of blood infused. It would seem more sensible to check calcium levels routinely with the other electrolytes and treat only if indicated. A spontaneous recovery from the coagulation defect is to be expected once the uterus is empty and well contracted, provided that blood volume is maintained by adequate replacement, monitored by central venous pressure and urinary output.

The single most important component of haemostasis, during delivery in normal circumstances, is contraction of the myometrium stemming the flow from the placental site. No excess of clotting factors will stop haemorrhage if the uterus remains flabby. It follows that vaginal delivery will make a less severe demand on the haemostatic mechanism than delivery by Caesarean section which requires the same haemostatic competence as any other major surgical procedure. Should DIC be established with the fetus in utero it is better to wait for spontaneous delivery, if possible, or stimulate vaginal delivery, avoiding episiotomy or other soft tissue damage, rather than to embark on heroic abdominal delivery.

We next consider defects of haemostasis in certain specific conditions.

Abruptio placentae

Premature separation of the placenta—abruptio placentae—is the commonest cause of coagulation failure in obstetrics. Many of the problems which confront the attendant in this situation are common to other conditions associated with DIC in obstetric practice, so that this will be used as the central focus to discuss some of the problems of management.

There is a wide spectrum in the severity of the haemostatic failure in this condition, which appears to be related to the degree of placental separation. In some cases of a small abruption, there is a minor degree of failure of haemostatic processes and the fetus does not succumb. When the uterus is tense and tender, and no fetal heart can be heard, then separation and retroplacental bleeding are extensive. The amount of vaginal bleeding is no guide to the severity of the haemorrhage or coagulation failure. There may be no external vaginal blood loss, even when the placenta is completely separated, the fetus dead, the circulating blood incoagulable, and there is five litres of concealed blood loss resulting in hypovolaemic shock. Haemostatic failure should be suspected if there is persistent oozing at the site of venepuncture or bleeding from the mucous membrane of mouth or nose. Simple rapid screening tests, as described below, will confirm the presence of DIC. There will be a low platelet count, greatly prolonged thrombin time and low fibrinogen, together with raised FDPs, due to secondary fibrinolysis stimulated by the intravascular deposition of fibrin. The mainstay of treatment is to maintain the circulating blood volume. This not only prevents renal shutdown and further haemostatic failure caused by hypovolaemic shock, but also helps clearance of FDPs, which in themselves act as potent anticoagulants. It has also been suggested that FDPs inhibit myometrial activity, since serious postpartum haemorrhage in women with abruptio placentae was found to be associated with high levels of FDP (Basu 1969). There is some suggestion that high levels of FDPs may also inhibit myocardial contractility (Pritchard 1973).

If the fetus is dead the aim should be prompt vaginal delivery, avoiding soft tissue damage. Once correction of hypovolaemia is underway, measures to speed up delivery should be instituted. Amniotomy may be performed or, if this fails, prostaglandin or oxytocin stimulation can be used. There is no evidence that the use of oxytoxic agents aggravates thromboplastin release from the uterus (Bonnar 1978). Following emptying of the uterus, myometrial contraction will greatly reduce bleeding from the placental site and spontaneous correction of the haemostatic defect usually occurs shortly after delivery, if the measures recommended below have been taken. However, postpartum haemorrhage is a not infrequent complication and is the commonest cause of death in abruptio placentae.

In cases where the abruption is small and the fetus is still alive, prompt Caesarean section may save the baby, if vaginal delivery is not imminent. Fresh frozen plasma, bank red cells and platelet concentrates should be available to correct the potentially severe coagulation defect in the maternal circulation (*see* above). In rare situations where vaginal delivery cannot be stimulated and haemorrhage continues, Caesarean section may be indicated even in the presence of a dead fetus. In all these circumstances, normal haemostasis should be restored as far as possible by the administration of fresh frozen plasma and platelet concentrates, if necessary, as well as red cells before surgery is undertaken.

Despite extravasation of blood throughout the uterine muscle its function is not necessarily impaired, and good contraction can follow removal of fetus, placenta and retroperitoneal clot. Hysterectomy should be avoided as delayed internal bleeding may occur, and regional anaesthesia or analgesia is contraindicated. Expansion of the lower limb vascular bed resulting from regional block can add to the problem of uncorrected hypovolaemia; furthermore in the presence of haemostatic failure there is the additional hazard of bleeding into the epidural space (Bonnar 1981).

In recent years, heparin has been used to treat all kinds of disseminated intravascular coagulation, whatever their cause. There is, however, no objective evidence to demonstrate that its use in abruptio placentae decreases morbidity and mortality, and very good results have been achieved without it (Pritchard 1973). With an intact circulation, its use would be sensible and logical to break the vicious circle of DIC, but in the presence of already defective haemostasis with a large bleeding placental site, it may prolong massive local and generalised haemorrhage. Treatment with antifibrinolytic agents such as EACA or trasylol can result in blockage of the small vessels of vital organs (such as the kidney or brain) with fibrin, therefore they are contraindicated, although Bonnar (1981) suggests that delayed severe and prolonged haemorrhage from the placental site, several hours postdelivery, may respond to their use if all other measures fail.

Amniotic fluid embolism

This obstetric disaster (recently reviewed by Morgan (1979)) usually occurs during or shortly after a vigorous labour with an intact amniotic sac, and can occur during a Caesarean section. It is thought that amniotic fluid enters the maternal circulation via lacerations of membranes and placenta. Platelet fibrin thrombi are formed and trapped within the pulmonary blood vessels; profound shock follows, accompanied by respiratory distress and cyanosis. There is a high mortality at this stage from a combination of respiratory and cardiac failure. If the mother survives long enough, massive intravascular coagulation with almost total consumption of coagulation factors invariably follows. There is bleeding from venepuncture sites and severe haemorrhage from the placental site after delivery (Gregory and Clayton 1973).

Confirmation of diagnosis is usually made postmortem by finding histological evidence of amniotic fluid and fetal tissue within the substance of the maternal lungs; occasionally, similar material may be aspirated from a CVP catheter. It is, therefore, difficult to assess the value of therapeutic measures taken, in the few reports which have appeared, for the successful management of a clinical syndrome which can usually only be suggestive of amniotic fluid embolism (Bonnar 1973; Skjodt 1965; Chung and Merkatz 1973).

The major differential diagnoses of amniotic fluid embolism in the collapsed patient are primary cardiovascular catastrophes such as pulmonary embolus or aspiration in the anaesthetised patient. Apart from the bleeding and evidence of DIC associated with amniotic fluid embolism, pulmonary embolus has specific features. These and other medical causes of shock in obstetric patients are considered in Table 4.1. Aspiration is usually associated with bronchospasm which is very rare in amniotic fluid embolus (Morgan 1979). At any time, if there is doubt about the diagnosis, the rapid fluid infusion necessary for the treatment of amniotic fluid embolus should be controlled by careful assessment of the venous pressure by CVP line. Such rapid fluid infusion would cause a marked rise in CVP in patients with pulmonary embolus, and could well lead to fatal fluid overload. In addition, the presence of the CVP line will allow aspiration of fetal material from the great veins, for confirmation of the diagnosis of amniotic fluid embolus (Resnik *et al* 1976). Such material should also be sought in maternal sputum (Tuck 1972).

The object of the treatment is to sustain the circulation while the intravascular thrombin in the lungs is cleared by the fibrinolytic response of the endothelium of the pulmonary vessels. If bleeding from the placental site can be controlled by stimulation of uterine contraction, then the logical treatment is carefully monitored transfusion of FFP and packed red cells with heparin administration and, if necessary, ventilation (*see* Chapter 1, p. 22).

Retention of a dead fetus

There is a gradual depletion of coagulation factors following intrauterine fetal death, and the changes are not usually detectable in vitro until 3–4 weeks have passed. Thromboplastic substances released from the dead tissues in the uterus into the maternal circulation are thought to be the trigger of DIC in this situation, which occurs in about one-third of patients who retain the dead fetus for more than 4–5 weeks (Pritchard 1959). About 80 per cent of pregnant women with intrauterine fetal death will go into spontaneous labour within three weeks. Problems resulting from defective haemostasis are much less common nowadays because labour is induced within 3–4 weeks of fetal death, before clinically significant coagulation changes develop. Rupture of the membranes is recommended once induced labour is established in such patients, as there is a risk of precipitate labour, and amniotic fluid embolism has been known to occur (Bonnar 1978).

If the screening tests previously described indicate that there is defective haemostasis, the coagulation factors should be restored to normal before delivery is attempted. Where the circulation is intact, heparin is the logical treatment to block the activation of the coagulation system. Intravenous infusion of 1000 IU heparin hourly for up to 48 hours is usually sufficient to restore the number of platelets and the level of fibrinogen and Factors V and VIII to normal (Bonnar 1978). The heparin should then be discontinued and labour should be induced. There should be plenty of compatible red cells and fresh frozen plasma available to treat any haemorrhage at placental separation promptly. If the patient goes into spontaneous labour while heparin is being administered, the infusion should be stopped. It is not necessary to neutralise the heparin with protamine sulphate unless the patient is bleeding.

INDUCED ABORTION USING HYPERTONIC SOLUTIONS

Changes in haemostatic components consistent with DIC have been demonstrated in patients undergoing abortion induced with hypertonic solutions of saline and urea (Stander *et al* 1971; Spivak *et al* 1972; Van Royen 1974; MacKenzie *et al* 1975). The stimulus appears to be the release of tissue factor into the maternal circulation from the placenta which is damaged by the hypertonic solutions. The resulting haemorrhage may be massive and has ended in maternal deaths. Prompt restoration of the blood volume, and transfusions with red cells and fresh frozen plasma as described below should resolve the situation which is self-limiting, once the uterus is empty. This complication is one of the reasons why the use of hypertonic solutions to induce abortion has largely been replaced by the administration of prostaglandin.

INTRAUTERINE INFECTION

Endotoxic shock associated with septic abortion, antepartum or post partum intra-uterine infection can trigger DIC in pregnancy and the puerperium (Graeff *et al* 1976; Steichele and Herschlein 1968). Infection with Gram-negative microorganisms is the usual finding. Fibrin is deposited in the microvasculature due to endothelial damage by the endotoxin; secondary red cell intravascular haemolysis with characteristic fragmentation, so-called microangiopathic haemolysis, is characteristic of the condition.

As stated previously DIC is always a secondary phenomenon, and the mainstay of management is to remove the initiating stimulus if possible. In this situation, elimination of the uterine infection remains the most important aspect of management (Studdiford and Douglas 1956). The differential diagnosis of endotoxin shock is discussed in Chapter 4 and in Chapter 7, where the renal complications are also considered. Claims that therapy with heparin has decreased maternal mortality in septic abortion are in doubt and the use of heparin remains controversial (Beller and Uszynski 1974). On the other hand purpura fulminans, a rare complication of puerperal infection, should be treated with heparin early in the disease. Haemorrhage occurs into the skin, in association with DIC. The purpuric patches have a jagged and erythematous border. The lesions become necrotic and gangrenous associated with shock, tachycardia and fever. Without treatment the mortality rate is high. Survival is currently much improved because of better supportive treatment for the shocked patient, effective control of infection, and heparin therapy.

Acquired primary defects of haemostasis

THROMBOCYTOPENIA

A low platelet count is seen most frequently in pregnancy in association with DIC (as already described). Sometimes severe megaloblastic anaemia of pregnancy is accompanied by thrombocytopenia, but the platelet count rapidly returns to normal after therapy with folic acid (Bonnar 1981). Toxic depression of bone marrow megakaryo-cytes in pregnancy can occur in association with infection, certain drugs and alcoholism. Neoplastic infiltration may also result in thrombocytopenia. Probably the single most important cause of isolated thrombocytopenia is immune thrombocyto-penia purpura (ITP) which is a disease primarily of young women in the reproductive years (McMillan 1981). The diagnosis used to be made when severe thrombocytopenia was found to be associated with normal or increased numbers of megakaryocytes in the bone marrow. There are now more reliable tests for demonstrating the responsible IgG antibody which can also be performed (Van Leeuwen *et al* 1981; Hegde *et al* 1981). The antibody is directed against and coats the platelet, which is rapidly removed from the circulation by the reticuloendothelial system. It is possible with these new tests to distinguish between IgG antibodies which can cross the placenta and IgM antibodies which do not (Van Leeuwen *et al* 1981), and also to identify platelet-bound antibody and the more dangerous free IgG antibody in the maternal plasma (Hegde *et al* 1981; Cines *et al* 1982). Much of the published literature (Carloss *et al* 1980; Territo *et al* 1973; Terao *et al* 1981) consists of retrospective analyses of women suffering from ITP, managed throughout pregnancy without the advantage of these tests which identify specific platelet autoantibodies. However, there are still centres where these laboratory investigations are not freely available, so that management may have to be planned without their aid. The maternal platelet count should be checked regularly during pregnancy and if it falls below 20×10^9/l then steroids are indicated. These should be tapered to the lowest dose that provides safe platelet counts (McMillan 1981; Carloss *et al* 1980). The use of steroids in pregnancy is described in Chapter 1.

Splenectomy during pregnancy should be avoided because an appreciable maternal mortality rate has been reported (9–10 per cent) which does not exist outside pregnancy (Bell 1977). It also predisposes to premature labour, and the fetal loss rate is high.

Because the IgG antibody will cross the placenta the major risk to the fetus is that of intracranial bleeding during delivery. If there is any question that a vaginal delivery will be difficult because of cephalo-pelvic disproportion, premature delivery, etc., elective Caesarean section should be carried out. It has also been recommended by several authors (*see* Carloss *et al* 1980) that, if the maternal platelet count is less than 100×10^9/l, indicating active ITP, Caesarean section should be performed. McMillan (1981) states that this is indicated if the spleen is absent regardless of platelet count. If, however, one has access to reliable reproducible platelet antibody tests, and no appreciable IgG platelet-bound or free maternal autoantibody can be demonstrated, this rule need not apply. If an easy vaginal delivery is expected in a term baby this should present no more risk of intracranial bleeding than does a Caesarean section. It should be remembered that a Caesarean section in the presence of maternal thrombocytopenia carries considerable risk of haemorrhage from incisions (not from the placental site, which is protected by normal myometrial contraction). Although transfused platelets will have a short life in the maternal circulation due to the antibody, they will help to achieve haemostasis of the wound, and should be given to the mother at delivery. Whatever the mode of delivery, maternal soft tissue damage should be avoided as far as possible.

A method for direct measurement of the fetal platelet count in scalp blood, obtained transcervically prior to or early in labour, has recently been described (Scott *et al* 1980). The authors recommend that Caesarean section should be performed in all cases where the fetal platelet count is less than $5 \times 10^9/l$. This approach is more logical than a decision about the mode of delivery based on the maternal platelet count and splenectomy status, but it is not without risk and demands urgent action on the results obtained. We have found that if reliable platelet/antibody tests are available and have been performed throughout the antenatal period, the decision concerning the need for Caesarean section and its timing can be taken at leisure; this can be based on a rational assessment of disease activity and the risk to the mother and fetus.

Due to its common occurrence in women during the childbearing years, ITP is one of the most frequently encountered haematological disorders in pregnancy, apart from anaemia. However, even without the introduction of more recent aids to diagnosis of activity of disease, but with supportive therapy, the maternal death rate has fallen from 8–9 per cent in 1950 to virtually zero. The outlook for the fetus which previously had a death rate of up to 26 per cent is also much more promising (Epstein *et al* 1950; Terao *et al* 1981).

FACTOR VIII ANTIBODY

A rare but major bleeding disorder associated with pregnancy is a haemophilia-like disease resulting from the spontaneous development of an antibody to Factor VIII (O'Brien 1954; Marengo-Rowe *et al* 1972; Voke and Letsky 1977; Coller *et al* 1981). It is often associated with later development of autoimmune disease, such as SLE or rheumatoid arthritis. The Factor VIII antibody usually develops in the puerperium, and may be associated with life-threatening haemorrhage at various sites not necessarily related to parturition. Management is difficult because treatment with conventional amounts of Factor VIII may only enhance antibody formation and fail to control the bleeding. The natural history is for the antibody to disappear gradually, usually within two years. Women should be advised to avoid further pregnancy until coagulation returns to normal, although in the one documented case where this has occurred, the antibody disappeared during the course of the pregnancy (Voke and Letsky 1977).

Inherited primary defects of haemostasis

VON WILLEBRAND'S DISEASE

The defect in von Willebrand's disease is a combination of a variable lack of coagulation Factor VIII (antihaemophilic factor) and a defect of platelet function. It is inherited as an autosomal dominant so that there is an equal incidence both in men and women. In its usual form mucous membrane bleeding (due to the platelet defect) is more of a problem than lack of Factor VIII which rarely reaches the low levels seen in true haemophilia.

Menorrhagia is also a problem in some sufferers. During normal pregnancy Factor VIII levels rise and, provided that a non-traumatic vaginal delivery can be achieved, there is not much risk of haemorrhage at delivery. However, if a woman known to have von Willebrand's disease does bleed, or is thought to be at risk of haemorrhage, the recommended treatment or prophylaxis is either intravenous administration of fresh frozen plasma, or preferably cryo-precipitate which has higher concentrations of Factor VIII and also contains the factor which restores platelet function.

Following treatment with either component of whole blood, the Factor VIII rises more than expected and the rise is prolonged, unlike the short survival (half life 12 hours) observed in haemophilia. Treatment should be given to maintain haemostasis for 4 5 days postdelivery. Caesarean section can be carried out, provided that suitable prophylaxis is given prior to surgery and maintained for ten days to cover the acute stage of wound healing.

It is very difficult to make a positive diagnosis of von Willebrand's disease during pregnancy, because of the alteration in coagulation factors, especially towards term. Therefore it is essential that in a woman at risk, investigations are undertaken at an approved centre, and a firm diagnosis made when she is not pregnant. If the question arises during pregnancy, in a previously undiagnosed woman, it is wiser to give prophylaxis at delivery and then make arrangements for her to be investigated 3–6 months postpartum.

CARRIERS OF HAEMOPHILIA AND CHRISTMAS DISEASE

Factor IX deficiency is an X-linked disorder carried by females who transmit the clinically manifest condition to their male offspring. The female carriers of haemophilia are not usually clinically affected but, in rare instances, Factor VIII levels may be as low as 10–20 per cent, levels which are not unusual in von Willebrand's disease and sometimes seen in the so-called 'mild' male haemophiliac. However, haemophilia is never mild once surgery is undertaken. Under these circumstances, Factor VIII levels must be maintained above 80 per cent until would healing is complete, in the same way as for a severe haemophiliac who has no detectable Factor VIII coagulation activity. This is achieved by infusing cryo-precipitate or Factor VIII concentrates for at least ten days postdelivery if Caesarean section is performed. The number of infusions should be monitored by daily Factor VIII assay. Normal vaginal delivery, avoiding soft tissue trauma, is not usually accompanied by significant haemorrhage, and this should be the aim if at all possible. Carriers of haemophilia can be diagnosed antenatally in more than 70 per cent of cases by examining Factor VIII-related antigen (Factor VIIIRAg) compared to the Factor VIII coagulant activity (Factor VIIIC). The ratio of VIIIC to VIIIRAg is usually reduced in haemophilia carriers. Because of elevations in the amount of VIIIC during pregnancy, investigations of carrier status are unreliable. The diagnosis should be established before pregnancy in women at risk, particularly since prenatal diagnosis of haemophilia in male fetuses is now possible (*see* below).

Christmas disease is indistinguishable clinically from haemophilia, and, as yet, there is no laboratory test which will identify the carrier. Of course, daughters of male sufferers of haemophilia or Christmas disease are obligate carriers of the conditions. Specific management of carriers of Christmas disease is rarely necessary, since Factor IX levels tend to rise during pregnancy and haemorrhage is unusual. Where abnormal bleeding does occur, the treatment of choice is fresh frozen plasma. The alternative, Factor IX concentrate, contains concentrated Factors II, VII and X in addition and carries a thrombogenic hazard (Urbaniak and Cash 1977) which would add to the already increased risk in pregnancy. Women suffering from these rare coagulation defects should give birth in hospitals which have the facilities to treat and monitor them and with an experienced coagulation expert on hand to give advice.

Prenatal diagnosis of coagulation defects

The major development of fetal blood sampling for prenatal diagnosis of the haemoglobinopathies (*see* Chapter 2) also made possible the diagnosis of other conditions, in particular the haemophilias.

There are between 3000 and 4000 people with haemophilia in Great Britain today. There is a high mutation rate and approximately one-third of cases have no known family history. Haemophilia is an X-linked inherited condition, the disease being manifest in the male and carried by the female. Advice on family planning has been based on identification of the carrier state and conventional genetic counselling for a sex-linked disorder—contraception or, if acceptable and safe, fetal sexing by amniocentesis and termination of male pregnancies. The defective coagulation factor in classical haemophilia A is antihaemophilic factor, Factor VIII. The coagulation activity in a bioassay is found to be severely depressed or absent, whereas the antigenic determinants of Factor VIII-related antigen are normal or increased.

Since the VIIIC:VIIIRAg ratio may be reduced in haemophilia carriers, this, together with family studies and discriminant functional analysis, has aided in their detection. This has not solved the problem for many putative carriers because they may wish to have a son, and object to the 50 per cent chance of losing a normal male fetus. Until recently prenatal diagnosis had not been thought possible because it requires the examination of fetal plasma. Most current methods of obtaining fetal blood provide amniotic fluid simultaneously. However, an absolutely pure sample of fetal blood is required because Factor VIIIC is labile, being destroyed when blood clots and is interfered with by amniotic fluid which has thromboplastic activity. The unit of Factor VIIIC would also be affected by the admixture of maternal plasma. Fetal plasma, unlike fetal red cells, cannot be separated from amniotic fluid or maternal plasma.

The discovery by Peake and Bloom (1978) in Cardiff, and almost simultaneously in the United States (Lazarchick and Hoyer 1978), of an VIIIC antigen, VIIIAg, detectable by immunoradiometric assay using an antibody raised in a treated haemophiliac, removed some of the problems. VIIICAg as apposed to VIIIRAg is reduced in haemophiliac plasma to the same extent or more than VIIIC. Unlike VIIIC it is stable, present in serum, and absent from and not affected by amniotic fluid. However, this method is not applicable to all cases because difficulties may arise where an affected member of the carrier's family has material which may cross-react with antibody to

VIIICAg. In severe haemophilia this is fortunately uncommon. In 1979 Firshein and colleagues in Connecticut published the results of prenatal diagnosis of six cases at risk for haemophilia using the estimation of Factor VIIICAg. Three cases had low values of Factor VIIICAg and normal levels of Factor VIIIRAg and the pregnancies were terminated, the diagnoses being confirmed in the abortuses. The other three cases had normal values, went to term, and the infants were normal at birth. These results depended on Factor VIIICAg levels corrected for considerable and inconstant dilution by amniotic fluid.

At the same time Rodeck at King's College Hospital was perfecting a technique of in utero blood sampling. He aspirates blood by placing a needle, under direct vision, into an umbilical blood vessel just above the attachmant of the cord to the chorionic plate (Rodeck and Campbell 1978). The advantage of this is that absolutely pure fetal blood, with no admixture of maternal blood or amniotic fluid, is obtained. There appears to be less bleeding following this method than after sampling blood from a fetal vessel on the surface of the placenta. No fetuses have been lost as a result of exsanguination following this procedure. In 1980 the results of investigations of fetuses at risk for haemophilia A, in which pure fetal blood was obtained using this technique, were published (Mibashan *et al* 1980). 38 of the 39 samples were pure fetal blood uncontaminated by amniotic fluid. The samples were taken at 18–20 weeks' gestation. Factor VIIIC was estimated by a modified, one stage bioassay at King's College Hospital in London and Factor VIIICAg was measured on the same samples by Professor Bloom in The University Hospital of Wales, Cardiff. There were no postoperative complications, spontaneous abortions or preterm labours. Eleven of the 39 fetuses at risk proved to be haemophiliac and the pregnancies were terminated, diagnosis being confirmed on the abortuses. The proportion is less than would be expected if all of the mothers seeking investigation were obligate carriers, but some of the mothers were only putative carriers. Five of the 12 fetuses of obligate carriers had haemophilia. The normal diagnosis has been confirmed in all those babies who have been born.

Prenatal diagnosis of Christmas disease—haemophilia B, Factor IX deficiency—has lagged behind that of haemophilia A, partly because it is less prevalent and also because the blood sampling and assay requirements are even more stringent in view of the normally low fetal levels of Factor IX. A sensitive immunoradiometric assay for Factor IX Ag has been reported (Holmberg *et al* 1980), capable of distinguishing the normally low levels in the fetus from those with Christmas disease. But this is not applicable to those families who have positive cross-reacting material, the incidence of which is much higher in Christmas disease than in haemophilia A.

Coagulant assays of Factor IX are not suitable for samples which are contaminated with amniotic fluid, but five cases at risk for Factor IX deficiency have been correctly diagnosed on pure fetal blood obtained by Rodeck's technique at King's College Hospital (Personal Communication); four were normal and confirmed in the newborn, and the fifth was found to be affected and the diagnosis verified in the abortus. The same arguments apply to the prenatal identification of von Willebrand's disease, a non X-linked inherited coagulation disorder of variable severity (*see* above). The diagnosis of the severe form depends on the demonstration of low Factor VIII coagulant activity.

This has been carried out on a fetus at risk using an immunoradiometric assay system (Homer *et al* 1979), but the analysis would be more reliable if pure fetal blood could be obtained without amniotic fluid contamination.

References

Basu H.K. (1969) Fibrinolysis and Abruptio Placentae. *Journal of Obstetrics and Gynaecology of the British Commonwealth* **76**, 481–96.

Bell W.R. (1977) Hematologic abnormalities in pregnancy. *Medical Clinics of North America* **61**, 1–165.

Beller F.K. & Uszynski M. (1974) Disseminated intravascular coagulation in pregnancy. *Clinics in Obstetrics and Gynecology* **17**, 264–78.

Biggs R., Denson K.W.E., Akman N., Borrett R. & Haddon, M.E. (1970) Antithrombin III, antifactor Xa and heparin. *British Journal of Haematology* **19**, 283–305.

Bonar J. (1973) Blood coagulation and fibrinolysis in obstetrics. *Clinics in Haematology* **2**, 213–33.

Bonnar J. (1978) Hemorrhagic disorders during pregnancy. In Hathaway W.E. and Bonnar J. (eds) *Perinatal Coagulation*, Monographs in Neonatology. Grune & Stratton, New York.

Bonnar J. (1981) Haemostasis and coagulation disorders. In Bloom A.L. and Thomas D.P. (eds) *Pregnancy. In Haemostasis and Thrombosis*, Churchill Livingstone, Edinburgh.

Bonnar J., Prentice C.R.M., McNicol G.P. & Douglas A.S. (1970) Haemostatic mechanism in uterine circulation during placental separation. *British Medical Journal* **2**, 564–7.

Carey L.C., Cloutier D.T. & Lowery B.D. (1970) The use of balanced electrolyte solution for resuscitation. In Fox Nahas (ed) *Body Fluid Replacement in the Surgical Patient*. Grune & Stratton, New York.

Carloss H.W., McMillan R. & Crosby W.H. (1980) Management of pregnancy in women with immune thrombocytopenia purpura. *Journal of the American Medical Association* **244**, 2756–8.

Cash J. (1981) Blood Replacement Therapy. In Bloom A.L. and Thomas D.P. (eds) *Haemostasis and Thrombosis*. Churchill Livingstone, Edinburgh.

Chung A.F. & Merkatz I.R. (1973) Survival following amniotic fluid embolism with early heparinisation. *Obstetrics and Gynecology* **42**, 809–14.

Cines D.B., Dusak B., Tomaski A., Mennuti M. & Schreiber A.D. (1982) Immune thrombocytopenic purpura and pregnancy. *New England Journal of Medicine* **306**, 826–31.

Coller B.S., Hultin M.B., Homer L.W., Miller F., Dobbs J.V., Dosik M.H. & Berger E.R. (1981) Normal pregnancy in a patient with a prior post-partum Factor VIII inhibitor: With observations on pathogenesis and prognosis. *Blood* **58**, 619–24.

Deblay M.F., Vert P., Andre M. & Marchal F. (1982) Transplacental vitamin K prevents haemorrhagic disease of infant of epileptic mother. *Lancet* **1**, 1247.

Doenicke A., Grote B. & Lorenz W. (1977) Blood and blood substitutes in management of the injured patient. *British Journal of Anaesthesia* **49**, 681–8.

Epstein R.D., Longer E.L. & Conbey J.T. (1950) Congenital thrombocytopenia purpura. Purpura haemorrhage in pregnancy and the newborn. *American Journal of Medicine* **9**, 44–56.

Fenton V., Saunders K. & Cavill I. (1977) The platelet count in pregnancy. *Journal of Clinical Pathology* **30**, 68–9.

Firschein S.I., Hoyer L.W., Lazarchick J., Forget B.G., Hobbins J.C., Clyne L.P., Pitzick F.A., Muir W.A., Merkatz I.R. & Mahoney M.J. (1979) Prenatal diagnosis of classic haemophilia. *New England Journal of Medicine* **300**, 937–41.

Fleming A.F. (1975) Haematological changes in pregnancy. *Clinics in Obstetrics and Gynaecology* **2**, 269–83.

Freeman M. (1979) Fatal reaction to Haemaccel. *Anaesthesia* **34**, 341.

Goldfarb A.W., Hochner-Celnikier D., Beller U., Menashe M., Dagan I. & Palti Z. (1982) A successful pregnancy in transfusion dependent homozygous B-thalassaemia: a case report. *International Journal of Gynaecology and Obstetrics* **20**, 319–22.

Graeff H., Ernst E., Bocaz J.A. *et al* (1976) Evaluation of hypercoagulability in septic abortion. *Haemostasis* **5**, 285–94.

Gregory M.G. and Clayton E.M.J. (1973) Amniotic fluid embolism. *Obstetrics and Gynecology* **42**, 236–44.

Hauser C.J., Shoemaker W.C., Turpin I. & Goldberg S.J. (1980) Oxygen transport responses to colloids and crystalloids in critically ill surgical patients. *Surgery, Gynecology and Obstetrics* **150**, 181–6.

Hedge U.M., Bowes A., Powell D.K. & Joyner M.V. (1981) Detection of platelet bound and serum antibodies in thrombocytopenia by enzyme linked assay. *Vox Sanguinis* **41**, 306–12.

Holmberg L., Bjorn C., Cordesius E., Kristofferson A.L., Ljung R., Löfberg L., Strömberg P. & Nilsson I.M. (1980) Prenatal diagnosis of haemophilia β by an immunoradiometric assay of Factor IX. *Blood* **56**, 397–401.

Homer L.W., Lindsten J., Blömbalk M., Hagenfeldt L., Cordesius E., Strömberg P. & Gustavii B. (1979) Prenatal evaluation of fetus at risk for severe von Willebrand's Disease. *Lancet* **ii**, 191–2.

Lazarchick J. & Hoyer L.W. (1978) Immunoradiometric measurement of the Factor VIII procoagulant antigen. *Journal of Clinical Investigation* **62**, 1048–52.

Lewis P.J. (1982) The role of prostacyclin in pre-eclampsia. *British Journal of Hospital Medicine* **28**, 393–50.

Lorenz W., Doenicke A., Messmer K., Reimann H.-J., Thermann M., Lahn K., Berr J., Schmal A., Dormann P., Regenfus P. & Hammelmann H. (1976) Histamine release in human subjects by modified gelatin (Haemaccel) and dextran: an explanation for anaphylactoid reactions observed under clinical conditions. *British Journal of Anaesthesia* **48**, 151.

McCann S.R., Lawlor E., McGovern M. & Temperley I.J. (1980) Severe megaloblastic anaemia of pregnancy. *Journal of the Irish Medical Association* **73**, 197–8.

MacKenzie I.Z., Sayers L., Bonnar J. *et al* (1975) Coagulation changes during second trimester abortion induced by intra-amniotic Prostaglandin E_2 and hypertonic solutions. *Lancet* **2**, 1066–9.

McMillan R. (1981) Chronic idiopathic thrombocytopenic purpura. *New England Journal of Medicine* **304**, 1135–47.

Marengo Rowe A.J., Murff G., Leveson J.E. & Cook J. (1972) Haemophilia-like disease associated with pregnancy. *Obstetrics and Gynecology*, **40**, 56.

Mibashan R.S., Rodeck C.H., Furlong R.A., Bains L., Peake I.R., Thumpston J.K., Corer R. & Bloom A.L. (1980) Dual diagnosis of prenatal haemophilia A by measurement of fetal Factor VIIIC and VIIIC Antigen (VIIICAg). *Lancet* **2**, 994–7.

Moncada M.D. & Vane J.R. (1979) Arachidonic acid metabolites and the interactions between platelets and blood-vessel walls. *New England Journal of Medicine* **300**, 1142–7.

Morgan M. (1979) Amniotic fluid embolism. *Anaesthesia* **34**, 20–32.

Moss G. (1972) An argument in favour of electrolyte solutions for early resuscitation. *Surgical Clinics in North America*, **52**, 3–17.

O'Brien J.R. (1954) An acquired coagulation defect in a woman. *Journal of Clinical Pathology* **7**, 22–5.

Peake I.R. & Bloom A.L. (1978) Immunoradiometric measurement of procoagulant Factor VIII antigen in plasma and serum and its reduction in haemophilia. *Lancet* **i**, 473–5.

Pritchard J.A. (1959) Fetal death in utero. *Obstetrics and Gynecology* **14**, 573–80.

Pritchard J.A. (1973) Haematological problems associated with delivery, placental abruption, retained dead fetus and amniotic fluid embolism. *Clinics in Haematology* , 563–86.

Rakoczi I., Tallian F., Bagdany S. & Gati I. (1979) Platelet life-span in normal pregnancy and pre-eclampsia as determined by a non-radioisotope technique. *Thrombosis Research* **15**, 533–6.

Redman C.W.G., Bonnar J. & Beilin L.J. (1978) Early platelet consumption in pre-eclampsia. *British Medical Journal* **i**, 467–9.

Remuzzi G., Misiani R., Marchesi D., Livio M., Mecca G., De Gaetano G. & Donati M.B. (1978) Haemolytic-uraemic syndrome. Deficiency of plasma factor(s) regulating prostacyclin activity? *Lancet* **2**, 871–2.

Resnik R., Swartz W.H., Plumer M.H., Ben Irschke K. & Stratthaus M.E. (1976) Amniotic fluid embolism with survival. *Obstetrics and Gynecology* **47**, 295.

Rodeck C.H. & Campbell S. (1978) Sampling pure fetal blood by fetoscopy in second trimester of pregnancy. *British Medical Journal* **ii**, 728–30.

Scott J.R., Cruickshank D.P., Kochenou R.M.D., Pitkin R.M. & Warenski J.C. (1980) Fetal platelet counts in the obstetric management of immunologic thrombocytopenia purpura. *American Journal of Obstetrics and Gynecology* **136**, 495–99.

Shaper A.G., Kear J., MacIntoch D.M., Kyobe J. & Njama D. (1968) The platelet count, platelet adhesiveness and aggregation and the mechanism of fibrinolytic inhibition in pregnancy and the puerperium. *Journal of Obstetrics and Gynaecology of the British Commonwealth* **75**, 433–41.

Sheppard B.L. & Bonnar J. (1974) The ultrastructure of the arterial supply of the human placenta in early and late pregnancy. *Journal of Obstetrics and Gynaecology of the British Commonwealth* **81**, 497–511.

Skjodt P. (1965) Amniotic fluid embolism—a case investigated by coagulation and fibrinolysis studies. *Acta Obstetrica et Gynecologica Scandinavica Supplement* **44**, 437–57.

Spivak J.L., Sprangler D.B. & Bell W.R. (1972) Defibrination after intra-amniotic injection of hypertonic saline. *New England Journal of Medicine* **287**, 321–3.

Stander R.W., Flessa H.C., Glueck H.C. *et al* (1971) Changes in maternal coagulation factors after intraamniotic injection of hypertonic saline. *Obstetrics and Gynecology* **37**, 660–6.

Steichele D.F. & Herschlein H.J. (1968) Intravascular coagulation in bacterial shock. Consumption coagulopathy and fibrinolysis after febrile abortion. *Medizinische Welt* **1**, 24–30.

Studdiford W.E. & Douglas G.W. (1956) Placental Bacteremia: a significant finding in septic abortion accompanied by vascular collapse. *American Journal of Obstetrics and Gynecology* **71**, 842–58.

Terao T., Oike J., Koboyashi T., Imai N., Manabe O., Koie K., Kamiya T. & Takamatsu J. (1981) Pregnancy complicated by idiopathic thrombocytopenia purpura. *Journal of Obstetrics and Gynaecology* **2**, 1–10.

Territo M., Finkelstein J. & Oh O. (1973) Management of autoimmune thrombocytopenia in pregnancy and the neonatal. *Obstetrics and Gynecology* **41**, 579–82.

Thomas A.N., Pattison C. & Serjeant G.R. (1982) Causes of death in sickle-cell disease in Jamaica. *British Medical Journal* **285**, 633–5.

Tuck C.S. (1972) Amniotic fluid embolus. *Proceedings of the Royal Society of Medicine* **65**, 94–5.

Tuck S.M. (1982) Sickle cell disease and pregnancy. *British Journal of Hospital Medicine* **28**, 125–7.

Urbaniak S.J. & Cash J.D. (1977) Blood replacement therapy. *British Medical Bulletin*, **33**, 273–82.

Van Dinh T., Boor P.J. & Garza J.R. (1982) Massive pulmonary embolism following delivery of a patient with sickle cell trait. *American Journal of Obstetrics and Gynecology* **143**, 722–4.

Van Leeuwen E.F., Helmerhorst F.M., Engelfriet C.P. & Von Dem Borne A.E.G. Kr. (1981)

Maternal autoimmune thrombocytopenia and the newborn. *British Medical Journal* **2, 283,** 104.

Van Royen E.A. (1974) Haemostasis in Human Pregnancy and Delivery. MD Thesis, University of Amsterdam.

Virgilio R.W., Rice C.L., Smith D.E., James D.R., Zarins C.K., Hobelmann F. & Perers R.M. (1979) Crystalloid versus Colloid resuscitation: is one better? *Surgery* **85,** 129–39.

Voke J. & Letsky E. (1977) Pregnancy and antibody to Factor VIII. *Journal of Clinical Pathology* **30,** 928–32.

4 Thromboembolism

Michael de Swiet

In this chapter we will consider deep vein thrombosis and pulmonary embolus complicating pregnancy, and the special case of antithrombin III deficiency as a risk factor. The importance of pulmonary embolus is as a cause of maternal mortality. If the patient does not die, she usually recovers completely, although a few patients subsequently have symptomatic pulmonary hypertension and rather more than might be expected have abnormal lung function tests (Sharma *et al* 1980). Deep vein thrombosis is important because it predisposes to pulmonary embolus. Also a considerable proportion of patients suffer from postphlebitic syndromes such as pain and swelling, particularly if they have had iliofemoral thrombosis.

Cerebral vein thrombosis is described in Chapter 14 and systemic thromboembolism arising from mitral valve disease and artificial heart valves is described in Chapter 5.

Incidence and significance

Pulmonary embolism is currently the most frequent cause of maternal mortality in England and Wales and is responsible for the deaths of about twelve women per year before or immediately after delivery (Department of Health & Social Security 1982). We can be reasonably confident of these data because death from pulmonary embolus is relatively easy to diagnose. Also, 99 per cent of all maternal deaths in England and Wales were analysed in the most recent report on confidential enquiries in maternal death (DHSS 1982). However, pulmonary embolus and deep vein thrombosis are not easy to diagnose in non-fatal cases and particularly in pregnancy (*see* below). It is therefore difficult to obtain accurate data for the incidence of non-fatal deep vein thrombosis and pulmonary embolus.

It appears that pregnancy increases the risk of thromboembolism sixfold (Royal

College of General Practitioners 1967) and the overall incidence is about 1.2 per cent of all pregnancies (Hellgren and Hygards 1981), with half the cases occuring antenatally (Henderson *et al* 1972). The incidence of pulmonary embolus in pregnancy is between 0.3 per cent (Friend and Kakkar 1972) and 1.2 per cent (Villasanta 1965). The incidence of deep vein thrombosis is between 0.2 per cent (Aaro *et al* 1966) and 0.5 per cent (Friend and Kakkar 1972), and this increases to 1.4 per cent if superficial thrombophlebitis is included (Aaro and Juergens 1974).

Risk factors

CLOTTING FACTORS (*see also* Chapter 3)

Any alteration in the balance between thrombosis due to activated clotting factors and lysis due to fibrinolytic mechanisms and thrombin inhibitors can precipitate blood clotting. During pregnancy, each of these systems is altered to change the balance towards clotting. After the first trimester, levels of Factors I (fibrinogen), II (prothrombin), VII, VIII, IX and X are increased (Bonnar 1975; Gallus 1976) and a further increase in the levels of Factors V, VII and X occurs in the first few days after delivery, even in normal pregnancy (Bonnar 1971); this further rise could account for the extra risk of thromboembolism at this time. The effect of an increase in clotting factors is added to by a decrease in the activity of the fibrinolytic system (Gallus 1976), although this returns to normal within a few hours of delivery (Bonnar 1970; Hellgren and Blombäck 1981). The level of antithrombin III also decreases in pregnancy (Zucker *et al* 1976).

VENOUS STASIS

Although the overall circulation time is reduced by the hyperdynamic circulation of pregnancy, venous return from the lower limbs is reduced because the pregnant uterus obstructs the inferior vena cava (Wright *et al* 1950; Clarke Pearson and Jelovsek 1981). A decrease in venous tone (Flessa *et al* 1974; McCausland *et al* 1961) may be another factor promoting venous stasis and thus increasing the risk of deep vein thrombosis.

BED REST

Venous stasis is the presumed mechanism whereby bed rest is associated with an increase in the risk of thromboembolism. This was noted in pregnancy by the confidential maternal mortality reports (DHSS 1982) which also drew attention to the particular risk in patients with severe pre-eclamptic toxaemia who are first rested in bed and then delivered by Caesarean section (DHSS 1979).

OPERATIVE DELIVERY

The current maternal mortality series (DHSS 1982) suggests that the risk of fatal thromboembolism following Caesarean section is markedly increased compared to that after vaginal delivery. In the 1976–78 series, there were nine deaths following Caesarean section, compared to 22 following vaginal delivery. The overall Caesarean section rate is likely to be between 5 and 10 per cent; therefore the extra risk associated with Caesarian section is between fourfold and eightfold in the patients of the confidential series. Finnerty & MacKay (1962) found that Caesarean section increased the overall risk of thromboembolism to 0.66 per 100 deliveries compared to 0.26 per 100 deliveries for vaginal delivery. Hiilesma (1960) showed a similar increase from 1.1. per cent to 2.2 per cent. Bergquist *et al* (1979) performed strain gauge plethysmography on 169 women following Caesarean section and showed that the incidence of deep vein thrombosis was 1.8 per cent. It is likely that the increased risk of operative delivery is not specific to Caesarean section, since Aaro and Juergens (1974) found that 25 per cent of cases of thromboembolism occurred in complicated pregnancies which included difficult forceps deliveries and prolonged labour, as well as Caesarean section, pre-eclamptic toxaemia and haemorrhage.

OTHER FACTORS

Other risk factors include age and parity, which operate independently of each other. The risk of fatal thromboembolism is 20 times greater in women over the age of 40 having their fifth or more pregnancy, compared with women of 20 in their first pregnancy (DHSS 1979). Oestrogen treatment to suppress lactation was shown to increase the risk of thromboembolism by Daniel *et al* (1967) and Jeffcoate *et al* (1968); if any drug treatment is necessary for suppression of lactation, bromocriptine should be used rather than oestrogen. Sickle cell anaemia is probably a risk factor for pulmonary embolus, since a high proportion of mortalities, due to sickle cell disease, have been reported to occur in pregnancy, usually due to pulmonary embolus (Thomas *et al* 1982). Van Dinh *et al* (1982) have also reported massive pulmonary embolus in a patient with sickle cell trait.

Obesity, congestive heart failure, dehydration, disseminated cancer and anaemia are all said to increase the risk of thromboembolism (Laros and Alger 1979) and probably do, but this has not been documented in obstetric practice. Similar risk factors have been demonstrated by Kimball *et al* (1978) for deaths caused by pulmonary embolus following legally induced abortion.

The 10 per cent risk of repeat thromboembolism in pregnancy in patients who have had thromboembolism in the past is considered on p. 107. The presence of blood group O is associated with a decreased incidence of thromboembolism. To have a blood group other than group O is therefore a positive risk factor (Jick *et al* 1969). This too is confirmed in the Confidential Maternal Mortality Series from 1963 to 1975: the expected frequency of blood group O in the general population in England and Wales is 46 per cent, but only 38 per cent of those with pulmonary emboli had blood group O (DHSS 1982).

Diagnosis of thromboembolism

DEEP VEIN THROMBOSIS

The history and physical signs of this condition are well described in the standard textbooks. However, it is clear that it is very difficult to make an accurate diagnosis based on physical signs alone (Simpson *et al* 1980), since perhaps 50 per cent of patients who have an acutely tender swollen calf do not have deep vein thrombosis. Ramsay (1983) has estimated that if venography is not used for the diagnosis of deep vein thrombosis, two patients are treated unnecessarily for every one treated correctly. It is possible that women who do not have a typical history are unlikely to have a deep vein thrombosis, and asymptomatic deep vein thrombosis is probably much rarer in pregnancy than after gynaecological surgery. This is supported by the study of Bergquist *et al* (1979) who showed by occlusion plethysmography that the incidence of deep vein thrombosis was only 1.8 per cent even after Caesarean section in comparison to the 10–20 per cent found after major gynaecological surgery (Bonnar and Walsh 1972; Friend and Kakkar 1972).

The non-invasive investigations available are based on the demonstration of blood clotting, by beta thromboglobulin elevation (Ludlam *et al* 1975), and of reduced blood flow in the femoral vein of the affected limb by Doppler flow studies (Preston Flanigan *et al* 1978) and impedance plethysmography (Hull *et al* 1977); the blood clot may be shown by I^{125} fibrinogen uptake (Browse 1978) and venography. If venous occlusion plethysmography is used, allowance should be made for the normal reduction in venous outflow that occurs in pregnancy (Clarke Pearson and Jelovsek 1981). Studies should be performed in the left lateral position before delivery in order to reduce the additional reduction in venous return caused by the obstruction of the gravid uterus.

Radioactive iodine should not be used in pregnancy. In the antenatal period it is trapped by the fetal thyroid and may cause hypothyroidism (Excess and Graeme 1974) or subsequent carcinoma. It is also secreted in high concentration in breast milk and the same risks apply to the breast-fed infant. At present, none of the diagnostic techniques available outside the specialised vascular laboratory approach the precision of venography, although it is possible that subsequent modifications or combinations of techniques will do so (Preston Flanigan *et al* 1978; Hull *et al* 1977). Because of the problems of treatment in the index and future pregnancies (*see* below), venography is therefore recommended in all patients who are considered to have deep vein thrombosis in pregnancy, unless the clinical diagnosis seems overwhelmingly certain. This occurs in severe proximal iliac vein thrombosis where the whole limb is markedly swollen. Venography of the femoral and more distal veins can be performed in pregnancy. With adequate shielding of the uterus, the direct radiation dose is very small, and less than in pelvimetry (Laros and Alger 1979), although there will be some additional scattered radiation.

PULMONARY EMBOLUS

Patients with major pulmonary emboli collapse with hypotension, chest pain, breathlessness and cyanosis. On further examination, they are also found to have a third heart sound, parasternal heave and elevated jugular venous pressure. It is the latter that helps to distinguish them from most of the other relatively common causes of collapse in pregnancy, where the diagnosis is not obvious, as in, for example, ante- or postpartum haemorrhage, ruptured or inverted uterus. These causes of collapse and some differentiating features are shown in Table 4.1. Most of the other causes are also considered elsewhere in this book: pulmonary aspiration in Chapter 1, amniotic fluid embolus in Chapter 3, myocardial infarction in Chapter 5, Gram-negative septicaemia in Chapters 3, 7 and 15.

The diagnosis of major pulmonary embolus is rarely in doubt. However, it is often preceded by smaller emboli, and a high index of clinical suspicion is essential to diagnose these. Warning signs and symptoms of small pulmonary emboli that are often ignored are unexplained pyrexia, syncope, cough, chest pain and breathlessness. Unless the patient has a high temperature or is producing quantities of purulent sputum, pleurisy should not be considered to be due to infection until pulmonary embolism has been excluded. It may be necessary to treat the patient with both antibiotics and anticoagulants until the diagnosis becomes clear.

Chest radiograph, electrocardiograph and blood gases

In considering the diagnosis of pulmonary embolus, it should be emphasised that the chest radiograph may be normal and that the electrocardiograph may be normal or may show features such as a deep S wave in lead I and Q wave and inverted T wave in lead III that can be caused by pregnancy alone. Blood gas measurement can be helpful, although false-positive and false-negative results may occur (Robin 1977). If the patient is hypoxaemic, with Pao_2 less than 70 mmHg and $Paco_2$ normal or reduced, it is likely that pulmonary embolus is the cause of chest symptoms, providing there is no radiological evidence of diffuse pulmonary disease or any other cause of reduced cardiac output. Such arterial samples should always be taken with the patient sitting, not supine (*see* p. 2).

Lung scans

Since it is so important to make an accurate diagnosis of thromboembolism in pregnancy, lung scans should be obtained, preferably with ventilation/perfusion imaging in all suspicious cases. The isotopes used in these scans, krypton-81m for ventilation and technetium-99m for perfusion, have very short half lives and the radiation to the fetus is therefore minimal. Even if the mother is breast feeding the quantities of technetium secreted in milk after the injection of technetium-99m macroaggregated albumen are negligible (Tribukait and Swedjemark 1978).

The lung scan is particularly helpful in cases where the chest X-ray is normal. A

Table 4.1   Features of some 'occult' causes of collapse in pregnancy.*

	Predisposing circumstances	*Common* presenting features	Helpful diagnostic features in *acute* stage†	
			Clinical	Laboratory
Amniotic fluid embolism (Chapter 3)	Labour, not necessarily precipitate	Respiratory distress cyanosis		Squames in SVC or sputum
Aspiration of gastric contents (Chapter 1)	Anaesthesia, not necessarily with vomiting	Respiratory distress cyanosis	Bronchospasm	
Pulmonary embolus (Chapter 4)	Increasing age, multiparity, previous thromboembolism, operative delivery, bedrest, oestrogens haemoglobinopathy	Respiratory distress cyanosis, chest pain	JVP +; 3rd heart sound, Parasternal heave	ECG, Chest X-ray, lung scan, blood gas, pulmonary angiography
Myocardial infarction (Chapter 5)	Increasing age	Chest pain, respiratory distress cyanosis	Pain character JVP +; crepitations	ECG
Intra-abdominal bleeding	Labour, though may occur spontaneously	Abdominal pain	JVP not +; signs in abdomen, laparotomy, paracentesis, culdocentesis	
Gram-negative sepsis (Chapters 3, 7, 15)	Previous infection (not necessarily)	Fever, rigors	Fever, rigors	Gram stain on blood sample. Blood culture positive

* This table excludes more obvious causes, such as ante- or postpartum haemorrhage, and ruptured or inverted uterus.
† These features are not absolute. For example, it is possible to have pulmonary crepitations in patients with pulmonary embolus and Gram-negative sepsis, without fever or rigors.

normal lung scan then excludes a pulmonary embolus. In contrast, false positives may occur but a large perfusion defect in the presence of a normal chest X-ray is likely to be due to pulmonary embolus. If the chest X-ray is abnormal, ventilation scanning is helpful. A reduction in perfusion with maintenance of ventilation indicates pulmonary embolus. If ventilation is reduced as well as perfusion, the condition is likely to be infective if the X-ray changes are acute.

Treatment

Patients with massive pulmonary embolus present with a catastrophic reduction in cardiac output and the immediate treatment should be the standard cardiac arrest procedure. If it is thought likely that the cause of the arrest is pulmonary embolus, i.v. heparin 20 000 units should be given to reverse the bronchoconstriction and vasoconstriction caused by the release of serotonin from platelets (Hume *et al* 1970). In addition, prolonged cardiac massage is advisable since this may break up the original clot, permitting an increase in pulmonary blood flow (Heimbecker *et al* 1973). After emergency resuscitation for pulmonary embolus, the treatment of both deep vein thrombosis and pulmonary embolus may be divided into an initial acute phase which lasts for up to a week and a subsequent chronic phase lasting for several months, where the aim of therapy is to prevent further incidents of thromboembolism.

Uncontrolled studies by Villasanta (1965) indicate that the maternal mortality associated with pulmonary embolus and deep vein thrombosis is reduced from 13 to 1 per cent by anticoagulant therapy. A similar mortality (1 in 113 patients) was found by Moseley and Kerstein (1980) in a literature search of anticoagulant-treated patients. It is generally accepted that anticoagulation is the treatment of choice in pulmonary embolism without shock (Morris and Mitchell 1978) and therefore it would not now be ethical to compare an anticoagulant and placebo treatment in thromboembolism, whether associated with pregnancy or not. The only controlled trial of anticoagulation versus placebo therapy in pulmonary embolus was abandoned because of very high mortality in the placebo group (Barritt and Jordan 1960).

Treatments used in the acute phase are heparin, surgery and thrombolytic agents such as streptokinase (Ludwig 1973). Treatment in the chronic phase is with warfarin or heparin.

ACUTE PHASE TREATMENT

Heparin

The majority of cases of venous thromboembolism are treated initially with heparin. Heparin, because it is so strongly polar, has particular advantages in pregnancy, since it does not cross the placenta for which lipid solubility is necessary. The object of heparin therapy in the initial phase of treatment of venous thromboembolism is to prevent further, possibly fatal, episodes. It is not believed that heparin increases the reabsorption of the original thrombus. In order confidently to prevent further clot formation, relatively high blood levels of heparin must be achieved; it has been suggested that particularly large doses are necessary in the presence of a large initial thrombus (Bonnar 1975). Although up to 40 000 units per day of heparin have been given subcutaneously (Bonnar 1976), this is not usually practical because of bruising and irregular absorption, and the initial treatment should be with i.v. heparin: 40 000 units per day by continuous infusion, aiming to achieve a level of 0.6–1.0 unit per ml as assayed by the protamine sulphate neutralisation test (Dacie 1975). Although many texts (e.g. Laros and Alger 1979) suggest monitoring heparin treatment by the partial thromboplastin test, the protamine sulphate neutralisation test appears to be more useful; a control sample taken from the patient before treatment is not necessary, and the test seems to reflect the patient's risk of bleeding more accurately than the partial thromboplastin time. In the acute phase, the heparin should be given by intravenous infusion (Salzman *et al* 1975). Heparin is not stable in dextrose and should therefore be given in saline (Jacobs *et al* 1973) preferably made up in a small volume of 20 ml and very slowly infused with a constant infusion pump. If this is not practical, the same total dose of heparin may be given by repeated intravenous infections, but no less frequently than every three hours. The half life of heparin is only about $1\frac{1}{2}$ hours (Estes 1970) and if the drug is given by large, infrequent intravenous injections, this produces unacceptable swings between hyper- and hypocoaguability (Sasahara 1974). The only side-effect of *acute* heparin administration is bleeding (*see* p. 108 for side effects of prolonged therapy). If it is necessary to reverse heparin therapy, cessation of infusion alone will be sufficient for most patients given intravenous heparin. There will be undetectable levels in the blood six hours after therapy has stopped. In the more urgent situation the patient can be given protamine 1 mg per 100 units of administered heparin. When using a continuous infusion of heparin, twice the quantity of protamine should be given to neutralise the hourly dose. No more than 50 mg of protamine should be given in a ten minute period, since protamine itself can cause bleeding (Laros and Alger 1979). A better alternative is to calculate the quantity of protamine needed from the protamine sulphate neutralisation test (Dacie 1975). If there is any doubt about the efficacy or desirability of protamine reversal, fresh frozen plasma should restore blood clotting to normal.

Because of the risk of haematoma formation in patients who are fully anticoagulated, other injections such as antibiotics should be given intravenously rather than intramuscularly. Arterial blood sampling should be from an intra-arterial canula or by needling a superficial artery, such as the radial artery rather than the deeper femoral artery.

Initial phase, high-dose intravenous heparin therapy is continued for an arbitrary period of 3–7 days; the length of treatment depends on the severity of the initial episode of venous thromboembolism and whether there is any evidence of recurrence. The alternatives to high dose intravenous therapy in the initial phase of treatment are surgery and thrombolytic therapy. Both these alternatives have the advantage of therapy directed towards removing the initial clot. Both should be considered in the nonpregnant state for initial treatment in patients with major pulmonary embolus or massive iliofemoral deep vein thrombosis.

Thrombolytic therapy

Thrombolytic agents are probably underused in the nonpregnant state (National Institute of Health Consensus Conference 1980), since there is evidence that patients who have had a deep vein thrombosis are much less likely to develop postphlebitic leg symptoms after being given thrombolytic therapy than after conventional treatment with heparin and warfarin (Elliot *et al* 1979). Browse (1977) also suggests that thrombolytic therapy is preferable to conventional anticoagulation to minimise the risk of massive pulmonary embolus in patients with extensive iliofemoral thrombosis where the proximal end is floating free; but this has not been proven.

Comparison of therapies

In a comparison of heparin and oral anticoagulants with urokinase in the treatment of pulmonary embolus in the nonpregnant state, urokinase therapy was associated with earlier resolution as shown by pulmonary angiography (Urokinase Pulmonary Embolism Trial Study Group 1970). It has also been shown that, after a pulmonary embolus, the pulmonary capillary blood volume and pulmonary diffusing capacity are normal in patients treated with thrombolytic therapy, whereas they usually remain abnormal in patients treated with heparin and warfarin, even if they are asymptomatic at follow-up one year later (Sharma *et al* 1980).

Pfeifer (1970a) claimed successful treatment of deep vein thrombosis in twelve pregnant patients with streptokinase given as a loading dose (250 000 units by intravenous infusion in over 20 minutes) followed by an infusion of 160 000 units per hour for four hours, with subsequent alteration of the infusion rate depending on the plasma thrombin time. Bell and Meek (1979) discount the necessity for adjusting the dosage schedule and would recommend a maintenance therapy of 100 000 i.u. per hour for 24–72 hours after the initial loading dose. Although Pfeifer (1970b) suggests that very little streptokinase crosses the human placenta, pregnancy is considered a minor contraindication to the use of thrombolytic therapy, and subsequent delivery within ten days is a major contraindication to thrombolytic therapy (National Institute of Health Consensus Conference 1980). Since it is possible that thrombolytic therapy may precipitate premature labour by an increase in circulating plasminogen levels (Amias 1977), there is a risk that the relatively minor contraindication will become the major contraindication. However, it has also been suggested that streptokinase therapy will cause relative uterine atony because of the interference of fibrin degradation products with uterine contraction (Hall *et al* 1972). If it is necessary to reverse thrombolytic therapy in pregnancy, aprotinin, which has large molecules and does not cross the placenta, should be used rather than aminocaproic acid. However, apart from the twelve patients treated in pregnancy by Pfeiffer (1970a), other studies are only case reports (McTaggart and Ingram 1977; Amias 1977; Hall *et al* 1972) and therefore there is really still not sufficient experience to recommend the use of thrombolytic agents in pregnancy except in exceptional circumstances (Flute 1976). Thus, the only currently acceptable alternative to heparin for initial phase treatment in pregnancy is surgery.

Surgery

Surgical removal of the thrombus (thrombectomy) may be indicated in massive iliofemoral deep vein thrombosis because of the suggestion that this too reduces the incidence of postphlebitic leg symptoms (Mayor 1969); however, this has not been substantiated in follow-up studies (Lansing and Davics 1968). There may be a place for surgery (venous plication or insertion of a 'vena caval umbrella') in recurrent pulmonary embolus following iliofemoral embolus (Sautter 1975) or thrombectomy where limb swelling is so great as to cause venous gangrene (Sautter 1975; Gurll *et al* 1971). However, with adequate anticoagulation, caval interruption is very rarely required (Silver and Sabiston 1975).

In cases of pulmonary embolus, patients who are shocked at the time of the initial event should also be considered for pulmonary embolectomy under cardiopulmonary bypass, as should those who have any of the following criteria one hour later: systolic blood pressure less than 90 mmHg, Pao_2 less than 60 mmHg, urine output less than 20 ml per hour (Sasahara and Barsamian 1973). The decision whether to operate will usually be supported by pulmonary angiography.

CHRONIC PHASE TREATMENT

Warfarin

It is established that there is a definite, though low, incidence of teratogenesis associated with the use of warfarin in the first trimester of pregnancy (Abbot *et al* 1977; Becker *et al* 1975; Kerber *et al* 1968; Pettifor and Benson 1975). The most common syndrome is chondrodysplasia punctata, in which cartilage and bone formation is abnormal (Becker *et al* 1975; Shaul *et al* 1975), although warfarin is not the only cause of this abnormality (Sheffield *et al* 1976). Warfarin embryopathy has also been described in two surviving siblings, where warfarin was taken in each pregnancy, but not in a third sibling that had not been exposed to warfarin in utero (Harrod and Sherrod 1981). The asplenia syndrome has also been reported (Cox *et al* 1977). It has also been recognised that the use of warfarin in late pregnancy after 36 weeks' gestation is associated with serious retroplacental and intracerebral fetal bleeding (Villasanta 1965) since, unlike heparin, warfarin crosses the placenta. As premature infants have low levels of factors XI and XII (Andrew *et al* 1981), it is likely that the fetus has low levels of clotting factors; therefore the fetus will be excessively anticoagulated if the mother's prothrombin time is within the normal therapeutic range. For these reasons Hirsh *et al* (1970) recommended that after the initial period of heparinisation in the acute attack, heparin should continue to be used for the first trimester, followed by warfarin between 13 and 36 weeks, reverting to heparin for the last weeks of pregnancy. These recommendations have been widely followed (de Swiet *et al* 1980; *British Medical Journal* 1975; Henderson *et al* 1972; Pridmore *et al* 1975; Szekely *et al* 1973) and indeed 73 per cent of currently practising obstetricians would follow them (de Swiet *et al* 1980). However, the question has arisen as to whether oral anticoagulants should be used even after the first trimester (*British Medical Journal* 1975) because of the risk of fetal malformation. Sherman and Hall (1976) described a case of microcephaly in a patient who had taken warfarin for the last six months of pregnancy, and this stimulated further reports (Hall 1976; Hall *et al* 1980), including one by Holzgreve *et al* (1976) in which five cases of microcephaly occurring in California were described. It has been suggested that warfarin causes repeated small intracerebral haemorrhages and that these are the causes of the optic atrophy, microcephaly and mental retardation that have been described (Shaul and Hall 1977).

These teratogenic risks may not be so great as anecdotal reports would suggest. Chen *et al* (1982) studied the outcome of 22 pregnancies, where the mother had taken warfarin in the first trimester, and 20 pregnancies where warfarin had been taken between 13 and 36 weeks. Warfarin was being used in the management of artificial heart valves. Although the spontaneous abortion rate was high (36 per cent in those taking warfarin) there were no cases of chondrodysplasia punctata or microcephaly. In another study in which we compared the infants of 20 patients who had taken warfarin in the second and third trimesters with those of well-matched controls, there was no difference in intellectual attainment at a mean age of four years (Chong *et al* 1984). Microcephaly is therefore unlikely to be common in the children of women taking warfarin.

Bleeding does appear to be more of a problem in pregnant women treated with warfarin than in those treated with heparin, even if the patients have prothrombin times within the normal therapeutic range (de Swiet *et al* 1977). Even if patients are not anticoagulated, they are at risk from antepartum and postpartum haemorrhages in pregnancy, and this risk seems to be increased by warfarin therapy. For these reasons I, and others (Laros and Alger 1979), believe that warfarin should not be used in the chronic phase of treatment of *venous* thromboembolism in pregnancy, or in the first week of the puerperium. The only situation where warfarin therapy is recommended in pregnancy is in the management of patients with mitral valve disease or artificial heart valves (*see* Chapter 5). The risk of genital tract bleeding is much less by seven days after delivery, and it is therefore reasonable to use warfarin at that time as an alternative to subcutaneous heparin. Patients may continue to breast feed (Brambel and Hunter 1950) since there is no detectable secretion of warfarin in breast milk (Orme *et al* 1977). This is not so for phenindione where maternal therapy has caused severe haemorrhage in a breast fed infant (Eckstein and Jack 1970).

HEPARIN

Subcutaneous, self-administered heparin is our preferred chronic phase treatment for venous thromboembolism in pregnancy, since it does not have the risks of warfarin. The half life of heparin injected subcutaneously is about 18 hours in comparison to intravenous heparin which has a half life of $1\frac{1}{2}$ hours. The possible complications of long-term heparin therapy are described in the following section.

After high dose intravenous heparin therapy for 3–7 days, the patient is given subcutaneous heparin, initially 10 000 units twice daily. This is monitored by the heparin assay (Denson and Bonnar 1973). The small doses of heparin used do not affect the whole blood-clotting system, and are below the limits of detection of more conventional tests, such as the partial thromboplastin time or protamine sulphate neutralisation test. Provided there is detectable heparin activity, the dose of heparin is not increased above 10 000 units every twelve hours. If the heparin assay exceeds 0.4 units per ml, the dose is reduced, since such levels are associated with excessive bleeding (Bonnar 1975).

Heparin levels are stable in patients who are taking subcutaneous heparin, but because of pregnancy-induced changes in blood volume and renal handling of heparin, and because treatment with heparin may continue for up to six months, heparin assays are made as frequently as the patient attends for normal antenatal visits. The onset of pre-eclamptic toxaemia may be preceded by a decrease in heparin requirements, possibly due to impaired renal excretion of heparin (Bonnar 1975) but this suggestion is only based on isolated clinical observations. Although patients show initial reluctance, the majority can be taught to give themselves subcutaneous heparin and can therefore be discharged home. Patients should use the concentrated heparin solution of 50 000 units per ml. We have not found any difference in bruising between sodium and calcium heparins. The heparin should be drawn up in a tuberculin syringe because of the small volumes used, and injected subcutaneously through a short (16 mm) 25 gauge needle. The injections should be made perpendicular to the skin surface to minimise the risk of trauma to skin blood vessels. Possible sites are the thighs, abdominal wall and upper arms.

Because of the high incidence of thromboembolism in the days following labour and delivery (DHSS 1982), subcutaneous heparin administration should be continued through labour. The heparin assay is checked in the week preceding delivery, since patients attend the hospital weekly at this time in pregnancy. There is no increased risk of postpartum haemorrhage in these patients (de Swiet *et al* 1981). However, epidural anaesthesia is contraindicated in all patients taking anticoagulants including subcutaneous heparin, because of the risk of epidural haematoma formation (Crawford 1978).

After delivery, the dose of subcutaneous heparin is empirically reduced to 8000 units b.d., because of the contraction in circulating blood volume and because the clotting factors return to normal levels during the puerperium. The heparin assay is checked at least once after delivery if the patient continues to take subcutaneous heparin for the recommended six weeks postpartum.

Therapy with heparin initiated in pregnancy or warfarin if introduced after seven days postpartum, is continued for an arbitrary period of six weeks postpartum, at which time the extra risk of thromboembolism associated with pregnancy is considered to have passed. Patients who develop venous thromboembolism in the pureperium should be treated as above, except that, after the acute phase, warfarin may be used alone in chronic phase treatment if it is not given for the first seven days after delivery. The total length of anticoagulant treatment should be at least six weeks.

Prophylaxis of thromboembolism

There are two groups of patients in whom prophylaxis might be considered: those who are at high risk because of age, parity, obesity or operative delivery (DHSS 1982) and those who have had thromboembolism in the past (Badaracco and Vessey 1974). With regard to the former group, it is generally believed (although not proven) that the risk of thromboembolism is greatest in the puerperium and therefore that any prophylaxis need only be used during this period and to cover labour. The Confidential Maternal Mortality Series very clearly shows that the risks of thromboembolism are increased markedly with high parity and increasing age, and that these risks are independent of each other (DHSS 1979). Applying these data, there is a case for using some form of prophylaxis in all patients undergoing operative delivery over the age of 30 years, and also in those over the age of 35, even if they have a spontaneous vaginal delivery. Subcutaneous heparin which has been widely used in other forms of surgery might not be the best choice. Because of the danger of epidural haematoma (Crawford 1978) its use would preclude epidural anaesthesia, and to be effective, it probably has to be given before the period of risk, i.e. before labour. Intravenous dextran given during labour or Caesarean section might be a better choice of prophylactic treatment. Although there has been no systematic evaluation of its efficacy and risks in pregnancy, Bergquist *et al* (1979) found no cases of deep vein thrombosis when they screened 19 patients given dextran 70 during Caesarean section, whereas three out of 150 patients that did not have dextran did have deep vein thrombosis following Caesarean section. These figures were based on a plethysmographic study of all patients following Caesarean section.

The second group of patients are those who have had thromboembolism in the past; they are considered to be at risk throughout pregnancy. Badaracco and Vessey (1974) in a retrospective study estimated that there was about a 12 per cent risk of developing pulmonary embolism or deep vein thrombosis in pregnancy if a patient had had thromboembolism in the past. The risk was not affected by the circumstances of the original event, i.e. whether it was associated with the contraceptive pill or not. The risk is likely to be exaggerated; the study was based on a postal survey, and information is not available as to how the thromboembolism was diagnosed in pregnancy. If a patient has had thromboembolism in the past, there is a particularly strong tendency to diagnose it again even on rather flimsy evidence.

Most British obstetricians (88 per cent) would use prophylactic anticoagulants for such patients if the index thromboembolism had previously occurred during pregnancy. Some (73 per cent) would use prophylaxis if the thromboembolism had occurred when taking the pill, and fewer (50 per cent) would use prophylaxis if the original thromboembolism had occurred ten years previously when the patients were taking neither the pill nor were pregnant (de Swiet *et al* 1980).

Although most obstetricians would still use the modified Hirsh regime of warfarin (Hirsh *et al* 1970) until 36 weeks' gestation for venous thromboembolism prophylaxis (de Swiet *et al* 1980), this seems unacceptable because of the maternal and fetal complications of warfarin therapy outlined above. The alternative is to use subcutaneous heparin throughout pregnancy. However, since these patients are asymptomatic at the beginning of treatment and treatment is only being used prophylactically, the safety of such therapy for mother and fetus must be established even more rigorously than in the treatment of established venous thromboembolism.

Hall and colleagues (1980) performed a retrospective study of the outcome of pregnancies associated with anticoagulant therapy, based on literature reports. Such a study is likely to be biased towards the reporting of complications, but they found that of 135 fetuses, 13 per cent were stillborn, 14 per cent were born prematurely, and 7 per cent died in the neonatal period. A comparative study performed at Queen Charlotte's Maternity Hospital of antenatal heparin prophylaxis compared to no antenatal prophylaxis did not show such a high perinatal mortality, but did suggest a slight increase in fetal morbidity associated with maternal heparin therapy (Howell *et al* 1983).

The most obvious maternal complication is bruising at the injection site. This can be reduced by good injection technique but rarely eliminated. Although this is undoubtedly an inconvenience, and at times painful, most mothers tolerate a degree of bruising. A further maternal complication of prolonged heparin therapy is a form of bone demineralisation described as osteopenia (Avioli 1975; Jaffee and Willis 1965; Squires and Pinch 1979). This occurred in one of our patients, and presented as severe backache which was much worse in the puerperium (Wise and Hall 1980). Radiography in the puerperium showed that the patient had three collapsed vertebrae. Griffith *et al* (1965) report that heparin-induced osteopenia only occurs in patients receiving more that 15 000 units per day for at least six months. The cause of the osteopenia is unknown, although it has been attributed to a deficiency of 1,25-dihydrotachysterol (Aarskog *et al* 1980). A follow-up study of our patients taking subcutaneous heparin suggests that even those patients who are asymptomatic may have some degree of bone demineralisation (de Swiet *et al* 1983). It has also been reported that heparin may cause thrombocytopenia with subsequent bleeding (Cines *et al* 1980) or thrombotic complications (Chong *et al* 1982), alopecia and allergic reactions. These have not been problems in our experience.

Because of the fetal and maternal complications of prolonged subcutaneous heparin therapy, I believe that it should no longer be used as a routine for prophylaxis throughout pregnancy in all patients who have had thromboembolism in the past. Since there are even more problems with warfarin therapy, there is no form of prophylaxis that can be considered harmless and effective. Alternative approaches are to use subcutaneous heparin in those patients who are particularly at risk, having had thromboembolism in more than one pregnancy or having antithrombin III deficiency (see below), or to use subcutaneous heparin at times when patients are most at risk, such as during admission to hospital for surgery or bedrest. Our present policy is to use dextran in labour, thus permitting epidural anaesthesia, and to give subcutaneous heparin for six weeks after delivery in all patients who have had thromboembolism in the past. However, this is an unsatisfactory compromise, since this regime does not provide any cover during the antenatal period before labour. Another option would be to use antiplatelet agents, such as dipyridamole. However, these drugs have not yet been evaluated in pregnancy, and there is also doubt about their efficacy as prophylactics in thromboembolic disease in general (Morris and Mitchell 1978).

Antithrombin III deficiency

Antithrombin III is a naturally occurring substance produced by the liver which inhibits the actions of thrombin and other clotting factors (*Lancet* 1983). Since thrombin promotes blood clotting by forming fibrin from fibrinogen, antithrombin III decreases the tendency of blood to clot. Antithrombin III deficiency, where the level of antithrombin III is 25–70 per cent of normal, is therefore associated with an increased risk of blood clotting. The condition is inherited as a mendelian dominant trait (Mackie *et al* 1978) in the 40 or so families that have been described (Brandt and Stenbjerg 1979). In some families the condition is due to gene deletion; in others it is not (Prochownik 1983). It often presents for the first time after oestrogen exposure either to the contraceptive pill or in pregnancy, where the risk of thromboembolism is about 70 per cent (32 of 47 pregnancies), if no prophylaxis is used (Hellgren 1981). This risk is so great that some form of prophylaxis must be considered. These patients are usually treated for life with warfarin because of the risk of fatal pulmonary embolism. However, for the reasons given above, warfarin should not be used in pregnancy. Although subcutaneous heparin treatment may be associated with a paradoxical decrease in antithrombin III levels (Marciniak and Gockerman 1977), Hellgren (1981) has shown that only one of seven patients treated with subcutaneous heparin and antithrombin III concentrate in pregnancy had an episode of thromboembolism; this must therefore be the treatment of choice. Hellgren used high-dose heparin 20 000–45 000 units every 24 hours to give a 5–10 second prolongation of the activated partial thromboplastin time, equivalent to 0.8–1.0 units of heparin per ml of plasma. In addition, she gave antithrombin III concentrate at the time of labour (Hellgren 1981) when heparin levels should be reduced to avoid the risk of bleeding. A similar approach was suggested by Brandt and Stenbjerg (1979). Fresh frozen plasma may be a suitable alternative source of antithrombin III rather than antithrombin III concentrate (Zucker *et al* 1976).

Thrombosis is a recognised complication of venography to which patients with antithrombin III deficiency are particularly susceptible (Winter *et al* 1981). Such patients should either not have venography or, as Winter *et al* (1981) recommended, have venography using the less thrombogenic contrast medium, metrizamide (Albrechtsson and Olsson 1979) washed through with heparin.

Septic pelvic thrombophlebitis

This is a diagnosis made by exclusion. The patient has fever, usually following Caesarean section, for which no cause can be found and which does not remit with appropriate antibiotic therapy. The more diligently the cause for a fever is sought, and the better the judgement in choice of antibiotic, the lower incidence of 'septic pelvic thrombophlebitis'. Malkamy (1980) found eleven patients in 1263 Caesarean deliveries (0.9 per cent) over a $2\frac{1}{2}$ year period. In those cases where a laparotomy or venography has been performed, the thrombosis is often seen to start in the ovarian vein(s) and may extend into the inferior vena cava (Raja Rao *et al* 1980). The fever remits with continuing antibiotics and a short course of heparin lasting ten days (Ledger and Peterson 1970). Some patients have septic pulmonary emboli and require full anticoagulation for six weeks to three months.

References

Aaro L.A., Johnson T.R. & Juergens J.L. (1966) Acute deep venous thrombosis associated with pregnancy. *Obstetrics and Gynecology* **28**, 553–8.

Aaro K.A. & Juergens J.L. (1974) Thrombophlebitis and pulmonary embolism as a complication of pregnancy. *Medical Clinics of North America* **58**, 829.

Aarskog D., Aksnes L. & Lehmann V. (1980) Low 1, 25-Dihydroxyvitamin D in heparin-induced osteopenia. *Lancet* **2**, 650–1.

Abbott A., Sibert J.R. & Weaver J.B. (1977) Chondrodysplasia punctata and maternal warfarin treatment. *British Medical Journal* **1**, 1639–40.

Albrechtsson U. & Olsson C.G. (1979) Thrombosis after phlebography: a comparison of two contrast media. *Cardiovascular Radiology* **2**, 9–18.

Amias A.G. (1977) Streptokinase, cerebral vascular disease—and triplets. *British Medical Journal* **1**, 1414–15.

Andrew M., Bhogal M. & Karpatkin M. (1981) Factors XI & XII and prekallikrein in sick and healthy premature infants. *New England Journal of Medicine* **305**, 1130–3.

Avioli L.V. (1975) Heparin-induced osteopenia: an appraisal. *Advances in Experimental Medicine and Biology* **52**, 375–87.

Badaracco M.A. & Vessey M. (1974) Recurrence of venous thromboembolism disease and use of oral contraceptives. *British Medical Journal* **1**, 215–17.

Barritt D.W. & Jordan S.C. (1960) Anticoagulant drugs in the treatment of pulmonary embolism: A controlled trial. *Lancet* **1**, 1309–12.

Becker M.H., Genieser N.B. & Feingold M. (1975) Chondrodysplasia punctata: is maternal warfarin therapy a factor? *American Journal of Disease in Childhood* **129**, 356–9.

Bell W.R. & Meek A.G. (1979) Guidelines for the use of thrombolytic agents. *New England Journal of Medicine* **301**, 1266–70.

Bergquist A., Bergquist D. & Hallbröök T. (1979) Acute deep vein thrombosis (DVT) after Caesarean section. *Acta Obstetrica et Gynecologica Scandinavica Supplement* **58**, 473–6.

Bonnar J., McNichol G.P. & Douglas A.S. (1970) Coagulation and fibrinolytic mechanisms during and after normal childbirth. *British Medical Journal* **2**, 200–3.

Bonnar J. (1971) The blood coagulation and fibrinolytic systems in the newborn and the mother at birth. *British Journal of Obstetrics and Gynaecology* **78**, 355.

Bonnar J. & Walsh J. (1972) Prevention of thrombosis after pelvic surgery by British dextran 70. *Lancet* **2**, 614.

Bonnar J. (1975) Thromboembolism in obstetric and gynaecological patients. In Nicolaides A.N. (ed) *Thromboembolism Aetiology, Advances in Prevention and Management*, pp. 311–41. Medical and Technical Publishing Co. Ltd., Lancaster.

Bonner J. (1976) Longterm self-administered heparin therapy for prevention and treatment of thromboembolic complications in pregnancy. In Kakkar V.V. and Thomas D.P. (eds) *Heparin Chemistry and Clinical Usage*. Academic Press, New York.

Brambel C.E. & Hunter R.E. (1950) Effect of dicoumarol on the nursing infant. *American Journal of Obstetrics and Gynecology* **59**, 1153–9.

Brandt P. & Stenbjerg A. (1979) Subcutaneous heparin for thrombosis in pregnant women with hereditary antithrombin deficiency. *Lancet* 1, 100–1.

British Medical Journal (1975) Editorial. Venous thromboembolism and anticoagulants in pregnancy. *British Medical Journal* 2, 421–2.

Browse N.L. (1977) Personal views on published facts. What should I do about deep vein thrombosis and pulmonary embolism? *Annals of the Royal College of Surgeons of England*, 59, 138–42.

Browse N. (1978) Diagnosis of deep vein thrombosis. *British Medical Bulletin* 34, 163–7.

Chen W.W.C., Chan C.S., Lee P.R., Wang R.Y.R. & Wong V.C.W. (1982) Pregnancy in patients with prosthetic heart valves: An experience with 45 pregnancies. *Quarterly Journal of Medicine* 51, 358–65.

Chong B.H., Pitney W.R. & Castaldi P.A. (1982) Heparin-induced thrombocytopenia: Association of thrombotic complications with heparin-dependent IgG antibody that induces thromboxane synthesis and platelet aggregation. *Lancet* 2, 1246–8.

Chong M.K.B., Harvey D. & de Swiet M. (1984) Follow-up study of children whose mothers were treated with warfarin during pregnancy. *British Journal of Obstetrics and Gynaecology* (in press).

Cines D.B., Kaywin P., Bina M., Tomaski A. & Schreiber A.D. (1980) Heparin-associated thrombocytopenia. *New England Journal of Medicine* 303, 788–95.

Clarke Pearson D.L. & Jelovsek F.R. (1981) Alterations of occlusive cuff impedance plethysmography in the obstetric patient. *Surgery* 89, 594–8.

Cox D.R., Martin L. & Hall B.D. (1977) Asplenia syndrome after fetal exposure to warfarin. *Lancet* 2, 1134.

Crawford J.S. (1978) *Principles and Practice of Obstetric Anaesthesia*, 4th ed., pp. 182–3. Blackwell Scientific Publications, Oxford.

Dacie J. (1975) *Practical Haematology*, pp. 413–14. Churchill Livingstone, Edinburgh.

Daniel D.G., Campbell H. & Turnbull A.C. (1967) Puerperal thromboembolism and suppression of lactation. *Lancet* 2, 287.

Denson K.W.E. & Bonnar J. (1973) The measurement of heparin: a method based on the potentiation of anti-factor X a. *Thrombosis et Diathesis Haemorrhagica* 30, 471.

Department of Health & Social Security (1979) *Report on Confidential Enquiries into Maternal Deaths in England and Wales 1973–1975*. Her Majesty's Stationery Office, London.

Department of Health & Social Security (1982) *Report on Confidential Enquiries into Maternal Deaths in England and Wales 1976–1978*. Her Majesty's Stationery Office, London.

de Swiet M., Letsky E. & Mellows H. (1977) Drug treatment and prophylaxis of thromboembolism in pregnancy. In Lewis P.J. (ed) *Therapeutic Problems in Pregnancy*, pp. 81–9. MTP Press, Lancaster.

de Swiet M., Bulpitt C.J. & Lewis P.J. (1980) How obstetricians use anticoagulants in the prophylaxis of thromboembolism. *Journal of Obstetrics and Gynaecology* 1, 29–32.

de Swiet M., Fidler J., Howell R. & Letsky E. (1981) Thromboembolism in pregnancy. In Jewell D.P. (ed) *Advanced Medicine 17*, pp. 309–17. Pitman Medical, Tunbridge Wells.

de Swiet M., Dorrington Ward P., Fidler J., Horsman A., Katz D., Letsky E., Peacock M. & Wise P.H. (1983) Prolonged heparin therapy in pregnancy causes bone demineralisation (heparin-induced osteopenia). *British Journal of Obstetrics and Gynaecology*. 90.

Eckstein H. & Jack B. (1970) Breast feeding and anticoagulant therapy. *Lancet* 1, 672–3.

Elliot M.S., Immelman E.J., Jeffery P., Benatar S.R., Funston M.R., Smith J.A., Shepstone B.J., Ferguson A.D., Jacobs P., Walker W. & Louw J.H. (1979) A comparative trial of heparin versus streptokinase in the treatment of acute proximal venous thrombosis: an interim report of a prospective trial. *British Journal of Surgery* 66, 838–43.

Estes J.W. (1970) Kinetics of the anticoagulant effect of heparin. *Journal of the American Medical Association* **212**, 1492.

Excess R. & Graeme B. (1974) Congenital athyroidism in the newborn infant from intrauterine radioactive action. *Biology of the Neonate* **24**, 289–91.

Finnerty J.J. & MacKay B.R. (1962) Antepartum thrombophlebitis and pulmonary embolism. *Obstetrics and Gynecology* **19**, 405.

Flessa H.C., Glueck H.I. & Dritshilo A. (1974) Thromboembolic disorders in pregnancy. *Clinical Obstetrics and Gynaecology* **17**, 195.

Flute P.T. (1976) Thrombolytic therapy. *British Journal of Hospital Medicine* **16**, 135–42.

Friend J.R. & Kakkar V.V. (1972) Deep vein thrombosis in obstetric and gynaecological patients. In Kakkar V.V. and Kakkar A.J. (eds) *Thromboembolism: Diagnosis and Treatment*, pp. 131–8. Churchill Livingstone, Edinburgh.

Gallus A.S. (1976) Venous thromboembolism; incidence and clinical risk factors. In Madden J.L. and Hume M. (eds) *Venous Thromboembolism.* Appleton-Century-Crofts, New York.

Griffith G.C., Nichols G., Asher J.D. & Hanagan B. (1965) Heparin osteoporosis. *Journal of the American Medical Association* **193**, 91–4.

Gurll W., Helfand Z., Salzman E.F. & Silen W. (1971) Peripheral venous thrombophlebitis during pregnancy. *American Journal of Surgery* **121**, 449–53.

Hall J.G. (1976) Warfarin and fetal abnormality. *Lancet* **1**, 1127.

Hall R.J.C., Young C., Sutton G.C. & Cambell S. (1972) Treatment of acute massive pulmonary embolism by streptokinase during labour and delivery. *British Medical Journal* **4**, 647–9.

Hall J.G., Pauli R.M. & Wilson K.M. (1980) Maternal and fetal sequelae of anticoagulation during pregnancy. *American Journal of Medicine* **68**, 122–40.

Harrod M.J.E. & Sherrod P.S. (1981) Warfarin embryopathy in siblings. *Obstetrics and Gynecology* **57**, 673–6.

Heimbecker R.O., Keon W.J. & Richards K.U. (1973) Massive pulmonary Embolism: A new look at surgical management. *Archives of Surgery* **107**, 740–6.

Hellgren M. (1981) Thromboembolism and pregnancy. MD Thesis, Karolinska Institute, Stockholm.

Hellgren M. & Blombäck M. (1981) Studies on blood coagulation and and fibrinolysis in pregnancy, during delivery and in the pueperium. 1. Normal condition. *Gynecologic and Obstetric Investigation* **12**, 141–54.

Hellgren M. & Nygards E.B. (1981) Long term therapy with subcutaneous heparin during pregnancy. *Gynecologic Obstetric Investigation* **13**, 76–89.

Henderson S.R., Lund C.J. & Creasman W.T. (1972) Antepartum pulmonary embolism. *American Journal of Obstetrics and Gynecology* **112**, 476–86.

Hiilesma (1960) Occurrence and anticoagulant treatment of thromboembolism in gravidas, parturients and gynecologic patients. *Acta Obstetrica et Gynecologica Scandinavica Supplement (2)* **39**, 5.

Hirsh J., Cade J.F. & O'Sullivan E.F. (1970) Clinical experience with anticoagulant therapy during pregnancy. *British Medical Journal* **1**, 270–3.

Holzgreve W., Carey J.C. & Hall B.D. (1976) Warfarin-induced fetal abnormalities. *Lancet* **2**, 914–15.

Howell R., Fidler J., Letsky E. & de Swiet M. (1983) The risks of antenatal subcutaneous heparin prophylaxis: a controlled trial. *British Journal of Obstetrics and Gynaecology* **90**.

Hull R., Hirsh J. & Sackett D.L. (1977) Combined use of leg scanning and impedance plethysmography in suspected venous thrombosis. An alternative to venography. *New England Journal of Medicine* **296**, 1497–1500.

Hume M., Sevitt S. & Thomas D.P. (1970) *Venous Thrombosis and Pulmonary Embolism.* Harvard University Press, Cambridge, Massachusetts.

Jacobs J., Kletter I., Superstine E., Hill K.R., Lynn B. & Webb R.A. (1973) Intravenous infusions of heparin and penicillins. *Journal of Clinical Pathology* **26**, 742–6.

Jaffe M.D. & Willis P.W. (1965) Multiple fractures associated with long-term sodium heparin therapy. *Journal of the American Medical Association* **193**, 152–4.

Jeffcoate T.N.A., Miller J., Ros R.F. & Tindall V.R. (1968) Puerpural thromboembolism in relation to the inhibition of lactation by oestrogen therapy. *British Medical Journal* **4**, 19.

Jick H., Slone D., Westerholm B., Inman W.H.W., Vessey M.P., Shapiro S., Lewis G.P. & Worcester J. (1969) Venous thromboembolic disease and ABO blood type. A cooperative study. *Lancet* **1**, 539–42.

Kerber I.J., Warr O.S. III & Richardson C. (1968) Pregnancy in a patient with a prosthetic mitral valve associated with a fetal anomaly attributed to warfarin sodium. *Journal of the American Medical Association* **203**, 223–5.

Kimball A.M., Hallum A.V. & Cates W. (1978) Deaths caused by pulmonary thromboembolism after legally induced abortion. *American Journal of Obstetrics and Gynecology* **132**, 169–74.

Lancet (1983) Familial Antithrombin III deficiency. *Lancet* **i**, 1021–2.

Lansing A.M. & Davies W.M. (1968) Five year follow-up study of ilio femoral venous thromboectomy. *Annals of Surgery* **168**, 620–8.

Laros R.K. & Alger L.S. (1979) Thromboembolism and pregnancy. *Clinical Obstetrics and Gynecology* **22**, 871–3.

Ledger W.J. & Peterson E.P. (1970) The use of heparin in the management of pelvic thrombophlebitis. *Surgery and Obstetrics* **131**, 1115.

Ludlam C.A., Bolton A.E., Moore S. & Cash J.D. (1975) New rapid method for diagnosis of deep vein thrombosis. *Lancet* **2**, 259–60.

Ludwig H. (1973) Results of streptokinase therapy in deep vein thrombosis during pregnancy. *Postgraduate Medical Journal* (Suppl. 5) **49**, 65–7.

McCausland A.M., Hyman C., Winsor T. & Trotter A.D. (1961) Venous distensibility during pregnancy. *American Journal of Obstetrics and Gynecology* **81**, 472–9.

Mackie M., Bennett B., Ogston D. & Douglas A. (1978) Familial thrombosis: inherited deficiency of antithrombin III. *British Medical Journal* **1**, 136–8.

McTaggart D.R. & Engram T.G. (1977) Massive pulmonary embolism during pregnancy treated with streptokinase. *Medical Journal of Australia* **1**, 18–20.

Malkamy H. (1980) Heparin therapy in post Caesarean septic pelvic thrombophlebitis. *International Journal of Gynaecology and Obstetrics* **17**, 564–6.

Marciniak E. & Gockerman J.P. (1977) Heparin-induced decrease in circulating antithrombin III. *Lancet* **2**, 581–4.

Mayor G.E. (1969) Deep vein thrombosis—surgical management. *British Medical Journal* **4**, 680–2.

Morris G.K. & Mitchell J.R.A. (1978) Clinical management of venous thromboembolism. *British Medical Bulletin* **34**, 169–75.

Moseley P. & Kerstein M.D. (1980) Pregnancy and thrombophlebitis. *Surgery, Gynecology and Obstetrics* **150**, 593–7.

National Institute of Health Consensus Conference (1980) Thrombolytic therapy in treatment. *British Medical Journal* **280**, 1585–7.

Orme M. L'E., Lewis P.J., de Swiet M., Serlin M.J., Sibeon R., Baty J.D. & Breckenbridge A.M. (1977) May mothers given warfarin breast-feed their infants? *British Medical Journal* **1**, 1564–5.

Pettifor J.M. & Benson R. (1975) Congenital malformations associated with the administration of oral anticoagulants during pregnancy. *Journal of Pediatrics* **86**, 459–62.

Pfeifer G.W. (1970a) The use of thrombolytic therapy in obstetrics and gynaecology. *Australian Annals of Medicine* (Suppl. 28–31).

Pfeifer G.W. (1970b) Distribution and placental transfer of [131]I Streptokinase. *Australian Annals of Medicine* (Suppl. 17–18).

Preston Flanigan D., Goodreau J.J., Burnham S.J., Bergan J.J. & Yao J.S.T. (1978) Vascular laboratory diagnosis of clinically suspected acute deep vein thrombosis. *Lancet* **1**, 331–4.

Pridmore B.R., Murray K.H. & McAllen P.M. (1975) The management of anticoagulant therapy during and after pregnancy. *British Journal of Obstetrics and Gynaecology* **82**, 740–4.

Prochownik E.V., Antonarakis S. & Bauer K.A. (1983) Molecular heterogenicity of inherited antithrombin III deficiency. *New England Journal of Medicine* **308**, 1549–52.

Raja Rao A.K., Zucker M. & Sacks D. (1980) Right ovarian vein thrombosis with extension to the inferior vena cava. *British Journal of Radiology* **53**, 160–1.

Ramsay L.E. (1983) Impact of venography on the diagnosis and management of deep vein thrombosis. *British Medical Journal* **286**, 698–9.

Robin E.D. (1977) Overdiagnosis and overtreatment of pulmonary embolism: The emperor may have no clothes. *Annals of Internal Medicine* **87**, 775–81.

Royal College of General Practitioners (1967) Oral contraception and thrombo-embolic disease. *Journal of the Royal College of General Practitioners* **13**, 267–79.

Salzman E.W., Deykin D., Shapiro R.M. & Rosenberg R. (1975) Management of heparin therapy—Controlled prospective trial. *New England Journal of Medicine* **292**, 1046–50.

Sasahara A.A. & Barsamian E.M. (1973) Another look at pulmonary embolectomy. *Annals of Thoracic Surgery* **16**, 317–20.

Sasahara A.A. (1974) Therapy for pulmonary embolism. *Journal of the American Medical Association* **229**, 1795–8.

Sautter R.D. (1975) In Fratantoni J. and Wessler S. (eds) *Prophylactic Therapy of Deep Vein Thrombosis and Pulmonary Embolism*, pp. 137–142. National Institutes of Health, Bethesda.

Sharma G.U.R.K., Burlesco U.A. & Sasahara A.A. (1980) Effect of thrombolytic therapy on pulmonary-capillary blood volume in patients with pulmonary embolism. *New England Journal of Medicine* **303**, 842–5.

Shaul W.L., Emery H. & Hall J.G. (1975) Chondodysplasia punctata and maternal warfarin use during pregnancy. *American Journal of Diseases in Children* **129**, 360–2.

Shaul W.L. & Hall J.G. (1977) Multiple congenital anomalies associated with anticoagulants. *American Journal of Obstetrics and Gynecology* **127**, 191–8.

Sheffield L.J., Danks D.M., Mayne V. & Hutchinson L.A. (1976) Chondodysplasia punctata—23 cases of a mild and relatively common variety. *Journal of Pediatrics* **89**, 916–23.

Sherman S. & Hall B.D. (1976) Warfarin and fetal abnormality. *Lancet* **1**, 692.

Silver D. & Sabiston D.C. (1975) The role of vena caval interruption in the management of pulmonary embolism. *Surgery* **77**, 3–10.

Simpson F.G., Robinson P.J., Bark M. & Losowsky M.S. (1980) Prospective study of thrombophlebitis and "pseudo thrombophlebitis". *Lancet* **1**, 331–3.

Squires J.W. & Pinch L.W. (1979) Heparin induced spinal fractures. *Journal of the American Medical Association* **241**, 2417–18.

Szekely P., Turner R. & Snaith L. (1973) Pregnancy and the changing pattern of rheumatic heart disease. *British Heart Journal* **35**, 1290–1303.

Thomas A.N., Pattison C. & Serjeant G.R. (1982) Causes of death in sickle-cell disease in Jamaica. *British Medical Journal* **285**, 633–5.

Tribukait B. & Swedjemark G.A. (1978) Secretion of ^{99m}Tc in breast milk after intravenous injection of marked macroaggregated albumin. *Acta Radiologica Oncology* **17**, 379–82.

Urokinase Pulmonary Embolism Trial Study Group (1970) Urokinase pulmonary embolism trial: Phase 1. *Journal of the American Medical Association* **214**, 2163–72.

Van Dinh T., Boor P.J. & Gazra J.R. (1982) Massive pulmonary embolism following delivery of a patient with sickle cell trait. *American Journal of Obstetrics and Gynecology* **143**, 722–4.

Villasanta U. (1965) Thromboembolic disease in pregnancy. *American Journal of Obstetrics and Gynecology* **93**, 142–60.

Winter J.H., Fenech A., Bennett B. & Douglas A.S. (1981) Thrombosis after venography in familial antithrombin III deficiency. *British Medical Journal* **283**, 1436–7.

Wise P.H. & Hall A.J. (1980) Heparin induced osteopenia in pregnancy. *British Medical Journal* **281**, 110–11.

Wright H.P., Osborn S.B. & Edmonds D.G. (1950) Changes in the rate of flow of venous blood in the leg during pregnancy, measured with radioactive sodium. *Surgery, Gynecology and Obstetrics* **90**, 481–5.

Zucker M.L., Gomperts E.D. & Marcus R.G. (1976) Prophylactic and therapeutic use of angiocoagulants in inherited ante thrombin III deficiency. *South African Medical Journal* **50**, 1743–8.

5 Heart Disease in Pregnancy

Michael de Swiet

Heart disease is a worrying problem for the obstetrician. As we shall see, it is uncommon, with an overall incidence of less than 1 per cent of all pregnancies; thus any one obstetrician is unlikely to acquire much experience in the management of heart disease in pregnancy. But heart disease is important, since it causes about ten maternal deaths per million maternities in England and Wales, making it equal to haemorrhage as a cause of maternal mortality (DHSS 1982). However, although the overall incidence is less than 1 per cent, symptoms such as breathlessness or signs such as an ejection systolic murmur that are suggestive of heart disease, may be present in up to 90 per cent of the pregnant population as a consequence of the physiological changes induced by pregnancy itself. There is the problem of diagnosis, therefore, as well as that of management of a relatively rare condition. In this chapter, we review first the physiological changes that occur in pregnancy, then consider the incidence, effects and management of heart disease in general. Sections follow, where relevant, on specific congenital and acquired conditions.

PART 1   GENERAL CONSIDERATIONS

Physiology

In normal individuals, pregnancy is associated with a rise in cardiac output of approximately 40 per cent, i.e. from about 3.5 l/min to 6.0 l/min when at rest. Such data derived from the cardiac catheter laboratory must be viewed with objectivity, and too much reliability must not be placed on individual measurements. There is considerable variation between individuals, and the experimental conditions under which investigations have been made are not always relevant to the situations of clinical importance, such as labour or other forms of exercise. The timing of this rise in cardiac output is also open to discussion. However, those investigators that have measured cardiac output early in pregnancy find that it is already markedly elevated in the first trimester, and suggest that the maximum elevation in resting cardiac output may occur by 30 weeks. The general consensus is that cardiac output then does not fall until some unspecified time after delivery, but Crawford *et al* (1971) and Ueland *et al* (1972) have suggested that there may be a fall before labour. The study of Crawford, based on pulmonary electrical impedance, is open to methodological criticism, because this technique has not been sufficienctly validated in pregnancy. It is difficult to understand why cardiac output should fall before labour. Other earlier investigators were in error in believing that cardiac output fell before labour because they did not realise that, when they measured cardiac output with their patients in the supine position, the gravid uterus would obstruct the venous return from the lower limbs.

The increase in cardiac output is caused partly by an increase in heart rate, and partly by an increase in stroke volume. Since blood pressure does not rise in pregnancy, and usually falls, the increase in cardiac output is associated with a marked fall in peripheral vascular resistance. Indeed, it is likely that the fall in peripheral resistance is one major factor that causes the rise in cardiac output. Only part of the change in peripheral vascular resistance could be accounted for by blood flow through the low resistance shunt of the pregnant uterus since cardiac output is elevated during the first trimester, at a time when there is very little change in uterine blood flow. Oestrogens and prostaglandins, including prostacyclin, are the likely mediators of the alterations in haemodynamics caused by pregnancy. (For further reviews of these changes, *see* de Swiet 1980.)

In contrast to the considerable volume of studies of the haemodynamics of pregnancy in normal individuals, there is little information concerning patients with heart disease. However, Ueland and his colleagues have shown that patients with asymptomatic mitral valve disease are unable to increase their cardiac outputs on exercise in pregnancy to the same level as normal patients at rest (Ueland *et al* 1972).

Natural history

INCIDENCE

The prevalence and incidence of all heart disease in pregnancy varies between 0.5 per cent (Sugrue *et al* 1981) and 3.5 per cent (Mendelson 1956). Other studies include those of Etheridge (1969) who found a prevalence of 0.5 per cent in Australia, Rush *et al* (1979) 0.8 per cent in South Africa, Buemann *et al* (1962) 0.9 per cent in Scandinavia and de Swiet and Fidler (1981) 0.5 per cent to 1.8 per cent in London. These figures probably do vary because of a genuine difference in the prevalence of heart disease in different communities. For example, the incidence of rheumatic fever varies considerably between countries, and is strongly related to their relative affluence. In addition, diagnostic criteria change with time and with the different referral populations of different hospitals. Fig. 5.1 shows the incidence of rheumatic and congenital heart disease at Queen Charlotte's Maternity and Hillingdon Hospitals, 1947–71, and at Queen Charlotte's Maternity Hospital, 1972–79. The steady fall in the incidence of rheumatic heart disease is probably genuine (*see also* Szekely *et al* 1972). However, the apparent rise in the incidence of congenital heart disease in the latter part of the series is unlikely to represent a true rise in the whole population. It relates to the figures for Queen Charlotte's Maternity Hospital alone which has a high referral rate from cardiology centres with a strong paediatric interest. Also many cases of mitral

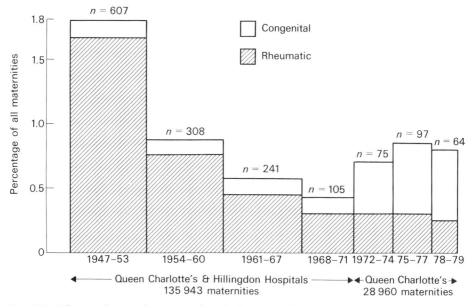

Fig. 5.1 The incidence of congenital and rheumatic heart disease at Queen Charlotte's Maternity and Hillingdon Hospitals, 1947–79. (Courtesy of the Editor, *Journal of the Royal College of Physicians.*)

valve abnormality which would have been considered rheumatic before 1972 are now diagnosed as congenital, particularly on the basis of echocardiographic data.

Nevertheless, it is likely that we will see a genuine change in the pattern of congenital heart disease in pregnancy following from the increase in paediatric cardiac surgery which occurred between 1965 and 1975. These patients will start to become pregnant in significant numbers from the age of 18 years onwards so that we should expect to see the change from 1983 and it is likely to be much more obvious by the end of the 1980s.

In all series the dominant lesion in rheumatic heart disease has been mitral stenosis (Szekely *et al* 1973; Etheridge 1966, 1969; Mendelson 1960; Metcalfe 1968; Sugrue *et al* 1981; Gleicher *et al* 1979). In 1048 patients with rheumatic heart disease reported from Newcastle, Szekely *et al* (1973) found dominant mitral stenosis in 90 per cent, mitral regurgitation in 6.6 per cent, aortic regurgitation in 2.5 per cent, and aortic stenosis in 10 per cent.

At present, the experience of congenital heart disease in pregnancy is limited to relatively simple defects which have usually not been corrected. Four representative series are shown in Table 5.1. Although the total numbers in each series are very different, the overall pattern is similar. The most common lesions are atrial septal defect and patent ductus arteriousus, together accounting for about 50 per cent of cases; followed by ventricular septal defect, pulmonary stenosis and Fallot's tetralogy which, together, contribute another 20 per cent. Isolated lesions such as coarctation of the aorta, aortic stenosis and Ebstein's anomaly account for the remainder (Neilson *et al* 1970; Ong and Puraviappan 1975; Copeland *et al* 1963; Sugrue *et al* 1981). It is likely that these data reflect no more than the incidence of congenital heart disease in the general female population. However, three of the series are quite old and date from 1963–75. In the more modern series from Dublin (1969–78) we see the effect of surgery and more cases of patent ductus arteriosus and atrial septal defect have been corrected.

Table 5.1   Incidence (%) of various forms of congenital heart disease in Ohio, Queensland, Malaysia and Dublin.

	Ohio[1] (n=125)	Queensland[2] (n=93)	Malaysia[3] (n=28)	Dublin[4] (n=47)
Patent ductus arteriosus	24	27	32	9
Atrial septal defect	29	26	29	38
Pulmonary stenosis	4	12	18	6
Ventricular septal defect	22	14	11	13
Fallot's tetralogy	4	4	7	13
Coarctation of the aorta	10	6	4	6
Aortic valve disease	3	4		6
Other	2	2		
Unclassified	5	5		

[1] Copeland *et al* (1968); [2] Neilson *et al* (1970); [3] Ong and Puraviappan (1975); [4] Sugrue *et al* (1981).

Other conditions, such as coronary artery disease or symptomatic arrhythmias, are so rarely associated with pregnancy that it is difficult to give a true incidence. However, Rush *et al* (1979) reported coronary artery disease in 0.4 per cent of 697 patients with heart disease in pregnancy. The same authors found an incidence of 17 cases of arrhythmia in 697 patients with heart disease in pregnancy. Szekely *et al* (1973) found that 69 of 1048 cases of rheumatic heart disease were complicated by atrial fibrillation. The incidence of cardiomyopathy of pregnancy is discussed later in the chapter.

MATERNAL MORTALITY

Although sporadic fatalities will be seen in all forms of heart disease in pregnancy, maternal mortality is most likely in those conditions where pulmonary blood flow cannot be increased (Jewett 1979). This occurs because of obstruction, either within the pulmonary blood vessels or at the mitral valve. The situation is documented clearly in Eisenmenger's syndrome, where up to now there has been no effective treatment and where the maternal mortality is between 30 per cent and 50 per cent (Pitts *et al* 1977; Neilson *et al* 1970; Morgan Jones and Howitt 1965; Gleicher *et al* 1979). The Confidential Enquiries into Maternal Mortality in England and Wales indicate that Eisenmenger's syndrome was the most frequent form of congenital heart disease associated with maternal mortality and was responsible for 17 of the 47 cases of death due to congenital heart disease between 1961 and 1975 (DHSS 1982). Only Batson (1976) has reported a series of 23 pregnancies with no maternal deaths; the reason for this unusual success is not clear. An elevation in pulmonary vascular resistance is also seen, though less frequently, in primary pulmonary hypertension when the reported maternal mortality is 50 per cent (Morgan Jones and Howitt 1965; Sinnenberg 1980). One fatality has been recorded in cor pulmonale (Rush *et al* 1979).

In contrast, in Fallot's tetralogy where the pulmonary vascular resistance is normal, the reported maternal mortality varies between 4 per cent and 20 per cent (Morgan Jones and Hewitt 1965; Mendelson 1960; Jacoby 1964). Furthermore, the figure of 20 per cent is only based on one maternal death in five pregnancies in the study of Jacoby. Espino Vela and Alvarado-Toro (1971) have reported a series of 105 patients with atrial septal defect (confirmed by catheter in 41 patients) who had up to ten or more pregnancies with no maternal mortality.

In Ehlers–Danlos syndrome the arterial and classic forms have also been associated with a high mortality, due to arterial dissection and bleeding (Barabas 1967; Pearl and Spicer 1981). More recently Ehlers–Danlos syndrome has been characterised on the basis of the specific collagen defect, and in Ehlers–Danlos syndrome type IV, the maternal mortality is said to be as high as 25% in North America (Rudd *et al* 1983). This high mortality has been disputed by Pope and Nicholls (1983) in a different series from the UK implying a different referral series or genetic heterogeneity.

In rheumatic heart disease the maternal mortality can now be very low. Szekely *et al* (1973) reported 26 mortalities in 2856 pregnancies (about 1 per cent) complicated by rheumatic heart disease between 1942 and 1969. Half of the deaths were due to pulmonary oedema, which became much less common once mitral valvotomy was freely available. These authors reported no maternal deaths in about a thousand pregnancies occurring after 1960. Rush *et al* (1979) also reported a maternal mortality of 0.7 per cent in 450 mothers with rheumatic heart disease in South Africa.

Although the prognosis is good in patients with rheumatic heart disease in pregnancy, many clinicians still believe that '. . . every pregnancy was so many nails in the coffin of a woman with heart disease' (Webster 1913). Chesley (1980) has reported a group of 38 patients with 51 pregnancies occurring after they were diagnosed as having severe heart disease. These were compared with a group of 96 women with equally severe rheumatic heart disease who did not have any pregnancies after diagnosis. The mean survival time (14 years) was no less and, in fact, was greater in the group that did have further pregnancies compared to the group that did not (12 years). I would agree with Chesley (1980) that pregnancy does not affect the long-term survival of a woman with rheumatic heart disease, providing that she survives pregnancy itself.

FETAL OUTCOME

The fetal outcome in rheumatic heart disease in pregnancy is usually good, and little diffrent from that in patients who do not have heart disease (Sugrue *et al* 1981; Rush *et al* 1979). However, the babies are likely to be lighter (Ueland *et al* 1972), by about 200 g in the study of Ho *et al* (1980).

In the four series of patients with congenital heart disease in pregnancy cited in Table 5.1, there was no excess fetal mortality except in the group with cyanotic congenital heart disease, whether associated with pulmonary hypertension or not. Here the babies are generally growth retarded (Batson 1974; Schafer *et al* 1968), and the fetal loss including abortion may be as high as 40 per cent (Batson 1974; Copeland *et al* 1963; Gleicher *et al* 1979). Even in the tetralogy of Fallot, which does not have a particularly high maternal mortality, the fetal loss rate may be as high as 57 per cent (Copeland *et al* 1963) and the majority of the babies are growth retarded (Jacoby 1964). This is hardly surprising, in view of the inefficient mechanisms of placental exchange which cannot compensate for the maternal systemic hypoxaemia. It is likely that the fetus dies because of inadequate oxygen supply or because of prematurity (Gleicher *et al* 1979) which may be iatrogenic. In contrast, the fetal results in 40 pregnancies following 27 cases of total correction of Fallot's tetralogy were excellent (Singh *et al* 1982).

Uncorrected coarctation of the aorta has also been associated with a 13 per cent fetal loss rate (Burwell and Metcalfe 1958), and intrauterine growth retardation (Benny *et al* 1980), presumably because of inadequate placental perfusion. However, severe aortic occlusion requiring axillary-femoral grafting may be compatible with a normally grown fetus (Socol *et al* 1981).

Management

All pregnant patients with heart disease should be managed in a combined obstetric/cardiac clinic by one obstetrician and one cardiologist. In this way, the number of visits that the patient makes to the hospital is kept to a minimum, and the obstetrician and cardiologist obtain the maximum experience in the management of relatively rare conditions.

HISTORY

As in all forms of medicine, the history is of paramount importance in the assessment of patients with heart disease. In the UK, most patients with heart disease know that they have it, or that they have a heart murmur. It is now rare to make the diagnosis of heart disease *de novo* in pregnancy. In all developed countries, women have frequent medical examinations from the time they are babies, and attend infant welfare clinics, to when they visit family planning clinics or attend for examination prior to employment. The exceptions are recent immigrants and patients from deprived social classes.

The most frequent symptom of heart disease in pregnancy is breathlessness. This is difficult to assess because it is a variable feature of all pregnancy (Milne *et al* 1978). Some patients are aware of increasing their ventilation; others are not. Breathlessness arising in pregnancy does not therefore necessarily indicate heart disease, and it is important to consider whether the patients were breathless before they became pregnant. The New York Heart Association classification of heart disease is largely based on limitation of physical activity and associated symptoms of heart disease such as shown below.

Class 1—no resulting limitation of physical activity. Ordinary physical activity does not cause undue fatigue, palpitation, dyspnoea or anginal pain.

Class 2—slight limitation of physical activity. Patients are comfortable at rest. Ordinary physical activity results in fatigue, palpitation, dyspnoea and anginal pain.

Class 3—marked limitation of physical activity. Patients are comfortable at rest. Less than ordinary activity causes fatigue, palpitation, dyspnoea or anginal pain.

Class 4—inability to carry on any physical activity without discomfort. Symptoms of cardiac insufficiency or of the anginal syndrome may be present even at rest. If any physical activity is undertaken, discomfort is increased (Mendelson 1960).

However, such a classification is only of value if it indicates the severity of the condition at the time of classification, and if it is reliable in predicting the outcome of pregnancy. Both these criteria may not be met with regard to the New York Heart Association classification. We have seen that symptoms of breathlessness are unreliable in pregnancy, and it is also well recognised that patients with mitral stenosis may have no symptoms at the beginning of pregnancy (Class 1) yet be in pulmonary oedema by the end of pregnancy (Class 4) (Szekely *et al* 1973; Howitt 1971). Indeed, Sugrue *et al* (1981) reported that 39 per cent of 38 patients with rheumatic heart disease, who developed heart failure in pregnancy, were originally classified as grade 1. Therefore a precise anatomical diagnosis supported by a pathophysiological assessment of the severity of the condition is preferable.

Syncope is also a very common feature of normal pregnancy, particularly in the middle trimester. Presumably in these patients peripheral vascular resistance decreases more than cardiac output increases. However, syncope may also occur rarely in severe aortic stenosis, hypertrophic cardiomyopathy (HOCM, subaortic stenosis), Fallot's tetralogy and Eisenmenger's syndrome. Syncope, like chest pain, can occur because of dysrhythmias. The patient may also be aware of the dysrhythmia as a feeling of palpitation.

Chest pain is usually a feature of ischaemic disease, which is uncommon in pregnancy (*see* below) but chest pain may also occur in severe aortic stenosis or, more commonly in pregnancy, in HOCM.

PHYSICAL SIGNS

The hyperdynamic circulation of pregnancy causes alterations in the cardiovascular system which mimic heart disease. Thus 20 per cent of patients originally thought to have rheumatic heart disease may have none at all, following a reassessment performed up to 30 years later (Gleicher *et al* 1979). Premature atrial and ventricular ectopic beats are common in pregnancy (Szekely *et al* 1973) and the peripheral pulse is increased in volume, suggesting aortic valve disease to the unwary. The neck veins pulsate more vigorously in pregnancy, but the mean right atrial pressure is unchanged—10 mmHg—(Bader *et al* 1955) and therefore the height of the jugular venous pressure is also unchanged. The heart apex beat is more forceful and because of the increase in cardiac output, may suggest cardiomegaly in normal patients. However, if the apex beat is more than 2 cm outside the midclavicular line, this should be considered definitely abnormal.

The ausculatory changes in normal pregnancy have been well documented in a phonocardiographic study by Cutforth and MacDonald (1966). The first heart sound is loud and the third heart sound is audible in 84 per cent of patients. This is the single greatest cause of confusion, since the third heart sound is interpreted as a diastolic murmur or opening snap. An ejection systolic murmur can be heard in 96 per cent of apparently normal pregnant women (Cutforth and MacDonald 1966). The murmur is very widely conducted, and can even be heard over the back. Although it is said that a diastolic murmur can arise in normal patients, due to high blood flow across the tricuspid valve (Cutforth and MacDonald 1966), this should be a diagnosis based on exclusion after echocardiography. Murmurs may be heard over the right or left second intercostal space, about 2 cm from the sternal edge. They may be systolic or continuous, and can be modified by pressure of the stethoscope. They are thought to be due to blood flow in mammary vessels (Cutforth and MacDonald 1966). Venous hums—continuous murmurs usually audible in the neck and modified by posture—may also be heard in pregnancy as in the nonpregnant state.

Any other murmurs or additional heart sounds should be considered significant. Particular difficulty occurs with systolic murmurs, since they are so common in normal pregnancy. Those that are significant are pansystolic murmurs (VSD, mitral regurgitation, tricuspid regurgitation), late systolic murmurs (mitral regurgitation, mitral valve prolapse), ejection systolic murmurs that are louder than grade 3/6 (aortic stenosis), or vary with respiration (pulmonary stenosis), or are associated with other abnormalities, e.g. ejection clicks (valvar pulmonary and aortic stenosis). The clinical signs of heart disease are briefly discussed with the individual conditions below, but an assessment of the patient's cardiac status should also include the signs of heart failure, whether the patient is cyanosed or has finger clubbing, the presence of pulse deficits and other peripheral signs of endocarditis such as splinter haemorrhages.

INVESTIGATIONS

Chest radiography

The increase in cardiac output and pulmonary blood volume causes slight cardiomegaly, increased pulmonary vascular markings and distension of the pulmonary veins. These return to normal after delivery, and they do not necessarily indicate that the patient has heart disease. The chest radiograph is unhelpful in the diagnosis of minor degrees of heart disease but will, of course, show typical changes in those that have haemodynamically significant heart disease.

Electrocardiography

Oram and Holt (1961) reported innocent depression of the S-T segment and flattening of the T wave in the left-sided precordial leads in 14 per cent of normal pregnant women. They state that such changes would normally lead one to suspect cardiomyopathy. Boyle and Lloyd-Jones (1966) disputed these findings, but most physicians would accept that even T wave inversion and Q waves in lead III (Carr *et al* 1933), which would normally by considered pathologic, may be seen in healthy pregnant women. Although a change in the electrical axis of the heart during pregnancy may be part of the explanation (Carruth *et al* 1981), it does not account for all these findings. Indeed, pregnancy itself does not account for all the findings, and there may be more variability in the electrocardiograph of healthy nonpregnant women than had previously been realised (Oram and Holt 1961). As a consequence, in pregnancy the electrocardiograph is more helpful in the diagnosis of dysrhythmias than in the demonstration of a structural abnormality of the heart.

Echocardiography

Recent studies in nonpregnant individuals have shown that the majority of structural cardiac abnormalities can be detected by echocardiography (St John Sutton *et al* 1981), and this would appear to be the technique of choice in pregnancy, since there is no radiation hazard, and because of the detailed information available in skilled hands. Rubler *et al* (1977), in an echocardiographic study designed to look at changes in cardiac output, also established normal values for chamber size in pregnancy, but more studies are required of the clinical application of echocardiography in patients with heart disease in pregnancy.

CLINICAL MANAGEMENT

Patients should be seen in a combined clinic and the nature and severity of their heart lesion assessed. Many patients will have no evidence of any lesion at all, and no further follow-up will be required. Some may only have a mild lesion with no haemodynamic problems, such as congenital mitral prolapse which has an excellent prognosis (Rayburn and Fontana 1981). Again, no further follow-up is necessary although, in my opinion, they should receive antibiotic prophylaxis in labour (*see* below). The remainder do have a condition with real or potential haemodynamic implications. They must first be assessed as to the need for termination, if seen early enough in pregnancy, and secondly the need for surgery. In patients with well managed heart disease, these decisions should have been made before the patient becomes pregnant (Burch 1980), but inevitably some patients present for the first time in pregnancy or have been lost to follow-up before pregnancy.

Because of the mortality statistics indicated above, only Eisenmenger's syndrome and primary pulmonary hypertension are absolute indications for termination of pregnancy. Termination may also be indicated very rarely in patients with such severe pulmonary disease that they have pulmonary hypertension. Under these circumstances, pulmonary artery pressure, if not known, should be measured directly by Swan–Ganz catheter (*see* Chapter 2). In all other cases, the decision whether the pregnancy should continue depends on an individual assessment of the risk of pregnancy compared to the patient's desire to have children.

In general, the indications for surgery in pregnancy are similar to those in the nonpregnant state: failure of medical treatment with either intractable heart failure or intolerable symptoms. However, because of the bad reputation of severe mitral stenosis in pregnancy, mitral valvotomy is performed relatively commonly in patients with suitable heart valves, whereas open heart surgery is done with reluctance because of worries about the fetus. Szekely *et al* (1973) reported 69 mitral valvotomies during pregnancy after 1951, although only five were performed between 1966 and 1969; presumably after 1966 the majority of patients with mitral stenosis had their valvotomies performed before pregnancy. The indications for valvotomy are pulmonary congestion not responding rapidly to drugs, any episode of pulmonary oedema before pregnancy (likely to recur in pregnancy) and profuse haemoptysis. In patients considered for closed valvotomy, there should be no significant mitral regurgitation, the mitral valve should not be calcified, and there should not be other significant valve involvement. The operation is usually performed in the middle trimester, but may be done at any time in pregnancy. Szekely *et al* (1973) reported only two operative deaths, with good fetal results (two spontaneous abortions, and six perinatal deaths) in 69 valvotomies in pregnancy. Nevertheless, mitral valvotomy has become rare in the UK. None have been performed in patients referred to Queen Charlotte's Maternity Hospital in the last ten years, and Sugrue *et al* (1981) only reported three cases from Dublin in 387 pregnancies complicated by rheumatic heart disease. Since very few cardiac surgeons now perform closed mitral valvotomies, preferring the improved control offered by open heart surgery, this trend seems likely to continue.

A review of open heart surgery during pregnancy by Zitnik *et al* (1969) indicates that, although maternal results are reasonable (5 per cent mortality in a group of 22 women with severely affected hearts), the fetal results are not, with a perinatal mortality of 33 per cent. There has been speculation that these poor figures are due to inadequate perfusion of the placenta during cardiopulmonary bypass, either because of relative hypotension or because of lack of pulsatile blood flow (Page and Toung 1975). These speculations have been supported by several recent reports of lack of beat-to-beat variation and bradycardia recorded by external cardiotocography during cardiopulmonary bypass (Levy *et al* 1980; Eilen *et al* 1981; Lamb *et al* 1981; Trimkas *et al* 1979; Bahary *et al* 1980). Alternatively, some of these findings may be accounted for by the artifically-induced hypothermia occurring during cardiopulmonary bypass. The earlier reports summarised by Zitnik (1969) were all of surgery performed early in pregnancy with a high abortion rate. More recently, Eilen *et al* (1981) have reviewed the literature and found no fetal losses in patients operated on after the first trimester. Nevertheless, the indication for open heart surgery in pregnancy is usually life-threatening pulmonary oedema that cannot be managed medically.

Although the first case of open heart surgery in pregnancy involved a woman with Fallot's tetralogy (Dubourg 1959) cardiac surgery in pregnancy is rarely considered in congenital heart disease. In coarctation of the aorta, the risk of dissection in pregnancy has probably been exaggerated (*see* below). Repair would therefore not be advised unless hypertension could not be controlled medically. Valve replacement with an additional aortic prosthesis might be considered in some cases of Marfan's syndrome; the risks would be those already discussed of open heart surgery.

ROUTINE ANTENATAL CARE

After the initial assessment of the patient, the remainder of medical management during pregnancy is associated with avoiding, if possible, those factors which increase the risk of heart failure, and treating heart failure vigorously if it occurs. Risk factors for heart failure include infections (particularly urinary tract infection in pregnancy), hypertension (both pregnancy-associated and pregnancy-induced), obesity, multiple pregnancy, anaemia, the development of arrhythmias and, very rarely, the development of hyperthyroidism.

ADMISSION FOR BED REST

One cannot make recommendations that all patients with a certain degree of heart disease should be admitted at a certain gestation. Each patient must be considered individually. For some, particularly those with other children, the emotional stress of separation from the rest of their families may cause more harm than the rest does good.

Other patients will benefit, and the gain may be more to the fetus at risk from intrauterine growth retardation than to its mother. All patients with heart failure must be treated in hospital, and few can be discharged for long before delivery.

TREATMENT OF HEART FAILURE AND DYSRHYTHMIAS DURING PREGNANCY

The principles of treatment of heart failure in pregnancy are the same as in the nonpregnant state.

Digoxin

The indications for the use of digoxin are to control the heart rate in atrial fibrillation and some other supraventricular tachycardias, and to increase the force of contraction when given acutely in heart failure. If patients do develop atrial fibrillation in pregnancy, consideration should be given to anticoagulation with warfarin (see below) because of the risk of systemic embolism (Szekely and Snaith 1953). Supraventricular tachycardia in the fetus arising in utero has also been managed by maternal digoxin therapy both successfully (Harrigan *et al* 1981) and unsuccessfully (Newburger and Keane 1979). Propranolol has also been given to the mother for this purpose (Teuscher *et al* 1978; Klein *et al* 1979).

Dosage requirements for digoxin are believed to be the same in pregnancy as in the nonpregnant state (Conradsson and Werkö 1974). Both digoxin (Rogers *et al* 1972) and digitoxin (Okita *et al* 1956) cross the placenta, and produce similar drug levels in the fetus to those seen in the mother (Rogers *et al* 1972; Saarikosi 1976). Digoxin enters the umbilical circulation within five minutes of intravenous administration to the mother (Saarikosi 1976). In general, there is no evidence that therapeutic maternal drug levels of digoxin affect the neonatal electrocardiograph (Rogers *et al* 1972; Mendelson 1960) or cause any harm to the fetus, although Szekely and Snaith (1974) reported one case of transient junctional rhythm in the newborn infant of one of a series of mothers who had been digitalized in pregnancy. Although therapeutic maternal drug levels do not harm the fetus, toxic levels do, as was shown in one case of maternal digitoxin poisoning where electrocardiograph changes of digitalis toxicity were demonstrated in the neonate which died aged three days (Sherman and Locke 1960).

Weaver and Pearson (1973) have reported that the shorter labours generally believed to occur in patients with heart disease were confined to those patients who took digoxin and they postulated a direct stimulating effect of digoxin on the myometrium. But the babies born to the digoxin-treated mothers were smaller and born more prematurely and these factors may have been the cause of the more rapid labours.

There may be a place for prophylactic digoxin therapy in selective patients who are not in heart failure. This is most likely to be of value to those patients who are at risk from developing atrial fibrillation, i.e. those with rheumatic mitral valve disease who have an enlarged left atrium, and possibly those who have paroxysmal atrial fibrillation or frequent atrial ectopic beats. But this form of treatment has not been subjected to formal clinical trial, and there is certainly no case for digitalisation of all patients with heart disease in pregnancy. Digoxin is also secreted in breast milk, but since the total daily excretion in the mother with therapeutic blood levels would not exceed 2 μg (Levy *et al* 1977) this too is unlikely to cause any harm to the neonate unless it has any other predisposing causes of digitalis toxicity such as hypokalaemia.

Diuretic therapy

Frusemide is the most commonly used and rapidly acting loop diuretic for the treatment of pulmonary oedema. Ethacrynic acid has also been used successfully in the management of pulmonary oedema associated with mitral stenosis in labour (Young and Haft 1970). In congestive cardiac failure where speed of action is not so important, oral thiazides are usually used in the first instance, although the extra potency of the loop diuretics may be necessary in a minority of cases. Andersen (1970) showed that the use of thiazide in late pregnancy was not associated with any significant salt or water depletion in the neonate.

There are no risks to the use of diuretics in the treatment of heart failure that are specific to pregnancy, but, as in the nonpregnant state, hypokalaemia is an important complication in a patient who may also be taking digoxin.

Treatment of pulmonary oedema should also include opiates such as morphine, which reduces anxiety and decreases venous return by causing venodilation, and also aminophylline if there is associated bronchospasm. Life-threatening pulmonary oedema that does not respond to drug therapy may be helped by mechanical ventilation. If this is successful, and in other cases which do not respond to medical treatment, cardiac surgery should be considered, if the patient has a potentially operable lesion.

Dysrhythmias

Most 'malignant' dysrhythmias are due to ischaemic heart disease which usually presents in women after their childbearing years, and is rare in pregnancy (Ginz 1970; Husaini 1971), therefore, there is limited experience in the treatment of dysrhythmias during pregnancy. Nevertheless, the problem does exist, particularly in patients who have non-ischaemic abnormalities of cardiac-conducting tissue, such as are believed to occur in the Wolff–Parkinson–White and Lown–Ganong–Levine syndromes. Furthermore, paroxysmal atrial tachycardia is said to occur more frequently in pregnancy than in the nonpregnant state (Szekely and Snaith 1953). The successful management of pregnancy in a patient with autosomal dominant ventricular dysrhythmia has been reported by Sachs and Van Idekinge (1979).

The antidysrhythmic drugs that have been used most frequently in pregnancy are digoxin (discussed above), quinidine and beta-adrenergic blocking agents, in particular propranolol and oxprenolol. The indications for the use of these drugs are unaltered by pregnancy. Although there are isolated case reports of intrauterine growth retardation, acute fetal distress in labour and hypoglycaemia in the neonate, in patients taking beta-adrenergic blocking agents (Cotrill *et al* 1977; Gladstone *et al* 1975; Habib and McArthy 1977), these have not been confirmed in clinical trial of oxprenolol when used for hypertension in pregnancy (Gallery *et al* 1978, Fidler *et al* 1983) (*see* Chapter 6). It would seem reasonable therefore to use propranolol or oxprenolol in both the acute and long-term treatment of supraventricular and ventricular tachycardia in pregnancy. Furthermore the dose of oxprenolol received by infants breast fed by mothers taking oxprenolol is very small (0.1 mg/kg/24 hrs) (Fidler *et al* 1983).

Quinidine is used to maintain or induce sinus rhythm in patients either after DC conversion or taking digoxin. It is well tolerated in pregnancy (Ueland *et al* 1981) and has only minimal oxytocic effect (Mendelson 1956). There is much less experience of other antidysrhythmic drugs such as verapimil, bretylium tosylate, disopyramide or amiodarone. However, a case report has suggested that mexiletine is safe in pregnancy for the treatment of ventricular, dysrhythmia and shown that mexilitene levels in cord blood and breast milk are similar to those in maternal plasma (Timmis *et al* 1980). The use of disopyramide has been associated with hypertonic uterine activity on one occasion (Leonard *et al* 1978) but not in others (Finlay & Edmunds 1979); therefore disopyramide should be used in pregnancy with caution. The long-term risks of phenytoin are well known, and are described in Chapters 2 and 14; however, this drug is only likely to be used in the acute treatment of dysrhythmias, particularly those induced by digitalis intoxication. Szekely and Snaith (1974) have also used procainamide successfully to abolish atrial fibrillation in pregnancy. Pitcher *et al* (1983) have reported the successful use of amiodarone in pregnancy in one case of resistant atrial tachycardia, with no obvious adverse effects in the fetus. The cord blood levels were only 10–25 per cent of maternal plasma levels after therapy for three weeks before delivery. Amiodarone contains substantial quantities of iodine, but neonatal thyroid function was normal. On the basis of this one report, it would seem reasonable to use amiodarone for resistant arrhythmias in late pregnancy.

DC conversion for tachyarrhythmias is safe in pregnancy and does not harm the fetus (Finlay and Edmunds 1979).

The difficulty arises in considering long-term prophylactic treatment with antidysrhythmic drugs which have not been extensively used in pregnancy. Here each case must be considered on its own merits, paying particular attention to the frequency and severity of the attacks of the dysrhythmia. A single short episode of supraventricular tachycardia associated with no other symptoms does not require prophylactic treatment. Frequent attacks of ventricular tachycardia associated with syncope would require prophylaxis—whatever the outcome in the fetus.

ANTICOAGULANT THERAPY

This is a major problem in the management of patients with heart disease in pregnancy. Anticoagulant therapy may be necessary in patients with congenital heart disease who have pulmonary hypertension due to pulmonary vascular disease, those who have artificial valve replacements, and those with atrial fibrillation. Limet and Crondin (1977) have reported two patients with embolic problems following artificial valve replacement when the patients were either not anticoagulated, or anticoagulated inadequately during pregnancy. They calculated from their own series that the risk of a woman having an embolic episode if she had an artificial valve and did not take anticoagulants was 1 per 100 months of exposure. Their literature search suggested that the risk of thromboembolism in such patients is higher (25 per cent per pregnancy) and that this risk can be reduced to 5 per cent, if the patients did take anticoagulants.

For conditions such as pulmonary embolus, subcutaneous heparin is safer than warfarin (*see* Chapter 4). There appears to be less maternal bleeding and less fetal risk of congenital abnormalities, such as chondrodysplasia punctata or optic atrophy. However, where there is a risk of systemic thromboembolism as in heart disease, subcutaneous heparin treatment does not seem to be adequate and indeed there are reports of Starr Edwards aortic and Björk–Shiley mitral valves that thrombosed during pregnancy when the mothers were either managed with subcutaneous heparin (Bennett & Oakley 1968; Mcleod *et al* 1978) or were not anticoagulated (Chen *et al* 1982).

Ahmad *et al* (1976) and Biale *et al* (1980) have reported one and four cases respectively, where patients with artificial heart valves have been treated with dipyridamole alone during pregnancy. There were no incidents of thromboembolism, but since the data of Limet and Crondin (1977) suggest that risk is only one in ten pregnancies if no anticoagulants are used, larger series are necessary to establish the effectiveness of this form of treatment. There is no ideal solution to this problem. Even though the risk of fetal malformations such as optic atrophy may persist after 16 weeks' gestation (Shaul and Hall 1977), warfarin should be used until about 37 weeks' gestation because subcutaneous heparin does not give adequate protection. Furthermore even subcutaneous heparin therapy has the risk of bone demineralisation (Chapter 4) and the risks of warfarin have probably been overestimated (Chapter 4). At 37 weeks, when the risk of fetal bleeding associated with labour seems to be too great, the patient should be admitted to hospital and given continuous intravenous heparin to produce a heparin level as assayed by protamine sulphate neutralisation of 0.4–0.6 units per ml (Dacie 1975). Heparin does not cross the placenta and therefore will not cause bleeding in the fetus. It is believed that the clotting system of the fetus will return to normal after warfarin has been withheld for one week. At that time, maternal heparin therapy should be reduced to give a heparin level of less than 0.4 units per ml and labour should be induced. If the patient inadvertently goes into labour taking warfarin she should be given vitamin K to reverse the action of warfarin in the fetus and started on heparin therapy as above. In extreme cases, vitamin K has been given intramuscularly to the fetus in utero by transamniotic injection (Larsen *et al* 1978).

After delivery, because of the risk of maternal postpartum haemorrhage, the patient should continue to receive heparin for seven days; then warfarin may be recommended. This is not a contraindication to breast feeding, since insignificant quantities of warfarin are secreted in breast milk (Orme *et al* 1977). However, Dindevan is excreted in breast milk (Eckstein & Jack 1970) and patients taking Dindevan should not breast feed.

LABOUR

Labour should not be induced because of heart disease; indeed, the risks of failed induction and of possible sepsis are relative contraindications. Nevertheless, these risks are slight, and induction should not be withheld if it is necessary for obstetric reasons. Furthermore, induction near term may be justified to plan delivery in daylight hours, in complicated cases requiring optimal medical support.

Patients with significant heart disease require care concerning fluid balance in labour. Many women in labour are given copious quantities of intravenous fluid. If they have normal hearts, they can cope with the resultant increase in circulating blood volume. Patients with heart disease cannot and may easily develop pulmonary oedema.

Patients with heart disease are also particularly sensitive to aorto-caval compression by the gravid uterus in the supine position, causing marked hypotension with maternal and fetal distress. The risk of this is even greater after epidural anaesthesia (Ueland *et al* 1968). Wedges to maintain the patient in the left lateral position can be helpful (Redick 1979).

Most patients with heart disease do have quite rapid, uncomplicated labours, particularly if they are taking digoxin (Weaver and Pearson 1973). In the majority, analgesia is best given by epidural anaesthesia which decreases cardiac output and heart rate, since it is an effective analgesic, and also decreases cardiac output by causing peripheral vasodilation and decreasing venous return. However, the use of epidural anaesthesia is questioned in Eisenmenger's syndrome and contraindicated in hypertrophic cardiomyopathy (*see* below). Most obstetric emergencies arising in labour, including the need for Caesarean section, can be managed using epidural anaesthesia. However, if this is not available, or if elective Caesarean section is advised, general anaesthesia probably causes less haemodynamic derangement than does epidural anaesthesia. But there are few adequate comparisons of these forms of anaesthesia in comparable patients, and more depends on the skill and preference of the anaesthetist.

It would seem sensible to keep the second stage of labour short in order to decrease maternal effort in patients with heart disease, but there is obviously no advantage in performing a forceps delivery in a woman who is going to push the baby out easily herself. The use of oxytocic drugs in the third stage of labour is much debated. The theoretical disadvantage is that ergometrine and Syntocinon will cause a tonic contraction of the uterus, expressing about 500 ml of blood into a circulation whose capacitance has also been made smaller by associated venoconstriction. However the management of postpartum haemorrhage in a patient with heart disease is not easy. I would suggest using Syntocinon in all patients in the third stage, unless they are in heart failure, since it has less effect on blood vessels and can be given by infusion. This infusion can be accompanied by intravenous frusemide.

ENDOCARDITIS AND ITS PREVENTION IN PREGNANCY

The Confidential Enquiries into Maternal Death in England and Wales show that there have been ten such deaths from endocarditis in England and Wales between 1970 and

1975 (DHSS 1982). However, the case for antibiotic prophylaxis in labour has not been proven. There are several large series of patients with heart disease in pregnancy where no antibiotics have been given, and where no endocarditis has been observed (Smith *et al* 1976; Fleming 1977; Sugrue *et al* 1981). It is difficult to document bacteraemia in labour (Burwell and Metcalfe 1958; Redleaf and Farell 1959). Several authors have argued persuasively against antibiotic prophylaxis (Fleming 1977; Sugrue *et al* 1980, 1982). A recent British Working Party recommended antibiotic prophylaxis in labour only in women with artificial heart valves, who are a particularly high-risk group if they do contract endocarditis (Working Party 1982).

Yet, from the data of the Confidential Maternal Mortality series, it would seem that women are at increased risk from endocarditis in pregnancy. What is not clear from the data of the Confidential Maternal Mortality reports is whether endocarditis was contracted during labour, and was potentially preventable by antibiotics, or whether it arose at some other time. The one case that is described in detail in the 1973–75 report did appear to develop endocarditis during a normal delivery, and other similar non-fatal cases have been reported (de Swiet *et al* 1975). Until more details are available, I will continue to use antibiotic prophylaxis, ampicillin 500 mg i.m. and gentamycin 80 mg i.m., three injections given every eight hours at the onset or induction of labour (Durack 1975). The patient who is penicillin sensitive receives one i.v. injection of vancomycin 500 mg (Durack 1975; Garrod 1962).

PULMONARY OEDEMA AND OTHER CARDIOVASCULAR SIDE-EFFECTS OF BETA-SYMPATHOMIMETIC DRUGS

Those obstetricians and physicians who practice in Western communities are more likely to see pulmonary oedema related to treatment of other conditions in pregnancy, than to structural heart disease. Although adverse cardiovascular side-effects of salbutamol and other beta-sympathomimetic agents given in premature labour have been reported, there is still a general lack of awareness of their importance. Whitehead *et al* (1979) reported the occurrence of chest pain and ischaemic *ECG* changes in one patient treated for five hours with intravenous salbutamol (4.2 mg), and subsequently reported pulmonary oedema in another patient given salbutamol 2.2 mg i.v. over six hours (Whitehead *et al* 1980). They suggested that vasodilation caused by concurrent administration of hydralazine and methyldopa for hypertension might be an additional factor in increasing circulating blood volume, and cited one similar maternal death reported to the Committee of Safety of Medicines after the use of salbutamol and methyldopa. Davies and Robertson (1980) reported another case of pulmonary oedema after the use of higher infusion rates of salbutamol (20 μg per minute) over a longer period (56 hours). In this case, betamethasone was used, and this may also have increased the circulating blood volume. These authors suggested that ergometrine given after delivery may have decreased the venous capacitance and thus contributed to the development of pulmonary oedema.

In North America, terbutaline (Bricanyl) is used to treat premature labour. It has the advantage that it can be given subcutaneously. Stubblefield (1978) reported one case of pulmonary oedema in which dexamethasone administration was an additional risk factor. Rogge *et al* (1979) reported three similar cases and cited knowledge of six other cases occurring in California. Pulmonary oedema has also been reported with the use of fenoterol (Kubli 1977) and ritodrine (Elliott *et al* 1978; Tinga and Aarnoudse 1979).

Beta-sympathomimetics are widely used for the treatment of premature labour (Lewis *et al* 1980) even though there are contradictory reports concerning their efficacy (Hemminki and Starfield 1978). They cause tachycardia both directly and reflexly because of associated vasodilitation. Both the tachycardia and the increased blood volume associated with vasodilation may contribute to the risk of pulmonary oedema, particularly if the vascular capacitance is suddenly reduced by ergometrine (Davies and Robertson 1980). In addition, beta-sympathomimetic agents have metabolic effects. They cause a rise in blood glucose by increasing glycogenolysis and decreasing glucose uptake (*see also* p. 373). Free fatty acid and lactate concentrations increase, and hypokalaemia has also been reported (Hastwell and Lambert 1978). These factors may further impair myocardial function in a situation which is already haemodynamically unfavourable. Although it has been suggested that tachycardia alone (Poole Wilson 1980) and/or circulatory overload (Davies 1980; Fogarty 1980) are the real causes of pulmonary oedema in these patients, this seems unlikely. Pulmonary oedema is a rare complication of modern obstetrics, and its occurrence on so many occasions with the use of beta-sympathomimetics suggests that there is specific interaction.

Since there is no universal belief in the efficacy of beta-sympathomimetics, and because of the maternal risk, the following guidelines are suggested concerning their use for the treatment of premature labour. Beta-sympathomimetic infusions should not be given for more than 24 hours, except in exceptional circumstances. The risk of cardiovascular side-effects increases in infusions given for more than 24 hours. Beta-sympathomimetic drugs should be given with great care to patients with pre-existing heart disease. The nature and severity of the heart disease are obviously critical (e.g. there would probably be no additional risk of giving salbutamol to a patient with mild mitral regurgitation, whereas such therapy could be fatal in a patient with severe mitral stenosis). If beta-sympathomimetric drugs are used, the obstetrician should be aware of the risk of other therapies. Glucocorticoids will exacerbate hyperglycaemia as well as causing an increase in circulating blood volumes due to associated mineralocorticoid activity. This will be exacerbated by vasodilator drugs, so scrupulous attention must also be paid to fluid balance and the maternal heart rate.

PART 2   SPECIFIC CONDITIONS OCCURRING DURING PREGNANCY

Many specific conditions have already been mentioned in this chapter. However, some give particular management problems and are considered further below.

Acquired heart disease

CHRONIC RHEUMATIC HEART DISEASE

As already indicated, this form of heart disease has been commonest in pregnancy in the UK and still is in many parts of the world. Szekely and his colleagues from Newcastle have given exhaustive accounts of rheumatic heart disease in pregnancy (Szekely *et al* 1973; Szekely and Snaith 1974). By far the most important lesion is mitral stenosis, which may be the only lesion or the dominant abnormality amongst several others. Women with mitral stenosis are particularly likely to develop pulmonary oedema in pregnancy because of the increase in cardiac output, the increase in heart rate preventing ventricular filling and the increase in pulmonary blood volume (Burwell and Metcalfe 1958). Mitral stenosis is the lesion that is most likely to require treatment for pulmonary oedema, or heart failure (*see above*) and also to require surgery during pregnancy. Mitral regurgitation puts a volume load on the left atrium and left ventricle, but it does not cause pulmonary hypertension until late in the condition, and heart failure is rare in pregnancy; it usually occurs in older women. Endocarditis is more common in patients with mitral regurgitation, particularly if they are in sinus rhythm. It is now realised that many patients who were thought to have rheumatic mitral regurgitation do in fact have congenital abnormalities of the mitral valve. Although such abnormalities may be associated with arrhythmias and endocarditis, this is uncommon, particularly in pregnancy.

Rheumatic aortic valve disease is much less common in women than in men, and much less common than mitral valve disease in pregnancy. Severe aortic regurgitation causes pulmonary oedema; aortic stenosis may be associated with chest pain, syncope and sudden death, but both conditions are usually not severe enough to be a problem in pregnancy.

Disease of the tricuspid valve almost never occurs in isolation. Also, tricuspid valve disease rarely requires specific treatment; the patient improves when the rheumatic disease of the other valves is treated, either medically or surgically. Although there are case reports of successful pregnancy following triple valve replacement (aortic, mitral and tricuspid) it is unusual for such surgery to be necessary in patients within the reproductive age group (Nagorney and Field 1981).

ACUTE RHEUMATIC FEVER

Because of the overall decline in incidence of rheumatic fever, acute rheumatic fever is now very uncommon in pregnancy. The diagnosis may often be missed in patients who only complain of non-specific malaise and joint pains, and who, on investigation, only have fever and anaemia that does not respond to haematinics. The more florid signs of swollen joints, rheumatic nodules and skin rashes do not necessarily occur in adults. The diagnosis may be made on the basis of a history of previous sore throat, elevated ASO titre, and ECG evidence of prolonged PR and QT_c intervals. The ESR should be elevated to more than 80 mm per hour, since levels of 60 mm per hour are common in pregnancy. If rheumatic fever does develop in pregnancy, it is likely to be severe with a high risk of heart failure from the myocarditis, which is part of the triad of pericarditis and endocarditis. Treatment should be with bedrest, salicylates, steroids, and penicillin therapy (for any residual streptococcal infection). The patient should then receive a prolonged period of prophylactic penicillin therapy. Chorea, another manifestation of the rheumatic process, is described in Chapter 14.

PREGNANCY IN PATIENTS WITH ARTIFICIAL HEART VALVES

As described earlier, anticoagulation is the major problem in these patients. Those patients who have successful isolated aortic or mitral valve replacements usually have near normal cardiac function and do not incur haemodynamic problems in pregnancy (Oakley 1983). Even those patients with multiple valve replacements usually have sufficient cardiac reserve for a successful pregnancy (Andrinopoulos and Arias 1980).

The problem of anticoagulation is shown in series from Hammersmith Hospital, London (Oakley and Doherty 1976), the National Maternity Hospital, Dublin (O'Neil *et al* 1983) and Hong Kong (Chen *et al* 1982). In the Dublin series of 18 pregnancies, all the patients were anticoagulated and there were eight fetal losses, and one case of warfarin embryopathy. In the Hammersmith series, 24 pregnancies, not treated with anticoagulants (usually because they had biological valves) resulted in 23 normal babies. Fifteen pregnancies treated with oral anticoagulants resulted in only seven healthy babies. In the Hong Kong series there were ten fetal losses in 30 pregnancies treated with anticoagulants but only one fetal loss in the group not treated with anticoagulants. Although it is clear that the long-term outlook is not so good for patients with artificial heart valves (Kirklin 1981), there is no doubt that these are superior in pregnancy.

MYOCARDIAL INFARCTION

Myocardial infarction is rare in pregnancy and in young women in general. Only 1 per cent of admissions for myocardial infarction occur in women younger than 45 years (Peterson *et al* 1972). Cortis *et al* (1979) cite only 76 cases of myocardial infarction in pregnancy in the literature since 1922. Most of these cases were in women aged 30–40 years. The immediate mortality was 26 per cent; some women died up to four years after the original event, making the overall mortality 32 per cent. In contrast to myocardial infarction occurring during pregnancy, myocardial infarction in the puerperium occurs in younger, often primigravid women. Their pregnancies have frequently been complicated by pre-eclampsia (Beary *et al* 1979). The precise mechanism of myocardial infarction is open to speculation in all patients. Women have a particularly high incidence of coronary spasm, and atypical mechanisms seem to be common in pregnancy. Beary *et al* (1979) suggest that the group of patients with mycocaridal infarction occurring in the puerperium are those that are most likely to have spasm or coronary artery thrombosis unassociated with atherosclerotic narrowing as documented by Ciraulo and Markovitz (1979). Another possible cause is primary dissection of the coronary arteries (Bulkley and Roberts 1973).

The diagnosis of myocardial infarction in pregnancy will be made on the basis of chest pain, with possible pericardial friction rub and fever. Only serial electrocardiographic changes are meaningful, because of the ECG changes induced by pregnancy itself. Moderate elevations of the white cell count and ESR are seen in normal pregnancy, when the level of lactic acid dehydrogenase may also be raised (Stone *et al* 1960). However, elevation of serum glutamic acid transaminase level would indicate myocardial infarction in the appropriate clinical setting (Stone *et al* 1960). During the puerperium even this enzyme will not be helpful, because it is liberated by the associated tissue destruction. The differential diagnosis of other occult causes of collapse in pregnancy is considered on p. 100 and in Table 4.1.

It is difficult to be dogmatic about management, since there is little experience and the pathology may be diverse. It would be sensible to treat the initial episode in a coronary care unit, with conventional opiate analgesics and medication for complications such as dysrhythmias. Because of the possibility of coronary spasm, nitroglycerine or other vasodilators should be used early in patients with continuing pain. Once the patient has been delivered, there is a good case for coronary arteriography to delineate the pathology which may be atypical. The angiographic demonstration of coronary embolus would be an indication for anticoagulation, but otherwise, the benefits of anticoagulation in myocardial infarction unassociated with pregnancy do not seem great enough to justify the considerable extra risks imposed on the pregnancy. Patients should be allowed a spontaneous vaginal delivery, unless there are good obstetric reasons for interfering. However, as in other cases of heart disease, the second stage should be limited by forceps delivery. Syntocinon infusion should be used rather than ergometrine in the third stage, since ergometrine is more likely to cause coronary artery spasm. There is no evidence that pregnancy predisposes to myocardial infarction. Unless it is thought that the patient has had a coronary embolus, pregnancy should not be discouraged in patients who have had myocardial infarction in the past.

CARDIOMYOPATHY IN PREGNANCY (HOCM)

Cardiomyopathy may arise *de novo* during pregnancy, and there is probably at least one form of cardiomyopathy (pregnancy cardiomyopathy, *see below*) that is specific to pregnancy. Alternatively, any form of cardiomyopathy due to other causes may complicate pregnancy. By far the most common of these other causes is hypertrophic obstructive cardiomyopathy (HOCM, subaortic stenosis) and even this condition is relatively rare. The cause is not known, but the pathological features are hypertrophy and disorganisation of cardiac muscle, particularly that of the left ventricular outflow tract. The patients present with chest pain, syncope, arrhythmias, or the symptoms of heart failure.

Extensive experience of the management of this condition in pregnancy has been reported by Oakley and colleagues from the Hammersmith Hospital (Oakley *et al* 1979). These authors originally advocated beta-adrenergic blockade in all cases to reduce the risk of syncope, due to obstruction of left ventricular outflow tract (Turner *et al* 1968); this is now reserved for symptomatic patients only. Patients should not be allowed to become hypovolaemic, since this too increases the risk of obstruction of the left ventricular outflow tract. Particular care should be taken to give adequate fluid replacement if these patients have an antepartum haemorrhage and also to avoid postpartum haemorrhage. During labour, patients with hypertrophic obstructive cardiomyopathy should not have epidural anaesthesia, since this causes relative hypovolaemia by increasing venous capacitance in the lower limbs.

PREGNANCY CARDIOMYOPATHY

This condition was first described by Hull & Hafkesbring (1937) and was extensively reviewed by Stuart (1968) and Meadows (1957) whose papers should be consulted for further references. The patient presents with heart failure, usually right sided, either at the end of pregnancy or more commonly in the puerperium. If the condition does arise in the puerperium, the patient is almost invariably breast feeding (Stuart 1968). There is no predisposing cause for the heart failure and the heart is grossly dilated. The patients are usually multiparous, black, relatively elderly and of poor social class. Pregnancy has often been complicated by hypertension. Pulmonary, peripheral and particularly cerebral embolisation is a major cause of morbidity and mortality. Apart from conventional antifailure treatment, these patients should also receive anticoagulant therapy until the heart size has returned to normal, and until they have no further dysrhythmias. Assuming that the patients recover from the initial episode, the long-term prognosis is good, but the conditions may re-occur in future pregnancies.

The pathogenesis is unknown; therefore some authors have denied that pregnancy cardiomyopathy is a specific entity (Brown *et al* 1967) and considered the condition to be another form of congestive cardiomyopathy caused by hypertension (Benchimol *et al* 1959). Rand *et al* (1975) on the basis of antibodies to heart muscle present in cord blood and serum from the mother in a case of pregnancy cardiomyopathy, postulate an immunological cause. Alternatively, the combination of multiparity and low social class has suggested that the condition is due to an undefined nutritional defect. Melvin *et al* (1983) have recently described three cases of peripartum cardiomyopathy due to myocarditis, proven by endomyocardial biopsy at cardiac catheterisation, and these authors propose that infection may be an important cause.

Davidson and Parry (1978) have described a specific form of peripartum cardiac failure occurring in the Hausa tribe in Northern Nigeria. They were able to document 224 cases and claimed that in the peak season, in summer, half the female medical beds in Zaria are occupied by patients with this condition. The peak incidence is four weeks postpartum. During this period, for up to 40 days after delivery, the Hausa woman spends 18 hours per day lying on a mud bed, heated so that the ambient temperature reaches 40°C. She also increases her sodium intake to 450 mmol/day by eating *kanwa* salt from Lake Chad. Many of the patients are hypertensive, but the condition regresses rapidly with diuretic and digoxin therapy, which causes a weight loss of 29 per cent in 15 days. The contribution of hypertension to the heart failure is debated (Sanderson 1977) but this would seem an extreme example of the instability of the cardiovascular system in the first few weeks of the puerperium. Blood volume and cardiac output must fall while peripheral resistance rises after delivery. The practices of the Hausa tribe will cause a marked rise in circulating blood volume, which would probably be sufficient to produce clinical cardiac failure. The high incidence of heart failure in the Hausa tribe demonstrates the vulnerability of the cardiovascular system in the puerperium, and perhaps explains why so many of Stuart's cases presented at this time. If peripheral vascular resistance rises very rapidly, before cardiac output falls, systemic hypertension will ensue, as is occasionally seen in patients who have no history of antecedent hypertension in pregnancy before delivery.

Congenital heart disease

EISENMENGER'S SYNDROME

As indicated above, Eisenmenger's syndrome has a very high maternal mortality. Only recently has there been any form of surgical treatment and this, heart and lung transplantation, must be considered experimental (Reitz *et al* 1982). Most patients with Eisenmenger's syndrome that die, do so in the puerperium. Although deaths are occasionally sudden, due to thromboembolism, this is not usually so. More frequently, these patients die due to a slowly falling systemic Pao_2 with associated decrease in cardiac output. A consideration of the haemodynamics involved (Fig. 5.2) suggests how this might occur and how it could be managed. In a defect, such as a large ventricular septal defect, the blood is freely mixed in the right and left ventricles, and the ratio of blood flows in the pulmonary circuit (Q_p) to systemic circuit (Q_s) is inversely proportional to the ratio of the pulmonary resistance (R_p) to the systemic resistance (R_s), i.e.

$$Q_p/Q_s \propto R_s/R_p$$

Pulmonary blood flow is also proportional to cardiac output (CO) so

$$Q_p \propto CO \times R_s/R_p$$

Thus any fall in the ratio R_s/R_p will cause a fall in pulmonary blood flow. For example, in pre-eclamptic toxaemia, the pulmonary vascular resistance increases and the cardiac output falls (Littler *et al* 1973). These factors would therefore decrease pulmonary blood flow and this could account for the observed deterioration in Eisenmenger's syndrome, associated with hypertensive pregnancy (Morgan Jones & Howitt 1965).

What can be offered to the pregnant patient with Eisenmenger's syndrome? Unfortunately, abortion would appear to be the answer. The maternal mortality

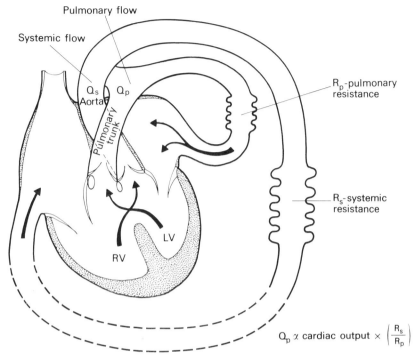

Fig. 5.2 Pulmonary and systemic blood flows and resistances in Eisenmenger's syndrome associated with ventricular septal defect (*see* text). (Courtesy of the Editor, *Journal of the Royal College of Physicians.*)

associated with abortion is only 7 per cent in comparison to 30 per cent for continuing pregnancy (Gleicher *et al* 1979). However, if the patient decides to continue with pregnancy, prophylactic anticoagulation, probably with subcutaneous heparin, should be offered, because of the risk of thromboembolism, both systemic and pulmonary. Labour should not be induced unless there are good obstetric reasons. Induced labour carries a higher risk of Caesarean section which is associated with a particularly high maternal mortality in Eisenmenger's syndrome (Gleicher *et al* 1979).

There is controversy concerning the place of epidural anaesthesis for the management of labour. Although epidural anaesthesia could decrease the Q_p/Q_s ratio by decreasing the systemic vascular resistance, this does not occur, at least in the one case studied by Midwall *et al* (1978). On balance, a carefully administered elective epidural anaesthetic at the beginning of labour is probably preferable to emergency epidural or general anaesthesia if it is suddenly decided that instrumental delivery is necessary (Gleicher 1979; Crawford 1971).

If the patient does become hypotensive with increasing cyanosis and decreasing cardiac output, it has been shown that high inspired oxygen concentrations will decrease pulmonary vascular resistance, increase the Q_p/Q_s ratio and increase peripheral oxygen saturation (Midwall *et al* 1978). In addition, alpha-sympathomimetic agents, such as phenylephrine, methoxamine and noradrenaline, will increase R_s and thus increase pulmonary blood flow (Devitt and Noble 1980). However, drugs such such as tolazoline, phentolamine, nitroprusside and isoprenaline, which have been used to decrease pulmonary vascular resistance in other clinical situations, probably should not be given, since they will also decrease the systemic vascular resistance (Devitt and Noble 1980). If R_s decreases more than R_p, pulmonary blood flow will decrease rather than increase. The same problem occurs with dopamine and beta-sympathomimetic drugs which have been given to increase cardiac output. They too will decrease R_s and if R_s decreases more than the cardiac output increases, pulmonary blood flow will fall. In summary, the management of the deteriorating patients with Eisenmenger's syndrome depends on giving oxygen and alpha-sympathomimetic amines.

COARCTATION OF THE AORTA AND MARFAN'S SYNDROME

In both these conditions, the maternal risk is of dissection of the aorta associated with the hyperdynamic circulation of pregnancy and possibly with an increased risk of medial degeneration due to the hormonal environment of pregnancy (Konishi *et al* 1980). The maternal mortality in coarction has been stated to be as high as 17 per cent (Mendelson 1940). It has therefore been suggested that all patients with coarctation presenting in pregnancy should either be aborted or have the defect repaired before delivery. However, Mendelson's series dates from 1858 to 1939, and there have only been 14 maternal deaths reported in the whole literature, none of which occurred in the 83 patients studied since 1960 (Deal and Wooley 1973). The risk of dissection has therefore probably been exaggerated and good obstetric care and effective antihypertensive therapy would decrease the risk still further. It is probable that we no longer see the patients similar to those of Mendelson's series, since most patients with severe coarctation are operated on in infancy. Only those patients who already have evidence of dissection should have the coarctation repaired in pregnancy. Any upper limb hypertension should be treated aggressively with antihypertensive drugs (Benny *et al* 1980). If there is gross widening of the ascending aorta suggesting intrinsic disease of the aorta, the patient should be delivered by elective Caesarean section to reduce the risk of dissection associated with labour.

Some authors also consider the risk of dissection to be so high in Marfan's syndrome that they advise avoidance of pregnancy or termination if there is any degree of aortic dilation (Pyeritz and McKusick 1979). Again, this seems an extreme attitude, which Pyeritz has modified to suggest that dilation of the aorta to more than 40 mm (as determined echocardiographically) should be the limit at which pregnancy is contraindicated (Pyeritz 1981). Some patients and families with Marfan's syndrome have *formes frustes* of the condition where there may be arachnodactyly, a high arch palate, lens abnormalities and long patella tendons with no evidence of disease of the aorta or aortic valves; there may only be minor mitral valve abnormalities, if there is any cardiac disease at all. The families tend to 'breed true', and pregnancy would confer no extra risk. Therefore, there cannot be an overall condemnation of pregnancy in all cases of Marfan's syndrome (Beighton 1982). Even if the patient does have involvement of the aorta, the number of cases of dissection reported in pregnancy is extemely small. It is therefore unlikely that the risk is very high, and I believe that pregnancy should be allowed to continue in all but the most severe cases.

Pyeritz (1981) has recently reported a series of pregnancies in 26 women with Marfan's syndrome. There was only one fatality and that patient died from endocarditis. As in coarctation of the aorta, any associated hypertension should be treated aggressively, and delivery should be by Caesarean section if there is evidence of aortic disease. Spontaneous uterine inversion has been reported in one case of Marfan's syndrome in pregnancy, possibly due to a generalised abnormality of connective tissue (Quinn and Mukerjee 1982).

CONGENITAL HEART BLOCK

This is usually no problem in pregnancy. Although part of the normal response to pregnancy includes an increase in heart rate to increase the cardiac output, this is not obligatory. There are many records of successful pregnancy in patients with heart block, both paced (Ginns and Holinrake 1970) and not paced (Szekely and Snaith 1974). Presumably, they are able to increase stroke volume sufficiently to cope with the increased demands of pregnancy. A few patients are unable to increase cardiac output sufficiently at the end of pregnancy or during labour (Bowman and Millar-Craig 1980). Therefore, patients with heart block who are not paced, or those where there is any question of pacemaker failure, should be managed in obstetric units where there is access to pacing facilities.

References

Ahmad R., Rajah S.M., Mearns A.J. & Deverall P.B. (1976) Dipyridamole in successful management of pregnant women with prosthetic heart valve. *Lancet* **2**, 1414–15.

Andersen J.B. (1970) The effect of diuretics in late pregnancy on the new born infant. *Acta Paediatrica Scandinavica* **59**, 659–63.

Andrinopoulos G.C. & Arias F. (1980) Triple heart valve prosthesis and pregnancy. *Obstetrics and Gynaecology* **55**, 762–4.

Bader R.A., Bader M.E., Rose D.J. & Braunwald E. (1955) Haemodynamics at rest and during exercise in normal pregnancy as studied by cardiac catheterization. *Journal of Clinical Investigation* **34**, 1524–36.

Bahary C.M., Ninio A., Gorodesky I.G. & Weri A. (1980) Tococardiography in pregnancy during extra corporeal bypass for mital valve replacement. *Israel Journal of Medical Science* **16**, 395–7.

Barabas A.B. (1967) Heterogeneity of the Ehlers–Danlos syndrome: description of three clinical types and a hypothesis to explain the basic defect(s). *British Medical Journal* **2**, 612–13.

Batson G.A. (1974) Cyanotic congenital heart disease and pregnancy. *British Journal of Obstetrics and Gynaecology* **81**, 549–53.

Beary J.F., Sumner W.R. & Bulkley B.H. (1979) Postpartum acute myocardial infarction: A rare occurrence of uncertain etiology. *American Journal of Cardiology* **43**, 158–60.

Beighton P. (1982) Pregnancy in the Marfan syndrome. *British Medical Journal* **285**, 464.

Benchimol A.B., Carneiro R.D. & Schlesinger P. (1959) Post-partum heart disease. *British Heart Journal* **21**, 89–100.

Bennett G.G. & Oakley C.M. (1968) Pregnancy in a patient with a mitral valve prosthesis. *Lancet* **1**, 616–19.

Benny P.S., Prasao J. & MacVicar J. (1980) Pregnancy and coarctation of the aorta. Case Report. *British Journal of Obstetrics and Gynaecology* **87**, 1159–61.

Biale Y., Cantor A., Lewenthal H. & Gueron M. (1980) The course of pregnancy in patients with artificial heart valves treated with dipyridamole. *International Journal of Obstetrics and Gynaecology* **18**, 128–32.

Boyle D.McC. & Lloyd-Jones R.L. (1966) The electrocardiographic S–T segment in pregnancy. *Journal of Obstetrics and Gynaecology of the British Commonwealth* **73**, 986–7.

Bowman P.R. & Millar-Craig M.W. (1980) Congenital heart block and pregnancy: a further case report. *Journal of Obstetrics and Gynaecology* **1**, 98–9.

Brown A.K., Doukas N., Riding W.D. & Wyn Jones E. (1967) Cardiomyopathy and pregnancy. *British Heart Journal* **29**, 387–93.

Buemann B. & Kragelund E. (1962) Clinical assessment of heart disease during pregnancy. *Acta Obstetrica et Gynecologica Scandinavica Supplement* **41**, 57–79.

Bulkley B.H. & Roberts W.C. (1973) Dissecting anneyrysm (haematoma) limited to coronary artery. *American Journal of Medicine* **55**, 747–56.

Burch G.E. (1980) Certain principles in the management of heart disease and pregnancy. *American Heart Journal* **100**, 775–7.

Burwell C.S. & Metcalfe J. (1958) *Heart Disease and Pregnancy; Physiology and Management.* Little Brown, Boston, Mass.

Carr F.B., Hamilton B.E. & Palmer R.S. (1933) The significance of large Q in lead III of the electrocardiogram during pregnancy. *American Heart Journal* **8**, 519.

Carruth S.E., Mirvis S.B., Brogan D.R. & Wenger N.K. (1981) The electrocardiogram in normal pregnancy. *American Heart Journal* **102**, 1075–8.

Chen W.W.C., Chan C.S., Lee P.K., Wang Ryc & Wong V.C.W. (1982) Pregnancy in patients with Prosthetic Heart Valves: an experience with 45 pregnancies. *Quarterly Journal of Medicine* **51**, 358–65.

Chesley L.C. (1980) Severe rheumatic cardiac disease and pregnancy: The ultimate prognosis. *American Journal of Obstetrics and Gynecology* **136**, 552–8.

Ciraulo D.A. & Markovitz A. (1979) Myocardial infarction in pregnancy associated with a coronary artery thrombosis. *Archives of Internal Medicine* **139**, 1046–7.

Conradsson T.B. & Werkö L. (1974) Management of heart disease in pregnancy. *Progress in Cardiovascular Disease* **16**, 407–19.

Copeland W.E., Wooley C.F., Ryan J.M., Runco V. & Levin H.S. (1963) Pregnancy and congenital heart disease. *American Journal of Obstetrics and Gynecology* **86**, 107–10.

Cortis B.S., Freese E., Luisada A.A., Motto S. & Zummo B. (1979) Precordial pain and myocardial infarction in pregnancy. *Gionale Italiano Cardiologica* **9**, 532–4.

Cotrill C.M., McAllister R.G. Jr., Gettes L. & Noonan J.A. (1977) Propranolol therapy during pregnancy, labor and delivery: evidence for transplacental drug transfer and impaired neonatal drug disposition. *Journal of Pediatrics* **91**, 812–14.

Crawford J.S., Mills W.G. & Pentecost B.L. (1971) A pregnant patient with Eisenmenger's Syndrome. *British Journal of Anaesthesia* **43**, 1091–4.

Cutforth R. & MacDonald C.B. (1966) Heart sounds and murmurs in pregnancy. *American Heart Journal* **71**, 741–7.

Dacie J. (1975) *Practical Haematology*, pp. 413–14. Churchill Livingstone, Edinburgh.

Davidson N. McD. & Parry E.H.O. (1978) Peri-partum cardiac failure. *Quarterly Journal of Medicine* **47**, 431–61.

Davies A.E. & Robertson M.J.S. (1980) Pulmonary oedema after the administration of intravenous salbutamol and ergometrine. *British Journal of Obstetrics and Gynaecology* 87, 539–41.

Deal K. & Wooley C.F. (1973) Coarctation of the Aorta and Pregnancy. *Annals of Internal Medicine* 78, 706–10.

Department of Health & Social Security (1982) *Report on Confidential Enquiries into Maternal Deaths in England and Wales 1976–1978.* HMSO, London.

de Swiet M (1980) The cardiovascular system. In Hytten F. and Chamberlain G. (eds) *Clinical Physiology in Obstetrics.* Blackwell Scientific Publications, Oxford.

de Swiet M. & Fidler J. (1981) Heart disease in pregnancy: Some controversies. *Journal of the Royal College of Physicians* 15, 183–6.

de Swiet M., de Louvois J. & Hurley R. (1975) Failure of cephalosporins to Prevent Bacterial endocarditis during labour. *Lancet* 2, 186.

Devitt J.H. & Noble W.H. (1980) Eisenmenger's syndrome and pregnancy. *New England Journal of Medicine* 302, 751.

Dubourg G. (1959) Correction complete d'une triade de Fallot en circulation extra-corporelle chez une femme enceinte. *Archives des Maladies du Coeur, des Vaisseux et du Sang* 52, 1389–91.

Dumesic D.A., Silverman N.H., Tobias D. & Golbus M.S. (1982) Transplacental cardioversion of fetal supraventricular tachycardia with procainamide. *New England Journal of Medicine* 307, 1128–31.

Durack D.T. (1975) Current practice in prevention of bacterial endocarditis. *British Heart Journal* 37, 478–81.

Eckstein H. & Jack B. (1970) Breast feeding and anticoagulant therapy. *Lancet* 1, 672–3.

Eilen B., Kaiser I.H., Becker R.M. & Cohen M.N. (1981) Aortic valve replacement in the third trimester of pregnancy: Case report and review of the literature. *Obstetrics and Gynecology* 57, 119–21.

Elliott H.R., Abdulla U. & Hayes P.J. (1978) Pulmonary oedema associated with ritodrine infusion and betamethasone administration in premature labour. *British Medical Journal* 2, 799–800.

Espino Vela J. & Alvarado-Toro A. (1971) Natural history of atrial septal defect. *Cardiovascular Clinics* 2, 104–25.

Etheridge M.J. (1966) Heart disease and pregnancy. *Medical Journal of Australia* 2, 1172.

Etheridge M.J. (1969) Heart disease and pregnancy. *Australian and New Zealand Journal of Obstetrics and Gynecology* 9, 7–11.

Fidler J., Smith V. & de Swiet M. (1983) Randomised controlled comparative study of methyl dopa and oxprenolol for the treatment of hypertension in pregnancy. *British Medical Journal* 286, 1927–30.

Fidler J., Fayers P.M.F., Smith V. & de Swiet M. (1983) The excretion of oxprenolol and timolol in breast milk. *British Journal of Obstetrics and Gynaecology* 90, 961–5.

Finlay A.Y. & Edmunds V. (1979) DC Cardioversion in pregnancy. *British Journal of Chemical Practice* 33, 88–94.

Fleming H.A. (1977) Antibiotic prophylaxis against infective endocarditis after delivery. *Lancet* 1, 144–5.

Fogarty A.J. (1980) Cardiac failure in a hypertensive woman receiving salbutamol for premature labour. *British Medical Journal* 281, 226.

Gallery E.D.M., Saunders D.M., Hunyor S.N. & Györy A.Z. (1978) Improvement in fetal growth with treatment of maternal hypertension in pregnancy. *Clinical Science and Molecular Medicine* 55, 359s–361s.

Garrod L.P. & Waterworth P.M. (1962) The risks of dental extraction during penicillin treatment. *British Heart Journal* **24**, 39–46.

Ginns H.M. & Holinrake K. (1970) Complete heart block in pregnancy treated with an internal cardiac pacemaker. *Journal of Obstetrics and Gynaecology of the British Commonwealth* **77**, 710.

Ginz B. (1970) Myocardial infarction in pregnancy. *Journal of Obstetrics and Gynaecology of the British Commonwealth* **77**, 610.

Gladstone G.R., Hordof A. & Gersony W.M. (1975) Propranolol administration during pregnancy: effects on the fetus. *Journal of Pediatrics* **86**, 962–4.

Gleicher N., Knutzen V.K., Elkayam U., Loew S. & Kerenyi T.D. (1979) Rheumatic heart disease diagnosed during pregnancy: A 30-year follow up. *International Journal of Gynaecology and Obstetrics* **17**, 51–7.

Habib A. & McArthy J.S. (1977) Effects on the neonate of propranolol administered during pregnancy. *Journal of Pediatrics* **91**, 808–11.

Hall J.G. (1981) Disorders of connective tissue and skeletal dysplasia. In Simpson J.L. and Shulman J.D. (ed.) pp. 57–87. *Genetic Disorders in Pregnancy*, Academic Press, New York.

Harrigan J.T., Kangos J.J., Sikka A., Spisso K.R., Natarajan N., Rosenfeld D., Leiman S. & Korn D. (1981) Successful treatment of fetal congestive heart failure secondary to tachycardia. *New England Journal of Medicine* **304**, 1527–1529.

Hastwell C. & Lambert B.E. (1978) The effect of oral salbutamol on serum potassium and blood sugar. *British Journal of Obstetrics and Gynaecology* **85**, 767–9.

Hemminki E. & Starfield B. (1978) Prevention and treatment of premature labour by drugs: Review of clinical trials. *British Journal of Obstetrics and Gynaecology* **85**, 411–17.

Ho P.C., Chen T.Y. & Wong V. (1980) The effect of maternal cardiac disease and digoxin administration on labour, fetal weight and maturity at birth. *Australia and New Zealand Journal of Obstetrics and Gynecology* **20**, 24–7.

Howitt G. (1971) Heart disease and pregnancy. *Practitioner* **206**, 765–72.

Hull E. & Haf Kesbring E. (1937) 'Toxic' postpartal heart disease. *New Orleans Medical and Surgical Journal* **89**, 550.

Husaini M.H. (1971) Myocardial infarction during pregnancy: report of two cases and review of the literature. *Postgraduate Medical Journal* **47**, 660.

Jacoby W.J. (1964) Pregnancy with tetralogy and pentalogy of Fallot. *American Journal of Cardiology* **14**, 866–73.

Jewett J.F. (1978) Two dissecting coronary artery aneurysms post partum. *New England Journal of Medicine* **278**, 1255–6.

Jewett J.F. (1979) Pulmonary hypertension and pre-eclampsia. *New England Journal of Medicine* **301**, 1063–4.

Kirklin J.W. (1981) The replacement of cardiac valves. *New England Journal of Medicine* **304**, 291–2.

Klein A.M., Holzman I.R. & Austin E.M. (1979) Fetal tachycardia prior to the development of hydrops—attempted pharmacological cardioversion: case report. *American Journal of Obstetrics and Gynecology* **134**, 347–8.

Konishi Y., Tatsuta N., Kumada K., Minami K., Matsuda K., Yamasato A., Usui N., Muraguchi T., Hikasa Y., Okamoto E. & Watanabe R. (1980) Dissecting aneurysm during pregnancy and the puerperium. *Japanese Circulation Journal* **44**, 726–32.

Kubli F. (1977) In Anderson A., Beard R., Brudenell M. and Dunn P.M. (eds) *Pre Term Labour*, pp. 218–20. Proceedings of the Fifth Study Group of the Royal College of Obstetricians and Gynaecologists. RCOG, London.

Lamb M.P., Ross K., Johnstone A.M. & Manners J.M. (1981) Fetal heart monitoring during open heart surgery. *British Journal of Obstetrics and Gynaecology* **88**, 669–74.

Larsen J.F., Jacobsen B., Holm H.H., Pedersen J.F. & Mantoni M. (1978) Intrauterine injection of vitamin K before the delivery during anticoagulant treatment of the mother. *Acta Obstetricia et Gynecologica Scandinavica Supplement* **57**, 227–30.

Leonard R.F., Braun T.E. & Levy A.M. (1978) Initiation of uterine contractions by disopyramide during pregnancy. *New England Journal of Medicine* **299**, 84.

Levy M., Grait L. & Laufer N. (1977) Excretion of drugs in human milk. *New England Journal of Medicine* **297**, 789.

Levy D.L., Warringer R.A. & Burgess G.E. (1980) Fetal response to cardiopulmonary bypass. *Obstetrics and Gynecology* **56**, 112–15.

Lewis P.J., de Swiet M., Boylan P. & Bulpitt C.J. (1980) How obstetricians in the United Kingdom manage preterm labour. *British Journal of Obstetrics and Gynaecology* **87**, 574–7.

Limet R. & Crondin C.M. (1977) Cardiac valve prothesis, anticoagulation and pregnancy. *Annals of Thoracic Surgery* **23**, 337–431.

Littler W.A., Redman C.W.G., Bonnar J., Berkin L.S. & Lee G.de.J. (1973) Reduced pulmonary arterial compliance in hypertensive pregnancy. *Lancet* **1**, 1274–8.

McLeod A.A., Jennings K.P. & Townsend E.R. (1978) Near fatal puerperal thrombosis on Björk-Sliley mital valve prosthesis. *British Heart Journal* **40**, 934–7.

Meadows W.R. (1957) Myocardial failure in the last trimester of pregnancy and the puerperium. *Circulation* **15**, 903–14.

Melvin K.R., Richardson P.J., Olsen E.G.J., Daly K. & Jackson G. (1982) Peripartum cariomyopathy due to myocarditis. *New England Journal of Medicine* **307**, 731–4.

Mendelson C.L. (1940) Pregnancy and coarctation of the aorta. *American Journal of Obstetrics and Gynecology* **39**, 1014–21.

Mendelson C.L. (1956) Disorders of the heart beat during pregnancy. *American Journal of Obstetrics and Gynecology* **72**, 1268.

Mendelson C.L. (1960) *Cardiac Disease in Pregnancy.* E.A. Davis Co., Philadelphia.

Metcalf J. (1968) Rheumatic heart disease in pregnancy. *Clinical in Obstetrics and Gynecology* **11**, 1010–25.

Midwall J., Jaffin H., Herman M.V. & Kuper Smith J. (1978) Shunt flow and pulmonary haemodynamics during labor and delivery in the Eisenmenger Syndrome. *American Journal of Cardiology* **42**, 299–303.

Milne J.A., Howie A.D. & Pack A.I. (1978) Dyspnoea during normal pregnancy. *British Journal of Obstetrics and Gynaecology* **85**, 260–3.

Morgan Jones A. & Howitt G. (1965) Eisenmenger Syndrome in pregnancy. *British Medical Journal* **1**, 1627–31.

Nagorney D.M. & Field C.S. (1981) Successful pregnancy 10 years after triple cardiac valve replacement. *Obstetrics and Gynecology* **57**, 386–8.

Neilson G., Galea E.G. & Blunt A. (1970) Congenital heart disease and pregnancy. *Medical Journal of Australia* **1**, 1086–8.

Newburger J.W. & Keane J.F. (1979) Intrauterine supraventricular tachycardia. *Journal of Pediatrics* **95**, 780–6.

Oakley C. (1983) Pregnancy in patients with prosthetic heart valves. *British Medical Journal* **286**, 1680–2.

Oakley C.M. & Doherty P. (1976) Pregnancy in patients after valve replacement. *British Heart Journal* **38**, 1140–8.

Oakley G.D.G., McGarry K., Limb D.G. & Oakley C.M. (1979) Management of pregnancy in patients with hypertrophic cardiomyopathy. *British Medical Journal* **1**, 1749–50.

Okita G.T., Plotz E.J. & Davis M.E. (1956) Placental transfer of radioactive digitoxin in pregnant woman and its fetal distribution. *Circulation Research* **4**, 376–80.

O'Neill H., Blake S., Sugrue D. & MacDonald D. (1983) Problems in the management of patients with artificial heart valves during pregnancy. *British Journal of Obstetrics and Gynaecology* (in press).

Ong H.C. & Puraviappan A.P. (1975) Congenital heart disease and pregnancy in the tropics. *Australia and New Zealand Journal of Obstetrics and Gynecology* **15**, 99–103.

Oram S. & Holt M. (1961) Innocent depression of the S.T. segment and flattening of the T-wave during pregnancy. *Journal of Obstetrics and Gynaecology of the British Commonwealth* **68**, 765–70.

Orme M. L'E., Lewis P.J., de Swiet M., Serlin M.J., Sibeon R., Baty J.D. & Breckenbridge A.M. (1977) May mothers given warfarin breast-feed their infants? *British Medical Journal* **1**, 1564–5.

Page P.A. & Toung T. (1975) A new probe for measurement of muscle PO_2 and its use during cardiopulmonary bypass. *Surgery, Gynecology and Obstetrics* **141**, 579–81.

Pearl W. & Spicer M. (1981) Ehlers–Danlos Syndrome. *Southern Medical Journal* **74**, 80–1.

Peterson D.R., Thomson D.J. & Chinn N. (1972) Ischaemic heart disease prognosis. A community-made assessment (1966–1969). *Journal of the American Medical Association* **219**, 1423–7.

Pitcher D., Leather H.M., Storey G.C.A. & Holt D.W. (1983) Amiodarone in pregnancy. *Lancet* **i**, 597–8.

Pitts J.A., Crosby W.M. & Basta L.C. (1977) Eisenmenger's syndrome in pregnancy. *American Heart Journal* **93**, 321–6.

Poole Wilson P.A. (1980) Cardiac failure in a hypertensive woman receiving salbutamol for premature labour. *British Medical Journal* **281**, 226.

Pope F.M. & Nicholls A.C. (1983) Pregnancy and Ehlers–Danlos syndrome type IV. *Lancet* **i**, 249–50.

Pyeritz R.E. (1981) Maternal and fetal complications of pregnancy in the Marfan syndrome. *American Journal of Medicine* **71**, 784–90.

Pyeritz R.E. & McKuisick V.A. (1979) The Marfan syndrome: diagnosis and management. *New England Journal of Medicine* **300**, 772–7.

Quinn R.J. & Mukerjee B. (1982) Spontaneous uterine inversion in association with Marfan's syndrome. *Australian and New Zealand Journal of Obstetrics and Gynaecology* **22**, 163–4.

Rand R.J., Jenkins D.M. & Scott D.G. (1975) Maternal cardiomyopathy of pregnancy causing stillbirth. *British Journal of Obstetrics and Gynaecology* **82**, 172–5.

Rayburn W.F. & Fontana M.E. (1981) Mitral valve prolapse and pregnancy. *American Journal of Obstetrics and Gynecology* **141**, 9–11.

Redick L.F. (1979) An inflatable wedge for prevention of aortocaval compression during pregnancy. *American Journal of Obstetrics and Gynecology* **133**, 458–9.

Redleaf P.D. & Farell E.J. (1959) Bacteremia during parturition—Prevention of subacute bacterial endocarditis. *Journal of the American Medical Association* **169**, 1284–5.

Reitz B.A., Wallwork J.L., Hunt S.A., Pennock J.L., Billingham M.E., Oyer P.E., Stinson E.B. & Shumway N.E. (1982) Heart–Lung transplantation. Successful therapy with pulmonary vascular disease. *New England Journal of Medicine* **306**, 557–64.

Report of a Working Party of the British Society for Antimicrobial Chemotherapy. (1982) The antibiotic prophylaxis of infective endocarditis. *Lancet* **ii**, 1323–6.

Rogers M.E., Willerson J.T., Goldblatt A. & Smith T.W. (1972) Serum digoxin concentrations in the human fetus, neonate and infant. *New England Journal of Medicine* **287**, 1010–13.

Rogge P., Young S. & Goodlin R. (1979) Post-partum pulmonary oedema associated with preventive therapy for premature labour. *Lancet* **1**, 1026–7.

Rubler S., Prabod Kumar M.D. & Pinto E.R. (1977) Cardiac size and performance during pregnancy estimated with echocardiography. *American Journal of Cardiology* **40**, 534–40.

Rudd N.L., Nimrod C., Holbrook K.A. & Byers P.H. (1983) Pregnancy complications in Type IV Ehlers–Danlos syndrome. *Lancet* **i**, 50–3.

Rush R.W., Verjand M. & Spracklen F.H.N. (1979) Incidence of heart disease in pregnancy. A study done at Peninsular Maternity Services Hospital. *South African Medical Journal* **55**, 808–10.

Saarikoski S. (1976) Placental transfer and fetal uptake of 3H-digoxin in humans. *British Journal of Obstetrics and Gynaecology* **83**, 879–84.

Sachs B.T. & Van Idekinge B. (1979) Successful pregnancy in a patient with autosomal dominant ventricular dysrhythmia. *American Journal of Obstetrics and Gynecology* **133**, 932–3.

St. John Sutton M.G., St. John Sutton M., Oldershaw P. *et al* (1981) Valve replacement without preoperative cardiac catheterization. *New England Journal of Medicine* **305**, 1233–8.

Sanderson J.E. (1977) Oedema and heart failure in the tropics. *Lancet* **2**, 1159–61.

Schaefer G., Arditi L.I., Solomon H.A. & Ringland J.E. (1968) Congenital heart disease and pregnancy. *Clinical Obstetrics and Gynecology* **11**, 1048–63.

Shaul W.L. & Hall J.G. (1977) Multiple congenital anomalies associated with oral anticoagulants. *American Journal of Obstetrics and Gynecology* **127**, 191–8.

Sherman J.L. & Locke R.V. (1960) Transplancental neonatal digitalis intoxication. *American Journal of Cardiology* **6**, 834.

Singh H., Bolton P.J. & Oakley C.M. (1982) Pregnancy after surgical correction of tetralogy of Fallot. *British Medical Journal* **285**, 168–70.

Sinneberg R.J. (1980) Pulmonary hypertension in pregnancy. *Southern Medical Journal* **73**, 1529–31.

Smith R.J., Radford D.J., Clark R.A. & Julian D.G. (1976) Infective endocarditis: a summary of cases in the South-East Region of Scotland 1969–72. *Thorax* **31**, 373–9.

Socol M.L., Conn J. & Frederiksen M.C. (1981) Pregnancy associated with partial aortic occlusion. *American Journal of Obstetrics and Gynecology* **139**, 965–7.

Stone M.L., Lending M., Slobody L.B. & Mestern J. (1960) Glutamine oxalacetic transaminase and lactic dehydrogenase in pregnancy. *American Journal of Obstetrics and Gynecology* **80**, 104.

Stuart K.L. (1968) Cardiomyopathy of pregnancy and the puerperium. *Quarterly Journal of Medicine* **37**, 463–78.

Stubblefield P.G. (1978) Pulmonary edema occurring after therapy with dexamethasone and terbutaline for premature labor: A case report. *American Journal of Obstetrics and Gynecology* **132**, 341–2.

Szekely P. & Snaith L. (1953) Paroxysmal tachycardia in pregnancy. *British Heart Journal* **15**, 195.

Szekely P., Turner R. & Snaith L. (1973) Pregnancy and the changing pattern of rheumatic heart disease. *British Heart Journal* **35**, 1293–1303.

Szekely P. & Snaith L. (1974) *Heart Disease and Pregnancy.* Churchill Livingstone, Edinburgh.

Sugrue D., Blake S., Troy P. & MacDonald D. (1980) Antibiotic prophylaxis against infective endocarditis after normal delivery—is it necessary? *British Heart Journal* **44**, 299–502.

Sugrue D., Blake S. & MacDonald D. (1981) Pregnancy complicated by maternal heart disease at the National Maternity Hospital, Dublin, Ireland, 1969 to 1978. *American Journal of Obstetrics and Gynecology* **139**, 1–6.

Sugrue D.D., Blake S. & MacDonald D. (1982) Infective endocarditis during pregnancy. *Journal of Obstetrics and Gynaecology* **2**, 210–14.

Teuscher A., Bossi E., Imhof P., Erb E., Stocker F.P. & Weber J.W. (1978) Effect of propranolol on fetal tachycardia in diabetic pregnancy. *American Journal of Cardiology* **42**, 304–7.

Timmis A.D., Jackson G. & Holt O.W. (1980) Mexiletine for control of ventricular dysrhythmias in pregnancy. *Lancet* **2**, 647–8.

Tinga D.H. & Aarnoudse J.G. (1979) Post-partum pulmonary oedema associated with preventative therapy for premature labour. *Lancet* **1**, 1026.

Trimkas A.P., Maxwell K.D., Berkay S., Gardner T.J. & Achuff S.C. (1979) Fetal monitoring during cardiopulmonary bypass for removal of a left atrial myxoma during pregnancy. *The Johns Hopkins Medical Journal* **144**, 156–60.

Turner G.M., Oakley C.M. & Dixon H.G. (1968) Management of pregnancy complicated by hypertrophic obstructive cardiomyopathy. *British Medical Journal* **4**, 281–4.

Ueland K., Gills R. & Hansen J.M. (1968) Maternal cardiovascular dynamics. I. Cesarean section under subarachnoid block anesthesia. *American Journal of Obstetrics and Gynecology* **100**, 42–53.

Ueland K., McAnulty J.H., Ueland F.R. & Metcalfe J. (1981) Special considerations in the use of cardiovascular drugs. *Clinical Obstetrics and Gynecology* **24**, 809–23.

Ueland K., Novy M.J. & Metcalfe S. (1972) Hemodynamic responses of patients with heart disease to pregnancy and exercise. *American Journal of Obstetrics and Gynecology* **113**, 47–59.

Weaver J.B. & Pearson J.F. (1973) Influence on time of onset and duration of labour in women with cardiac disease. *British Medical Journal* **2**, 519–20.

Webster J.C. (1913) The conduct of pregnancy and labor in acute and chronic affections of the heart. *Transactions of the American Gynecological Society* **38**, 223.

Whitehead M.L., Mander A.M., Hertogs K., Williams R.M. & Pettingale K.W. (1980) Acute congestive cardiac failure in a hypertensive woman receiving salbutamol for premature labour. *British Medical Journal* **1**, 1221–2.

Whitehead M.I., Mander A.M., Hertogs K. & Rothman M.T. (1979) Myocardial ischaemia after withdrawal of salbutamol for pre-term labour. *Lancet* **2**, 904.

Young B.K. & Haft J.I. (1970) Treatment of pulmonary edema with ethacrynic acid during labour. *American Journal of Obstetrics and Gynecology* **107**, 330–1.

Zitnik R.S., Brandenburg R.O., Sheldon R. & Wallace R.B. (1969) Pregnancy and open heart surgery. *Circulation* (Suppl) **39**, 257.

6   Hypertension in Pregnancy

Chris Redman

Cardiovascular changes in pregnancy

Cardiac output increases by about 40 per cent during the first trimester; measurements made in the lateral position show that this increase in the cardiac output is maintained during the third trimester (Lees *et al* 1967b; Ueland *et al* 1969). If measurements are made in the supine position, cardiac output declines during the third trimester (Ueland *et al* 1969; Bader *et al* 1955; Walters *et al* 1966), because in this position venous return to the heart is obstructed by the gravid uterus. This acutely reduces cardiac output by 20 per cent or more (Lees *et al* 1967a).

Arterial pressure begins falling in the first trimester, when the cardiac output is already rising, and continues to a nadir in midpregnancy (MacGillivray *et al* 1969) (Fig. 6.1). It is exclusively determined by total peripheral resistance and cardiac output, so these observations indicate a profound fall in arterial resistance (Bader *et al* 1955) beginning in the first trimester. This must be a systemic change, because at this time the uteroplacental circulation is not large enough to affect total peripheral resistance. During the third trimester both systolic and diastolic readings slowly rise to about the prepregnant levels (MacGillivray *et al* 1969). At this stage the measurements are peculiarly dependent on posture. In the supine position, with vena-caval compression and reduced venous return, arterial pressure is maintained by reflex peripheral vasoconstriction (Lees *et al* 1967a), which causes a narrowing of the pulse pressure

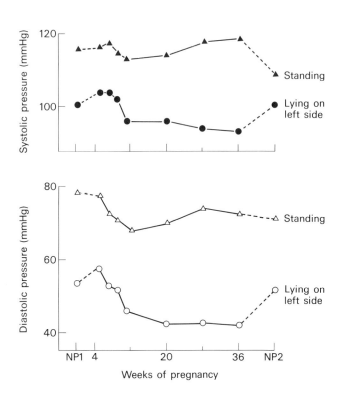

Fig. 6.1   The arterial pressures of ten women were measured using a London School of Hygiene sphygmomanometer to reduce observer bias. Readings were taken in the right arm and phase IV of the Korotkoff sounds defined the diastolic pressures. Pressures taken before conception (NP1), during pregnancy, and six weeks after delivery (NP2) are shown, both standing (▲,△) and supine on the left side (●,○). The fall in both systolic and diastolic pressures in the first trimester is clearly seen.

(Holmes 1960). Nevertheless, the systolic pressure may fall in 10 per cent of cases by more than 30 per cent (Holmes 1960). Signs and symptoms of 'supine hypotension' may then occur, including restlessness, faintness, hyperpnoea and pallor. There may also be aortic compression in the supine position (Bienarz *et al* 1968), which can mimic a minor degree of aortic coarctation causing higher arterial pressures in the arm than in the leg. At least some cases of late gestational hypertension may be caused by this change alone (Scanlon 1974).

The reduced peripheral resistance of normal pregnancy is associated with relative arterial refractoriness to the constrictor actions of exogenous angiotensin II but not noradrenaline (Gant *et al* 1973; Raab *et al* 1956). Reduced reactivity to angiotensin II can be detected at eight weeks' gestation and is maximal at midpregnancy (Gant *et al* 1973). The mechanism of this blunted responsiveness has not been elucidated but it may be prostaglandin dependent.

Prostaglandin E_2 enhances the arterial refractoriness to angiotensin II in pregnant (but not non-pregnant) women (Broughton Pipkin *et al* 1982), whereas prostaglandin synthetase inhibitors have the opposite effect (Everett *et al* 1978a). Oestrogens and progesterone have no effect (Chesley and Tepper 1967) but a metabolite of progesterone, 5 α-dihydroprogesterone which is present in pregnancy plasma at high concentrations, also enhances arterial refractoriness to angiotensin II (Everett *et al* 1978b).

FACTORS INFLUENCING BLOOD PRESSURE IN NORMAL PREGNANCY

In non-gravid individuals, blood pressure levels are influenced by age, sex, race, body-build and many other factors, particularly the circumstances under which the measurement is taken. Pregnant women are usually young and fit. The range of their blood pressures therefore tends to be narrower than in the general population; it is distributed around mean levels which change at different stages of gestation but which in midpregnancy are lower than in a comparable non-pregnant population.

The term 'hypertension in pregnancy' carries three implications:

1   That it is possible to measure blood pressure accurately.

2   That a gravid woman's status can be characterised by one or more blood pressure readings.

3   That there is a threshold above which hypertension can be diagnosed.

Errors in the measurement of blood pressure

The indirect method of measuring blood pressure gives an approximate estimate of the true intra-arterial pressure. There is no agreement as to the cause or magnitude of the discrepancies between direct and indirect measurements even in non-pregnant subjects (Pickering 1968a). In two studies of simultaneous measurements in pregnant women the direct readings differed on average from indirect readings by $-6/-15$ and $+5/-7$ mmHg respectively (Ginsberg and Duncan 1969; Raftery and Ward 1968). The discrepancies were not related to the level of blood pressure, arm skinfold thickness or arm circumference (Raftery and Ward 1968). Nevertheless, it is generally agreed that hypertension in obese individuals is overdiagnosed if a cuff is used which is too small in relation to the patient's arm circumference. The discrepancy becomes important for individuals with arm circumferences over 35 cm for whom either a larger arm cuff (15×33 cm) or even a thigh cuff (18×36 cm) should be used in preference to a regular cuff (12×23 cm) (Maxwell *et al* 1982). The mean arm circumference of chronically hypertensive pregnant women is 27.5 cm, exceeding 35 cm in less than 5 per cent of this group, so the problem of a large arm is not a common one. The effect of body weight on the blood pressure in pregnant women at the time that they booked for antenatal care is shown in Fig. 6.2.

Indirect blood pressure measurements should be made with the cuff at the level of the heart. If it is above or below this position the pressure in the brachial artery will fall or rise because of hydrostatic forces. Thus a pressure in the right (uppermost) arm with the patient lying on her left side will seem to be lower than the same reading when she lies flat on her back (Fig. 6.3). This is relevant when the lateral position is used in the third trimester to avoid the 'supine hypotension syndrome'. If the patient sits or stands peripheral resistance increases by vasoconstriction in the lower extremities to maintain systolic pressure, with the effect of increasing diastolic pressure (Fig. 6.3); thus standardisation of posture and arm position is crucial. The semiprone position is recommended by the author; if lateral tilt is needed (i.e. in the third trimester) the cuff must be positioned level with the heart.

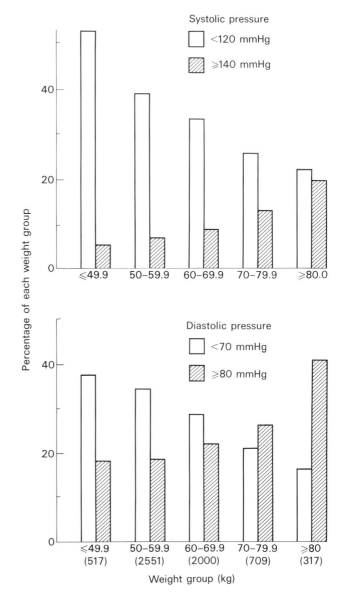

Fig. 6.2   The arterial pressures of 6094 women who booked for antenatal care at 10–20 weeks have been studied. The effect of maternal weight is shown in terms of the preponderance of small women with low pressures, and heavy women with high pressures. The numbers in parentheses are the totals for each weight group.

Phase I of the Korotkoff sounds defines the systolic pressure. In non-gravid individuals, phase V (extinction of Korotkoff sounds) is recommended as the diastolic end-point rather than phase IV (muffling) (Kirkendall *et al* 1981). However, phase V not uncommonly does not exist in pregnancy—the Korotkoff sounds being audible down to zero cuff pressure. For this reason, phase IV has to be used as the diastolic end-point, even though phase V, when present, is slightly better correlated with the

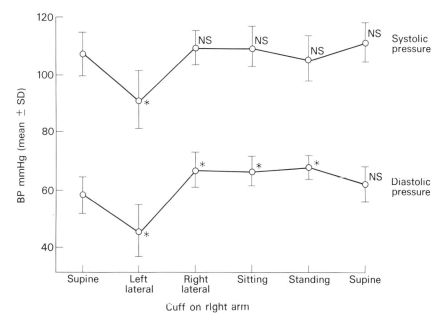

Fig. 6.3 Twenty normal women were studied in mid-pregnancy. Their arterial pressures were taken in the right arm using a London School of Hygiene sphygmomanometer. The diastolic pressures were taken at phase IV of the Korotkoff sounds. The effect of different positions is clearly shown, particularly the reduced pressure in the uppermost arm when the subject lies on her left side. (Difference from supine positions: NS not significant, * *P*<0.05).

directly measured diastolic pressure (Raftery and Ward 1968). For most individuals phases IV and V are within one or two beats of each other.

Can a pregnant woman be categorised by her blood pressure?

Fig. 6.4 shows a 24 hour blood pressure record of a hospitalised woman having mild chronic hypertension in the third trimester, classified by conventional clinical criteria. Her blood pressure varies from 130/85 to 70/40. The major differences (as in non-gravid individuals) are determined by sleep (Redman *et al* 1976a). However, even whilst awake, the patient's blood pressure fluctuates from 100/50 to 130/85. This well-known variability of blood pressure means that any one reading, however carefully and accurately taken, may deviate significantly from what is representative or average for an individual. In other words, there are large sampling errors which are distinct from the possible technical errors of measurement. These can be reduced by averaging a large number of readings taken under standard conditions. In clinical practice, and in most clinical investigations, this ideal is never approached. Comparisons are made between individuals based on unstandardised and grossly restricted samples of their blood pressure measurements. Furthermore these unsatisfactory readings are used to define 'normotension' and 'hypertension', giving an illusion of precision where none exists.

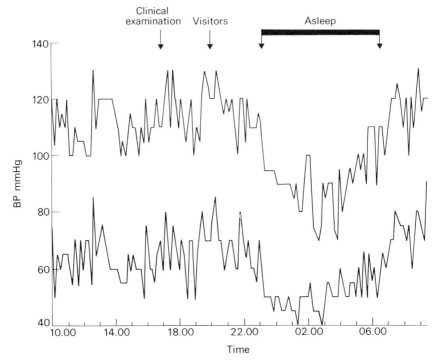

Fig. 6.4 The circadian pattern of the arterial pressure of a pregnant woman with mild chronic hypertension at rest in bed during the third trimester is shown. The major change in the levels is the normal fall which occurs during sleep.

What is hypertension in pregnancy?

Many years ago Pickering emphasised that high blood pressure is a 'sign not a disease'; that arterial pressure is 'distributed continuously in the population at large'; and that the dividing line between normotension and hypertension is 'nothing more than an artefact' (Pickering 1968b). These observations are as true for pregnant women as for the general population. Hypertension in pregnancy is an artificial concept. An arbitrary threshold is used which divides the population quantitatively but not qualitatively—an important but frequently forgotten distinction. A very high blood pressure may be unusual, but not necessarily abnormal.

The average blood pressure of over 6000 women booking before 20 weeks for delivery in Oxford was 120/70. Two and three standard deviations above this mean were 144/87 and 156/95 respectively. The actual distribution of the readings are shown in Table 6.1. Later in pregnancy the blood pressure rises. A maximum antenatal reading (excluding those taken in labour) of 140/90 or more was found in 21.6 per cent of all women; of 170/110 or more in 1.2 per cent. However, a maximum reading is a biased statistic, because the greater the number of available readings the greater the chance of an 'atypical' freak level. Nevertheless, these data describe the blood pressures observed in a unit serving an unselected obstetric population. By convention, the

Table 6.1   Distribution by parity of booking blood pressures at 10–20 weeks of pregnancy.

	% Distribution	
	Primigravidae (2861)	Multiparae (3581)
Booking systolic pressure (mmHg)		
≤109	8.7%	11.6%
110–119	23.7%	26.8%
120–129	33.3%	32.1%
130–139	25.1%	21.3%
140–149	6.4%	5.9%
150–159	2.5%	1.7%
160–169	0.3%	0.4%
≥170	0.1%	0.1%
Booking diastolic pressure (mmHg)		
≤69	29.4%	31.1%
70–79	48.2%	47.2%
80–89	19.0%	18.9%
90–99	3.1%	2.6%
100–109	0.4%	0.2%
≥110	0.0%	0.0%

threshold for 'diagnosing' hypertension in pregnancy is 140/90 mmHg. In the first half of pregnancy this identifies a small group (< 2.0 per cent) of hypertensive individuals. In the second half, a much greater proportion (21.6 per cent) exceeds this limit at least once. So, although 140/90 is an appropriate limit to begin with, in the second half of pregnancy it would be better to use a cut-off of 170/110 (maximum antenatal reading) to identify the extreme end of the distribution in populations which resemble the Oxford population.

Summary of the definition of hypertension in pregnancy

1   Blood pressure should be measured in the semirecumbent position with a cuff which is large enough for the patient's arm.
2   Phases I and IV of the Korotkoff sound identify the systolic and diastolic pressures respectively.
3   A single reading cannot characterise an individual's blood pressure status accurately.
4   Hypertension is not a disease but one end of the continuous distribution of all individuals' blood pressures.
5   A blood pressure of 140/90 is the conventional dividing line for obstetric hypertension. In the first half of pregnancy this is appropriate.

6   In the second half of pregnancy a maximum reading of 170/110 or more would be better for defining a small hypertensive group.

7   All classifications of individuals as normotensive and hypertensive are crude and to some extent arbitrary simplifications.

Terminology

In this chapter the term 'hypertension' is used to describe a blood pressure deemed to be higher than average. Hypertension in pregnancy has three possible aetiologies: (a)   it may be caused by the pregnancy itself; (b)   it may be a long-term problem present before the pregnancy began; (c)   much more rarely, it may be a new medical problem, coinciding with pregnancy by chance.

Pre-eclampsia, pre-eclamptic toxaemia (PET), gestosis, pregnancy-induced hypertension (PIH) or gestational hypertension are terms used to describe hypertension caused by pregnancy itself. It is not known if pregnancy-specific hypertension is one or several disorders. In this chapter the single term pre-eclampsia is used because it identifies the end-point of the problem(s), namely eclampsia. Toxaemia is an obsolete expression, previously used to describe any hypertension or proteinuria in pregnancy, whether pregnancy-induced or not. 'Chronic hypertension' is used to describe the condition of long-term high blood pressure. The usual cause is 'essential hypertension', meaning an inherited condition with no underlying pathology. There are other rarer causes—discussed later. Superimposed pre-eclampsia describes a mixed syndrome comprising pre-eclampsia in an individual with pre-existing or chronic hypertension.

THE DEFINITION OF PRE-ECLAMPSIA

The commonly used definitions of pre-eclampsia have been devised primarily for use in epidemiological studies (Nelson 1955, Rippmann 1968, Chesley 1978a). They are not so useful to the clinician who has to make individual diagnoses. In different ways they emphasise three features—hypertension, oedema and proteinuria—not because these are known to be the most important but because, historically, they were the first to be defined and because they happened to be signs which are easily accessible to clinicians. Pre-eclampsia is a disorder of the second half of pregnancy which regresses after delivery. Its cause is not yet known but must lie within the gravid uterus. Therefore although pre-eclampsia is conventionally defined by hypertension it is not primarily a hypertensive disease. The raised blood pressure and other maternal signs by which it is recognised are secondary features, mere reflections of an intrauterine problem. Because pre-eclampsia is a disorder of pregnancy and not simply a maternal problem, the fetus is invariably involved and may suffer its own morbidity or mortality. The signs of pre-eclampsia are best considered, therefore, as the consequence of a more fundamental pathological process, affecting specific maternal target systems. The targets include the maternal arterial, renal, coagulation and hepatic systems. The widespread systemic nature of the maternal disturbances is all too often not recognised. Many clinicians wrongly conceive of pre-eclampsia as only the aggregate of its conventionally defined signs of hypertension, oedema and proteinuria.

Pre-eclampsia once established is relentlessly progressive until delivery. Throughout almost all its course the patient is asymptomatic—a critical feature where diagnosis and management are concerned. Terminally the patient feels ill with headaches, visual disturbances, nausea, vomiting, epigastric pain and neurological irritability— including clonus and shaking. At this point convulsions may occur and the illness has progressed to its end-point of eclampsia.

Pathophysiology

INVOLVEMENT OF THE MATERNAL ARTERIAL SYSTEM

Hypertension is an early feature of pre-eclampsia. It is caused by vasoconstriction of unknown aetiology associated with a reduced circulating plasma volume (Blekta *et al* 1970; Chesley 1972; Gallery *et al* 1979a), and a normal or reduced cardiac output (Assali *et al* 1964; Smith 1970). Arterial reactivity is altered so that the normal refractoriness to angiotensin II is lost, and this may be detectable before the onset of the hypertension itself (Chesley 1966). Basal blood pressure becomes characteristically unstable with sudden spikes unrelated to any external stimuli (Chesley 1978b), while the usual nocturnal fall of the blood pressure beomes attenuated (Seligman 1971). In advanced pre-eclampsia, the circadian blood pressure pattern may even be reversed, with the highest pressures occurring at night during sleep (Redman *et al* 1976a). The hypertension is important for two reasons: first it is a key early diagnostic sign; second, if extreme, it can cause direct arterial injury.

Hypertension as a diagnostic sign

Pre-eclampsia is detected by a rise in the blood pressure during the second half of pregnancy which is abnormal in magnitude relative to the time of pregnancy at which it occurs. Thus a diastolic rise of about 10 mmHg is normal for the last 12 weeks of pregnancy (MacGillivray *et al* 1969) (Fig. 6.5) but a rise of only 5 mmHg between weeks 20 and 30 is associated with significantly higher rates of maternal proteinuria, prematurity and perinatal death (MacGillivray 1961). Hence to separate pre-eclampsia from other forms of hypertension by blood pressure readings it is necessary to refer to a change from a baseline rather than an absolute level (e.g. the American College of Obstetricians requires that the systolic and diastolic pressures increase by at least 30 mmHg and 15 mmHg respectively (Chesley 1978a)).

A high blood pressure reading by itself does not necessarily signify pre-eclampsia. Before 20 weeks it indicates hypertension which preceded pregnancy; after 20 weeks it may represent a continuation of chronic hypertension or a de novo (i.e. pre-eclamptic) problem. Given the technical and sampling errors of blood pressure measurement, small increases of pre-eclamptic origin are difficult to detect. Diagnostic accuracy may be improved by standardisation of the methods of measurement (Gallery *et al* 1977).

It has been claimed that the increased arterial sensitivity to angiotensin II of

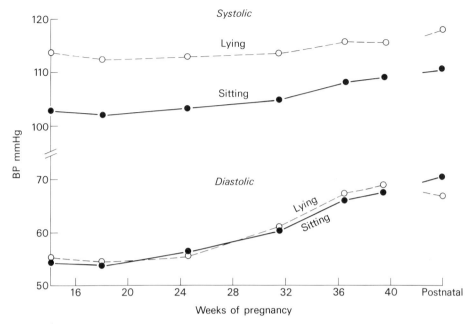

Fig. 6.5   Serial arterial pressures in 226 primigravidae taken both lying and sitting. (Courtesy of MacGillivray *et al* 1969.)

pre-eclampsia correlates with an exaggerated increase in diastolic pressure when the pregnant woman moves from the left side to supine—the roll-over test (Gant *et al* 1974). Angiotensin infusion tests cannot be used for clinical screening and diagnosis, so the roll-over test has been proposed as a simpler alternative. Its predictive value has been confirmed by some (Karbhari *et al* 1977; Marshall and Newman 1977; Peck 1977), but not by others (Campbell 1978; Kassar *et al* 1980; Poland *et al* 1980). The false positive rates have ranged from 6.3 per cent (Gant *et al* 1974) to 90.9 per cent (Poland *et al* 1980); and the false negative rates from 3.9 per cent (Phelan *et al* 1977) to 29.6 per cent (Kassar *et al* 1980). None of these reports has analysed the roll-over test in relation to clinical outcomes other than eventual hypertension. These data indicate that the roll-over test is of unproven value, and clinical practice should depend instead on carefully standardised blood pressure readings.

Complications of the hypertension

In general, a sudden increase of blood pressure above a critical threshold causes acute arterial damage and loss of vascular autoregulation. This has been demonstrated both experimentally, for example in rats (Goldby and Beilin 1972), and clinically (Johansson *et al* 1974). These factors explain the pathogenesis of malignant hypertension, hypertensive encephalopathy and hypertensive cerebral haemorrhage. Antihypertensive treatment prevents these problems which gives further proof of their aetiology (Pickering 1968c).

Table 6.2   The similarities and differences between malignant hypertension and eclampsia.

	Malignant hypertension	Eclampsia
Convulsion	+	+
Cerebral haemorrhage	+	+
Retinal haemorrhage	+	Rarely
Heart failure	+	+
Proteinuria	+	+
Renal failure	+	+
Disseminated intravascular coagulation	+	+
Microangiopathic haemolysis	+	+
Hepatic pathology	0	+
Renal artery intimal proliferation	+	0

Pre-eclampsia may cause blood pressures which are well above the level (i.e. a mean arterial pressure of about 140 mmHg) at which arterial and arteriolar damage would be expected. It is not surprising, therefore, that malignant hypertension and eclampsia are similar, although not identical conditions (Redman 1980a) (Table 6.2). Nor is it surprising that the commonest cause of maternal death from pre-eclampsia and eclampsia is cerebral haemorrhage, the pathology of which is similar to that seen in other hypertensive states (Sheehan and Lynch 1973a). In England and Wales maternal death from hypertensive cerebral injury exceeds the sum of all other causes of death from pre-eclampsia and eclampsia (*Report on Confidential Enquiries into Maternal Deaths 1973–75* (1979), *1976–78* (1982)) (Table 6.3). Similar findings have been reported from Australia (National Health and Medical Research Council 1981).

In summary, hypertension is an early secondary sign of pre-eclampsia. Severe hypertension is the main cause of maternal death from this disorder.

Table 6.3   Causes of maternal death from pre-eclampsia and eclampsia in England and Wales.

Complications	1973–75[1]	1976–78[2]
Cerebral	23	21
Anaesthetic	5	0
Hepatic	4	0
Cardiopulmonary	3	3
Hepato-renal	1	1
Other	3	3
Inadequate information	0	1
Total	39	29

[1] *Report on Confidential Enquiries into Maternal Deaths in England and Wales, 1973–1975* (1979).
[2] *Report on Confidential Enquiries into Maternal Deaths in England and Wales, 1976–1978* (1982).

THE MATERNAL RENAL SYSTEM AND FLUID RETENTION

Proteinuria is the conventionally recognised but late sign of renal involvement in pre-eclampsia. Once present, it indicates a poorer prognosis for both mother and baby (Taylor *et al* 1954; Butler and Bonham 1963; Naeye and Friedman 1979). On average it appears about three weeks before intrauterine death or mandatory delivery (Redman *et al* 1976b). It is moderately selective in terms of the molecular size of the filtered proteins (MacLean *et al* 1972; Simanowitz *et al* 1973), and may be heavy (greater than 5.0 g per day). Overall, pre-eclampsia is the commonest cause of nephrotic syndrome in pregnancy (Fisher *et al* 1977).

Proteinuria is one of several signs of involvement of the renal glomerulus in pre-eclampsia. Renal biopsy has shown a characteristic non-inflammatory lesion, primarily of swelling of the glomerular endothelial cells, which encroach on and occlude the capillary lumina—'glomerular endotheliosis'. The epithelial cells are also swollen but the foot processes are intact (Pollak and Nettles 1960). It should be noted that renal biopsy is never indicated for the diagnosis or management of pre-eclampsia. Renal function is also impaired. The changes are biphasic involving first tubular function and later glomerular function. An early feature of pre-eclampsia is a reduced uric acid clearance, reflecting altered tubular function (Chesley and Williams 1945), and causing a reciprocal rise in plasma urate. Later, at about the time that proteinuria develops, glomerular filtration becomes impaired. Rising plasma urate is thus an early sign of pre-eclampsia which precedes a later rise in plasma creatinine or urea (Redman *et al* 1976b). It is also the biochemical change which best correlates with the renal biopsy appearances of pre-eclampsia (Pollak and Nettles 1960).

Oedema and fluid retention

Eighty-five per cent of women with proteinuric pre-eclampsia have oedema (Thomson *et al* 1967). However, pre-eclampsia without oedema—'dry pre-eclampsia'—has long been recognised as a particularly dangerous variant (Eden 1922) (e.g. the perinatal mortality is higher than if oedema is present (Chesley 1978c)). The oedema fluid is an ultra-filtrate of plasma. The oedema is associated with reduced plasma albumin (Horne *et al* 1970) and hence with a lower oncotic pressure as well as reduced plasma volume (*see* above). Thus although there is fluid retention, the extracellular fluid is distributed abnormally between intra- and extravascular compartments. This should imply a change in capillary permeability, but this has not been demonstrated; nor does the protein concentration in the oedema fluid suggest that capillary permeability is grossly altered (MacGillivray 1967).

The cause of pre-eclamptic oedema is not yet known. It is associated with renal retention of both sodium and potassium. The pre-eclamptic patient excretes a sodium load more slowly than normal pregnant women. In part, this is because the filtered load of sodium is reduced by the lower glomerular filtration rate, in part because net tubular reabsorption of sodium tends to be increased (Chesley *et al* 1958). It is likely but not proven that the renal changes are secondary to the oedema-forming process.

Diagnostic value of oedema and changes in renal function

The pathological oedema of pre-eclampsia is easily confused with the physiological oedema found in 80 per cent of normal pregnant women (Robertson 1971). Physiological oedema has not been shown to be the precursor of pathological oedema, but will appear to be so, if definitions of pre-eclampsia are used which emphasise oedema, even in the absence of hypertension (such as those of the American Committee on Maternal Welfare (Chesley 1978a)). In the best prospective study of pregnant women with no oedema, or early or late onset oedema, all had a similar incidence of hypertension (Robertson 1971). For all these reasons the detection of oedema is not useful clinically, nor should oedema be included in the definition of pre-eclampsia (Vosburgh 1976). Development of oedema is associated with a higher rate of weight gain, hence the numerous reports associating excessive weight gain with the development of pre-eclampsia (Abitbol 1969). However, excessive weight gain—if it can be defined—is no more useful as a clinical sign than is the demonstration of oedema.

An elevated plasma uric acid is a useful diagnostic feature of early pre-eclampsia (Lancet and Fisher 1956; Connon and Wadsworth 1968; McFarlane 1963). It precedes the development of proteinuria and is the only simple investigation which can confirm the diagnosis in non-proteinuric pre-eclampsia. Two standard deviations above the mean of the plasma concentrations at 16, 28, 32 and 36 weeks are 0.28, 0.29, 0.34 and 0.39 mmol/l respectively (Redman, unpublished observations). Levels above these values in the third trimester are suggestive of pre-eclampsia. However, as with all other signs of pre-eclampsia, hyperuricaemia is non-specific and may instead result from renal impairment, diuretic use, or merely reflect a long-term constitutional characteristic of the gravid woman. Women with chronic hypertension without pre-eclampsia have normal plasma urate levels (Redman *et al* 1976b). Thus an elevated plasma urate should distinguish pre-eclamptic hypertension, with a poor fetal outcome, from chronic hypertension with a normal fetal outcome. This has been demonstrated (Redman *et al* 1976): for a given blood pressure level a plasma urate above 0.35 mmol identified a sub-group with a tenfold increase in perinatal mortality. A raised plasma creatinine ($\geqslant 90$ μmol/l) or blood urea ($\geqslant 6.0$ mmol/l) is usual only with proteinuric pre-eclampsia. In this situation these measurements are essential not for diagnosis but to anticipate increasing renal impairment which might precede acute renal failure.

Complications of the fluid retention and renal impairment

Ascites is not uncommon (e.g. affecting 13 of 99 women seen personally with severe pre-eclampsia). Pulmonary oedema is a rare but life-threatening complication presenting before or after delivery (Szekely and Snaith 1947; Strauss *et al* 1980). Laryngeal oedema may cause respiratory obstruction as well as difficulties if a general anaesthetic is required (Jouppila *et al* 1980). Acute renal failure with tubular, partial cortical or total cortical necrosis are terminal complications, more common previously than in current medical practice (*see also* Chapter 7). The latter two events are more likely in the context of an abruptio placentae complicating pre-eclampsia or eclampsia (Smith *et al* 1968).

INVOLVEMENT OF THE MATERNAL COAGULATION SYSTEM (*see also* Chapter 3)

The coagulation system is another target for the pre-eclamptic process. Normal pregnancy is a 'hypercoagulable' state, meaning that the blood response to clotting stimuli is brisker and that the natural 'turnover' of the system is enhanced. The latter change is detected by the increased circulating levels of soluble fibrin monomer complexes in the third trimester (Beller *et al* 1979). The turnover is further exaggerated in early pre-eclampsia. At this time the platelet count is moderately reduced (Redman *et al* 1978), indicating increased consumption with a reduced platelet lifespan (Rakoczi *et al* 1979; Boneu *et al* 1980). Platelet activation has been confirmed by the higher circulating levels of the platelet-specific protein, beta-thromboglobulin (Redman *et al* 1977; Douglas *et al* 1982) which is a product of the platelet release reaction; and by the overall loss of the platelet content of 5-hydroxytryptamine and the platelet responsiveness to various aggregating agents (Whigham *et al* 1978) indicating abnormal platelet aggregation and disaggregation *in vivo*. Relative macrothrombocytosis in pre-eclampsia shows that there is increased entry of young (i.e. large) platelets into the circulation (Giles and Inglis 1981).

In early pre-eclampsia there is also indirect evidence for increased Factor VIII consumption (Redman *et al* 1977). Urinary fibrinolytic activity is increased (Chen *et al* 1980) presumably indicating clearance of fibrin from the renal glomeruli. This is a chronic fully compensated process which cannot be labelled as a pathological disseminated intravascular coagulation (DIC). Of the three major inhibitors of the coagulation pathway: α_2 macroglobulin is increased (Horne *et al* 1972), α_1 antitrypsin is unchanged (Clarke *et al* 1971), and antithrombin III is reduced (Büller *et al* 1980; Weiner and Brandt 1982), relative to normal pregnancy.

DIC is a late and inconstant feature of pre-ictal pre-eclampsia. It is particularly severe if there is concomitant hepatic involvement (Killam *et al* 1975). Consumption of coagulation factors—fibrinogen Factors VII and VIII—and elevated serum fibrin/fibrinogen degradation products, are associated with the severe systemic disturbances of fibrin deposition in the microcirculation (Galton *et al* 1971; Bonnar *et al* 1971). Thus the coagulation disturbances proceed through two phases: **1** An early abnormal but fully compensated activation. **2** Later decompensation when the fibrinolytic system is overwhelmed by widespread fibrin deposition.

Diagnostic value of changes in the coagulation system

Although a declining platelet count is an early feature of pre-eclampsia (Redman *et al* 1978), it has limited diagnostic value because of the large variability between individuals in normal pregnancy. Prospective serial counts in selected high-risk patients are more useful when the patient's own baseline is established early in pregnancy. The ratio of Factor VIII-related antigen to Factor VIII activity also increases in early pre-eclampsia (Redman *et al* 1977). However, this is an expensive investigation which most hospital laboratories could not routinely undertake. The early detection of clotting disturbances in pre-eclampsia is not a simple aid to diagnosis; in comparison the renal changes are easier to detect (Dunlop *et al* 1978). The more profound disturbances of advanced pre-eclampsia are more readily observed, correlate with an adverse outcome, and can be used to monitor the course of the disease (Howie *et al* 1976). A diminished platelet count and raised fibrin/fibrinogen degradation products are the most easily detected changes. In severe pre-eclampsia it is essential to know the degree of the clotting disturbance because if DIC is present it indicates a much more serious situation.

Complications of the clotting disturbances

It has been suggested that fibrin deposition may cause the renal glomerular disease of pre-eclampsia, especially as infusion of thromboplastin into rabbits causes similar renal lesions (Vassalli *et al* 1963b). Fibrinogen derivatives are found within the swollen endothelial cells' cytoplasm at renal biopsy (Vassalli *et al* 1963a). The DIC of terminal pre-eclampsia and eclampsia undoubtedly contributes to the gross pathology of widespread fibrin deposition, tissue haemorrhage and necrosis in the viscera and brain (McKay *et al* 1953). Specific lesions include renal cortical necrosis, adrenal and pituitary haemorrhage and necrosis, and periportal hepatic necrosis. Microangiopathic haemolysis is a rare but well-defined consequence of pre-eclamptic DIC causing haemoglobinaemia, a sudden decline in haemoglobin, a reduced haptoglobin level and evidence of red cell fragmentation in the blood film (Pritchard *et al* 1954; Vardi and Fields 1974; Weinstein 1982).

INVOLVEMENT OF THE LIVER IN PRE-ECLAMPSIA

Liver dysfunction is a feature of pre-eclampsia detected by elevations of circulating hepatic enzymes (Shukla *et al* 1978), later progressing to jaundice and severe hepatic impairment (Long *et al* 1977; Killam *et al* 1975; Davies *et al* 1980). There is periportal haemorrhage and necrosis (Sheehan and Lynch 1973b), associated with widespread capillary thrombosis (Arias and Mancilla-Jimenez 1976). Coagulation disturbances are prominent (Killam *et al* 1975, Weinstein 1982) and the case mortality is high. There may well be an overlap between the liver involvement in pre-eclampsia and acute fatty liver of pregnancy (*Lancet* 1983) (*see* Chapter 9).

A rare terminal complication of pre-eclampsia—not necessarily preceded by jaundice—is hepatic rupture which presents as epigastric pain and circulatory collapse usually in pre-eclamptic multipara (Bis and Waxman 1976). The maternal mortality is 60 per cent.

Placental pathology

In pre-eclampsia the terminal segments of the uterine spiral arteries become blocked by accumulations of lipophages, fibrin and platelet aggregates—so-called 'acute atherosis'

(Zeek and Assali 1950). These lesions explain the reduced uteroplacental blood flow of pre-eclampsia (McClure Browne and Veall 1953; Johnson and Clayton 1957), as well as the increased incidence of placental infarcts (Little 1960), and the placental dysfunction which causes the fetal asphyxia and nutritional failure. It is probable that the maternal signs of pre-eclampsia are secondary to placental ischaemia. Experimental models of pre-eclampsia in baboons, dogs, rabbits or rats all depend on procedures which reduce placental blood flow (Cavanagh *et al* 1977; Abitbol 1977a; Wardle and Wright 1973; Douglas and Langford 1969). The cause of acute atherosis is not known. The lesions are not the consequence of hypertensive injury but may have an immune aetiology (Redman 1980b).

Summary of the features of pre-eclampsia

Pre-eclampsia is probably a placental disorder which causes secondary changes in different maternal target systems by which the disease is recognised. Hypertension is one of many aspects of pre-eclampsia. It is neither its primary feature nor its only significant sign. A list of some of the maternal complications of pre-eclampsia is given in Table 6.4.

Diagnosis of pre-eclampsia

None of the signs of this disorder is specific—not even the convulsions of eclampsia— therefore it must be diagnosed by demonstrating the presence of more than one

Table 6.4   Complications of pre-eclampsia.

Central Nervous System
    Eclamptic convulsions
    Cerebral haemorrhage
    Cerebral oedema
    Retinal oedema
    Retinal detachment

Renal system
    Renal cortical necrosis
    Renal tubular necrosis

Respiratory system
    Laryngeal oedema
    Pulmonary oedema

Hepatic system
    Jaundice
    Hepatic rupture

Coagulation system
    Disseminated intravascular coagulation
    Microangiopathic haemolysis

Placenta
    Placental infarction
    Retroplacental bleeding and abruptio placenta

component. Any of the following—isolated hypertension, proteinuria, hyperuricaemia or convulsions—cannot establish a firm diagnosis; but hypertension combined with hyperuricaemia, or proteinuria, or convulsions makes the diagnosis much more certain. Diagnosis must take account of the following factors. There are all gradations of disease from barely discernible to gross. The condition is highly variable in presentation, both with respect to the speed at which it evolves, and the extent to which different maternal target systems are involved. The diagnosis of mild pre-eclampsia at term is always uncertain because delivery prevents the appearance of the corroborative signs of more advanced disease. Hypertension and hyperuricaemia are early signs. Proteinuria, major coagulation disturbances, significant hepatic dysfunction and placental impairment are late signs. Diagnosis must be made in asymptomatic women by screening. Given that pre-eclampsia can begin at any time after 20 weeks' gestation and progress to a dangerous extent within a two week period, how often should a mother be screened for this condition? Current routines of care for primigravidae consist of monthly visits to 28 weeks, fortnightly visits to 36 weeks and weekly visits thereafter. The infrequent checks between 20 and 28 weeks make this a vulnerable period during which pre-eclampsia can progress easily, undetected. Therefore antenatal screening should be more intensive if the mother is known to have a high risk of developing pre-eclampsia.

Maternal risk factors

Primigravidae are fifteen times more likely to develop proteinuric pre-eclampsia than parous women (MacGillivray 1958). Even secundiparae with an affected first pregnancy have a lower overall incidence, which, nevertheless, is forty times higher than for secundiparae with a previously normal pregnancy (MacGillivray 1958). The risk increases slightly with age but is not affected by social class (Baird 1977). Pre-eclampsia may be inherited (Cooper and Liston 1979) so that a positive family history is a risk factor: the daughters of eclamptic women are eight times more likely to have pre-eclampsia than would be expected (Chesley *et al* 1968).

It is widely believed that overweight women are more susceptible to the disorder (Stewart and Hewitt 1960; MacGillivray 1961), although there are few data to support this contention. The usual diagnostic criteria for pre-eclampsia mean that a gravid population so defined will, in part, have the characteristics of chronically hypertensive individuals, including the tendency to be heavier than average (Pickering 1968d). This bias was recognised by Lowe (1961), who found that by applying more specific diagnostic criteria for 'toxaemia' the association with maternal weight disappeared. Instead, the affected women were, if anything, lighter than average.

Chronically hypertensive women are 3–7 times more likely to develop higher blood pressures combined with proteinuria or 'superimposed pre-eclampsia', than are normotensive women (Chesley *et al* 1947; Butler and Bonham 1963; Harley 1966; Walters 1966), therefore, a correlation between obesity and pre-eclampsia would be expected as a secondary association. A much more significant combination is renal disease and hypertension, when the incidence of complicating pre-eclampsia is very high (Felding 1969).

Pre-eclamptic women tend to be shorter (Baird 1977). Predisposing fetal factors include multiple pregnancy (MacGillivray 1958), hydatidiform mole (Chun *et al* 1964) and hydrops fetalis (Jeffcoate and Scott 1959), with rhesus isoimmunisation, or due to other causes such as fetal alpha thalassaemia (*see* Chapter 2). Although maternal smoking is associated with other major perinatal problems, nearly all authors agree that gravidae who smoke have a lower incidence of pre-eclampsia (Zabriskie 1963; Underwood *et al* 1965; Duffus and MacGillivray 1968). It is not known whether all these risk factors can be formally combined to give clinically useful predictions of the onset of pre-eclampsia.

Clinical management

Pre-eclampsia is the commonest cause of curable hypertension; delivery always reverses the problem. Therefore the principles of management are: screening of the asymptomatic patient, early diagnosis, and well-timed delivery. Interposed between diagnosis and delivery is the need for hospital admission. This achieves two objectives: bedrest and close monitoring of the mother's condition. Conventionally the first objective is given greater emphasis than the second. The evidence that bedrest is beneficial is not reliable, and is derived circumstantially from the dramatic improvements in outcome when early admission to hospital was introduced in an uncontrolled way for the management of pre-eclampsia (Hamlin 1952). Other justifications for bedrest include the theoretical benefit of a lower blood pressure, the possibility of increased cardiac output (Ueland *et al* 1969), and increased sodium excretion (Redd *et al* 1968).

Equally valid counterarguments suggest that, as a result of pressure by the enlarged uterus on the great vessels, supine recumbency in gravidae may significantly reduce cardiac output (Lees *et al* 1967a), alter renal function in a way that exacerbates abnormalities due to pre-eclampsia (Lindheimer 1970) and reduce uteroplacental blood flow (Abitbol 1977b). Only two controlled trials of bedrest have been conducted: both of them were small, thus rendering the results difficult to interpret. Bedrest was beneficial in pregnancies complicated by severe albuminuric hypertension with hyperuricaemia and a fetus grossly small for dates (Mathews *et al* 1982). In a controlled trial of bedrest for non albuminuric hypertension, there was no evidence for benefit (Mathews 1977).

If the value of bedrest can be questioned, it nevertheless cannot be disputed that as pre-eclampsia develops, admission to hospital becomes essential for the correct timing and management of pre-emptive delivery. What is in question is not *if* but *when* the pre-eclamptic patient should be admitted. Once the diagnosis has been made, critical decisions about management depend on an assessment of the speed with which the condition is progressing. There are only rudimentary data to help the clinician make this estimate: the major resource is continuing close observation, which necessitates hospital admission. In hospital, it is possible to keep track of this dangerous, unpredictable and changeable condition; at home it is not. In general symptomatic pre-eclampsia (symptoms, hypertension and proteinuria) justifies an emergency admission. Asymptomatic proteinuric pre-eclampsia demands urgent admission on the day of diagnosis. Aproteinuric pre-eclampsia which has been confirmed by biochemical testing (e.g. hyperuricaemia) is usually best managed in hospital after elective admission. Mild hypertension with no other complicating factor can be managed conservatively from routine clinics. In the United States the cost of inpatient treatment has prevented the extensive use of hospital admission for managing pre-eclampsia. Paradoxically, now that inpatient management is being questioned in Great Britain (Mathews *et al* 1978), reports from the USA are beginning to extol its benefits (Hauth *et al* 1976).

Antihypertensive drugs

Antihypertensive treatment will prevent only those problems directly caused by maternal hypertension. From the preceding discussion it will be apparent that pre-eclamptic hypertension is a secondary or peripheral feature of a more fundamental problem—that extreme pre-eclamptic hypertension causes direct arterial injury and the cerebral haemorrhages which make pre-eclampsia a potentially lethal disorder. Pre-eclamptic patients must be managed to avoid hypertension of a degree which can cause arterial injury. The threshold at which this occurs is at about a mean arterial pressure of 140 mmHg (180–190/120–130). Definitive treatment is delivery, but antihypertensive agents may need to be used to protect the mother before, during and after parturition. Our aim is to keep all blood pressure readings below 170/110; thus, treatment is started if maximum blood pressures repeatedly reach these limits in any period.

Treatment of extreme pre-eclamptic hypertension

The vasospasm responds best to the drugs that directly relax vascular smooth muscle, namely diazoxide and hydralazine. These are the agents of choice for acute hypertensive emergencies in pregnancy. Both are usually used in the immediate peripartum period, but neither has been tested in adequately controlled trials.

Hydralazine has probably been used more extensively in pregnancy than has diazoxide (Assali *et al* 1953; De Alvarez 1955; Joyce and Kenyon 1972). It is best reserved for transient rises in blood pressure which are treated with intermittent i.m. or s.c. administration of 10–20 mg. Side effects, because they comprise headaches, vomiting, shakiness and even hyper-reflexia, can mimic impending eclampsia, and are likely to be more troublesome with a continuous i.v. infusion. Hydralazine has a weak and transient action, its effectiveness being enhanced by concurrent sympathetic inhibition, which blocks the reflex tachycardia that develops as the blood pressure falls. In pregnancy this is achieved if the patient is already taking methyl dopa. Fetal side effects have not been reported. However, it should not be used indiscriminately or at levels exceeding 300 mg in 24 hours.

Diazoxide has been used mainly for intrapartum hypertensive emergencies (Barden and Keenan 1971; Pennington and Picker 1972; Morris *et al* 1977; Neuman *et al* 1979). The standard dose of 300 mg by rapid i.v. injection is excessive and can cause serious hypotension (Neuman *et al* 1979), a tendency which is probably aggravated by the plasma volume depletion of pre-eclampsia. Titration by intermittent administration of small bolus doses of 30–60 mg is preferable and effective (Ram and Kaplan 1979; Thien *et al* 1980). Diazoxide relaxes uterine muscle and usually inhibits labour (Morishima *et al* 1976; Wilson *et al* 1974). The advantages of using diazoxide have been queried (Perkins 1977). There is no doubt that it is a drug to be reserved for the most extreme situations (in our practice less than 0.05 per cent of all maternities). Apart from hypotension and shock, neonatal hyperglycaemia after acute administration in labour has been reported (Neuman *et al* 1979). On the other hand, diazoxide is the drug most likely to control dangerous hypertension successfully, and if used cautiously, is probably the safest option in these circumstances. Clonidine (Turnbull and Ahmed 1969) and labetalol (Lamming *et al* 1980) have both been used in the treatment of severe hypertension in pregnancy, but there is not enough experience to recommend them for routine practice.

Agents that inhibit the renin-angiotensin system might, in the future, be a useful part of treatment. In the immediate postpartum period an angiotensin converting enzyme inhibitor did not lower the blood pressure of five pre-eclamptic women (Sullivan *et al* 1978). Experimental administration of captopril (an angiotensin converting enzyme inhibitor used for the treatment of hypertension in non-pregnant patients), causes a high fetal mortality in pregnant sheep and rabbits (Broughton-Pipkin and Turner 1982), and for this reason it is contraindicated in clinical use.

Lowering the blood pressure and placental perfusion

Perfusion of the human placenta, and how it is controlled, is poorly understood because of the obvious ethical problems of measurement and experimentation. Whether or not acute hypotensive treatment causes reduced placental perfusion cannot be answered directly, nor do clinical studies of fetal morbidity or mortality after treatment provide useful information, because there are no controlled observations. Blood flow in a vascular bed depends on resistance as well as arterial pressure, therefore a lowered blood pressure does not necessarily mean a reduction of flow. One set of uncontrolled observations indicates that hypotensive treatment of severely pre-eclamptic gravidae with hydralazine was associated with changes in fetal heart rate patterns, suggesting aggravation of fetal compromise (Vink *et al* 1980). If perfusion of the pre-eclamptic placenta can only be maintained by a blood pressure that directly threatens maternal well being, then urgent delivery is the main priority. In practice this is a rare circumstance.

Conservative treatment of severe pre-eclampsia (B.P. > 170/110)

The earlier the presentation, the more justified it is to attempt conservative management of pre-eclampsia, in order to allow fetal maturation and enhance neonatal survival. The patient must be asymptomatic, have adequate renal function, and be under constant inpatient supervision. In these circumstances, parenteral therapy is inappropriate, and oral agents need to be used. Methyldopa is the first choice.

The safety of methyldopa in pregnancy has been established by case-control studies (Leather *et al* 1968; Redman *et al* 1976; Redman *et al* 1977). No serious adverse fetal effects have yet been documented. Methyldopa crosses the placenta and accumulates in relatively high concentrations in amniotic fluid (Jones and Cummings 1978). Fetal heart rate variability is unaffected (Redman *et al* 1983, unpublished observations); however, there is a slight but discernible slowing of the fetal heart rate, and neonatal blood pressure is transiently reduced for a short period after delivery (Whitelaw 1981); yet none of these effects is clinically important. Its use not only relieves the patient of the problems of parenteral therapy, but if, at a later time, diazoxide or hydralazine is needed, their action is potentiated, because the sympathetic reflex tachycardia, which these agents induce, is inhibited.

Although methyldopa can be given i.v., oral administration can achieve an adequate therapeutic response within twelve hours provided a large initial loading dose of 750–1000 mg is used. This can be followed by 1–2 g per day which is rapidly adjusted to 3–4 g per day as needed. A satisfactory drop in the blood pressure tends to provoke transient oliguria, which may cause anxiety about pre-eclamptic renal failure—a complication discounted by measuring the plasma urea and creatinine. Despite good blood pressure control, the other changes of pre-eclampsia (abnormalities of renal, coagulation and placental function) remain unchanged. Thus, hypotensive treatment is merely suppressing one dangerous manifestation of this disorder. The treatment regimen of hypertension in pre-eclampsia may need to anticipate nocturnal hypertension (Redman *et al* 1976a) by a variable schedule, with the largest doses at night.

Escape from blood pressure control

While pregnancy continues, pre-eclampsia is a relentlessly progressive disorder; sooner or later, escape from blood pressure control can be expected. In general, the maternal and fetal condition deteriorate together and it is not difficult to see when the limits of conservative management have been reached and delivery is indicated. Oral vasodilators, however, may be usefully added to the medical regimen to prevent loss of blood pressure control. Oral hydralazine, which on its own is a weak hypotensive agent, effectively augments methyldopa given at doses of 25–75 mg every six hours. The long-term use of oral diazoxide, for periods of 19–69 days, has been reported in eight pregnancies (Pohl and Thurston 1972; Redman 1980a). Diazoxide was detected in cord blood and amniotic fluid, and excreted in the neonates' urine for the first week of life. Neonatal blood pressure was not affected, but transient glucose intolerance requiring neonatal insulin administration was observed in one case (Smith *et al* 1982). Alopecia has been another neonatal side-effect.

Treatment of mild to moderate pre-eclamptic hypertension (140–170/90–110)

In medical practice the objectives of treating moderate hypertension are long-term and are not transferrable to young women for the brief period of pregnancy; nor do non-obstetric studies provide any guidelines as to how treating moderate hypertension might affect the fetus. The argument for treating moderate hypertension in pregnancy comes from the well-documented association between maternal hypertension and increased perinatal mortality: the higher the arterial pressure, the higher are the chances of perinatal death (Page and Christianson 1976). It has been assumed that this means that maternal hypertension is the cause of the perinatal problem, that is, that association implies causation. There is now considerable evidence that this is incorrect, as has already been discussed in this chapter. Therefore, for pre-eclamptic hypertension, treatment should be reserved for more extreme hypertension, starting at a level (170/110) which allows a wide margin of safety.

PREVENTION AND TREATMENT OF ECLAMPTIC FITS

Eclampsia is now rare and few obstetricians, and even fewer general practitioners, have extensive experience of its presentation and management. The differential diagnosis of generalised seizures occurring in pregnancy is considered in Chapter 14. A number of case series have been published recommending management protocols, many of which use drugs and methods which are now considered outmoded. No controlled trials have been reported. The aim of management is to protect the maternal airway, control convulsions, control extreme hypertension and expedite delivery. A recent report emphasises how confused practitioners can be when trying to achieve these objectives because of their lack of practice (Wightman *et al* 1978). In the USA magnesium sulphate is used as an anticonvulsant, on the grounds that it causes the least neonatal problems (Chesley 1978a). In England various regimens dependent on heavy sedation have evolved into the intravenous use of either chlormethiazole (Duffus *et al* 1969) or benzodiazepines (Lean *et al* 1968). It is meaningless to claim that one regimen is superior to the other, because they have never been compared. A controlled trial would not now be possible in Britain because of the lack of cases.

Indications for prophylactic anticonvulsant treatment include all symptomatic pre-eclampsia, and proteinuric pre-eclampsia with excessive jitteriness, particularly clonus (more than three beats). A typical regimen would be a loading dose of 20 mg of diazepam intravenously and 10 mg per hour to keep the patient asleep but fully rousable. If a patient is bad enough to need anticonvulsant therapy, then immediate delivery is required. Prolonged use of diazepam will adversely effect the neonate causing depression at birth, hypotonia, poor feeding and inadequate temperature control (Cree *et al* 1973).

OTHER MEASURES FOR THE TREATMENT OF PRE-ECLAMPSIA AND ITS
COMPLICATIONS

Sedatives

It is not easy to determine why sedatives came to be part of the standard management of
pre-eclampsia and eclampsia. There seem to be three reasons. First, anticonvulsants
and sedatives have been curiously confused. To treat impending or actual eclampsia
with paraldehyde (Williams 1964), barbiturates (Menon 1953), parenteral benzodiazepines (Lean *et al* 1968), chlormethiazole (Duffus *et al* 1969) or magnesium sulphate
(Chesley 1978d) is logical—although not necessarily safe—because these preparations
have anticonvulsant action. To treat with tribromethol or phenothiazines (Menon
1961), opiates (Theobald 1956) or oral benzodiazepines is illogical because these
sedatives have no anticonvulsant action. Indeed, phenothiazines (which lower the
threshold for convulsions), and opiates (which cause vomiting and respiratory
depression) can only exacerbate the problems of the convulsing patient.

Second, it has been assumed that acute sedation of the pre-ictal patient should be
extended to chronic sedation of milder cases of pre-eclampsia, so it is not uncommon to
find domiciliary patients treated with phenobarbitone. This is illogical: if the patient is at
immediate risk of convulsing she needs to be in hospital; if she is not, she does not need
phenobarbitone. Finally, it is misconceived by obstetric practitioners that the
hypertension of pre-eclampsia is a direct consequence of anxiety, which will be relieved
by sedation. In this respect sedatives are occupying '. . . a time honoured place among
the magical drugs used in the treatment of hypertension' (Pickering 1968e), despite
well-designed trials which have shown them to be useless (Cooper and Cranston 1957;
Chesrow *et al* 1966). The hypertension of pre-eclampsia responds to delivery, not relief
of anxiety. To make a patient feel that her anxiety is compounding her problems is both
unkind and unnecessary.

Treatment of fluid disturbances and excessive weight gain; volume expansion

The symptom of pre-eclamptic oedema has been extensively treated by both salt
restriction and the use of diuretics. Salt restriction is still an important part of the
management of hypertension in non-pregnant patients and is widely used for the
treatment of pre-eclampsia in some countries, although not in the United Kingdom. Salt
restriction in pregnancy has been tested in only one controlled trial (Robinson 1958).
Perinatal mortality in the salt restricted group was significantly increased by nearly
twofold, and was associated with more 'toxaemia', both in nulliparous and parous
patients. While none of the other 'trials' have been sufficiently well-designed to refute
these data, at least they are in agreement that a high salt diet is not detrimental (Chesley
and Annitto 1943; Mengert and Tacchi 1961). Salt restriction is not without hazards.
It may aggravate renal impairment (Mulé *et al* 1957) to the point of iatrogenic acute
renal failure (Palomaki and Lindheimer 1970), and it may contribute to a puerperal
shock syndrome which used to be seen in severely pre-eclamptic patients (Tatum and

Mulé 1956). The evidence establishes no case for salt restriction in the prophylaxis or management of pre-eclampsia.

For a while after their introduction, the thiazide diuretics were prescribed widely for the prevention and treatment of pre-eclampsia. Their use achieves approximately the same end as salt restriction, so it is not surprising that the controlled trials agree that they confer no benefit (Flowers *et al* 1962; Weseley and Douglas 1962; Landesman *et al* 1965; Kraus *et al* 1966; Campbell and MacGillivray 1975). Two trials claimed a reduction in the final incidence of pre-eclampsia, but as oedema was included as a diagnostic sign, the improvement merely reflected the undoubted ability of diuretics to clear pre-eclamptic oedema (Cuadros and Tatum 1964; Menzies 1964). A massive improvement in perinatal mortality was reported by Finnerty and Bepko (1966). However, the treatment group was heavily biased by a composition in favour of a lower perinatal mortality because two high-risk groups—women with asymptomatic bacteriuria and treatment defaulters—were selectively deleted. The latter were moved to the control group for analysing the results which, because they are not the outcome of true randomisation, have to be discounted.

A number of serious side effects have been associated with the use of thiazide diuretics. These drugs aggravate the hypovolaemia of severe pre-eclampsia and may precipitate renal failure (Palomaki and Lindheimer 1970). The fetal consequences of their diabetogenic action have not been defined. Diuretics have caused maternal death from pancreatitis (Minkowitz *et al* 1964; Menzies and Prystowsky 1967) and from excessive ingestion (Schifrin *et al* 1969), and may cause hypokalaemia (Pritchard and Walley 1961) and hyperuricaemia, which obscures one of the more useful signs of early pre-eclampsia. There is indirect evidence for reduced placental perfusion following diuretic therapy (Gant *et al* 1975). For these reasons diuretics should not now be used in the management of pre-eclampsia, except for treating the rare complication of left ventricular failure. More recently, attention has been focused on the hypovolaemia of pre-eclampsia. It has been claimed that plasma volume expansion is beneficial (Goodlin *et al* 1978; Morris and O'Grady 1979) to correct poor renal and placental function. It has also been shown that plasma protein infusions lower blood pressure in pre-eclamptic women, but by a mechanism not dependent on plasma volume expansion (Gallery *et al*, personal communication). The evidence in favour of plasma volume expansion is circumstantial and not validated. The possibility that it could cause circulatory overload and pulmonary oedema makes the treatment potentially dangerous. It cannot therefore be considered to be a part of routine management.

It is still widely believed that dietary restriction of weight gain will prevent the onset of pre-eclampsia despite the absence of a rationale for this regimen and any evidence that it is effective. The best investigation has been a randomised controlled trial of calorie restriction in primigravidae with excessive weight gain (Campbell and MacGillivray 1975). Dieting did not alter the incidence of pre-eclampsia, but did cause a significant reduction in the birth weights. A partial follow up of the children at 4–6 years of age showed that the diet-treated cases were less well-grown than the controls (Blumenthal 1976).

Treatment of the coagulation disturbances

In general the only remedy for DIC is to correct the underlying problem. In pre-eclampsia this means delivery. With the knowledge that abnormal coagulation probably mediates at least some of the terminal complications of the disorder, various regimens of anticoagulation have been tried. Heparinisation failed to modify the course of severe pre-eclampsia (Howie *et al* 1975). Prostacyclin infusion corrected the hypertension in one case, but not the underlying fetal problems which necessitated premature delivery (Fidler *et al* 1980). Successful prophylactic anticoagulation with warfarin has been reported twice (Valentine and Baker 1977; Schramm 1979). More recently a prophylactic antiplatelet regimen (aspirin and dipyridamole) was associated with a significantly better perinatal outcome in a randomised controlled trial in high risk subjects (Beaufils *et al* 1982). The dangers of anticoagulation in patients at risk of cerebral haemorrhage need to be emphasised. Overall, in routine clinical practice, anticoagulation should not be used either prophylactically or therapeutically unless more definitive evidence is forthcoming.

Management of the pre-eclamptic patient during labour and delivery

The pregnancies of hypertensive women are more likely to be terminated by induction and delivered operatively, particularly by Caesarean section. Low doses of oxytocin (2–5 mu/min) are antidiuretic within 10–15 minutes of the start of the infusion (Abdul-Karim and Rizk 1970). If given intravenously with large volumes of 5 per cent dextrose and water, this can cause hyponatraemia and convulsions (McKenna and Shaw 1979). The drug causes peripheral vasodilatation with a reflex tachycardia which may stimulate significant increases in cardiac output. If cardiac function is already compromised, which may happen in rare cases of severe pre-eclampsia, myocardial failure may occur (Tepperman *et al* 1977).

The role of epidural analgesia in the acutely hypertensive patient prior to delivery is controversial (Hibbard and Rosen 1977; Gant and Worley 1980). It provides a valuable way of controlling hypertension in labour (Willocks and Moir 1968), but because pre-eclamptic women are vasoconstricted and hypovolaemic, there is some danger of precipitating severe hypotension; however, this can be anticipated and prevented by intravenous fluid loading. Anxieties about a possible adverse effect on uteroplacental blood flow have been allayed by the demonstration that, if given correctly, epidural analgesia neither reduces the cardiac output (Graham and Goldstein 1980) nor placental blood flow as measured by ^{133}Xe clearance (Jouppila *et al* 1979).

The drugs used for the management of pre-eclampsia do not interfere with the administration of general anaesthesia. Intubation causes intense reflex hypertension, imposing a transient increase in circulatory afterload. The risks of encountering laryngeal oedema when pre-eclamptic women are intubated have already been discussed.

In the management of the third stage, ergometrine should be avoided because it causes hypertension (Forman and Sullivan 1952), and syntocinon used instead. The pre-eclamptic patient is particularly prone to hypertension following ergometrine (Baillie 1963), and headaches, convulsions and death have been reported as major sequelae (Tepperman *et al* 1977).

A woman with a shrunken intravascular compartment is less tolerant of blood loss than is the normal pregnant woman (Tatum and Mulé 1956). Blood replacement must therefore be initiated sooner, at the same time very carefully, to guard against the dangers of underfilling and overfilling. Close monitoring of the central venous pressure is helpful, especially where there is oliguria.

SUMMARY OF TREATMENT OF PRE-ECLAMPSIA

The correct treatment for pre-eclampsia is delivery. Antihypertensive drugs should be used to ensure that the maternal blood pressure remains below 170/110. Anticonvulsant drugs will rarely be needed to prevent or treat eclamptic convulsions. No medical treatment has yet been conclusively shown to prevent or retard the development of pre-eclampsia.

Chronic hypertension (CHT) in pregnancy

This group comprises women with essential and renal hypertension, and hypertension caused by miscellaneous but rare conditions. The first condition is most commonly encountered. Women with essential hypertension tend to be older and therefore more likely to be parous, heavier and to have a family history of hypertension.

The physiological decline in the blood pressure in early pregnancy is exaggerated in women with CHT (Chesley 1978e) so that the underlying situation may be masked. Conversely in later pregnancy the normal rise in blood pressure is exaggerated. Thus an individual with CHT may appear normotensive when she starts antenatal care early in the second trimester and then show a rise in blood pressure in the third trimester of a degree which resembles pre-eclampsia. This has lead to considerable diagnostic confusion but explains why third trimester hypertension segregates into two groups: non-recurrent, affecting primigravidae, and with a raised perinatal mortality; recurrent, affecting multiparae, with a good perinatal outcome (Adams and MacGillivray 1961; MacGillivray 1982). The former group would have pre-eclampsia as defined in this chapter, the latter probably have CHT. Thus the only sure way to detect CHT in pregnancy is to refer to prepregnancy readings, or, if as is usual, these are not available, to reassess the blood pressure at a remote time after delivery. However, if blood pressures are consistently at or above 140/90 in the first half of pregnancy, then CHT can be inferred. Not uncommonly the presentation is of mild hypertension alone in the second half of pregnancy without any antecedent readings at all. It is not possible, in these circumstances, to distinguish CHT from pre-eclampsia with absolute certainty.

Chronic hypertension is one of the major predisposing factors to pre-eclampsia so that the two conditions, which in their pure forms are easily separable, may commonly occur together. Pre-eclampsia superimposed on chronic hypertension tends to be recurrent in later pregnancies whereas in a normotensive individual, pre-eclampsia tends not to recur. If a blood pressure of 140/90 in the first half of pregnancy is evidence of CHT then the affected individuals have an approximately fivefold increased risk of later pre-eclampsia compared to normotensive individuals (Butler and Bonham 1963). This close link between the two conditions led earlier clinicians to conclude that CHT is extremely dangerous when combined with pregnancy (Browne and Dodds 1942). It is now clear that the particular risks of chronic hypertension in pregnancy are entirely attributable to the increased chance of developing superimposed pre-eclampsia, and that the majority of chronically hypertensive women who do not get pre-eclampsia can expect a normal perinatal outcome (Chamberlain *et al* 1978).

The signs of pre-eclampsia in chronically hypertensive women are the same as in other women except that the blood pressure levels start from a higher baseline. Thus the demonstration of a rise in the blood pressure ($+30/+15$ mmHg from baseline) of a progressive hyperuricaemia, or abnormal activation of the clotting system is evidence of superimposed pre-eclampsia which will progress to proteinuria unless pre-empted by delivery. When proteinuria develops, intrauterine growth retardation is almost the rule. The easiest diagnostic guide is the maternal plasma urate level. Values below 0.30 mmol/l are not in favour of pre-eclampsia and in a hypertensive woman would suggest the diagnosis of a chronic problem. Overall the differential diagnosis of chronic from pre-eclamptic hypertension rests on the demonstration of the absence of pre-eclamptic features such as a change in the blood pressure from baseline, a rise in maternal plasma urate levels, and absence of proteinuria and activation of the clotting system.

TREATMENT OF CHRONIC HYPERTENSION IN PREGNANCY

If antihypertensive treatment has been started before conception, the patient may seek advice about the possible effects of her medications on the growth and development of her fetus. None of the commonly used antihypertensive drugs is known to be teratogenic. This does not preclude the possibility of subtle problems which are as yet unknown. For this reason it is appropriate that women with no more than moderate hypertension should stop treatment before conception, so that only those whose hypertension constitutes an immediate health hazard continue taking treatment throughout the first trimester. By the twelfth week the normal fall in blood pressure is such that the need for treatment is either temporarily diminished or no longer present. If chronic hypertension is diagnosed for the first time in pregnancy, it is necessary to treat those in whom it presents an immediate (as opposed to a long-term) hazard. The precise levels for treatment have not been agreed upon; we take a cut-off point at or above 170/110.

The problem of less severe chronic hypertension (i.e. 140–170/90–110 mmHg) needs to be considered. In general medical practice, the purpose of treating this degree of hypertension is to prevent long-term complications which are not relevant for the brief period of gestation. For this reason the only indication for antihypertensive treatment in these women would be if it could prevent the superimposition of pre-eclampsia which is the major short-term problem. There is clear evidence based on a large randomised control trial that the early control of moderate chronic hypertension does not lessen the eventual incidence of superimposed pre-eclampsia (Redman 1980a). Thus, there is no worthwhile fetal indication for the control of moderate hypertension in pregnancy—that is in patients with blood pressures less than 170/110. Consequently the medical management hinges entirely around considerations of maternal welfare.

Oral antihypertensive agents that are used in CHT

The choice of drugs is dictated by fetal considerations. Methyldopa is preferred because its fetal effects have been defined much more clearly than those of any other drug, and its antihypertensive action and side effects are the same as in non-pregnant individuals. Detailed developmental follow-ups of drug exposed fetuses, to the age of seven years, confirm the absence of any significant adverse drug reaction (Mutch *et al* 1977a, 1977b; Ounsted *et al* 1980; Cockburn *et al* 1982). Fetuses exposed in utero to methyldopa for the first time between 16 and 20 weeks' gestation, may have slightly reduced head circumferences (Moar *et al* 1978). The effect is of minor clinical relevance, because at 16–20 weeks, the blood pressure is at its gestational nadir, so there is little need to start treatment at this time. Second, the effect on the babies is so small as to be of doubtful importance—and the long-term follow-up of the affected children shows totally normal development (Redman and Ounsted 1982). The usual treatment schedule is 1–4 g per day in divided doses. The effect of methyldopa can be supplemented by low doses of oral hydralazine as for the treatment of pre-eclamptic hypertension.

Beta adrenergic blocking agents

These have been used less extensively in pregnancy, and their possible fetal effects have not been completely evaluated. Intrauterine growth retardation, respiratory difficulties at birth, neonatal bradycardia, and hypoglycaemia have all been reported as possible problems after long-term propranolol at levels of 20–240 mg per day (Tcherdakoff *et al* 1978; Pruyn *et al* 1979; Gladstone and Gersony 1975; Habib and McCarthy 1977; Cottrill *et al* 1977). However, neonatal hypoglycaemia or bradycardia was not noted in a large uncontrolled series of babies, born to 101 mothers who were treated for hypertension with metoprolol in various combinations with hydralazine or diuretics (Sandström 1978). Further, improved fetal outcome was observed in 26 hypertensive patients treated with long-term oxprenolol compared with 27 patients treated with methyldopa (Gallery *et al* 1979b). The investigators claimed that oxprenolol not only controlled maternal hypertension but promoted plasma volume expansion, causing the apparently better fetal growth in the oxprenolol treated groups. This apparently beneficial effect of oxprenolol has not been confirmed in a similar but larger trial (Fidler *et al* 1983). A further large, randomised, controlled trial of the combined alpha-beta adrenergic receptor antagonist labetalol, compared with methyldopa, likewise shows no significant short-term advantage in terms of fetal growth or survival (Redman 1982).

Adrenergic control of uterine activity is well established. Beta adrenergic blockade enhances uterine activity in experimental animals and in pregnant women in the second and third trimesters (Maughan *et al* 1967; Amy and Karim 1974; Barden and Stander 1968), therefore, premature or precipitate labour might be a complication of treatment, but the larger series are reassuring on this point. Acute experiments in the ewe suggest that propranolol reduces umbilical blood flow (Oakes *et al* 1976) and impairs the fetal lambs' ability to withstand acute anoxic stress. If these data can be applied to the human situation, then fetal problems might only be expected when there is already compromise in terms of pre-existing placental inadequacy; therefore beta adrenoceptor blocking agents should not be used indiscriminately in pregnancy, although it is now clear that in general they are safe.

Other drugs

If diuretics are essential for good blood pressure control, they can be continued throughout pregnancy, but their use carries certain disadvantages if pre-eclampsia should supervene. Bethanidine, clonidine (Turnbull and Ahmed 1969) and prazosin (Lubbe and Hodge 1981) have all been used in pregnancy, but their effect on the fetus has not been fully defined. Reserpine and captopril both have adverse fetal or neonatal side effects and so should not be used.

UNUSUAL CAUSES OF HYPERTENSION IN PREGNANCY

Phaeochromocytoma

This is a rare but dangerous complication of pregnancy, with a maternal mortality previously as high as 50 per cent (Blair 1963). The presentation frequently simulates severe pre-eclampsia with extreme but unstable hypertension, proteinuria and pre-eclamptic-like symptoms such as headaches (Schenker and Chowers 1971). For this reason, all patients with proteinuric hypertension in pregnancy should be screened for phaeochromocytoma, although even then the diagnosis can be missed by false-negative results (Coden 1972). Provided the condition can be identified and treated before delivery the maternal mortality is reduced (to zero in cases where alpha adrenergic blockade has been used). Methods of diagnosis are the same as in non-pregnant individuals, but radiological localisation is precluded because of the risks to the fetus. Treatment with alpha adrenergic blockade, with or without addition of beta adrenergic blockade, is compatible with normal fetal survival. Given adequate medical treatment tumour resection can be successfully accomplished at delivery by Caesarean section, or at a later elective date (Shenker and Chowers 1971). Both malignant and ectopic tumours have been reported in pregnancy (Fawcett and Kimbell 1971; Simanis *et al* 1972).

Coarctation of the aorta (*see* Chapter 5).

Previously this condition was associated with a high enough mortality in pregnancy for termination to be recommended (Deal and Wooley 1973). Maternal death was primarily from dissection or rupture of the aorta. Contemporary experience is more favourable and decisions about the advisability of a pregnancy may depend more on related factors such as associated cardiac malformation. Surgical resection during pregnancy is not advisable (Goodwin 1961), but a previous successful resection is not a contraindication to undertaking pregnancy.

Cushing's syndrome (*see* Chapter 12).

Amenorrhoea and menstrual irregularities are common features of Cushing's syndrome, so that the likelihood of conception is diminished. Many of the features of the syndrome—increased pigmentation, striae, weight gain, hyperglycaemia and hypertension—may occur during pregnancy in the absence of the disease. Difficulties of diagnosis are further compounded because normal pregnancy causes increased bound and unbound plasma cortisol with blunting of its diurnal variation, increased urinary free cortisol, and moderately increased 17-hydroxysteroids and 17-ketosteroids (Ramsay 1980). Suppression of cortisol production by dexamethasone is the appropriate diagnostic test, although normally this is less complete than in non-pregnant subjects. There is a relatively high incidence of primary adrenal tumours including carcinoma as rare instances (Kreines and DeVaux 1971). For these reasons surgical exploration and removal should be considered once the diagnosis is made. Adrenalectomy during pregnancy with a later successful outcome has been reported (Parra and Cruz-Krohn 1966). Fetal loss is high in Cushing's syndrome and there may be neonatal adrenal insufficiency (Kreines and DeVaux 1971).

Conn's syndrome

This is a rare cause of hypertension in pregnancy. It has usually been diagnosed either before or after pregnancy on the basis of hypokalaemia combined with hypertension (Crane *et al* 1964; Gordon *et al* 1967). During pregnancy both plasma concentrations and urinary excretion of aldosterone are increased which makes diagnosis difficult. Remission of the disorder may occur during pregnancy possibly caused by progesterone which antagonises the renal action of aldosterone (Aoi *et al* 1978). Successful pregnancies with and without medical treatment have been reported.

Neurofibromatosis, which may be complicated by hypertension in pregnancy, is considered on p. 470.

LONG-TERM SEQUELAE OF HYPERTENSION IN PREGNANCY

Severe pre-eclampsia and eclampsia can cause irreversible maternal damage, particularly acute renal and cortical necrosis or cerebral haemorrhage. In the absence of these complications there is no evidence at the present time that long-term health is impaired by a pre-eclamptic illness. However, in terms of life expectancy, pre-eclamptic women fall into two groups. Those who have an episode in the first pregnancy only and become normotensive soon after delivery, have a normal life expectancy. The second group have recurrent pre-eclampsia in several pregnancies, or blood pressures which remain elevated in the puerperium. They have a higher incidence of later cardiovascular disorders and a reduced life expectancy compatible with the diagnosis that the initial episode of pre-eclampsia was superimposed on pre-existing hypertension (Chesley *et al* 1976). In terms of long-term follow-up a remote postnatal reassessment is therefore desirable after a hypertensive pregnancy. This should include measurements of blood pressure and renal function. If there has been significant proteinuria an intravenous pyelogram is indicated. If the proteinuria persists, further investigation including a renal biopsy may be indicated.

Since the first report (Brownrigg 1962), oral contraceptives have been implicated as a cause of hypertension which may be severe and very rarely malignant (Zech *et al* 1975). For this reason chronic hypertension is a relative contraindication to their use. It has been suggested (Carmichael *et al* 1970) but not confirmed (Pritchard and Pritchard 1977) that pre-eclampsia may be associated with hypertension induced by oral contraceptives. The advice given to postpartum women should therefore be guided by whether or not hypertension persists as a chronic problem. If a pre-eclamptic woman's blood pressure returns to normal, there seems little reason to deny her the benefits of oral contraceptives provided adequate and continuing medical supervision is available.

Conclusions

1   Hypertension is an artificial concept.

2   A raised blood pressure is one of many secondary effects of pre-eclampsia on the maternal system.

3   In pre-eclampsia, the main differential diagnosis is from chronic hypertension which, in its pure form, does not share the renal, coagulation, hepatic and placental abnormalities of pre-eclampsia.

4   The perinatal risks of chronic hypertension in pregnancy are mediated through superimposed pre-eclampsia.

5   Extreme hypertension in pregnanacy is as dangerous as it is in any other medical situation, and demands urgent treatment.

6   The early treatment of mild CHT does not prevent the later superimposition of pre-eclampsia.

7   Methyldopa is the most thoroughly tested hypertensive agent in pregnancy. Apart from a possible effect on fetal head growth, if treatment was started between 16 and 20 weeks' gestation, no significant adverse reaction has been observed.

8   Beta blocking agents seem to be as safe, but the clinical trial data are less complete than for methyldopa.

9   Diuretics should primarily be reserved for the treatment of heart failure complicating pre-eclampsia.

References

Abdul-Karim R.W. & Rizk P.T. (1970) The effect of oxytocin on renal hemodynamics, water and electrolyte excretion. *Obstetrical and Gynaecological Survey* **25**, 805–13.

Abitbol M.M. (1969) Weight gain in pregnancy. *American Journal of Obstetrics and Gynecology* **104**, 140–56.

Abitbol M.M. (1977a) Hemodynamic studies in experimental toxemia of the dog. *Obstetrics and Gynecology* **50**, 293–8.

Abitbol M.M. (1977b) Aortic compression and uterine blood flow during pregnancy. *Obstetrics and Gynecology* **50**, 562–70.

Adams E.M. & MacGillivray I. (1961) Long-term effect of pre-eclampsia on blood pressure. *Lancet* **ii**, 1373–5.

Amy J.J. & Karim S.M.M. (1974) Intrauterine administration of L-noradrenaline and propranolol during the second trimester of pregnancy. *British Journal of Obstetrics and Gynaecology* **81**, 75–83.

Aoi, W., Doi Y., Tasaki S., Mitsuoka J., Suzuki S. & Hashiba K. (1978) Primary aldosteronism aggravated during peripartum period. *Japanese Heart Journal* **19**, 946–53.

Arias F. & Mancilla-Jimenez R. (1976) Hepatic fibrinogen deposits in pre-eclampsia. *New England Journal of Medicine* **295**, 578–82.

Assali N.S., Holm L.W. & Parker H.R. (1964) Systemic and regional hemodynamic alterations in toxemia. *Circulation* **29** and **30** (Suppl. II), 53–7.

Assali N.S., Kaplan S., Oighenstein S. & Suyemoto R. (1953) Hemodynamic effects of 1-hydrazinophthalazine in human pregnancy; results of intravenous administration. *Journal of Clinical Investigation* **32**, 922–30.

Bader R.A., Bader M.E., Rose D.J. & Braunwald E. (1955) Hemodynamics at rest and during exercise in normal pregnancy as studied by cardiac catheterisation. *Journal of Clinical Investigation* **34**, 1524–36.

Baillie T.W. (1963) Vasopressor activity of ergometrine maleate in anaesthetised parturient women. *British Medical Journal* **1**, 585–8.

Baird D. (1977) Epidemiological aspects of hypertensive pregnancy. *Clinics in Obstetrics and Gynaecology* **4**, 531–48.

Barden T.P. & Keenan W.J. (1971) Effects of diazoxide in human labour and the fetus-neonate. *Obstetrics and Gynecology* **37**, 631–2.

Barden T.P. & Stander R.W. (1968) Myometrial and cardiovascular effects of an adrenergic blocking drug in human pregnancy. *American Journal of Obstetrics and Gynecology* **101**, 91–9.

Beaufils M., Uzan S., Don Simoni R. & Colau J.C. (1982) A prospective controlled study of dipyridamole and aspirin in high risk pregnancy. Preliminary results in 57 cases. *Clinical and Experimental Hypertension* **B1**, 334.

Beller F.K., Ebert C. & Dame W.R. (1979) High molecular fibrin derivatives in pre-eclamptic and eclamptic patients. *European Journal of Obstetrics, Gynecology and Reproductive Biology* **9**, 105–10.

Bienarz J., Crottogini J.J., Curuchet E., Romero-Salinas G., Yoshida T., Poseiro J.J. & Caldeyro-Barcia R. (1968) Aortocaval compression by the uterus in late human pregnancy. *American Journal of Obstetrics and Gynecology* **100**, 203–17.

Bis K.A. & Waxman B. (1976) Rupture of the liver associated with pregnancy: a review of the literature and report of 2 cases. *Obstetrical and Gynecological Survey* **31**, 763–73.

Blair R.G. (1963) Phaeochromocytoma and pregnancy. *Journal of Obstetrics and Gynaecology of the British Commonwealth* **70**, 110–19.

Blekta M., Hlavaty V., Trnkova M., Bendl J., Bendova L. & Chytil M (1970) Volume of whole blood and absolute amount of serum proteins in the early stage of late toxemia of pregnancy. *American Journal of Obstetrics and Gynecology* **106**, 10–13.

Blumenthal I. (1976) Diet and diuretics in pregnancy and subsequent growth of offspring. *British Medical Journal* **2**, 733.

Boneu B., Fournie A., Sie P., Grandjean H., Bierme R. & Pontonnier G. (1980) Platelet production time, uricemia and some hemostasis tests in pre-eclampsia. *European Journal of Obstetrics, Gynecology and Reproductive Biology* **11**, 85–94.

Bonnar J., McNicol G.P. and Douglas A.S. (1971) Coagulation and fibrinolytic systems in pre-eclampsia. *British Medical Journal* **2**, 12–16.

Broughton Pipkin F., Hunter J.C., Turner S.R. and O'Brien P.M.S. (1982) Prostaglandin E_2 attenuates the pressor response to angiotensin II in pregnant subjects but not in nonpregnant subjects. *American Journal of Obstetrics and Gynecology* **142**, 168–76.

Broughton Pipkin F. and Turner S.R. (1982) The effect of antiotensin converting-enzyme inhibitor in pregnant animals. In Sammour M.B., Symonds E.M., Zuspan F.P. and El-Tomi N. (eds) *Pregnancy Hypertension*, pp. 507–13. Ain Shamo University Press, Cairo.

Browne F.J. and Dodds G.H. (1942) Pregnancy in the patient with chronic hypertension. *Journal of Obstetrics and Gynaecology of the British Empire* **49**, 1–17.

Brownrigg G.M. (1962) Toxemia in hormone-induced pseudopregnancy. *Canadian Medical Association Journal* **87**, 408–9.

Büller H.R., Weenink A.H., Treffers P.E., Kahle L.H., Otten H.A. & Ten Cate J.W. (1980) Severe antithrombin III deficiency in a patient with pre-eclampsia. Observations on the effect of human AT III concentrate transfusion. *Scandinavian Journal of Haematology* **25**, 81–6.

Butler N.R. & Bonham D.G. (1963) *Perinatal Mortality*, pp. 86–100. Edinburgh, E. and S. Livingstone.

Campbell D.M. (1978) The effect of posture on the blood pressure in pregnancy. *European Journal of Obstetrics, Gynecology and Reproductive Medicine* **8**, 263–8.

Campbell D.M. & MacGillivray I. (1975) The effect of a low calorie diet or a thiazide diuretic on the incidence of pre-eclampsia and on birthweight. *British Journal of Obstetrics and Gynaecology* **82**, 572–7.

Carmichael S.M., Taylor M.M. & Ayers C.R. (1970) Oral contraceptives, hypertension and toxemia. *Obstetrics and Gynecology* **35**, 371–6.

Cavanagh D., Rao P.S., Tsai C.C. & O'Connor T.C. (1977) Experimental toxemia in the pregnant primate. *American Journal of Obstetrics and Gynecology* **128**, 75–85.

Chamberlain G., Philipp E., Howlett B. & Masters K. (1978) *British Births 1970*, pp. 80–107. E. & S. Livingstone, London.

Chen H.F., Nakabayashi M., Satoh K. & Sakamoto S. (1980) Urinary fibrinolysis in toxemia of pregnancy. *Acta Obstetricia et Gynecologica Scandinavica Supplement* **59**, 499–504.

Chesley L.C. (1966) Vascular reactivity in normal and toxemic pregnancy. *Clinical Obstetrics and Gynecology* **9**, 871–81.

Chesley L.C. (1972) Plasma and red cell volumes during pregnancy. *American Journal of Obstetrics and Gynecology* **112**, 440–50.

Chesley L.C. (1978a) *Hypertensive Disorders in Pregnancy*, pp. 9–11. New York, Appleton-Century-Crofts.

Chesley L.C. (1978b) *Hypertensive Disorders in Pregnancy*, pp. 124–6. New York, Appleton-Century-Crofts.

Chesley L.C. (1978c) *Hypertensive Disorders in Pregnancy*, p. 210. New York, Appleton-Century-Crofts.

Chesley L.C. (1978d) *Hypertensive Disorders in Pregnancy*, pp. 318–24. New York, Appleton-Century-Crofts.

Chesley L.C. (1978e) *Hypertensive Disorders in Pregnancy*, p. 478. New York, Appleton-Century-Crofts.

Chesley L.C. & Annitto J.E. (1943) A study of salt restriction and of fluid intake in prophylaxis against pre-eclampsia in patients with water retention. *American Journal of Obstetrics and Gynecology* **45**, 961–71.

Chesley L.C., Annitto J.E. & Cosgrove R.A. (1968) The familial factor in toxemia of pregnancy. *Obstetrics and Gynecology* **32**, 303–11.

Chesley L.C., Annitto J.E. & Cosgrove R.A. (1976) The remote prognosis of eclamptic women. Sixth periodic report. *American Journal of Obstetrics and Gynecology* **124**, 446–59.

Chesley L.C., Annitto J.E. & Jarvis D.G. (1947) A study of the interaction of pregnancy and hypertensive disease. *American Journal of Obstetrics and Gynecology* **53**, 851–63.

Chesley L.C. & Tepper I.H. (1967) Effects of progesterone and estrogen on the sensitivity to angiotensin II. *Journal of Clinical Endocrinology and Metabolism* **27**, 576–81.

Chesley L.C., Valenti C. & Rein H. (1958) Excretion of sodium loads by non-pregnant and pregnant normal, hypertensive and pre-eclamptic women. *Metabolism* **7**, 575–88.

Chesley L.C. & Williams L.O. (1945) Renal glomerular and tubular functions in relation to the hyperuricaemia of pre-eclampsia and eclampsia. *American Journal of Obstetrics and Gynecology* **50**, 367–75.

Chesrow E.J., Bernstein M., Weiss D. & Marquardt G.H. (1966) Comparison of mebutamate, phenobarbital and placebo in the treatment of mild essential hypertension. *American Journal of Medical Sciences* **251**, 166–74.

Chun D., Braga C., Chow C. & Lok L. (1964) Clinical observations on some aspects of hydatidiform moles. *Journal of Obstetrics and Gynaecology of the British Commonwealth* **71**, 180–4.

Clarke H.G.M., Freeman T. & Pryse-Phillips W. (1971) Serum proteins in normal pregnancy and mild pre-eclampsia. *Journal of Obstetrics and Gynaecology of the British Commonwealth* **78**, 105–9.

Cockburn J., Moar V.A., Ounsted M. & Redman C.W.G. (1982) Final report of study on hypertension during pregnancy: the effects of specific treatment on the growth and development of the children. *Lancet* i, 647–9.

Coden J. (1972) Phaeochromocytoma in pregnancy. *Journal of the Royal Society of Medicine* **65**, 863.

Connon A.F. & Wadsworth R.J. (1968) An evaluation of serum uric acid estimations in toxaemia of pregnancy. *Australia and New Zealand Journal of Obstetrics and Gynaecology* **8**, 197–201.

Cooper D.W. & Liston W.A. (1979) Genetic control of severe pre-eclampsia. *Journal of Medical Genetics* **16**, 409–16.

Cooper E.H. & Cranston W. (1957) A comparison of the effects of phenobarbitone and reserpine in hypertension. *Lancet* **1**, 396–7.

Cottrill C.M., McAllister R.G., Gettes L. & Noonan J.A. (1977) Propranolol therapy during pregnancy, labour, and delivery: evidence for transplacental drug transfer and impaired neonatal drug disposition. *Journal of Paediatrics* **91**, 812–14.

Crane M.G., Andes J.P., Harris J.J. & Slate W.G. (1964) Primary aldosteronism in pregnancy. *Obstetrics and Gynecology* **23**, 200–8.

Cree J.E., Meyer J. & Hailey D.M. (1973) Diazepam in labour: its metabolism and effect on the clinical condition and thermogenesis of the newborn. *British Mecical Journal* **4**, 251–5.

Cuadros A. & Tatum H.J. (1964) The prophylactic and therapeutic use of bendroflumethiazide in pregnancy. *American Journal of Obstetrics and Gynecology* **89**, 891–7.

Davies M.H., Wilkinson S.P., Hanid M.A., Portmann B., Brudenell J.M., Newton J.R. & Williams R. (1980) Acute liver disease with encephalopathy and renal failure in late pregnancy and the early puerperium: a study of fourteen patients. *British Journal of Obstetrics and Gynaecology* **87**, 1005–14.

Deal K. & Wooley C.F. (1973) Coarctation of the aorta and pregnancy. *Annals of Internal Medicine* **78**, 706–10.

De Alvarez R.R. (1955) Use of hypotensive agents in treatment of pre-eclamptic toxemia of pregnancy. *Obstetrics and Gynecology* **6**, 55–62.

Douglas B.H. & Langford H.G. (1969) Post-term blood pressure elevation produced by uterine wrapping. *American Journal of Obstetrics and Gynecology* **97**, 231–4.

Douglas J.T., Shah M., Lowe G.D.O., Belch J.J.F., Forbes C.D. & Prentice C.R.M. (1982) Plasma fibrinopeptide A and beta-thromboglobulin in pre-eclampsia and pregnancy hypertension. *Thrombosis and Haemostasis* **47**, 54–5.

Duffus G. & MacGillivray I. (1968) The incidence of pre-eclamptic toxaemia in smokers and non-smokers. *Lancet* **1**, 994–5.

Duffus G.M., Tunstall M.E., Condie R.G. & MacGillivray I. (1969) Chlormethiazole in the prevention of eclampsia and the reduction of perinatal mortality. *Journal of Obstetrics and Gynaecology of the British Commonwealth* **76**, 645–51.

Dunlop W., Hill L.M., Landon M.J., Oxley A. & Jones P. (1978) Clinical relevance of coagulation and renal changes in pre-eclampsia. *Lancet* **2**, 346–50.

Eden T.W. (1922) Eclampsia: a commentary on the reports presented to the British Congress of Obstetrics and Gynaecology. *Journal of Obstetrics and Gynaecology of the British Empire* **29**, 386–401.

Everett R.B., Worley R.J., MacDonald P.C. & Gant N.F. (1978a) Oral administration of theophylline to modify pressor responsiveness to angiotensin II in women with pregnancy-induced hypertension. *American Journal of Obstetrics and Gynaecology* **132**, 359–62.

Everett R.B., Worley R.J., MacDonald P.C. & Gant N.F. (1978b) Modification of vascular responsiveness to angiotensin II in pregnant women by intravenously infused 5 α-dihydro-progesterone. *American Journal of Obstetrics and Gynaecology* **131**, 352–7.

Fawcett F.J. & Kimbell N.K.B. (1971) Phaeochromocytoma of the ovary. *British Journal of Obstetrics and Gynaecology* **78**, 458–9.

Felding C.F. (1969) Obstetric aspects in women with histories of renal disease. *Acta Obstetricia et Gynecologica Scandinavica* **48** (Suppl. 2), 1–43.

Fidler J., Bennett M.J., de Swiet M., Ellis C. & Lewis P.J. (1980) Treatment of pregnancy hypertension with prostacyclin. *Lancet* **ii**, 31–2.

Fidler J., Smith V. & de Swiet M. (1983) Randomised controlled comparative study of methyl dopa and oxprenolol for the treatment of hypertension in pregnancy. *British Medical Journal* **286**, 1927–80.

Finnerty F.A. & Bepko F.J. (1966) Lowering the perinatal mortality and the prematurity rate. *Journal of the American Medical Association* **195**, 429–32.

Fisher K.A., Ahuja S., Luger A., Spargo B. & Lindheimer M. (1977) Nephrotic proteinuria with pre-eclampsia. *American Journal of Obstetrics and Gynecology* **129**, 643–6.

Flowers C.E., Grizzle J.E., Easterling W.E. & Bonner O.B. (1962) Chlorothiazide as a prophylaxis against toxemia of pregnancy. A double-blind study. *American Journal of Obstetrics and Gynecology* **84**, 919–29.

Forman J.B. & Sullivan R.L (1952) The effects of intravenous injections of ergonovine and methergine on the post partum patient. *American Journal of Obstetrics and Gynecology* **63**, 640–4.

Gallery E.D.M., Hunyor S.N. & Gyory A.Z. (1979a) Plasma volume contraction: a significant factor in both pregnancy-associated hypertension (pre-eclampsia) and chronic hypertension in pregnancy. *Quarterly Journal of Medicine* **48**, 593–602.

Gallery E.D.M., Ross M., Hunyor S.N. & Gyory A.Z. (1977) Predicting the development of pregnancy-associated hypertension. *Lancet* **1**, 1273–5.

Gallery E.D.M., Saunders D.M., Hunyor S.N. & Gyory A.Z. (1979b) Randomised comparison of methyldopa and oxprenolol for treatment of hypertension in pregnancy. *British Medical Journal* 1, 1591 4.

Galton M., Merritt K. & Beller F.K. (1971) Coagulation studies on the peripheral circulation of patients with toxemia of pregnancy: a study for the evaluation of disseminated intravascular coagulation in toxemia. *Journal of Reproductive Medicine* 6, 89–100.

Gant N.F., Chand S., Worley R.J., Whalley P.J., Crosby U.D. & MacDonald P.C. (1974) A clinical test useful for predicting the development of acute hypertension in pregnancy. *American Journal of Obstetrics and Gynecology* 120, 1–7.

Gant N.F., Daley G.L., Chand S., Whalley P.J. & MacDonald P.C. (1973) A study of angiotensin II pressure response throughout primigravid pregnancy. *Journal of Clinical Investigation* 52, 2682–9.

Gant N.F., Madden J.D., Siiteri P.K. & MacDonald P.C. (1975) The metabolic clearance rate of dehydroisoandrosterone. III. The effect of thiazide diuretics in normal and future pre-eclamptic pregnancies. *American Journal of Obstetrics and Gynecology* 123, 159–63.

Gant N.F. & Worley R.J. (1980) *Hypertension in Pregnancy. Concepts and Management*, p. 121. Appleton-Century, Crofts, New York.

Giles C. & Inglis T.C.M. (1981) Thrombocytopenia and macrothrombocytosis in gestational hypertension. *British Journal of Obstetrics and Gynaecology* 88, 1115–19.

Ginsberg J. & Duncan S.B. (1969) Direct and indirect blood pressure measurement in pregnancy. *Journal of Obstetrics and Gynaecology of the British Commonwealth* 76, 705–10.

Gladstone G.R. & Gersony W.M. (1975) Propranolol administration during pregnancy: effects on the fetus. *Journal of Pediatrics* 86, 962–4.

Goldby F.S. & Beilin L.J. (1972) Relationship between arterial pressure and the permeability of arterioles to carbon particles in acute hypertension in the rat. *Cardiovascular Research* 6, 384–90.

Goodlin R.C., Cotton D.B. & Haesslein H.C. (1978) Severe edema-proteinuria-hypertension gestosis. *American Journal of Obstetrics and Gynecology* 132, 595–8.

Goodwin J.F. (1961) Pregnancy and coarctation of the aorta. *Clinical Obstetrics and Gynecology* 4, 645–64.

Gordon R.D., Fishman L.M. & Liddle G.W. (1967) Plasma renin activity and aldosterone secretion in a pregnant woman with primary aldosteronism. *Journal of Clinical Endocrinology and Metabolism* 27, 385–8.

Graham C. & Goldstein A. (1980) Epidural analgesia and cardiac output in severe pre-eclampsia. *Anaesthesia* 35, 709–12.

Habib A. & McCarthy J.S. (1977) Effects on the neonate of propranolol administered during pregnancy. *Journal of Pediatrics* 91, 808–11.

Hamlin R.H.J. (1952) The prevention of eclampsia and pre-eclampsia. *Lancet* 1, 64–8.

Harley J.M.G. (1966) Pregnancy in the chronic hypertensive woman. *Proceedings of the Royal Society of Medicine* 39, 835–8.

Hauth J.C., Cunningham F.G. & Whalley P.J. (1976) Management of pregnancy-induced hypertension in the nullipara. *Obstetrics and Gynecology* 48, 253–9.

Hibbard B.M. & Rosen M. (1977) The management of severe pre-eclampsia and eclampsia. *British Journal of Anaesthesia* 49, 3–9.

Holmes F. (1960) Incidence of the supine hypotensive syndrome in late pregnancy. *Journal of Obstetrics and Gynaecology of the British Empire* 67, 254–8.

Horne C.H.W., Briggs J.D., Howie P.W. & Kennedy A.C. (1972) Serum α-macroglobulins in renal disease and pre-eclampsia. *Journal of Clinical Pathology* 25, 590–3.

Horne C.H.W., Howie P.W. & Goudie R.B. (1970) Serum alpha$_2$-macroglobulin, transferrin, albumin and IgG levels in pre-eclampsia. *Journal of Clinical Pathology* 23, 514–16.

Howie P.W., Begg C.B., Purdie D.W. & Prentice C.R.M. (1976) Use of coagulation tests to predict the clinical progress of pre-eclampsia. *Lancet* **2**, 323–5.

Howie P.W., Prentice C.R.M. & Forbes C.D. (1975) Failure of heparin therapy to affect the clinical course of severe pre-eclampsia. *British Journal of Obstetrics and Gynaecology* **82**, 711–17.

Jeffcoate T.N.A. & Scott J.S. (1959) Some observations on the placental factor in pregnancy toxemia. *American Journal of Obstetrics and Gynecology* **77**, 475–89.

Johansson B., Strandgaard S. & Lassen N.A. (1974) On the pathogenesis of hypertensive encephalopathy. *Circulation Research* **34** (Suppl. 1), 167–71.

Johnson T. & Clayton C.G. (1957) Diffusion of radioactive sodium in normotensive and pre-eclamptic pregnancies. *British Medical Journal* **1**, 312–14.

Jones H.M.R. & Cummings A.J. (1978) A study of the transfer of α-methyldopa to the human fetus and newborn infant. *British Journal of Clinical Pharmacology* **6**, 432–4.

Jouppila R., Jouppila P. & Hollmen A. (1980) Laryngeal oedema as an obstetric anaesthesia complication: case reports. *Acta Anaesthesiologica Scandinavica* **24**, 97–8.

Jouppila R., Jouppila P., Hollmen A. & Koivula A. (1979) Epidural analgesia and placental blood flow during labour in pregnancies complicated by hypertension. *British Journal of Obstetrics and Gynaecology* **86**, 969–72.

Joyce D.N. & Kenyon V.G. (1972) The use of diazepam and hydrallazine in the treatment of severe pre-eclampsia. *Journal of Obstetrics and Gynaecology of the British Commonwealth* **79**, 250–4.

Karbhari D., Harrigan J.T. & Lamagra R. (1977) The supine hypertensive test as a predictor of incipient pre eclampsia. *American Journal of Obstetrics and Gynecology* **127**, 620–2.

Kassar N.S., Aldridge J. & Quirk B. (1980) Roll over test. *Obstetrics and Gynecology* **55**, 411–13.

Killam A., Dillard S., Patton R. & Pederson P. (1975) Pregnancy-induced hypertension complicated by acute liver disease and disseminated intravascular coagulation. *American Journal of Obstetrics and Gynecology* **123**, 823–8.

Kirkendall W.M., Feinleib M., Freis E.D. & Mark A.L. (1981) Recommendations for human blood pressure determination by sphygmomanometers. Sub-committee of the AHA postgraduate education committee. *Hypertension* **3**, 510A–19A.

Kraus G.W., Marchese J.R. & Yen S.S.C. (1966) Prophylactic use of hydrochlorothiazide in pregnancy. *Journal of the American Medical Association* **198**, 1150–4.

Kreines K. & Devaux W.D. (1971) Neonatal adrenal insufficiency associated with maternal Cushing's syndrome. *Pediatrics* **47**, 516–19.

Lamming G.D., Broughton Pipkin F. & Symonds E.M. (1980) Comparison of the alpha and beta blocking drug, labetalol, and methyl dopa in the treatment of moderate and severe pregnancy-induced hypertension. *Clinical and Experimental Hypertension* **3**, 865–95.

Lancet (1983) Acute fatty liver of pregnancy. *Lancet* **i**, 339.

Lancet M. & Fisher I.L. (1956) The value of blood uric acid levels in toxaemia of pregnancy. *Journal of Obstetrics and Gynaecology of the British Commonwealth* **63**, 116–19.

Landesman R., Aguero O., Wilson K., La Russa R., Campbell W. & Penaloza O. (1965) The prophylactic use of chlorthalidone, a sulfonamide diuretic in pregnancy. *Journal of Obstetrics and Gynaecology of the British Commonwealth* **72**, 1004–10.

Lean T.H., Ratnam S.S. & Sivasamboo R. (1968) The use of chlordiazepoxide in patients with severe pregnancy toxaemia. *Journal of Obstetrics and Gynaecology of the British Commonwealth* **75**, 853–5.

Leather H.M., Humphreys D.M., Baker P. & Chadd M.A. (1968) A controlled trial of hypotensive agents in hypertension in pregnancy. *Lancet* **2**, 488–90.

Lees M.M., Scott D.B., Kerr M.G. & Taylor S.H. (1967a) The circulatory effects of recumbent postural change in late pregnancy. *Clinical Science* **32**, 453–65.

Lees M.M., Taylor S.H., Scott D.B. & Kerr M.G. (1967b) A study of cardiac output at rest throughout pregnancy. *Journal of Obstetrics and Gynaecology of the British Commonwealth* **74**, 319–27.

Little W.A. (1960) Placental infarction. *Obstetrics and Gynecology* **15**, 109–30.

Lindheimer M.D. (1970) Further characterisation of the influence of supine posture on renal function in late pregnancy. *Gynecological Investigation* **1**, 69–81.

Long R.G., Scheuer P.J. & Sherlock S. (1977) Pre-eclampsia presenting with deep jaundice. *Journal of Clinical Pathology* **30**, 212–15.

Lowe C.R. (1961) Toxaemia and pre-pregnancy weight. *Journal of Obstetrics and Gynaecology of the British Commonwealth* **68**, 622–7.

Lubbe W.F. & Hodge J.V. (1981) Combined α- and β-adrenoceptor-antagonism with prazosin and oxprenolol in control of severe hypertension in pregnancy. *New Zealand Medical Journal* **94**, 169–72.

McClure Browne J.C. & Veall N. (1953) The maternal placental blood flow in normotensive and hypertensive women. *Journal of Obstetrics and Gynaecology of the British Empire* **60**, 141–47.

McFarlane C.N. (1963) An evaluation of the serum uric acid level in pregnancy. *Journal of Obstetrics and Gynaecology of the British Commonwealth* **70**, 63–8.

MacGillivray I. (1958) Some observations on the incidence of pre-eclampsia. *Journal of Obstetrics and Gynaecology of the British Commonwealth* **65**, 536–9.

MacGillivray I. (1961) Hypertension in pregnancy and its consequences. *Journal of Obstetrics and Gynaecology of the British Commonwealth* **68**, 557–69.

MacGillivray I. (1967) The significance of blood pressure and body water changes in pregnancy. *Scottish Medical Journal* **12**, 237–45.

MacGillivray I. (1982) Pregnancy hypertension—is it a disease? In Sammour M.B., Symonds E.M., Zuspan F.P. and El-Tomi N. (eds) *Pregnancy Hypertension*, pp. 1–15. Ain Sharns University Press, Cairo.

MacGillivray I., Rose G.A. & Rowe B. (1969) Blood pressure survey in pregnancy. *Clinical Science* **37**, 395–407.

McKay D.G., Merrill S.J., Weiner A.E., Hertig A.T. and Reid D.E. (1953) The pathologic anatomy of eclampsia bilateral renal corticol necrosis, pituitary necrosis, and other acute fatal complications of pregnancy, and its possible relationship to the generalised Shwartzman phenomenon. *American Journal of Obstetrics and Gynecology* **66**, 507–39.

McKenna P. & Shaw R.W. (1979) Hyponatremic fits in oxytocin—augmented labours. *International Journal of Gynaecology and Obstetrics* **17**, 250–2.

Maclean P.R., Paterson W.G., Smart G.E. Petrie J.J.B., Robson J.S. & Thomson P. (1972) Proteinuria in toxaemia and abruptio placentae. *Journal of Obstetrics and Gynaecology of the British Commonwealth* **79**, 321–6.

Marshall G.W. & Newman R.L. (1977) Roll-over test. *American Journal of Obstetrics and Gynecology* **127**, 623–5.

Mathews D.D. (1977) A randomised controlled trial of bed rest and sedation or normal activity and non-sedation in the management of non-albuminuric hypertension in late pregnancy. *British Journal of Obstetrics and Gynaecology* **84**, 108–14.

Mathews D.D., Agarwal V. & Shuttleworth T.P. (1982) A randomised controlled trial of complete bed rest versus ambulation in the management of proteinuric hypertension during pregnancy. *British Journal of Obstetrics and Gynaecology* **89**, 128–31.

Mathews D.D., Shuttleworth T.P. & Hamilton E.F.B. (1978) Modern trends in management of non-albuminuric hypertension in late pregnancy. *British Medical Journal* **2**, 623–5.

Maughan G.B., Shabanah E.H. & Toth A. (1967) Experiments with pharmacologic sympatholysis in the gravid. *American Journal of Obstetrics and Gynecology* **97**, 764–76.

Maxwell M.H., Waks A.U., Schroth P.C., Karam M. & Dornfield L.P. (1982) Error in blood-pressure measurement due to incorrect cuff size in obese patients. *Lancet* **2**, 33–5.

Mengert W.F. & Tacchi D.A. (1961) Pregnancy toxemia and sodium chloride. *American Journal of Obstetrics and Gynecology* **81**, 601–5.

Menon M.K.K. (1953) Some observations on the treatment of eclampsia with sodium thiopentone. *Journal of Obstetrics and Gynaecology of the British Empire* **60**, 710–14.

Menon M.K.K. (1961) The evolution of the treatment of eclampsia. *Journal of Obstetrics and Gynaecology of the British Commonwealth* **68**, 417–26.

Menzies D. & Prystowsky A. (1967) Acute hemorrhagic pancreatitis during pregnancy and the puerperium associated with thiazide therapy. *Journal of the Florida Medical Association* **54**, 564–5.

Menzies D.N. (1964) Controlled trial of chlorothiazide in treatment of early pre-eclampsia. *British Medical Journal* **1**, 739–42.

Minkowitz S., Soloway H., Hall E.J. & Yermakov V. (1964) Fatal hemorrhagic pancreatis following chlorothiazide administration in pregnancy. *American Journal of Obstetrics and Gynecology* **24**, 337–41.

Moar V.A., Jefferies M.A., Mutch L.M.M., Ounsted M.K. & Redman C.W.G. (1978) Neonatal head circumference and the treatment of maternal hypertension. *British Journal of Obstetrics and Gynaecology* **85**, 933–7.

Morishima H.O., Caritis S.N., Yeh M.-N. & James L.S. (1976) Prolonged infusion of diazoxide in the management of premature labor in the baboon. *Obstetrics and Gynecology* **48**, 203–7.

Morris J.A., Arce J.J., Hamilton C.J., Davidson E.C., Maidman J.E., Clark J.H. & Bloom R.S. (1977) The management of severe pre-eclampsia and eclampsia with intravenous diazoxide. *Obstetrics and Gynecology* **49**, 675–80.

Morris J.A. & O'Grady J.P. (1979) Volume expansion in severe edema-proteinuria-hypertension gestosis. *American Journal of Obstetrics and Gynecology* **135**, 276.

Mulé J.G., Tatum H.J. & Sawyer R.E. (1957) Nitrogenous retention in patients with toxemia of pregnancy—an unusual complication of salt restriction. *American Journal of Obstetrics and Gynecology* **74**, 526–37.

Mutch L.M.M., Moar V.A., Ounsted M.K. & Redman C.W.G. (1977a) Hypertension during pregnancy, with and without specific hypotensive treatment. I. Perinatal factors and neonatal morbidity. *Early Human Development* **1**, 47–57.

Mutch L.M.M., Moar V.A., Ounsted M.K. & Redman C.W.G. (1977b) Hypertension during pregnancy, with and without specific hypotensive treatment. II. The growth and development of the infant in the first year of life. *Early Human Development* **1**, 59–67.

Naeye R.L. & Friedman E.A. (1979) Causes of perinatal death associated with gestational hypertension and proteinuria. *American Journal of Obstetrics and Gynecology* **133**, 8–10.

National Health and Medical Research Council (1981) *Report on Maternal Deaths in Australia 1976–1978*. Australian Government Publishing Service, Canberra.

Nelson T.R. (1955) A clinical study of pre-eclampsia. *Journal of Obstetrics and Gynaecology of the British Empire* **62**, 48–57.

Neuman J., Weiss B., Rabello Y., Cabal L. & Freeman R.K. (1979) Diazoxide for the acute control of severe hypertension complicating pregnancy: a pilot study. *Obstetrics and Gynecology* **53** (Suppl.), 50S–55S.

Oakes G.K., Halker A.M., Ehrenkranz R.A. & Chez R.A. (1976) Effect of propranolol infusion on the umbilical and uterine circulations of pregnant sheep. *American Journal of Obstetrics and Gynecology* **126**, 1038–42.

Ounsted M.K., Moar V.A., Good F.J. & Redman C.W.G. (1980) Hypertension during pregnancy with and without specific treatment; the children at the age of 4 years. *British Journal of Obstetrics and Gynaecology* **87**, 19–24.

Page E.W. & Christianson R. (1976) The impact of mean arterial pressure in the middle trimester upon the outcome of pregnancy. *American Journal of Obstetrics and Gynecology* **125**, 740–6.

Palomaki J.F. & Lindheimer M.D. (1970) Sodium depletion simulating deterioration in a toxemic pregnancy. *New England Journal of Medicine* **282**, 88–9.

Parra A. & Cruz-Krohn J. (1966) Intercurrent Cushing's syndrome and pregnancy. *American Journal of Medicine* **40**, 961–6.

Peck T.M. (1977) A simple test for predicting pregnancy-induced hypertension. *Obstetrics and Gynecology* **50**, 615–17.

Pennington J.C. & Picker R.H. (1972) Diazoxide and the treatment of the acute hypertensive emergency in obstetrics. *Medical Journal of Australia* **2**, 1051–4.

Perkins R.P. (1977) Treatment of toxemia of pregnancy. *Journal of the American Medical Association* **238**, 2143–4.

Phelan J.P., Everidge G.J., Wilder T.L. & Newman C. (1977) Is the supine pressor test an adequate means of predicting acute hypertension in pregnancy? *American Journal of Obstetrics and Gynecology* **128**, 173–6.

Pickering G. (1968a) *High Blood Pressure*, pp. 9–12. London, J. and A. Churchill Ltd.

Pickering G. (1968b) *High Blood Pressure*, pp. 1–5. London, J. and A. Churchill Ltd.

Pickering G. (1968c) *High Blood Pressure*, pp. 414–25. London, J. and A. Churchill Ltd.

Pickering G. (1968d) *High Blood Pressure*, pp. 215–16. London, J. and A. Churchill Ltd.

Pickering G. (1968e) *High Blood Pressure*, p. 412. London, J. and A. Churchill Ltd.

Pohl J.E.F. & Thurston H. (1972) The successful use of oral diazoxide in the treatment of severe toxaemia of pregnancy. *British Medical Journal* **2**, 568–70.

Poland M.L., Mariona F., Darga L., Laurent D. & Lucas C.P. (1980) The roll-over test in healthy primigravid subjects. In Bonnar J., MacGillivray I. and Symonds E.M. (eds) *Pregnancy Hypertension*, pp. 113–18. Lancaster, M.T.P.

Pollak V.E. & Nettles J.B. (1960) The kidney in toxemia of pregnancy: a clinical and pathologic study based on renal biopsies. *Medicine* **39**, 469–526.

Pritchard J.A. & Pritchard S.A. (1977) Blood pressure response to estrogen–progestin oral contraceptive after pregnancy-induced hypertension. *American Journal of Obstetrics and Gynecology* **129**, 733–9.

Pritchard J.A. & Walley P.J. (1961) Severe hypokalemia due to prolonged administration of chlorothiazide during pregnancy. *American Journal of Obstetrics and Gynecology* **81**, 1241–4.

Pritchard J.A., Weisman R., Ratnoff O.D. & Vosburgh G.J. (1954) Intravascular hemolysis, thrombocytopenia and other hematologic abnormalities associated with severe toxemia of pregnancy. *New England Journal of Medicine* **250**, 89–98.

Pruyn S.C., Phelan J.P. & Buchanan G.C. (1979) Long-term propranolol therapy in pregnancy: maternal and fetal outcome. *American Journal of Obstetrics and Gynecology* **135**, 485–9.

Raab W., Schroeder G., Wagner R. & Gigee W. (1956) Vascular reactivity and electrolytes in normal and toxemic pregnancy. *Journal of Clinical Endocrinology* **16**, 1196–1216.

Raftery E.B. & Ward A.P. (1968) The indirect method of recording blood pressure. *Cardiovascular Research* **2**, 210–18.

Rakoczi I., Tallian F., Bagdany S. & Gati I. (1979) Platelet life-span in normal pregnancy and pre-eclampsia as determined by a non-radioisotope technique. *Thrombosis Research* **15**, 553–6.

Ram C.V.S. & Kaplan N.M. (1979) Individual titration of diazoxide dosage in the treatment of severe hypertension. *American Journal of Cardiology* **43**, 627–30.

Ramsay I.D. (1980) The adrenal gland. In Hytten F. and Chamberlain G. (eds) *Clinical Physiology in Obstetrics*, pp. 415–16. Blackwell Scientific Publications, Oxford.

Redd J., Mosey L.M. & Langford H.G. (1968) Effect of posture upon sodium excretion in pre-eclampsia. *American Journal of Obstetrics and Gynecology* **100**, 343–7.

Redman C.W.G. (1980a) Treatment of hypertension in pregnancy. *Kidney International* **18**, 267–78.

Redman C.W.G. (1980b) Immunological aspects of eclampsia and pre-eclampsia. In Hearn J.P. (ed.) *Immunological Aspects of Reproduction and Fertility Control*, pp. 83–104. Lancaster, M.T.P.

Redman C.W.G. (1982) A controlled trial of the treatment of hypertension in pregnancy: labetalol compared with methyldopa. In Riley A. and Symonds E.M. (eds) *The Investigation of Labetalol in the Management of Hypertension in Pregnancy*, pp. 101–10. Excerpta Medica, International Congress Series 591.

Redman C.W.G., Allington M.J., Bolton F.G. & Stirrat G.M. (1977) Plasma β-thromboglobulin in pre-eclampsia. *Lancet* **2**, 248.

Redman C.W.G., Beilin L.J. & Bonnar J. (1976a) Variability of blood pressure in normal and abnormal pregnancy. In Lindheimer M.D., Katz A.I. and Zuspan F.P. (eds) *Hypertension in Pregnancy*, pp. 53–60. New York, John Wiley.

Redman C.W.G., Beilin L.J. & Bonnar J. (1976b) Renal function in pre-eclampsia. *Journal of Clinical Pathology* **10** (Suppl. Royal College of Pathologists), 91–4.

Redman C.W.G., Beilin L.J. & Bonnar J. (1977) Treatment of hypertension in pregnancy with methyldopa: blood pressure control and side effects. *British Journal of Obstetrics and Gynaecology* **84**, 419–26.

Redman C.W.G., Beilin L.J., Bonnar J. & Ounsted M.K. (1976) Fetal outcome in trial of antihypertensive treatment in pregnancy. *Lancet* **2**, 753–6.

Redman C.W.G., Beilin L.J., Bonnar J. & Wilkinson R.H. (1976) Plasma-urate measurements in predicting fetal death in hypertensive pregnancy. *Lancet* **1**, 1370–3.

Redman C.W.G., Bonnar J. & Beilin L.J. (1978) Early platelet consumption in pre-eclampsia. *British Medical Journal* **1**, 467–9.

Redman C.W.G., Denson K.W.E., Beilin L.J., Bolton F.G. & Stirrat G.M. (1977) Factor VIII consumption in pre-eclampsia. *Lancet* **2**, 1249–52.

Redman C.W.G. & Ounsted M.K. (1982) Safety for the child of drug treatment for hypertension in pregnancy. *Lancet* **i**, 1237.

Report on Confidential Enquiries into Maternal Deaths in England and Wales 1973–1975 (1979), pp. 21–29. London, HMSO.

Report on Confidential Enquiries into Maternal Deaths in England and Wales 1976–1978 (1982), pp. 19–25. London, HMSO.

Rippmann E.T. (1968) Gestosis of late pregnancy. *Gynaecologia* **165**, 12–20.

Robertson E.G. (1971) The natural history of oedema during pregnancy. *Journal of Obstetrics and Gynaecology of the British Commonwealth* **78**, 520–9.

Robinson M. (1958) Salt in pregnancy. *Lancet* **1**, 178–81.

Sandström B.O. (1978) Antihypertensive treatment with the adrenergic beta-receptor blocker metoprolol during pregnancy. *Gynecological and Obstetric Investigation* **9**, 195–204.

Scanlon M.F. (1974) Hypertension in pregnancy. *Journal of Obstetrics and Gynaecology of the British Commonwealth* **81**, 539–44.

Schenker J.G. & Chowers I. (1971) Phaeochromocytoma and pregnancy. *Obstetrical and Gynecological Survey* **26**, 739–47.

Schifrin B.S., Spellacy W.N. & Little W.A. (1969) Maternal death associated with excessive ingestion of a chlorothiazide diuretic. *Obstetrics and Gynecology* **34**, 215–20.

Schramm M. (1979) Prophylactic anticoagulation in the management of recurrent pre-eclampsia and fetal death. *Australia and New Zealand Journal of Obstetrics and Gynaecology* **19**, 230–2.

Seligman S.A. (1971) Diurnal blood-pressure variation in pregnancy. *British Journal of Obstetrics and Gynaecology* **78**, 417–22.

Sheehan H.L. & Lynch J.P. (1973a) *Pathology of Toxaemia of Pregnancy*, pp. 524–53. London, Churchill-Livingstone.

Sheehan H.L. & Lynch J.B. (1973b) *Pathology of Toxaemia of Pregnancy*, pp. 328–330. London, Churchill-Livingstone.

Shukla P.K., Sharma D. & Mandal R.K. (1978) Serum lactate dehydrogenase in detecting liver damage associated with pre-eclampsia. *British Journal of Obstetrics and Gynaecology* **85**, 40–42.

Simanis J., Amerson J.R., Hendee A.E. & Anton A.H. (1972) Unresectable phaeochromocytoma in pregnancy. *American Journal of Medicine* **53**, 381–5.

Simanowitz M.D., MacGregor W.G. & Hobbs J.R. (1973) Proteinuria in pre-eclampsia. *Journal of Obstetrics and Gynaecology of the British Commonwealth* **80**, 103–8.

Smith K, Browne J.C.Mc., Shackman R. & Wrong O.M. (1968) Renal failure of obstetric origin. *British Medical Bulletin* **24**, 49–58.

Smith M.J., Aynsley-Green A. & Redman C.W.G. (1982) Neonatal hyperglycaemia after prolonged maternal treatment with diazoxide. *British Medical Journal* **284**, 1234.

Smith R.W. (1970) Cardiovascular alterations in toxemia. *American Journal of Obstetrics and Gynecology* **107**, 979–83.

Stewart A. & Hewitt D. (1960) Toxaemia of pregnancy and obesity. *Journal of Obstetrics and Gynaecology of the British Empire* **67**, 812–18.

Strauss R.G., Keefer J.R., Burke T. & Civetta J.M. (1980) Hemodynamic monitoring of cardiogenic pulmonary edema complicating toxemia of pregnancy. *Obstetrics and Gynecology* **55**, 170–4.

Sullivan J.M., Palmer E.T., Schoeneberger A.A., Jennings J.L., Morrison J.C. & Ratts T.E. (1978) SQ 20,881: Effect on eclamptic–pre-eclamptic women with postpartum hypertension. *American Journal of Obstetrics and Gynecology* **131**, 707–15.

Szekely P. & Snaith L. (1947) The heart in toxaemia of pregnancy. *British Heart Journal* **9**, 128–37.

Tatum H.J. & Mulé J.G. (1956) Puerperal vasomotor collapse in patients with toxemia of pregnancy—A new concept of the etiology and a rational plan of treatment. *American Journal of Obstetrics and Gynecology* **71**, 492–501.

Taylor H.C., Tillman A.J. & Blanchard J. (1954) Fetal losses in hypertension and pre-eclampsia. *Obstetrics and Gynecology* **3**, 225–39.

Tcherdakoff P.H., Colliard M., Berrard E., Kreft C., Dupay A. & Bernailie J.M. (1978) Propranolol in hypertension during pregnancy. *British Medical Journal* **2**, 670.

Tepperman H.M., Beydoun S.N. & Abdul-Karim R.W. (1977) Drugs affecting myometrial contractility in pregnancy. *Clinical Obstetrics and Gynecology* **20**, 423–45.

Theobald G.W. (1956) *The Pregnancy Toxemias*, pp. 446–57. New York, Hoeber.

Thien Th., Koene R.A.P., Schijf Ch., Pieters G.F.F.M., Eskes T.K.A.B. & Wijdeveld P.G.A.B. (1980) Infusion of diazoxide in severe hypertension during pregnancy. *European Journal of Obstetrics, Gynecology and Reproductive Biology* **10**, 367–74.

Thomson A.M., Hytten R.E. & Billewicz W.Z. (1967) The epidemiology of edema during pregnancy. *Journal of Obstetrics and Gynaecology of the British Commonwealth* **74**, 1–10.

Turnbull A.C. & Ahmed S. (1969) Catapres in the treatment of hypertension in pregnancy. In Conolly M.E. (ed.) *Catapres in Hypertension*, pp. 237–45. London, Butterworths.

Ueland K., Novy M.J., Peterson E.N. & Metcalfe J. (1969) Maternal cardiovascular dynamics. IV. The influence of gestational age on the maternal cardiovascular response to posture and exercise. *American Journal of Obstetrics and Gynecology* **104**, 856–64.

Underwood P., Hester L.L., Lafitte T. & Gregg K.V. (1965) The relationship of smoking to the outcome of pregnancy. *American Journal of Obstetrics and Gynecology* **91**, 270–6.

Valentine B.H. & Baker J.L. (1977) Treatment of recurrent pregnancy hypertension by prophylactic anticoagulation. *British Journal of Obstetrics and Gynaecology* **84**, 309–11.

Vardi J. & Fields G.A. (1974) Microangiopathic hemolytic anemia in severe pre-eclampsia. *American Journal of Obstetrics and Gynecology* **119**, 617–22.

Vassalli P., Morris R.H. & McCluskey R.T. (1963a) The pathogenic role of fibrin deposition in the glomerular lesions of toxemia of pregnancy. *Journal of Experimental Medicine* **118**, 467–77.

Vassalli P., Simon G. & Rouiller C. (1963b) Production of ultra-structural glomerular lesions resembling those of toxaemia of pregnancy by thromboplastin infusion in rabbits. *Nature* **199**, 1105–6.

Vink G.J., Moodley J. & Philpott R.H. (1980) Effect of dihydralazine on the fetus in the treatment of maternal hypertension. *Obstetrics and Gynecology* **55**, 519–22.

Vosburgh G.J. (1976) Blood pressure, edema and proteinuria in pregnancy. 5. Edema relationships. *Progress in Clinical and Biological Research* **7**, 155–68.

Walters W.A.W. (1966) Effects of sustained maternal hypertension on fetal growth and survival. *Lancet* **ii**, 1214–17.

Walters W.A.W., MacGregor W.G. & Hills M. (1966) Cardiac output at rest during pregnancy and the puerperium. *Clinical Science* **30**, 1–11.

Wardle E.N. & Wright N.A. (1973) Role of fibrin in a model of pregnancy toxemia in the rabbit. *American Journal of Obstetrics and Gynecology* **115**, 17–26.

Weiner C.P. & Brandt J. (1982) Plasma antithrombin III activity: an aid in the diagnosis of pre-eclampsia–eclampsia. *American Journal of Obstetrics and Gynecology* **142**, 275–81.

Weinstein L. (1982) Syndrome of hemolysis, elevated liver enzymes, and low platelet count: a severe consequence of hypertension on pregnancy. *American Journal of Obstetrics and Gynecology* **142**, 159–67.

Weseley A.C. & Douglas G.W. (1962) Continuous use of chlorothiazide for prevention of toxemia of pregnancy. *Obstetrics and Gynecology* **19**, 355–8.

Whigham K.A.E., Howie P.W., Drummond A.H. & Prentice C.R.M. (1978) Abnormal platelet function in pre-eclampsia. *British Journal of Obstetrics and Gynaecology* **85**, 28–32.

Whitelaw A. (1981) Maternal methyldopa treatment and neonatal blood pressure. *British Medical Journal* **283**, 471.

Wightman H., Hibbard B.M. & Rosen M. (1978) Perinatal mortality and morbidity associated with eclampsia. *British Medical Journal* **2**, 235–7.

Williams B. (1964) Paraldehyde in the treatment of eclampsia. *Journal of Obstetrics and Gynaecology of the British Commonwealth* **71**, 621–3.

Willocks J. & Moir D. (1968) Epidural analgesia in the management of hypertension in labour. *Journal of Obstetrics and Gynaecology of the British Commonwealth* **75**, 225–8.

Wilson K.H., Lauersen N.H., Raghavan K.S., Fuchs F. & Niemann W.H. (1974) Effects of diazoxide and beta adrenergic drugs on spontaneous and induced uterine activity in the pregnant baboon. *American Journal of Obstetrics and Gynecology* **118**, 499–509.

Zabriskie J.R. (1963) Effect of cigarette smoking during pregnancy. Study of 2000 cases. *Obstetrics and Gynecology* **21**, 405–11.

Zech P., Rifle G., Lindner A., Sassard J., Blanc-Brunat N. and Traeger J. (1975) Malignant hypertension with irreversible renal failure due to oral contraceptives. *British Medical Journal* **4**, 326–7.

Zeek P.M. & Assali N.S. (1950) Vascular changes with eclamptogenic toxemia of pregnancy. *American Journal of Clinical Pathology* **20**, 1099–1109.

7 Renal Disease

John Davison

Women with renal problems often consult the clinician on the advisability of becoming pregnant or continuing a pregnancy already in progress. When counselling such women emotions must not be allowed to override objectivity and this requires knowledge of the physiological changes which occur during normal pregnancy and of the various pitfalls in the detection and diagnosis of obstetric renal problems. Therefore, this chapter first summarises the changes that occur in the urinary tract in pregnancy and then discusses the management of problems associated with chronic renal disease, infectious renal complications, pregnancy in haemodialysis and renal transplant patients and acute renal failure.

The kidney in normal pregnancy

ANATOMICAL CHANGES

The kidney increases approximately 1 cm in length during normal pregnancy. More striking, however, are the anatomical changes in the calyces, renal pelvis and ureter, which dilate markedly, often giving the erroneous impression of obstructive uropathy (Bailey and Rolleston 1971; Roberts 1976). These changes have important clinical implications:

1   Dilatation of the urinary tract may lead to collection errors in tests based on timed urine volume (e.g. 24 hour oestriol, creatinine or protein excretion).

2   Urinary stasis within the ureters may predispose pregnant women with asymptomatic bacteriuria to develop acute symptomatic pyelonephritis.

3   Acceptable norms of kidney size should be increased by 1 cm if estimated during pregnancy or immediately after delivery; since dilatation of the ureters persists into the puerperium, elective radiological examination of the urinary tract should be deferred until at least 16 weeks after delivery.

FUNCTIONAL CHANGES

Renal haemodynamics

Glomerular filtration rate (GFR) and effective renal plasma flow (ERPF) increase to levels about 50 per cent above nonpregnant values. These increases occur shortly after conception (Davison and Noble 1981), and all increments are present by the second trimester (Fig. 7.1) (Davison and Hytten 1974; Dunlop 1981). There is a reduction in GFR of about 15 per cent during the third trimester (measured as 24-hour creatinine clearance) and this must be taken into account, especially when assessing the course of pregnancy in a woman with known renal disease (Davison *et al* 1980) (Fig. 7.2).

Since GFR increases without substantial alterations in the production of creatinine and urea, plasma levels of these solutes decrease. Creatinine levels fall from a nonpregnant value of 73 μmol/l to 65 μmol/l in the first trimester and 51 μmol/l in the second trimester (Kuhlback and Widholm 1966).

Average plasma urea levels of 3.5, 3.3 and 3.1 mmol/l in successive trimesters, rising to 4.3 mmol/l six weeks postpartum, have been described (Robertson and Cheyne 1972). Urea levels can be reported in a number of different ways; results may be given as either plasma (or serum) or whole blood levels, the latter being 10 per cent below plasma levels. Some of the fall in plasma urea may be due to reduced protein degradation as well as increased clearance of this solute.

Awareness of these physiological changes is important since values considered normal in nonpregnant women may reflect decreased renal function during

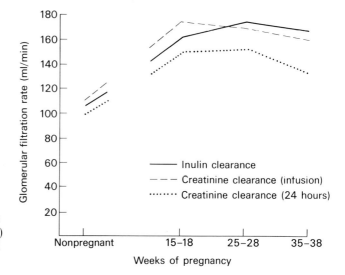

Fig. 7.1   Mean GFR in ten healthy women during pregnancy and 8–12 weeks after delivery (nonpregnant) (Modified from Davison and Hytten 1974).

pregnancy. Plasma levels of creatinine and urea exceeding 75 μmol/l and 4.5 mmol/l respectively, should alert the clinician to investigate renal function further.

A number of other changes in normal pregnancy may be due to augmented renal haemodynamics, including increased excretion of nutrients and protein (Davison 1975). With regard to nutrient excretion, particularly glucose, renal tubular reabsorption is also less efficient so that glycosuria does not necessarily signify hyperglycaemia (Davison and Dunlop 1980). Increased urinary protein excretion should not be considered abnormal until it exceeds 500 mg per 24 hours and increasing proteinuria in women with chronic renal disease does not necessarily signify deterioration.

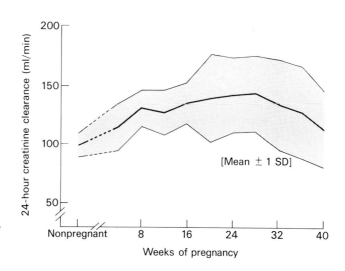

Fig. 7.2   Changes in 24-hour creatinine clearance throughout normal human pregnancy. Calculated from data of Davison and Hytten (1974), Davison *et al* (1980) and Davison and Noble (1981).

Volume homeostasis

Healthy women eating an unrestricted diet gain an average of 12.5 kg during their first pregnancy and 11.5 kg in subsequent pregnancies. Until fairly recently, clinicians regarded published averages as the upper limits of permissible weight gain, forgetting that there is a plus as well as a minus to deviations about a mean. Consequently many pregnant women were admonished for excessive weight gain and their intakes of calories, sodium or both were needlessly restricted.

The increase in weight is largely fluid, total body water increasing by 6–8 litres, 4–6 of which are extracellular (Chesley 1978; Lindheimer and Katz 1981b). There is also cumulative retention of approximately 900 mmol of sodium distributed between the products of conception and the maternal extracellular space. This accumulation occurs gradually and even in late pregnancy, the period of most rapid maternal weight gain, the amount retained is only 3–4 mmol per day, which is usually too small to be detected by conventional balance techniques.

Most of the maternally sequestered sodium is located in the extracellular space. Plasma volume increases by 40–50 per cent, starting in the first trimester, accelerating to a peak in the second and remaining elevated until near term (Chapter 2). However, increases in maternal interstitial volume (as well as fetal storage of sodium) are greatest in the third trimester. The increases in maternal plasma volume and interstitial space constitute a physiological hypervolaemia (Fig. 7.3). However, the mother's volume receptors sense these changes as normal; when salt restriction or diuretic therapy limits the expansion, the maternal response resembles that of salt-depleted nonpregnant subjects (Nolten and Ehrlich 1980). Whether or not the increases in the fluid spaces are 'necessary' remains to be elucidated, but this seems to be likely, since failure of plasma

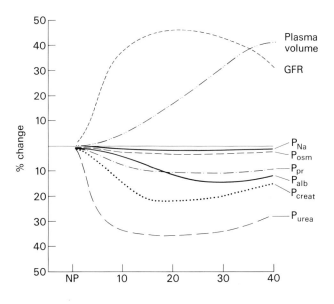

Fig. 7.3 Physiological changes induced by pregnancy. Increments and decrements in various parameters are shown in percentage terms with reference to the nonpregnant baseline. GFR glomerular filtration rate, P_{Na} plasma sodium, P_{osm} plasma osmolality, P_{pr} plasma proteins, P_{alb} plasma albumin, P_{creat} plasma creatinine, P_{urea} plasma urea, NP nonpregnant, 10–40 weeks of pregnancy.

volume to increase appropriately has been correlated with poor reproductive performance (Lindhcimcr and Katz 1981b).

BLOOD PRESSURE REGULATION

Mean blood pressure decreases early in pregnancy and, by the second trimester, diastolic levels are 10–15 mmHg lower than before the patient became pregnant (MacGillivray *et al* 1969). Blood pressure then increases slowly, approaching prepregnancy values shortly before delivery. Since cardiac output rises quickly in the first trimester (reaching values that are 40 per cent greater than those before pregnancy) and remains relatively constant thereafter, the decline in blood pressure must be due to a marked decrease in peripheral vascular resistance. This is greatest in the uterine vasculature, which eventually develops into a large, low resistance shunt. However, other organ systems, especially the kidneys and skin, participate in the generalised vasodilation which is characteristic of normal pregnancy. The rise of blood pressure toward nonpregnant levels after the second trimester suggests that increasing vasoconstrictor tone is a feature of late normal pregnancy (Gant *et al* 1980) and if the clinician is not aware of this pattern of change diagnostic errors may ensue.

Chronic renal disease and pregnancy

Pregnancy will usually end successfully if there is no significant hypertension or overt renal insufficiency prior to conception. There is no evidence that pregnancy accelerates the progress of renal disease.

PATHOPHYSIOLOGY OF RENAL DYSFUNCTION

To assess pregnancy and its altered renal physiology in the presence of chronic renal disease it is necessary to understand what happens when nephron mass has been lost. The relationship between plasma creatinine concentration, creatinine clearance (GFR) and nephron population shown in Fig. 7.4 reveals that an individual may lose about 50 per cent of renal function and still have a plasma creatinine of less than 130 μmol/l. However, if renal function is more severely compromised then a small decrease in GFR causes a marked increase in plasma creatinine. Nevertheless, a patient who has lost 75 per cent of her nephrons may have only lost 50 per cent of function and may have a deceptively normal plasma creatinine. Thus evaluation of renal function should be based on the clearance of creatinine rather than on its plasma concentration.

PREPREGNANCY COUNSELLING (*see* Table 7.1)

In patients with renal disease, pathology may be both clinically and biochemically silent. Most individuals remain symptom-free until their GFR falls to less than 25 per cent of its original level. Many plasma constituents are frequently normal until a late stage of the disease.

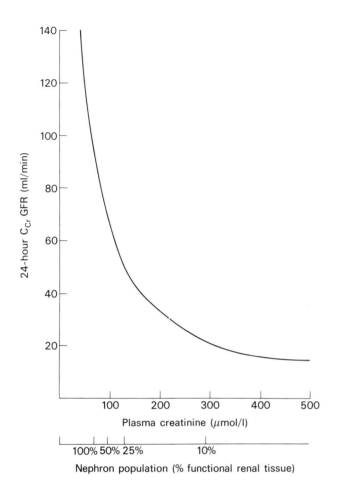

Fig. 7.4 Relationship of clearance of creatinine (GFR) in ml/min to plasma creatinine concentration (μmol/l) and nephron population (per cent) assuming a constant 24-hour creatinine excretion of about 11.5 mmol. (Nonpregnant data; Davidson, unpublished observations.)

As renal function declines so does the ability to conceive and to sustain a viable pregnancy. Degrees of impairment that do not cause symptoms or appear to disrupt homeostasis in nonpregnant individuals, can jeopardise pregnancy. Normal pregnancy is rare when nonpregnant plasma creatinine and urea levels exceed 275 μmol/l and 10 mmol/l, respectively. These increments above normal nonpregnant levels appear

Table 7.1 Prepregnancy counselling.

1. Type of chronic renal disease under consideration
2. General health considerations
3. Diastolic BP < 80 mmHg
4. Renal function:
    Plasma creatinine < 250 μmol/l
    Plasma urea < 10 mmol/l
    Presence or absence of proteinuria
5. Need to review prepregnancy drug therapy

trivial, but they represent decrements in function of more than 50 per cent (Fig. 7.4).

Assessment of a patient with chronic renal disease presents two basic and often conflicting issues: fetal prognosis and the maternal prognosis, both during pregnancy and in the long-term. These issues must be carefully weighed and this delicate 'balance' is illustrated in Fig. 7.5.

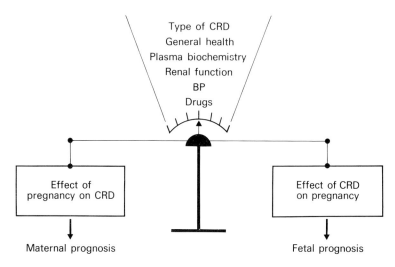

Fig. 7.5   Pregnancy and chronic renal disease (CRD) depicting the balance between maternal and fetal prognosis and the role of factors such as the type of CRD, the degree of renal insufficiency, the presence or absence of hypertension and the type of drug therapy that is needed.

THE COURSE OF PREGNANCY

There are conflicting views concerning the course of pregnancy in women with renal disease. This reflects the variability of populations studied and the lack of large prospective series in which diagnosis had been established by renal biopsy and the pathology correlated with observations of fetal outcome. To some extent this situation has recently been remedied by a large collaborative study in women with a variety of renal diseases, all biopsy proven (Katz *et al* 1980; 1981).

The effect of pregnancy on renal function

The glomerular filtration rate in women with renal disease is usually lower than that of normal pregnant women but it still increases in pregnancy (Fig. 7.6). Towards term GFR tends to fall but in some instances renal function can decrease earlier than this, most often in women with diffuse glomerulonephritis. The decrement is usually mild to moderate and reverses after delivery.

Increased proteinuria is the most common effect of pregnancy on the kidney, reflecting the tendency to increased protein excretion seen in normal pregnancy. A

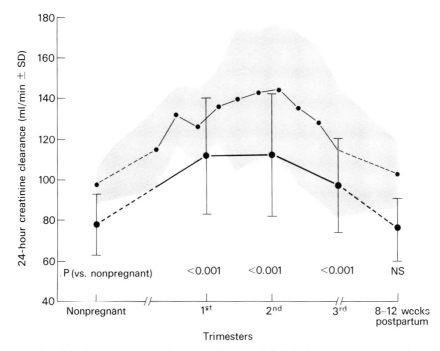

Fig. 7.6   Serial 24-hour creatinine clearances (mean ± 1 SD) during pregnancy complicated by chronic renal disease (solid line). Thirty-three pregnancies of 26 women studied pre-conception, in each trimester and 8–12 weeks after delivery. Measurements from ten healthy women (mean ± 1 SD) shown by shaded area. (From Katz *et al* 1980.)

marked increase in proteinuria occurs in about half the pregnancies complicated by renal disease, although this tends to be less common in women with chronic interstitial nephritis (invariably pyelonephritis). Massive protein excretion, exceeding 3 g per 24 hours, complicates 30 per cent of pregnancies and frequently leads to nephrotic oedema.

About 20 per cent of women with chronic pyelonephritis have one or more episodes of acute urinary tract infection during pregnancy, but this usually does not affect renal function adversely.

The effect of pregnancy on blood pressure in patients with renal disease

Hypertension, usually mild, occurs in about 25 per cent of pregnancies, but in half of these blood pressure is elevated before conception. Hypertension is more common and more severe in women with diffuse glomerulonephritis but is also prominent in women with focal glomerulonephritis and arteriolar nephrosclerosis.

More recently Brenner and his colleagues (1982) have suggested that the hyperfiltration of residual (intact) nephrons in the kidneys of patients with moderate renal insufficiency might cause further progressive loss of renal function. It is thought that the increased glomerular pressure and/or plasma flow leads to sclerosis of the glomerulus. They further claim that compensatory renal hypertrophy in the single kidneys of uninephrectomised subjects is another form of hyperfiltration which will lessen the lifespan of the remaining kidney over many years. This hypothesis is provocative and relevant to pregnancy in women with underlying renal disorders since these patients, like healthy women, experience physiological hyperfiltration of pregnancy. This caution is mainly theoretical at the moment but requires further study.

The incidence of pre-eclampsia

There is controversy about the incidence of pre-eclampsia in women with pre-existing renal disease. This is because the diagnosis cannot be made with certainty on clinical grounds, particularly in women with co-existent renal disorders. Hypertension and proteinuria may be manifestations of the underlying disease rather than signs of pre-eclampsia.

Obstetric outcome

Perinatal mortality and the incidence of preterm deliveries and small-for-dates infants may be considerably higher than in healthy pregnancies (Fig. 7.7). The data of Klockars *et al* (1980) are more reassuring (Table 7.2), but are based on a smaller series than that of Katz *et al* (1980). Further reductions in perinatal mortality are always possible with improvements in methods of fetal surveillance and further advances in perinatal care.

Table 7.2   Outcome of pregnancy in renal disease (Klockars *et al* 1980).

	Patients	Pregnancies	Live births	Abortions
Chronic glomerulonephritis	20	29	25*	4 (spontaneous)
Chronic pyelonephritis	3	3	3	1 (therapeutic)
Polycystic disease	2	3	3	—
Renal transplant	5	5	6*	—
Totals	30	40	37	5

* Including one pair of twins.

THE EFFECT OF PREGNANCY ON RENAL DISEASE

The majority view is that, with the exception of an increased risk of pyelonephritis, pregnancy has no adverse effect on the natural history of established renal parenchymal disease, provided that renal function is only moderately compromised and hypertension is absent (Werkö and Bucht 1956; Kaplan *et al* 1962; Felding 1969; Strauch and Hayslett 1974; Bear 1976; Leppert *et al* 1979; Klockars *et al* 1980; Katz *et al* 1980; 1981). A minority believe that pregnancy frequently results in progression of the renal lesions and further deterioration of renal function (Tenny and Dandrow

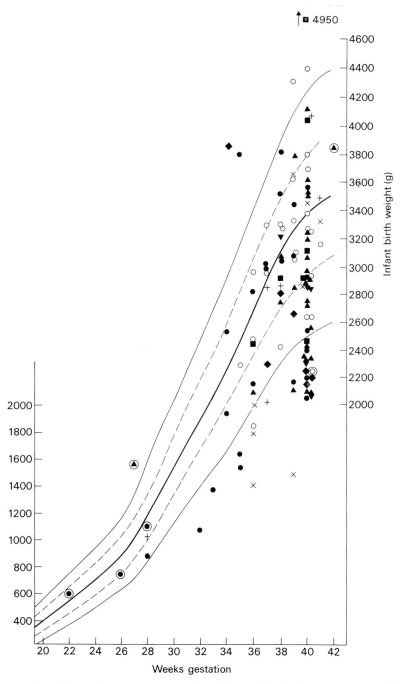

Fig. 7.7 Birthweight in relation to gestational age for 111 live births in women with chronic renal disease (Katz *et al* 1980). Lines represent mean weight ± 1 and 2 standard deviations of 25 608 live births at University Hospital of Cleveland, Ohio, USA (1958–68) compiled by Dr C. H. Hendricks. (From Katz *et al* 1980.) ● Diffuse glomerulonephritis; ▲ focal glomerulonephritis; ▼ membranoproliferative glomerulonephritis; ■ membranous nephropathy; ♦ lipoid nephrosis and FSGS; ○ interstitial nephritis; × arteriolar nephrosclerosis; + miscellaneous kidney disease; Ⓞ neonatal death. There is a high incidence of growth retardation.

1961; Kincaid-Smith *et al* 1967; Fairley *et al* 1973). Furthermore, these latter authors believe that fetal outlook is poor primarily because many of these pregnancies are complicated by the early appearance of pre-eclampsia. However, in many of these cases the deterioration of renal function may have resulted from dehydration and reduced renal perfusion secondary to diuretic therapy (inadvertent or not) and/or strict sodium restriction.

MANAGEMENT OF CHRONIC RENAL DISEASE IN PREGNANCY

Antenatal care

There is good evidence from the studies of Katz *et al* (1980, 1981) and Klockers *et al* (1980) that one of the main factors in reducing maternal and perinatal morbidity and mortality is good antenatal care. The value of such care is greatly enhanced by early and regular attendance so that trends may be detected and the significance of an abnormal observation assessed when taken in context with previous observations. Where patients have chronic renal disease the following factors are important:
1   Careful monitoring of blood pressure; detection of hypertension and assessment of its severity and long-term effects.
2   Assessment of renal function (by 24 hour creatinine clearance and protein excretion) and also nutritional status in heavily proteinuric patients.
3   Assessment of the size, developments and wellbeing of the fetus.
4   Early detection of asymptomatic bacteriuria or confirmation of urinary tract infection.

Criteria for hospital admission

As long as the antenatal course is uncomplicated the patient should be seen at two-weekly intervals until 32 weeks' gestation and then weekly thereafter. Immediate hospital admission is indicated in the following circumstances:
1   Deterioration of renal function as evidenced by decrements in creatinine clearance to 20 per cent and/or the onset of proteinuria or marked increases in proteinuria which persists.
2   Development of even moderate hypertension: i.e. blood pressure greater than 140/90 on two or more occasions separated by an interval of at least six hours.
3   Signs of intrauterine growth retardation and/or deterioration of placental function.
4   Change in rate of weight gain, either cessation or excess.
5   Symptoms of impending eclampsia.

DIAGNOSIS DURING PREGNANCY (*see* Table 7.3)

When the question of renal disease is raised for the first time during a pregnancy it is essential to try to establish a diagnosis and a course of management that will be helpful to both mother and fetus. When a patient presents with hypertension, proteinuria

Table 7.3   Diagnosis during pregnancy.

1. Type of chronic renal disease, if known
2. General health considerations
3. Effect of pregnancy on blood pressure
4. Effect of pregnancy on renal function and plasma biochemistry
5. Past obstetric history
6. Use of drug therapy

and/or abnormal renal function it is difficult to distinguish parenchymal renal disease from pre-eclampsia. A previous history of renal disorders, abnormal urine analysis, a family history of renal disease or a history of systemic illness known to involve the kidneys is obviously helpful, but even so parenchymal renal disease and pre-eclampsia may co-exist.

The assessment of the patient and subsequent blood and urine testing are similar to those of nonpregnant patients but the definitive diagnosis usually has to wait until after delivery. Such patients should be hospitalised and their pregnancies allowed to continue if renal function and blood pressure remain stable. However, since pre-eclampsia is so serious, the pregnancy should be terminated if deterioration occurs. The use of interim haemodialysis to 'buy time' has been advocated but this is not established practice (Mitra *et al* 1970; Goldsmith *et al* 1971; Naik *et al* 1979; Trebbin 1979).

The role of renal biopsy in obstetric practice

Experience with renal biopsy in pregnancy is sparse, mainly because clinical circumstances rarely justify the minimal risks of biopsy at this time and the procedure is usually deferred to the postpartum period (Lindheimer and Katz 1977). Reports of excessive bleeding and other complications in pregnant women have led some to consider pregnancy a relative contraindication to renal biopsy (Schewitz *et al* 1965), although others have not observed any increased morbidity (Lindheimer *et al* 1975). When the biopsy is performed in the immediate puerperium in subjects with well controlled blood pressure and normal coagulation indices, the morbidity is certainly similar to that reported in nonpregnant patients (Lindheimer *et al* 1981).

There are few indications for antepartum biopsy; one is the nephrotic syndrome of unknown aetiology occurring late in the second or early in the third trimester. A diagnosis of pre-eclampsia would suggest termination of pregnancy, while demonstration of other pathology by biopsy is helpful in selecting appropriate therapy. Renal biopsy should not be performed after 34 weeks' gestation since, by this time, the fetus can be delivered regardless of biopsy results.

Assessment of renal function in pregnancy

Serial data on renal function are needed to supplement routine antenatal observations. Tests that are available for use in routine clinical practice include the estimation of plasma urea and electrolytes and determination of the clearances of creatinine and urea. These tests are usually influenced by multiple mechanisms: for example, urea and creatinine clearances do not measure absolute GFR as urea is reabsorbed and creatinine secreted by the renal tubules. The assessment of renal function therefore requires serial surveillance of creatinine clearance and protein excretion.

When reporting renal function values it must be remembered that correcting data to a standard body surface area of $1.73m^2$ (and thus, by implication, to a standard kidney size) is not applicable in pregnancy (Chesley and Williams 1945). Serial renal function tests should be performed and where possible compared to prepregnancy values.

If renal function deteriorates during any stage of pregnancy, reversible causes should be sought such as urinary tract infection or obstruction and dehydration or electrolyte imbalance, which may be subtle, perhaps secondary to diuretic therapy. Failure to detect a reversible cause for the decrease is an indication for ending the pregnancy by elective delivery.

Near term, a 15 per cent decrement in function (which affects plasma creatinine minimally) is normal (Davison *et al* 1980). If hypertension accompanies any observed decrease in renal function the outlook is usually more serious and the fetus should be delivered.

DECISIONS REGARDING TREATMENT OF HYPERTENSION

This is perhaps the most controversial area in the management of renal disease during pregnancy and is also discussed in Chapter 6. Two surveys have attempted to determine how clinicians currently manage hypertension in pregnancy (Chamberlain *et al* 1978; Lewis *et al* 1982) and the results are quite revealing. Treatment of pre-eclampsia, especially when convulsions seem imminent, is markedly different in the UK compared to the USA. Furthermore, whilst obstetricians tend to condemn the use of diuretics, many nephrologists favour this therapy and there are disagreements about the level at which hypertension should be treated and about the role of antithrombotic and volume expansion therapy.

These arguments emphasise several issues. Most current practices have not been validated by controlled trials in pregnant patients so that many clinicians, not cognisant of pregnancy pathophysiology, prescribe therapy that has been determined to be appropriate by careful studies in nonpregnant populations but which may be unwise in pregnant women. Caution is certainly needed in treating pregnant women and, more important, there is a need for more concentrated and collaborative efforts in evaluating therapy in pregnancy.

In deciding what, if any, treatment is appropriate for hypertension several factors should be taken into consideration:

Level of hypertension under consideration

There is no widespread agreement concerning classification of hypertension. From the clinical point of view, it is a question of establishing a dividing line which is useful for management (Redman 1980). Moderate hypertension is usually defined as a blood pressure between 140/90 and 170/110. Severe hypertension is a blood pressure of 170/110 or greater, and may be a chronic state or of acute onset. These levels must be present on two or more occasions separated by an interval of at least six hours.

Raised blood pressure in nervous patients should not be ignored. Nervous patients with hypertension are at no less risk because of their nervousness (Tillman 1955). If lightly dismissed they may reappear with severe hypertension.

Underlying cause of the hypertension

When considering this problem it is difficult to distinguish clinically between the different aetiological categories: pre-eclampsia, hypertension secondary to the chronic renal disease, essential hypertension and combinations of these (Fisher *et al* 1981; Lindheimer and Katz 1981a). Except for the occasional availability of biopsy or autopsy material, reliance is placed on clinical assessment. The most common cause of severe hypertension in pregnancy is severe pre-eclampsia which may, of course, be superimposed on the chronic renal disease. Pre-eclampsia (more common in primigravidae) is characterised by hypertension, proteinuria, oedema and, at times, coagulation abnormalities, and is the most serious of the hypertensive complications of pregnancy. If it is neglected it may rapidly progress to the life-threatening convulsive phase, eclampsia.

Effect on maternal complication rate

Severe hypertension, as defined above, corresponds to a mean arterial pressure of 130 mmHg, the level at which acute vascular damage occurs experimentally (Goldby and Beilin 1972). Thus, on general principles, blood pressure at or above 170/110 should be treated for reasons of maternal wellbeing, reducing the increased risks of cerebral haemorrhage, cardiac failure and, occasionally, renal failure.

In long-term studies, reduction of arterial blood pressure by antihypertensive agents has proved to be of benefit in nonpregnant patients with chronic hypertension. It is not relevant, however, to make a comparison with moderate hypertension in pregnancy because pregnant women are young, the exacerbating stimulus is finite and the complications to be avoided are rare at these blood pressure levels. The risks of moderate hypertension in pregnancy are closely related to the fundamental question of how it predisposes to pre-eclampsia.

Effect on perinatal morbidity and mortality

Most of the specific risks of moderate hypertension appear to be mediated through superimposed pre-eclampsia. Without this complication, pregnancies have a similar or even better perinatal outcome than do normal pregnancies (Page and Christianson 1976; Leppert *et al* 1979).

Detrimental effects of treatment

It has been argued that hypertension is compensatory and necessary for an adequate blood flow to vital organs. Hypertension largely depends on arteriolar constriction and, if that is reduced specifically, then the resistance to flow decreases and perfusion is maintained at lower pressures. The effect on the uteroplacental circulation is an important consideration when deciding whether or not to reduce the blood pressure of a pregnant woman with hypertension.

There is little evidence with which to rationalise the use of antihypertensive agents on the basis of improvement of the lifeline to the fetus. Two approaches are followed. One view is that the uterine artery behaves like a rigid conduit and that reductions in maternal blood pressure concomitantly decrease uteroplacental perfusion; consequently large reductions in maternal blood pressure are guarded against, especially when acute hypertension develops near term (*see* Woods and Brinkman 1975; Lindheimer and Katz 1982). The other view is that uteroplacental blood flow autoregulates rapidly and completely, and therefore aggressive lowering of blood pressure should be the aim (*see* Ferris 1977; Slavin 1980).

Obviously, the best approach to treatment will not be known until there is resolution of this controversy. There have been detailed discussions of the effects of antihypertensive agents on uterine blood flow in experimental animals (Lindheimer and Katz 1981b) and it appears that most measurements include perfusion of uterine tissues (nonplacental flow) as well as the placental bed—thus it is difficult to decide if the changes observed were in the former, the latter, or both. If it is assumed that autoregulation does take place in humans, a critical but unanswered question is how quickly does it occur, because the fetus may be compromised by trivially brief periods of ischaemia.

There are very few controlled studies of the efficacy and side-effects of antihypertensive agents in pregnant women. The pharmacology and the role of a number of these agents in pregnancy is discussed in Chapter 6.

Effect on long-term maternal prognosis

In the absence of chronic pathology the ultimate prevalence of hypertension among primigravidae who develop severe pre-eclampsia is no greater than that in unselected women matched for age and race (Chesley 1978 and 1980). In multiparous women who have severe pre-eclampsia it is the antecedent hypertension that has predisposed them to it rather than the pre-eclampsia which led to chronic hypertension. Recurrent hypertension in pregnancy is indicative of a high risk of later chronic hypertension. Women who remain normotensive throughout successive pregnancies are at very low risk of developing chronic hypertension (Fisher *et al* 1980).

ANTIHYPERTENSIVE THERAPY IN PREGNANCY

It is evident that neither on maternal nor fetal grounds are there definite reasons for drug treatment of moderate hypertension in pregnancy. Nonspecific sedation does not control blood pressure and it is dangerous to resort to this approach. Rest is important and it is common to encounter patients whose blood pressure is controlled by hospitalisation alone, but who experience striking exacerbations upon discharge (Hauth *et al* 1976; Pritchard 1980).

The various antihypertensive drug regimes are given in detail in Chapter 6. In the present context there are three situations where decisions about therapy in pregnancy need to be made.

1. Control of blood pressure in severe chronic hypertension

This is invariably as a continuation of treatment started before conception. If a woman is stabilised effectively with drugs not specifically contraindicated in pregnancy, these drugs (with the exception of diuretics) should be continued during pregnancy. Hospitalisation is necessary for initiation or alteration of therapy.

2. Prevention of amelioration of superimposed pre-eclampsia in severe chronic hypertension

The earlier the presentation the more justified it is to attempt conservative management in order to allow fetal maturation, provided there are no other features necessitating delivery. If *de novo* treatment is indicated in pregnancy it must take place in hospital where the responses can be monitored. If the hypertension is not severe enough to require this, then it does not require treatment. If treatment is indicated for maternal reasons then hospital admission is mandatory. Antihypertensive therapy merely controls only one of the potentially dangerous problems but it allows further maturation before delivery becomes necessary for maternal and fetal reasons.

3. Control of acute severe hypertension

This is usually due to pre-eclampsia and includes hypertensive emergencies. Where such acute episodes occur early in the third trimester without marked deterioration in renal function, then some attempt might be made to control the blood pressure in the short-term to enhance neonatal survival. Despite lowering the blood pressure to protect the mother against dangerous consequences, the other changes of pre-eclampsia will progress. Blood pressure may prove increasingly difficult to control and, if blood pressure 'escapes', this is then an indication to end the pregnancy by elective delivery.

FETAL SURVEILLANCE

Assessment of fetal wellbeing is important because renal disease is associated with intrauterine growth retardation (Fielding 1969; Strauch and Hayslett 1974; Katz *et al* 1980). Also, when complications do arise, the judicious moment for intervention is influenced by fetal status.

The use of modern techniques for fetal surveillance should minimise death *in utero* and reduce neonatal morbidity and mortality. The use of 24-hour total urinary oestriol excretion in patients with renal disease is controversial, primarily because the main urinary oestriol metabolite, oestriol-16-glucosiduronate, is removed by glomerular filtration and tubular excretion (Marwood *et al* 1977). A more useful test is measurement of free or unconjugated oestriol. All other current antenatal monitoring precedures should be utilised: ultrasound, antenatal fetal heart monitoring and amniotic fluid assessment of gestational age and/or fetal pulmonary maturity (Godfrey 1981).

DECISIONS REGARDING DELIVERY

If pregnancy procedes satisfactorily it is probably advisable to induce labour at 38 weeks because prolonging the pregnancy beyond this time can be associated with a greater risk of placental failure and intrauterine death. Moreover, at this gestation, the fetus should be relatively free of risks if the expected date of delivery is correct.

Delivery before 38 weeks may be necessary if renal function deteriorates markedly, if there are signs of impending intrauterine death, if uncontrollable hypertension supervenes or if eclampsia occurs. Patients should be delivered where full facilities and personnel are available for fetal monitoring, operative delivery and neonatal resuscitation.

OTHER THERAPEUTIC CONTROVERSIES

Diuretics

The claim that prophylaxis with thiazides reduces the incidence of pre-eclampsia has not been confirmed in carefully controlled studies (Kraus and Marchese 1966). Diuretics may successfully reduce oedema in overt pre-eclampsia, but this therapy is controlling a sign without modifying the basic disorder and without ameliorating whatever causes the pre-eclampsia. Indeed, it has been observed that when some patients are given thiazides their condition deteriorates (Salerno *et al* 1959).

Any approach to diuretic therapy must be based on current concepts of volume homeostasis in pregnancy (*see* page 195) (Lindheimer and Katz 1981b). In view of the mechanisms involved in the control of tubular sodium reabsorption and the many haemodynamic and humoral alterations that occur during pregnancy, it is remarkable that problems related to sodium and water homeostasis do not affect pregnant women more frequently. Nevertheless, many pregnant women have asymptomatic oedema at some time during pregnancy, and in the absence of pre-eclampsia, infants borne of women with oedema of hands and face weigh more at birth than do infants of women without oedema (Hytten and Thomson 1976).

As diuretics do not prevent pre-eclampsia and do not have a favourable effect on the cause of the disorder they should not be used. Administration of these agents is not without risk: the occurrence of maternal pancreatitis, severe hypokalaemia, neonatal electrolyte imbalance, bleeding diatheses, cardiac arrhythmias and thrombocytopenia have all been related to the use of diuretics (Chesley 1978). This argument does not ignore the fact that oedema does occur in pre-eclampsia and therefore, in this context, is significant; it merely emphasises that, in the mild case, the differentiation between physiological and early pre-eclamptic oedema may not be possible. The only patients for whom diuretics should be prescribed unhesitatingly are pregnant women with heart failure.

Anticoagulation therapy

There have been isolated and conflicting reports on the use of heparin in the management of pre-eclampsia (Howie *et al* 1975). The risk of anticoagulants in patients where hypertensive disease can be associated with cerebral bleeding and subcapsular haematoma of the liver is too hazardous, especially when alternative treatment is available.

Volume expansion therapy

This has been suggested as a form of treatment where pre-eclampsia supervenes. The decrease in plasma volume, the occasional low central venous pressure and the possibility that vasoconstriction may be due to overcompensation of the sympathetic or other pressor systems to intravascular volume depletion, all provide the basis for a controversy. One view is that decreased intravascular volume is the primary event which may be responsible for the rise in blood pressure. Another view—that of the traditional hypertension experts—is that decrements in volume are secondary to vasoconstriction and they warn that treatment with volume expanders is dangerous.

Reviewing the literaure the findings are equivocal and unconvincing. The experience of Gallery and associates (1981) is the exception. These authors have carefully studied hospitalised hypertensive pregnant women whose blood pressure remained elevated despite 48 hours of bed rest. Plasma volume and extracellular spaces were measured with Evans' blue dye and mannitol, respectively, and the patients were infused with 500 ml of a commercial stable-protein-substitute over 15–20 minutes. Rapid decreases in both systolic and diastolic pressure occurred and persisted for about 48 hours. Remeasurement of intravascular and extracellular compartments demonstrated that the decrement in pressure was accompanied by restoration of an initially low plasma volume to values normal for pregnancy, the increment in intravascular volume being due to mobilisation of fluid from the interstitial space. The authors acknowledge the possibility that the decrement in pressure may be due to contamination of the plasma protein infusate with vasodilatory peptides (e.g. bradykinin) but believe that, if such were the case, the decrease in blood pressure should be transient while that observed by them persisted for 48 hours.

While the results of the elegant studies described above are impressive, most of the patients had only moderate hypertension. Myocardial performance may be compromised in severe pre-eclampsia and, if volume expansion (especially with saline) sensitises these patients' vasculature further to endogenous angiotensin and catecholamines, such therapy could induce pulmonary oedema. For the moment, there should be caution against plasma expansion therapy until much more carefully controlled data is available for analysis.

Use of epidural anaesthesia in labour

The role of epidural anaesthesia in the acutely hypertensive patient prior to delivery is controversial (Crawford 1977; Joyce *et al* 1979; Pritchard 1980). These patients are vasoconstricted and hypovolaemic. Although autonomic nervous system blockade may reverse the hypertension, a severe degree of hypotension may ensue because of the hypovolaemia. Avoidance or alleviation of this hypotension by intravenous fluid loading may help, but the effect of these manoeuvres on the uteroplacental circulation is not known. However, there is no doubt that epidural anaesthesia is an effective method of pain relief without significant transfer of central nervous system depressants to the fetus.

Blood transfusion policy in hypertensive emergencies

A woman with a shrunken intravascular compartment is less tolerant of blood loss than is the normal pregnant woman (Tatum and Mule 1956). Blood replacement must therefore be initiated sooner, though managed very carefully, to guard against the dangers of underfilling and overfilling. Close monitoring of the central venous pressure (CVP) is helpful, especially where there is oliguria.

SPECIFIC PROBLEMS IN RELATION TO CERTAIN TYPES OF RENAL DISEASE

Table 7.4 summarises the course of pregnancy in a number of specific diseases.

Acute and chronic glomerulonephritis

Acute poststreptococcal glomerulonephritis complicating pregnancy is very rare but does occur (Nadler *et al* 1969), and has been mistaken for pre-eclampsia. The prognosis of chronic glomerulonephritis during pregnancy is hard to evaluate primarily because most reports are poorly documented, often failing to list the degree of functional impairment, the blood pressure prior to conception and the histology of the 'glomerulonephritis'.

The Melbourne group (Kincaid-Smith *et al* 1967, 1980; Fairley *et al* 1973) have stated that pregnancy tends to aggravate most glomerular diseases due to the hypercoaguable state that accompanies pregnancy; in particular they claim that crescentric glomerular lesions occur more readily. They also indicate that such patients are more prone to superimposed pre-eclampsia or hypertensive crises early in pregnancy. Other experience (Katz *et al* 1980, 1981) is that renal function decreases most often in patients with diffuse glomerulonephritis in whom hypertension is invariably both more common and severe; nonetheless, most of the pregnancies are successful.

Table 7.4   Effects of pregnancy on pre-existing renal disease.

Chronic glomerulonephritis and non-infectious tubulointerstitial disease	Usually no adverse effect in the absence of hypertension Some believe that glomerulonephritis is adversely affected by coagulation changes in pregnancy Urinary tract infections may occur more frequently
Lupus nephropathy	Controversial; the prognosis is most favourable if the disease is in remission >6 months prior to conception. Steroid dosage should be increased in the puerperium
Diabetic nephropathy	Probably no adverse effect on the renal lesion, although the frequency of leg oedema, pre-eclampsia and infection is higher
Chronic pyelonephritis (infectious tubulo-interstitial disease)	Bacteriuria during pregnancy leads to more frequent exacerbation
Polycystic disease	Functional impairment and hypertension are usually minimal in childbearing years. Probably no adverse effect
Urolithiasis	Infections may be more frequent, otherwise ureteral dilatation and stasis do not seem to affect natural history
After nephrectomy; solitary and pelvic kidneys	Pregnancy is usually well tolerated. Dystocia has been rarely attributed to pelvic kidneys; it can be associated with other malformations of urogenital tract
Nephrotic syndrome	Tolerated well, infants may have low birthweight. Diuretics should not be used

Hereditary nephritis is an uncommon disorder which may first manifest or exacerbate during pregnancy (Grünfeld *et al* 1973). A variant of hereditary nephritis in which the patients have disordered platelet morphology and function can occur. Pregnancy in these women has been successful from a renal viewpoint but their pregnancies can be complicated by bleeding problems.

Collagen diseases (*see also* Chapter 8)

There are differing opinions about the effects of pregnancy on lupus nephropathy. Transient improvements, no change and a tendency to relapse have all been reported. Some patients have a definite tendency towards relapse (occasionally severe) in the puerperium and therefore it is prudent to prescribe or increase the use of steroids at this time.

Lupus nephropathy may sometimes become manifest during pregnancy and, when accompanied by hypertension and renal dysfunction in late pregnancy, may be mistaken for pre-eclampsia.

The majority of pregnancies succeed, especially if the maternal disease is in remission for at least six months prior to conception, even if the patient has severe pathological changes in her renal biopsy and heavy proteinuria in the early stages of her disease. However, continued signs of disease activity or increasing renal dysfunction reduce the likelihood of an uncomplicated pregnancy (Haslett and Lynn 1980; Houser *et al* 1980).

In contrast to lupus nephropathy, the outcome of pregnancy in women with renal involvement due to periarteritis nodosa and scleroderma is very poor, largely because of the associated hypertension which is frequently of a malignant nature. Not only is fetal prognosis dismal, but many of the cases reported ended with maternal deaths (Seigler and Spain 1965; Karlan and Cook 1970).

Diabetes mellitus (see also Chapter 10)

During pregnancy diabetic women have an increased prevalance of bacteriuria and may be more susceptible to symptomatic urinary tract infection. They also have an increased frequency of peripheral oedema and pre-eclampsia. Most women with diabetic nephropathy demonstrate the normal increments in renal function (Sims 1961) and pregnancy does not necessarily accelerate deterioration of diabetic nephropathy (Kitzmiller *et al* 1981).

Tubulointerstitial diseases

The prognosis of pregnancy in women with 'chronic pyelonephritis' is similar to that of patients with glomerular disease; its outcome is most favourable in normotensive patients with adequate renal function (Katz *et al* 1980, 1981). Women whose disease is of an infectious nature have a propensity to deteriorate during pregnancy, which may be minimised if the patient is well hydrated and rests frequently, lying in lateral recumbency (ureteral obstruction by the enlarged uterus does not occur in this position) (Lindheimer and Katz 1972). It has been suggested that these patients are more prone to hypertensive complications during pregnancy but recent reports indicate that they have a more benign antenatal course than do women with glomerular disease (Katz *et al* 1980, 1981).

Polycystic kidney disease

This condition may remain undetected during pregnancy, but careful questioning of pregnant women for a family history and the use of ultrasonography may lead to earlier diagnosis. These patients do well when functional impairment is minimal and hypertension absent, as is often the case during childbearing years.

This is a hereditary disease transmitted by a Mendelian dominant, and other congenital abnormalities may be present such as a cystic liver. Non-functioning infantile polycystic kidney disease affects 25 per cent of infants born to couples who are carriers and this condition is incompatible with extrauterine survival. With the improved resolution of grey scale ultrasound equipment and the availability of high resolution real-time instrumentation, visualisation of the urinary tract should be undertaken in fetuses of couples at risk.

Urolithiasis

Urolithiasis during pregnancy has a prevalence of between 0.03 and 0.35 per cent (Harris and Dunnihoo 1967). The course of the disease is unaffected by pregnancy although urinary tract infections are more common in such patients (Coe *et al* 1978; Lattanzy and Cook 1980). If nephrectomy has been performed because of nephrolithiasis, the remaining kidney may be infected and such patients should be carefully scrutinised by means of frequent urine cultures throughout pregnancy.

Renal calculi are one of the most common causes of non-uterine-related abdominal pain severe enough to require hospitalisation of pregnant patients (Folger 1955). When there are complications such as deteriorating renal function suggesting the need for surgical intervention, pregnancy should not be a deterrent to intravenous urography (Waltzer 1981).

Conservative management of pregnant patients with ureteric calculi consists of hydration and systemic analgesics (Strong *et al* 1978). Recently the application of continuous segmental epidural block (T11 to L2) to treat renal colic in pregnancy has been reported (Ready and Johnson 1981). This approach has been applied extensively in nonpregnant patients presenting with renal colic (Romagnoli and Batra 1973) and, in addition to providing pain relief, may also favourably influence spontaneous passage of the calculi. Whether or not this is the case in pregnancy is not known but compared to standard conservative treatment with potent narcotics, segmental blockade has many advantages for the mother and possibly for the fetus. Continuous epidural segmental blockade is already widely practised in modern obstetrical units and the personnel are therefore expert in the techniques and familiar with the care of patients. If the block is carefully confined to only the relevant segments for pain relief, patients should be able to move about without assistance and void without difficulty. Women who are comfortable and who are able to move with ease are at less risk of thromboembolism than those who are immobile in bed with severe pain, nausea and vomiting and drowsiness.

The solitary kidney

Some patients have either a congenital absence of one kidney or marked unilateral hypoplasia but the majority of cases have had a previous nephrectomy because of pyelonephritis with abscess, hydronephrosis, unilateral tuberculosis, congenital abnormalities or tumour. When counselling women with a single kidney, it is important to know the indication for and the time since nephrectomy. In patients who had an infectious and/or structural renal problem sequential prepregnancy investigation is needed to detect any persistent infection. If renal function is normal and stable a pregnancy may be considered.

It does not matter whether the right or left kidney remains as long as it is located in the normal anatomical position. Such women seem to tolerate pregnancy well (Davison 1978). Ectopic kidneys (usually pelvic) are more vulnerable to infection and are associated with decreased fetal salvage probably because of an association with other malformations of the urogenital tract. If infection occurs in a solitary kidney during pregnancy and does not quickly respond to antibiotics, termination may have to be considered to preserve renal function.

Nephrotic syndrome and pregnancy

The most common cause of nephrotic syndrome in late pregnancy is pre-eclampsia (First *et al* 1978; Fisher *et al* 1980). This form of pre-eclampsia has a poorer fetal prognosis than pre-eclampsia with less heavy proteinuria, but the maternal prognosis is similar.

Other causes of nephrotic syndrome in pregnancy include membranous nephropathy, proliferative or membranoproliferative glomerulonephritis, lipid nephrosis, lupus nephropathy, hereditary nephritis, diabetic nephropathy, renal vein thrombosis, amyloidosis and secondary syphilis (Lindheimer and Katz 1977). Some of these possibilities emphasise the importance of establishing a tissue diagnosis before initiating steroid therapy.

If renal function is adequate and hypertension is absent, there should be few complications during pregnancy; however, several of the physiological changes occurring during pregnancy may simulate aggravation or exacerbation of the disease. For example, increments in renal blood flow as well as increase in renal vein pressure may enhance protein excretion. Levels of serum albumin usually decrease by 5–10 g/l in normal pregnancy, and the further decreases that can occur in the nephrotic syndrome may enhance the tendency toward fluid retention. Therefore a high protein diet (3 g/kg/day) is important in these patients. Despite oedema, diuretics should not be given as these patients have a decreased intravascular volume and this therapy could further compromise uteroplacental perfusion or aggravate the increased tendency to thrombotic episodes.

While the majority of these pregnancies succeed and are maintained to term, there is evidence that the hypoalbuminaemia and the associated decreased intravascular volume may cause small-for-dates infants (Studd and Blainey 1969). Furthermore, there is a report that infants of normotensive mothers who had heavy proteinuria during pregnancy manifested impaired neurological and mental development (Rosenbaum *et al* 1969).

Asymptomatic bacteriuria

This is a condition where true bacteriuria exists but there are no symptoms or signs of acute urinary tract infection (*see also* Chapter 15)

DIAGNOSTIC PITFALLS

Pregnant women often complain of or will admit to symptoms of urgency, frequency, dysuria and nocturia, occurring singly or in combination. These symptoms are not in themselves diagnostic of urinary tract infection and can be elicited from women with sterile urine.

Urine collection and examination

The growth of bacteria on qualitative culture of a urine specimen may represent either true bacteria (the multiplication of bacteria within the urinary tract) or contamination of the urine with urethral or perineal organisms at the time of collection. True bacteriuria can be separated from contamination on the basis of colony counts from a freshly obtained midstream urine specimen (MSU), with 100 000 colonies per ml of urine as the dividing line (Kass 1956). Two consecutive clean-voided specimens containing the same organism in numbers greater than 100 000 colonies per ml of urine represents true bacteriuria, as does a single suprapubic aspiration with any bacterial growth (Norden and Kass 1968; McFadyen *et al* 1973).

The use of the clean-catch or clean-void technique is satisfactory provided each clinic determines the number of cultures needed to achieve a 95 per cent or greater level of confidence that bacteriuria exists (Cohen and Kass 1967). The use of antiseptic solutions for vulval cleansing should be avoided as contamination of the urine may result in a false-negative culture (Roberts *et al* 1967). A plain soap solution or distilled water is satisfactory.

A number of presumptive tests based on changes in chemical indicators are available but the dependability of these varies greatly (Mead and Gump 1976).

Site of infection

Asymptomatic bacteriuria is a heterogenous condition and several different approaches have attempted to differentiate between upper and lower urinary tract bacteriuria (Lindheimer and Katz 1981). Ureteral catheterisation, bladder washout techniques, renal biopsy, urinary concentration tests, determination of serum antibody titres and identification of antibody-coated bacteria in the urine have all been tried (Fairley *et al* 1966, 1967; Clark *et al* 1969; Heineman and Lee 1973; Turck 1975; Mundt and Polk 1979). No single test is sufficiently precise, however, to give complete confidence in localising infections.

CLINICAL IMPLICATIONS

Incidence

The reservoir of young women with asymtomatic bacteriuria acquired during childhood has been estimated at 5 per cent but only 1.2 per cent are infected at any one time (Kunin 1970). The incidence increases after puberty coincident with sexual activity and varies from 2 to 10 per cent depending on the techniques employed for testing and the socioeconomic status of the patients (Savage *et al* 1967; Norden and Kass 1968).

In pregnancy, true asymptomatic bacteriuria is invariably diagnosed at the first antenatal visit if tested for at that time and less than 1.5 per cent subsequently acquire bacteriuria in late pregnancy.

Importance of diagnosis

It is important to identify and treat the infected group because up to 40 per cent develop acute symptomatic urinary tract infection (Whalley 1967; Williams *et al* 1973). Treating this group will prevent approximately 70 per cent of all cases of acute urinary tract infection (Fig. 7.8).

However, about 2 per cent of those with negative cultures will also develop acute infections. Thus of the 90–98 per cent that do not have asymptomatic bacteriuria at the booking visit (and therefore will not be treated) the number actually at risk of developing an acute urinary tract infection is quite significant and accounts for about 30 per cent of all cases of acute urinary tract infection in pregnancy (Lawson and Miller 1971, 1973; Swann 1973).

A positive history of previous urinary tract infection may be almost as effective as screening in predicting urinary tract infection in pregnancy (Chng and Hall 1982). Furthermore, the combination of bacteriuria with a history of urinary tract infection gives the most accurate prediction. Such women are at ten times greater risk than those with neither feature, and four times greater risk than those with asymptomatic bacteriuria alone.

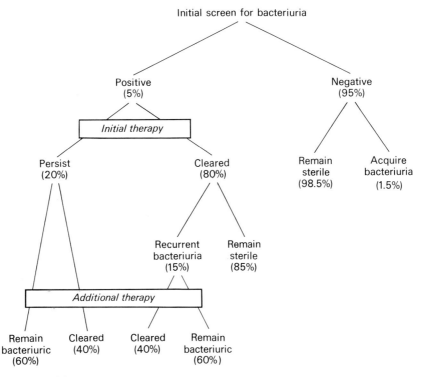

Fig. 7.8 Natural history of asymptomatic bacteriuria and affects of treatment in pregnancy. Approximate percentages are given in parentheses.

Any other postulated benefits of eradication of asymptomatic bacteriuria are unsubstantiated. The available data suggest that the association of asymptomatic bacteriuria and increased fetal loss, prematurity, pre-eclampsia, and anaemia are unproven (Williams *et al*, 1973; Condie *et al* 1973; Mead and Gump 1976; Brumfitt 1981; Lindheimer and Katz 1981).

Some 30–40 per cent of pregnant women with asymptomatic bacteriuria may have upper (renal) urinary tract infection and these women may be a special population at greatest risk of pregnancy problems as well as acute urinary tract infection. This assumption has recently been questioned by a study specifically designed to determine what adverse effects asymptomatic renal bacteriuria had on maternal and fetal wellbeing (Gilstrap *et al* 1981). In a prospective study pregnancy outcomes in women with treated asymptomatic bacteriuria of renal origin (diagnosed by the antibody-coated bacteria technique, with a 20 per cent false-positive rate, p. 215), were compared to outcomes in those with treated bladder bacteriuria as well as non-infected control subjects. Women with asymptomatic renal bacteriuria appeared to be at no greater risk than abacteriuric women of developing pregnancy problems, nor were their progeny at greater risk. Nevertheless, even though the impact of asymptomatic renal infection on ultimate pregnancy outcome is minimal, the need for screening for and eradication of asymptomatic bacteriuria in order to prevent pyelonephritis is still important. This study also reconfirmed the fact that symptomatic infections may be implicated in delivery of low birthweight infants when acute pyelonephritis complicates preterm labour, suggesting a causal role in its initiation.

Where underlying undiagnosed chronic pyelonphritis is present then this could be responsible for the reported obstetric complications and increased perinatal losses (Fig. 7.7).

Choice of drug

The choice of drug must be based on the sensitivity of the isolated organism(s). Short-acting sulphonamides or nitrofurantoin derivatives are often the initial therapy (Andrioli 1975; Mead and Gump 1976). Other drugs are reserved for treatment of failures and for symptomatic infection. Ampicillin and the cephalosporins can be safely used in pregnancy. Tetracyclines are contraindicated because of staining of the teeth of infants by binding with orthophosphates, as well as the rare maternal complication of acute fatty liver of pregnancy (*see* p. 304). If sulphonamides are prescribed in late pregnancy they should be withheld during the last 2–3 weeks since they compete with bilirubin for albumin-binding sites, increasing the risk of fetal hyperbilirubinaemia and kernicterus. Nitrofurantoin used during the last few weeks may precipitate haemolytic anaemia due to glucose-6-phosphate dehydrogenase deficiency in the newborn. Trimethoprim, a constituent of Bactrim and Septrin, is not recommended for use in pregnancy since it is a folic acid antagonist. Nevertheless it is extensively used and probably safe, though not a drug of first choice.

Duration of therapy

Opinions on optimal duration of therapy differ. Continuous antibiotic therapy from the time of diagnosis until after delivery has been recommended because of the belief that renal parenchymal involvement causes a high relapse rate. However, at least 60 per cent of patients have bladder involvement alone and the administration of short-term therapy (two weeks) should be satisfactory. Furthermore, if patient follow-up is meticulous, there is no advantage in using continuous long-term administration of antibiotics and the possible hazards of such therapy to the fetus are avoided. Urine cultures should be obtained one week after therapy is discontinued and then at regular intervals throughout the pregnancy.

Relapses and reinfections

Relapse is the recurrence of bacteriuria caused by the same organism, usually within six weeks of the initial infection. Reinfection is the recurrence of bacteriuria involving a different strain of bacteria, after successful eradication of the initial infection (Turck *et al* 1968). Most patients with reinfections have infections limited to the bladder, usually occurring at least six weeks after therapy.

Approximately 15 per cent of patients will have a recurrence during pregnancy and a second course of treatment should be given, based on a repeat culture with sensitivity testing. In the group of patients who relapse or who are resistant to the first course of therapy, only about 40 per cent will have the asymptomatic bacteriuria cleared with subsequent therapy (Leveno *et al* 1981). Since *Eschericia coli* causes the majority of initial infections as well as recurrences, it may be necessary to employ an *E. coli* serotyping system to precisely distinguish different stains, although this does not help in clinical management.

Long-term considerations

As the interval between treatment of bacteriuria in pregnancy and postpartum follow-up becomes longer, the influence of the initial course of treatment on the incidence of bactcriuria becomes less noticeable (Mead and Gump 1976). Ten or more years after an initial episode of bacteriuria of pregnancy, the prevalence of bacteriuria in women not treated during pregnancy (25 per cent) is virtually the same as in those women who were treated (29 per cent). In contrast, women who have never been bacteriuric during pregnancy have rates of bacteriuria of about 5 per cent. Thus a single course of treatment during the index pregnancy does not appear to protect against persistent or recurrent bacteriuria years later. There are few prospective studies available, but there is no evidence that persistent asymptomatic bacteriuria in women with normal urinary tracts causes long-term renal damage or that treatment reduces the incidence of chronic renal disease (Brumfitt 1981).

Postpartum intravenous urography

There is no consensus of opinion regarding the need for postpartum intravenous urography (IVU) in patients who have had bacteriuria. It is known that 20 per cent of all patients with asymptomatic bacteriuria have IVU abnormalities and this percentage is increased amongst patients with acute infections during pregnancy or with infections that have been difficult to eradicate (Gower *et al* 1968).

The significance of an IVU abnormality is not so certain (Briedahl *et al* 1972). It may signify a predisposition to infection; it may result from infection or it may be unrelated to infection. Most abnormalities are minor and probably do not result from or cause renal infection. Furthermore, the role of infection in childhood, as indicated by scars on the IVU, is controversial (Gower *et al* 1968).

In order to detect about 90 per cent of the women with major urinary tract abnormalities or to document a non-obstructed urinary tract, an IVU should be performed in women who have asymptomatic bacteriuria during pregnancy who fulfil the following additional criteria:

1 Difficulty in eradicating the bacteriuria during the pregnancy.
2 Episode(s) of acute symptomatic urinary tract infection during the pregnancy.
3 History of acute infection(s) prior to the index pregnancy.
4 Persistence/recurrence of asymptomatic bacteriuria or acute infection postpartum.

Those patients who do have major abnormalities demonstrated postpartum are more likely to require careful long-term follow-up for eradications of bacteriuria rather than surgery. However, a non-functioning kidney may be removed and major drainage anomalies may be corrected.

Acute symptomatic urinary tract infection

Acute pyelonephritis (*see also* Chapter 15), the most common renal complication of pregnancy, occurs in 1–2 per cent of all pregnancies. It has been blamed as a cause of intrauterine growth retardation, congenital abnormalities, fetal death and certainly causes premature labour (Condie *et al* 1973; Brumfitt 1981; Gilstrap *et al* 1981a & b).

CLINICAL IMPLICATIONS

Pyelonephritis must be distinguished from two other important conditions. Pneumonia on the affected side should present no difficulties if attention is paid to the type of respiration, the respiratory rate and the physical signs in the chest. Acute appendicitis is a difficult diagnosis to make, especially in late pregnancy, but usually at the onset pain of appendicitis is referred to the centre of the abdomen, vomiting is not a marked feature, the pyrexia is not so high as in pyelonephritis and rigors do not occur.

Once the diagnosis is considered, a midstream urine should be sent for culture and sensitivities. Antibiotic treatment should be aggressive and must be undertaken in a hospital setting. It should be started once the diagnosis has been made and before the sensititivies are available. If the patient is dehydrated, due to vomiting and sweating, then intravenous fluids should be given. Regular assessment of renal function should be undertaken: although the infectious attack is said to have little effect on renal function in nonpregnant patients, such attacks during pregnancy have been observed to cause transient but marked decrements in GFR (Whalley *et al* 1975). The use of tepid sponging and antipyretic drugs such as paracetamol may reduce the incidence of premature labour.

Choice and duration of therapy

Dogmatic statements cannot be justified regarding the type of antimicrobial therapy for acute urinary tract infection and the appropriate duration of regimens is also debatable (Mead and Gump 1976). Treatment should aim at giving the most effective drug to eradicate a particular infection without exposing the fetus to an unnecessarily harmful agent.

Antibiotics producing high blood levels and resultant high renal parenchymal concentrations are favoured, although the importance of these factors is still undetermined (Stamey *et al* 1965). Two suitable groups of antibiotics are the broad spectrum penicillins, e.g. ampicillin, and the cephalosporins; *E. coli* is the most common organism isolated in urinary infections and is usually sensitive to either of them. Trimethoprim/sulphonamide combinations, such as Septrin, are also used (p. 217). Aminoglycosides, such as kanamycin and gentamicin, can be given if there are problems with microbial resistance. Treatment should be monitored by blood levels. Whilst the patient is febrile, it is preferable to give intravenous antibiotics which can be continued orally when the pyrexia has settled. Antibiotic sensitivities should be reviewed within 48 hours.

The duration of treatment should be 2–3 weeks. In patients showing clinical deterioration or whose urine cultures reveal bacteria resistant to the selected antibiotic, repeat urine cultures are mandatory and alternative antibiotic therapy should be considered. In severely ill patients blood specimens should be taken for culture. After the completion of the course of treatment urine cultures should be taken at every antenatal visit for the rest of the pregnancy.

Gram-negative sepsis

This can occur in severely ill patients with acute pyelonephritis but the situation is commonly associated with instrumentation of an infected urinary tract. An aminoglycoside antibiotic is best because it is effective against nearly all of the Gram-negative urinary bacteria. Enterococci less commonly cause bacteraemia but because of resistance to aminoglycosides ampicillin can be used combined with an aminoglycoside until culture results are available. Patients who are sensitive to penicillin should receive a cephalosporin. Haematological aspects of the management of Gram-negative sepsis are considered on pp. 76–82.

ACUTE RENAL FAILURE AND PYELONEPHRITIS

This is discussed on pp. 234–46.

Haematuria during pregnancy

Spontaneous gross or microscopic haematuria can be due to a variety of causes (Texter *et al* 1980). Urinary tract infections, particularly those associated with congenital anomalies are difficult to eradicate and predispose to haematuria, especially if pyelonephritis is present. Rupture of small veins about the dilated renal pelvis may also cause bleeding. Spontaneous or traumatic rupture of the kidney can occur, usually where there are underlying anatomical abnormalities (Maresca and Kowcky 1981). Spontaneous nontraumatic renal rupture, however, is very rare. Acute glomerulonephritis has been discussed earlier (p. 210).

Haematuria may be secondary to any type of primary neoplasm, metastatic neoplasma, haemangiomas, calculi or fungal diseases involving the urinary system. Endometriosis, inflammatory bowel lesions, leukoplakia, amyloidosis and granulomas may involve the urinary tract and produce haematuria. The ureteral stump after a nephrectomy (for either benign or malignant disease) may be involved by any of the aforementioned pathology and should be investigated.

An aggressive approach to evaluation is needed. This may be deferred until after delivery but the clinician should assess all the circumstances to decide whether or not it takes absolute priority. In the absence of any demonstrable cause, haematuria can be classified as idiopathic and recurrences are unlikely in the current or subsequent pregnancy (Reid 1972).

Acute hydronephrosis and hydroureter

Very occasionally pregnancy can precipitate acute hydronephrosis or hydroureter. Obstruction may occur at varying levels at or above the pelvic brim. It has been suggested that the physiological changes of pregnancy may cause an underlying compensated pelviureteric junction obstruction to become decompensated and hence symptomatic.

The condition should be suspected when there are recurrent episodes of loin or low abdominal pain radiating to the groin and repeat midstream urine specimens are sterile. Diagnosis can be confirmed using excretory urography or ultrasound (no evidence of stone) and ureteral catheterisation. If positioning the patient on the unaffected side (with antibiotic therapy if appropriate) fails to relieve the situation, then ureteral catheterisation or nephrostomy may be required. Typically, the pain is immediately relieved by ureteric catheterisation and the urine can be sterile or infected (Schloss and Solomkin 1952). Corrective surgery is best delayed until the postpartum period (Meares 1978).

Pregnancy in renal transplant patients

Renal transplantation usually reverses the abnormal reproductive function and sexual disorders of haemodialysed women (*BMJ* Editorial 1982). The resumption of regular menstruation and ovulation correlate closely with the level of function achieved by the graft (Merkatz *et al* 1971). With the increase in the number of transplanted women of childbearing age clinicians must now both counsel such patients as to whether or not they should conceive and also manage the pregnancies of those already pregnant. Indeed, it has been estimated that one of every 50 women of childbearing age who have a functional renal transplant will become pregnant (*BMJ* Editorial 1976).

A recent review of 759 such pregnancies emphasised the difficulty in assessing the exact incidence of the various management problems because some of the data in the literature are incomplete and many more pregnancies than those reported have occurred (Davison and Lindheimer 1982a & b). Excluding the large Denver series (Penn *et al* 1980a & b) where 75 per cent of patients had received kidneys from living donors, only 20 per cent of births occurred in recipients of living donor grafts. Despite publication of numerous case reports, several series and registry data from the USA and Europe, little has been done to establish guidelines on the management of the transplant recipient who conceives. In some instances pregnancy is not diagnosed until the second or even the third trimester and many patients are under the impression that they could not conceive. Medical concern seems to be concerned with the management of the pregnancy rather than the advisability of the initial conception.

PREGNANCY COUNSELLING

Management should start by counselling all couples who want a child, with a discussion of the implications of pregnancy as well as long-term prospects.

Prepregnancy assessment

Patients should be assessed on the basis of the following general guidelines (Davison *et al* 1976) the absence of some of which (e.g. 1, 2, 6) is only a relative contraindication to pregnancy:
1   Good general health for two years after transplantation.
2   Stature compatible with good obstetric outcome.
3   No proteinuria.
4   No significant hypertension.
5   No evidence of graft rejection.
6   No evidence of pelvicalyceal distention on a recent excretory urogram.
7   Plasma creatinine of 180 μmol/l or less.
8   Drug therapy: prednisone, 15 mg/day or less and azathioprine 2 mg/kg/day or less.
    After full prepregnancy assessment advice can be given but it can only be advice, since patients must ultimately decide for themselves what degree of risk is acceptable. If the situation is tackled prospectively the final decision is more of an agreement than a judgement.

Long-term considerations

The major concern is that the mother may not survive or remain well enough to raise the child she bears. Average survival figures of large numbers of patients from all over the world indicate that between 60 and 80 per cent of recipients of kidneys from related living donors are alive five years after transplantation; and with cadaver kidneys the figure is 40–50 per cent (Renal Transplant Registry 1977; UK Transplant 1981). Functional survival of the allograft at five years is 45–65 per cent in recipients of living donor kidneys and 30–35 per cent in recipients of cadaver organs. Despite these statistics many patients will choose parenthood in an effort to renew a normal life and possibly in defiance of the sometimes negative attitudes of the medical establishment.

Based on a comparison of very small groups of renal cadaver transplant recipients (those who became pregnant and those who did not), Whetam and colleagues (1983) concluded that pregnancy had no effect on graft function or survival. More long-term studies are needed to assess this important area, so that counselling is thorough and based on recorded experience and not clinical anecdote.

GENERAL MANAGEMENT PLAN (*see* Table 7.5)

Pregnancy management

Patients must be monitored as high-risk cases. Management requires attention to serial assessment of renal function, diagnosis and treatment of rejection, blood pressure control, prevention or early diagnosis of anaemia, treatment of any infection as well as the meticulous assessment of fetal wellbeing.

Antenatal visits should be two-weekly up to 32 weeks and weekly thereafter. At each visit routine antenatal care should be supplemented with the following:
1 Full blood count, including platelets (Coulter counter analysis).
2 Urea and electrolytes.
3 24-hour creatinine clearance and protein excretion.
4 Midstream urine specimen for microscopy and culture.
5 Plasma protein, calcium and phosphate levels (Kobayashi *et al* 1981) and

Table 7.5 Pregnancy management.

1. Hospital-based antenatal care in conjunction with nephrologists
2. Surveillance of renal function
3. Graft rejection
4. Hypertension/pre-eclampsia
5. Maternal infection
6. Intrauterine growth retardation
7. Preterm labour
8. Effects of drug therapy on fetus and neonate
9. Decision on timing and route of delivery

cytomegalovirus (CMV) and herpes hominis virus (HHV) titres should be checked at 6-weekly intervals.

Immunosuppressive therapy is usually maintained at prepregnancy levels but adjustments may be needed if there are decreases in the maternal leucocyte and platelet counts. Haematinics and vitamin D and calcium supplements should be prescribed if indicated (Parsons *et al* 1979; Rabau-Friedman *et al* 1982). Metabolic bone disease in renal failure is mentioned on p 443.

Early pregnancy problems

Ectopic pregnancy can occur and the diagnosis can be difficult in these patients because irregular bleeding and amenorrhoea may be associated with deteriorating renal function as well as an intrauterine pregnancy (Davison and Lindheimer 1982). Transplant patients might be at slightly higher risk of ectopic pregnancy because of pelvic adhesions due to previous urological surgery, peritoneal dialysis, pelvic inflammatory disease or the overzealous use of intrauterine contraceptive devices. The main clinical problem is that symptoms secondary to genuine pelvic pathology are erroneously attributed to the transplant because of its location near the pelvis (Scott *et al* 1978).

Allograft function (Fig. 7.9)

Serial surveillance of creatinine clearance is essential and the following points are important:

1   The increase in GFR characteristic of early pregnancy and maintained thereafter, is

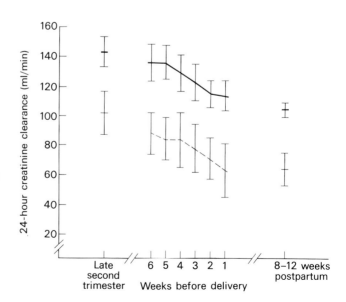

Fig. 7.9 Changes in 24-hour creatinine clearance in late pregnancy in ten healthy women (upper) compared to ten renal allograft recipients (lower) mean ± SEM. (Compiled from data of Davison *et al* (1980) and Davison and Lindheimer (1982a, 1982b).)

surprisingly also evident in transplant recipients even though the allograft is ectopic, denervated, possibly from an old donor, potentially damaged by previous ischaemia and immunologically different from both recipient and her fetus (Davison *et al* 1976; Coulam and Zincke 1981; Coulam *et al* 1982a).

2 The better the renal function before pregnancy the greater is the increment in GFR during pregnancy.

3 There can be a transient reduction in GFR during the third trimester (Merkatz *et al* 1971; Warren *et al* 1981) just as occurs in normal pregnancy (Davison *et al* 1980) and such a change does not necessarily represent a deteriorating situation with permanent impairment.

4 In 15 per cent of patients significant impairment of renal function develops during pregnancy and may persist following delivery (Merkatz *et al* 1971). As a gradual decline in allograft function is a common occurrence in nonpregnant patients, it is difficult to delineate the specific role of pregnancy. Subclinical chronic rejection, with declining renal function, may occur as a late result of tissue damage after acute rejection or when immunosuppression has not been adequate.

5 Proteinuria occurs near term in about 40 per cent of patients but disappears postpartum and in the absence of hypertension is not significant.

Allograft rejection

It has been reported that serious rejection episodes occur in 9 per cent of women with pregnancies lasting into the third trimester (Rudolph *et al* 1979). While the incidence of rejection is no greater than expected for nonpregnant transplant patients it might be considered unusual because it had always been assumed that the privileged immunological state of pregnancy would benefit the transplant. Furthermore, there are reports of reduction or cessation of immunosuppressive therapy during pregnancy without rejection episodes (Kauffman *et al* 1967; Rifle and Traeger 1975).

Chronic rejection may be a problem in all recipients and probably has a progressive subclinical course. If this is somehow influenced by pregnancy there do not appear to be any consistent factors serving to predict which patients will develop rejection episodes, as there is no relationship to prior rejection episodes, HLA types, the transplant–pregnancy time interval or problems in previous pregnancies (Guttman 1979). The following points are important: 1. Rejection at any time is difficult to diagnose. 2. If any of the clinical hallmarks such as fever, oliguria, deteriorating renal function associated with renal enlargement and tenderness are present, then the diagnosis must be considered. 3. Without renal biopsy, rejection cannot be distinguished from acute pyelonephritis, recurrent glomerulopathy and possibly severe pre-eclampsia. Renal biopsy is therefore indicated before embarking upon antirejection therapy. 4. Rejection occasionally occurs in the puerperium (Rifle and Traeger 1975; Parsons *et al* 1979) and this may be the result of the return to a normal immune state (despite immunosuppression) or possibly a rebound effect from the altered immunoresponsiveness associated with pregnancy.

Hypertension and pre-eclampsia

The appearance of hypertension and proteinuria in the third trimester and their relationship to deteriorating renal function, the possibility of chronic underlying pathology and pre-eclampsia are difficult diagnostic problems. Pre-eclampsia is diagnosed clinically in about 30 per cent of pregnancies and, interestingly, is not related to the chronological age of the donor organ (Coulam *et al* 1982a). Where eclampsia supervenes, its development may be rapid (Williams and Jelen 1979).

Infections

Although some reports describe an increased incidence of all types of infection, this is controversial (Horbach *et al* 1973; Sciarra *et al* 1975). Nevertheless, patients should be carefully monitored throughout pregnancy, particularly with regard to urinary tract infection. The occurrence of viral infections in immunosuppressed patients is always a potential hazard to mother and fetus (MacLean *et al* 1977; Spencer and Anderson 1979).

Fetal wellbeing

Meticulous monitoring of fetal growth is needed and is best performed by serial ultrasound studies. Measurement of maternal urinary oestriol excretion is of no value because the administration of steroids suppresses the synthesis of fetal adrenal steroid precursors and the transplanted kidney may not excrete oestriol normally (Sheriff *et al* 1978; Conlam *et al* 1982b). Human placental lactogen (hPL) levels are normal in these patients if the placenta is functioning well and may be used for monitoring fetal wellbeing. Where there is evidence of intrauterine growth retardation, the possibility of congenital CMV infection should be considered (Evans *et al* 1975).

Immunosuppressive therapy during pregnancy

A literature survey reveals no predominent or frequent developmental abnormalities. Azathioprine is teratogenic in animals but only in large doses (equivalent to more than 6 mg per kg body weight), so that the risks of modest doses (2 mg per kg per day or less) taken by patients with stable renal function may not be excessive. Also the fetus lacks the necessary enzyme (inosinate pyrophosphorylase) which converts azathioprine to its active form, thionosinic acid (Saarikoski and Seppala 1973; Williamson and Rann 1981). Similarly congenital abnormalities result from very large doses of steroids in experimental animals but the consensus is that the risk to the fetus from doses used after transplantation is small (Waltzer *et al* 1980) (*see also* p. 12). However, in one series (Registration Committee of EDTA 1980) where birth anomalies were present in 7 out of 103 offspring, the mothers of abnormal babies had been taking a significantly higher daily dose of azathioprine than those who had normal babies: 2.64 mg/kg vs. 2.02

mg/kg. This was based on a relatively small number of abnormal babies and could still be due to chance. There was no significant difference in the daily dose of prednisone between the two groups.

Changes in therapy must not jeopardise overall suppression even though there are some reports where therapy was reduced or stopped during pregnancy without invoking rejection (Kauffmann *et al* 1967; Rifle and Traeger 1975). At no point after transplantation barring serious drug toxicity is it prudent to stop all immunosuppressive therapy (Guttman 1979).

With the introduction of the new immunosuppressive agent cyclosporin A (European Multicentre Trial 1982), which is supposedly more effective than conventional therapy (azathioprine and/or steroids), new evaluations will be needed. cyclosporin A is a fungal metabolite which acts on the early part of the immune response, perhaps on the antigen recognition process or the release and action of interleukins (Hall 1982). Nephrotoxicity can be a major side-effect which makes its use in renal transplantation paradoxical but it is not myelosuppressive (Calen *et al* 1979) nor mutagenic on *in vitro* testing. The long-term efficacy and side-effects of cyclosporin A are unknown but liver impairment and lymphoma development have been reported.

To-date, there is only one report of a pregnancy in a transplant patient taking cyclosporin A (Lewis *et al* 1983). This patient had had two previous unsuccessful transplants and presumably the cyclosporin A had been given at the time of the third transplant rather than azathioprine and steroids in the hope of improving graft acceptance. The pregnancy was not complicated and the offspring's weight was appropriate for gestational age. As more data accrue important questions will be whether cyclosporin A should be used as a long-term maintenance immunosuppressive agent and whether or not it is a suitable agent in transplant recipients contemplating pregnancy.

DECISIONS REGARDING DELIVERY

Preterm delivery is common (45–60 per cent) because of intervention for obstetric reasons and the common occurrences of premature rupture of membranes and premature labour. Premature labour is commonly associated with poor renal function and this may be a contributory factor in transplant patients (Felding 1969). In some, however, there is no obvious explanation and it has been postulated that long-term steroid therapy may weaken connective tissues and contribute to the increased incidence of premature rupture of membranes (Rudolph *et al* 1979).

Augmentation of steroids is necessary to cover the stress of delivery. A reasonable dose would be hydrocortisone, 100 mg i.m. six-hourly during labour. Vaginal delivery should be the aim and there is no evidence that there is any extra risk of mechanical injury to the transplanted kidney. Unless there are problems or unusual circumstances (Salant *et al* 1976; MacLean *et al* 1980), the onset of labour should be spontaneous but of course induction should be undertaken if there are specific indications.

Management during labour

Careful monitoring of maternal fluid balance, cardiovascular status and temperature is essential. Aseptic technique is mandatory at all times (Myerowitz *et al* 1972): any surgical procedure, however trivial, such as an episiotomy, should be covered with prophylactic antibiotics (ampicillin and Flagyl). Indeed, surgical induction of labour by amniotomy might be considered to warrant antibiotic cover.

Pain relief is conducted as for healthy women. If there are problems with acute hypertension then management should be as discussed in Chapter 6.

Fetal electronic monitoring should be undertaken. If fetal scalp blood samples are taken then a fetal platelet count would help to exclude fetal thrombocytopenia, which increases the risk of fetal intracerebral haemorrhage and is an indication for Caesarean section (Scott *et al* 1980) (*see also* pp. 86–7).

Role of Caesarean section

Although obstructed labour due to the position of the graft has been reported (Nolan *et al* 1974), the kidney does not usually obstruct the birth canal. Caesarean section is only necessary for purely obstetrical reasons (Salant *et al* 1976; MacLean *et al* 1980). However, from the literature more Caesarean sections have been performed than might be expected, presumably reflecting fear of the unknown, rather than certainty that vaginal delivery would be hazardous for mother and/or child.

The following are important when making a final decision on the route of delivery:
1   Transplant patients may have pelvic osteodystrophy related to their previous renal failure (and dialysis) or prolonged steroid therapy, particularly before puberty (Huffer *et al* 1975). For instance, avascular necrosis, particularly of the femoral head, is a common problem, occurring in 20 per cent of all transplant patients (Ibels *et al* 1978; Elmstedt 1981). Patients with pelvic problems should be recognised antenatally and delivered by Caesarean section if there is cephalopelvic disproportion.
2   Some authors have recommended that if there is any question of disproportion or kidney compression then simultaneous intravenous urogram and X-ray pelvimetry should be performed at 36 weeks' gestation (Rifle and Traeger 1975).
3   When a Caesarean section is performed, a lower segment approach is usually feasible but previous urological surgery may make this difficult (Faber *et al* 1976; Coyne *et al* 1981).

PAEDIATRIC MANAGEMENT (*see* Table 7.6.)

Immediate problems

Over 50 per cent of liveborns have no neonatal problems. Preterm delivery is common (45–60 per cent), small-for-dates infants are delivered in about 15–20 per cent of cases and occasionally the two problems occur together (Fig. 7.10).

It is known that immunogenetic disparity between a conceptus and its mother

Table 7.6 Neonatal paediatric problems.

1. Preterm delivery
2. Respiratory distress syndrome
3. Depressed haematopoiesis
4. Septicaemia
5. Lymphoid hypoplasia
6. Andrenocortical insufficiency
7. CMV infection
8. Chromosome aberrations
9. Congenital abnormalities
10. HBsAg carrier state

actually results in some apparent reproductive advantages. Specifically, placentae and fetuses are larger when greater maternofetal histo-incompatibility exists. The nature of the maternal immune response producing these changes is still unclear but it might be anticipated that nonspecific depression of the immune system by immunosuppressive drugs could result in adverse effects such as fetal growth retardation (Scott 1977). The

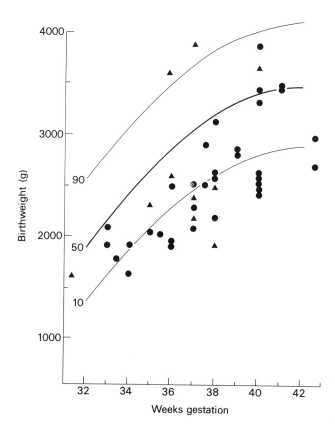

Fig. 7.10 Birthweight and gestational age of infants born to renal allograft recipients, who all received azathioprine prior to and throughout pregnancy (modified from Scott *et al* 1977). 10th, 50th and 90th centiles are shown. Ten cases managed in Newcastle upon Tyne (1976–82) are shown as ▲.

effect could also be explained by the cytotoxic action of azathioprine on the intrauterine contents (Rosenkrantz *et al* 1967; Gross *et al* 1976).

The neonatal paediatric management is the same as for babies of non-transplant mothers but there are some problems peculiar to the offspring of this group of patients (Rasmussen *et al* 1981). Thymic atrophy, transient leucopenia, bone marrow hypoplasia, reduced blood levels of IgG and IgM, septicaemia, chromosome aberrations in lymphocytes (Table 7.7), hypoglycaemia and hypocalcaemia have all been reported (*see* Davison and Lindheimer 1982b). Cord blood samples taken at delivery should aim at excluding any serious problems.

Adrenocortical insufficiency due to the maternal steroid therapy increases the risk of overwhelming neonatal infection. Occasionally the neonate collapses shortly after delivery with overwhelming infection, and adrenocortical insufficiency should be suspected (Penn *et al* 1980a). Once the diagnosis has been considered, the proper therapy consists of steroids, antibiotics, gammaglobulin and appropriate electrolyte solutions.

Table 7.7   Chromosome aberrations* (per cent) in cultured lymphocytes of two renal transplant mothers and their offspring compared to nonpregnant transplant patients and the normal population. (Modified from Price *et al* 1976.)

	Adult	Infant		
		birth	6 months	>6 months
Mother 1	25	16	8	10
Mother 2	12	18	14	0
Renal transplant patients (nonpregnant)	26			
Normal	2.5	0.5–1	0.5–1	0.5–1

* Gaps, fragments, deletions, rings, etc. studied in metaphase.

It is likely that children born to renal transplant mothers who are carriers of HBsAg (during and after pregnancy) become antigen carriers themselves (Skinhöj *et al* 1976; Rasmussen *et al* 1981). Of interest is the fact that any woman with acute hepatitis in late pregnancy or within two months after delivery transmits HBsAg to her offspring in at least 75 per cent of cases, whereas in asymptomatic carriers the risk of the children becoming antigen-positive is much less (*see* Chapter 9). Even if there is little effect on general health, however, serum aminotransferases may be elevated perhaps signifying chronic persistent hepatitis, which in some cases has been verified by biopsy (Gerety and Schweitzer 1977). The use of hyperimmunoglobulin against HBsAg given prophylactically to neonates has been investigated and it is known that the carrier state can be prevented in 75 per cent if newborns are given hepatitis B immunoglobulin immediately after birth (Recommendations of Immunization Practices Advisory Committee; Mulley *et al* 1982). (*See also* pp. 311–12.)

Breast feeding

In theory, if the baby has been exposed to azathioprine and its metabolites throughout pregnancy, it should be well accustomed to them and if their concentrations in breast milk are minimal then breast feeding would not be contraindicated. Despite the beneficial effects of breast feeding, more specific information is needed about whether the amounts of azathioprine and its metabolites are trivial or substantial from a biological point of view (Fagerholm *et al* 1980; Coulam *et al* 1982) and only then can sound advice be given.

Long-term problems

If azathioprine causes chromosome aberrations in fetal lymphocytes (*see* Table 7.7) (Price *et al* 1976)—however transient—the fear is that these anomalies may not be temporary in other somatic cells not studied and in the germ cells. The sequelae could be future development of malignancies or impairment of reproduction in the affected offspring. There is some evidence of this from animal studies (Reimers and Sluss 1978). The ovaries of female offspring of mothers treated with 6-mercaptopurine (the principal metabolite of azathioprine: equivalent to 3 mg/kg) contained fewer oocytes and ovarian follicles compared to offspring of mothers that had not received the drug. Furthermore, these mice had fertility problems when they were bred. Despite normal body weight and general appearance, many proved to be sterile or, if they became pregnant, had smaller litters and more dead fetuses.

   This effect was probably initiated while the offspring were developing in the uteri of their mothers during treatment. It is unlikely that such damage would be eliminated or repaired, as seems to happen in somatic cells, because synthesis of DNA stops when the germ cells are arrested in the prophase of the first meiotic division in utero, and no new DNA is synthesised until after fertilisation.

   Thus exposure of the fetus to low doses of potential mutagens may not cause immediate, obvious effects such as morbidity or birth defects, but may have severe consequences when otherwise normal female offspring reach puberty. As yet, there are no animal data on the reproductive performance of the male offspring.

   It is therefore imperative that any child exposed to immunosuppressive therapy in utero has a careful evaluation of the immune system and long-term follow-up.

POSTNATAL ASSESSMENT

These patients have the same problems that afflict healthy women. Moreover, because they are receiving immunosuppressive therapy, they have a risk of developing *de novo* malignancy that is 35 times greater than normal (Hoover and Fraumeni 1973) and the female genital tract is no exception. There are reports of cervical changes ranging from cellular atypia through carcinoma-in-situ to invasive squamous cell carcinoma (Porreco *et al* 1975). Consequently, a cervical smear is mandatory at the postnatal review and regular gynaecological assessment should be organised if it was not already underway before pregnancy.

All women should be routinely counselled about contraception. The choice depends on balancing the desirability of pregnancy prevention against the potential risks of the contraceptive method. Contraceptive steroids can produce subtle changes in the immune system (Keller *et al* 1976), but this is not necessarily a contraindication to their use. Low-dose oestrogen-progesterone preparations can be prescribed although some have avoided them because of the possibility of causing or aggravating hypertension or further increasing the incidence of thromboembolism (Taylor, 1975; Rao *et al* 1976). If the oral contraceptive is prescribed, careful and frequent surveillance is needed.

An intrauterine contraceptive device can aggravate any tendency towards menstrual problems and these in turn may confuse the signs and symptoms of abnormalities in early pregnancy, such as threatend abortion or ectopic pregnancy (Scott *et al* 1978). The risks of pelvic infection are increased and this could be disastrous in an immunosuppressed patient (Tatum 1976). Furthermore, it has been suggested that the antifertility action of an IUCD can be inhibited by immunosuppressive agents (Taylor *et al* 1975).

Pregnancy in haemodialysis patients

It is over ten years since the first documentation of conception and successful delivery in a patient undergoing chronic haemodialysis (Confortini *et al* 1971) and since then further case reports and registry data have been published (Unzelman *et al* 1973; Ackrill *et al* 1975; Sheriff *et al* 1978; Rigenbach *et al* 1978; Thomson *et al* 1978, Marwood *et al* 1979; Trebbin 1979; Registration Committee of EDTA 1980; Kobayashi *et al* 1981; Sardie *et al* 1982). In one of the cases reported (Unzelman *et al* 1973) the renal function was so good that success might have been achieved without dialysis.

Any optimism must be tempered by remembering that clinicians are reluctant to publish their failures and consequently the true incidence of unsuccessful pregnancies and their sequelae in women on haemodialysis cannot be determined. There is no doubt that the high surgical abortion rate in these patients indicates that those who become pregnant do so accidentally, probably because they are unaware that pregnancy is a possibility.

As yet there are no reports of pregnancies in patients undergoing the relatively new chronic ambulatory peritoneal dialysis (CAPD), but there are reports of gynaecological sequelae in these patients, such as reflux of menstrual blood through the intraperitoneal catheter due to possible endometriosis (Blumenkrantz *et al* 1981) and severe pelvic peritonitis (Rubin *et al* 1980), as well as psychosocial problems which could influence libido and potency (Borgeson 1982).

PREGNANCY COUNSELLING

In spite of irregular or absent menstruation (Lim *et al* 1980), decreased libido and potency, and impaired fertility, women undergoing haemodialysis should always use contraception if they wish to avoid pregnancy (Soffer 1980; BMJ Editorial 1982). *There are substantial arguments against pregnancy and these should be pointed out, not least the risks to the patient and the greatly reduced likelihood of successful outcome.*

GENERAL MANAGEMENT PLAN

Early pregnancy assessment

Early diagnosis of pregnancy can be a problem. Irregular menstruation is common and a missed period will usually be ignored (Emmanouel *et al* 1980). The big mistake the clinician may make is not even to consider the possibility of pregnancy. As urine pregnancy tests are unreliable (Hogan and Price 1967), even if there is any urine available, then early diagnosis and estimation of gestational age is best accomplished by ultrasound.

Management objectives

For a successful outcome scrupulous attention must be paid to blood pressure control, fluid balance, increased dialysis requirements and provision of good nutrition. It should be emphasised that this will place many demands on the hospital team as well as the patient's family. It might even be considered to be a misuse of scarce resources and manpower.

Dialysis strategy during pregnancy

Women with residual renal function and satisfactory daily urine volumes, in whom biochemical control is easier, are more likely to become pregnant. Some patients show increments in GFR even if the level of renal function is too poor to sustain life without haemodialysis. The dialysis strategy should have the following aims:

1   Maintain plasma urea at less than 20 mmol/l. It has been suggested that intauterine death is likely if levels are much in excess of 20 mmol/l (Tenney and Dandrow 1961), but in one case report (Ackrill *et al* 1975) success was achieved despite levels of 25 mmol/l for many weeks.

2   Ensure rigid control of blood pressure.

3   Avoid hypotension during dialysis. In late pregnancy the gravid uterus and the supine posture may aggravate this by decreasing venous return.

4   Ensure minimal fluctuations in fluid balance and limit volume changes. Regular uterine contractions often occur during dialysis (Ackrill *et al* 1975).

5   Limit interdialysis weight gain to 0.5 kg until late pregnancy.

Inevitably this strategy means increased length and frequency of dialysis—in some instances by as much as 50 per cent (Kobayashi *et al* 1981). There is no doubt that frequent dialysis renders dietary management and control of weight gain much easier but the domestic problems caused might require that a combination of home and hospital dialysis is used.

Anaemia

Increasing anaemia causes concern for maternal and fetal welfare. Patients are usually anaemic and blood transfusion may be needed, especially before delivery, for safe obstetric management (Rigenbach *et al* 1978; Kobayashi *et al* 1981). Caution is needed because transfusion may exacerbate hypertension and might also impair the ability to control circulatory overload, even with extra dialysis. Fluctuations in blood volume can be minimised, however, if nitrogen-frozen packed red cells are transfused during dialysis.

Unnecessary blood sampling should be avoided and, in any case, lack of venepuncture sites can be a problem. The protocol for the various routine tests performed in a particular unit should be followed meticulously, removing no more blood per venepuncture than is absolutely necessary. Screening for Australia antigen is mandatory.

Hypertension

Blood pressure can fluctuate wildly. These patients have such abnormal lipid profiles and accelerated atherogenesis that it is difficult to predict the ability of the cardiovascular system to tolerate the stresses of pregnancy. Normal blood pressure, however, is reassuring. Unfortunately, hypertension is a common problem, though it may be possible to control this by ultrafiltration, provided exacerbation does not occur between dialyses. Any other measures must be carefully assessed in the light of possible side-effects.

Attention to nutrition

Despite more frequent dialysis, free dietary intake should be discouraged. An oral intake of at least 70 g protein, 1500 mg calcium, 50 mmol potassium and 80 mmol sodium per day is advised and oral supplements of dialysable vitamins should be given. Vitamin D supplements can be difficult to judge in patients who have had a parathyroidectomy. It is not clear to what extent these dietary factors and maternal uraemia affect the fetus and its nutrition.

Fetal surveillance and delivery

The fetus should be monitored as already described in the section on chronic renal disease (p. 207). The greatly reduced clearance of conjugated oestrogens means that separate measurement of free or unconjugated oestriol is necessary (Sheriff *et al* 1978).

Caesarean section should only be necessary for purely obstetrical reasons, although it could be argued that an elective Caesarean section would always minimise potential problems of volume and blood pressure control during labour. In fact, preterm labour is generally the rule and the role of Caesarean section under these circumstances needs to be carefully considered (Lim and Fairweather 1981).

Acute renal failure

Acute renal failure is a clinical syndrome characterised by a sudden and marked decrease in glomerular filtration, rising plasma urea and creatinine levels, and usually by a decrease in urine output to below 400 ml in 24 hours. As a clinical diagnosis the term only describes *the functional state of the kidneys* without distinguishing between the different forms of underlying pathology. For the most part, acute renal failure occurs in persons with previously healthy kidneys but it may also complicate the course of patients with pre-existing renal disease.

Before anuria or oliguria are ascribed to acute renal failure, obstruction to the renal outflow must be excluded, usually by infusion urography, if investigation is needed. This is particularly pertinent in obstetric practice, since it is all too easy to unwittingly damage the urinary tract when performing emergency surgery for obstetric disasters, such as postpartum haemorrhage, which are themselves causes of acute renal failure (Table 7.8).

Twenty years ago the incidence of acute renal failure in pregnancy was 0.02–0.05 per cent (Kerr and Elliott 1963) and represented about 2 per cent of cases reported of renal failure of all causes (Kleinknecht and Ganeval 1965). At that time acute renal failure was a substantial cause of maternal mortality, as at least 20 per cent of women with this complication died (Smith *et al* 1968).

Table 7.8   Some causes of obstetric acute renal failure.

Volume contraction/hypotension	Antepartum haemorrhage due to placenta praevia Postpartum haemorrhage: from uterus or extensive soft tissue trauma Abortion Hyperemesis gravidarum Adrenocortical failure; usually failure to augment steroids to cover delivery in patient on long-term therapy
Volume contraction/hypotension and coagulopathy	Antepartum haemorrhage due to abruptio placentae Pre-eclampsia/eclampsia Amniotic fluid embolism Incompatible blood transfusion Drug reaction(s) Acute fatty liver Haemolytic uraemic syndrome
Volume contraction/hypotension, coagulopathy and infection	Septic abortion Chorioamnionitis Pyelonephritis Puerperal sepsis
Urinary tract obstruction	Damage to ureters: during Caesarean section and repair of cervical/vaginal lacerations Pelvic haematoma Broad ligament haematoma

Recently there has been a marked decline in cases of acute renal failure related to obstetrics, largely attributable to liberalisation of abortion laws and improvements in perinatal care which have reduced complications, such as sepsis, eclampsia, hypovolaemia and severe haemorrhage (Hawkins *et al* 1975). The current incidence is probably less than 0.01 per cent, but still has a bimodal distribution corresponding to septic abortion in early pregnancy and pre-eclampsia and bleeding problems in the third trimester (Lindheimer *et al* 1982). In contrast to the situation in developed countries, there are still parts of the world where the incidence of severe acute obstetric renal failure remains high and Chugh and his colleagues (1976) have reported that 22 per cent of 325 admissions to their unit in Northern India were related to pregnancy, and that 55 per cent of these women died.

PATHOLOGY

Within the kidney there are three common patterns of altered function and anatomy, which are probably part of a spectrum of increasing severity of the same pathological process, i.e. preglomerular vasoconstriction causing renal hypoperfusion with preferential cortical ischaemia (Steinhausen *et al* 1981).

Prerenal failure or vasomotor nephropathy

This is a relatively mild form of acute renal failure and is caused by moderate degrees of renal ischaemia. It is partly a functional disorder, in which there are no changes in renal morphology, and it is reversible if renal perfusion is improved.

Acute tubular necrosis

This occurs if renal ischaemia is more severe or persists longer. The damage is limited to the most metabolically active tubular cells. The blood vessels and glomeruli do not show significant alteration. It is also reversible after a variable period of renal shutdown.

Acute cortical necrosis

This is the result of extremely severe or protracted renal ischaemia or when there is intense intravascular coagulation. There is evidence of widespread morphological disruption with complete disintegration of glomeruli and tubules. The lesion is usually bilateral, involving the entire cortex, so that the clinical condition is irreversible. In a minority of cases, however, the necrosis may be more limited and patchy which accounts for the rare patient who recovers with a slight amount of residual renal function (Grünfeld *et al* 1980).

PHASES OF ACUTE RENAL FAILURE

Traditionally there are three consecutive phases and these have important management implications.

Oliguria

Urine volumes are less than 400 ml in 24 hours. This phase may last from a few days to several weeks. Complete anuria is uncommon in acute tubular necrosis and is usually a manifestation of massive acute cortical necrosis or complete obstruction. Non-oliguric forms of acute cortical necrosis may be occasionally encountered in which urine volumes seem adequate but renal function is severely impaired (Vertel and Knochel 1967).

Polyuria

Urine volumes increase markedly and can be up to 10 litres in 24 hours. The polyuria may last from several days to two weeks. The urine is dilute and, despite the large volumes excreted, metabolic waste products are not efficiently eliminated. Consequently plasma urea and creatinine levels will continue to rise for several days in parallel with increased urine output. Profound fluid and electrolyte losses can endanger survival if not adequately replaced.

Recovery

Urine volumes decrease towards normal. Renal function gradually improves, nearing the level before the acute renal failure developed.

DIAGNOSIS AND INVESTIGATION

A carefully taken history may reveal a background of abortion, severe hyperemesis gravidarum, haemorrhage, sensitisation to drugs, incompatible blood transfusion, pre-eclampsia and/or neglect of recent steroid intake (*see* Table 7.8). Once the diagnosis has been entertained then the possible causes must be pursued and, in conjunction with a nephrologist, a full initial assessment should be undertaken. The investigations should include the following:

1   Blood specimens: full blood count (Coulter counter analysis), urea, electrolytes and osmolality, glucose, liver function tests, amylase, plasma proteins, particular albumin, coagulation indices, acid-base status (arterial blood sample).

2   Urine specimens: specific gravity and osmolality, electrolyte concentrations, protein excretion.

3   Bacteriological assessment: blood cultures (aerobic and anaerobic), vaginal swabs, midstream urine specimen (MSU).

4 Electrocardiogram (ECG): Abnormalities do not necessarily correlate with the degree of hyper- or hypokalaemia. Initially, in hyperkalaemia, there are peaked T waves with QRS prolongation and then disappearance of P waves with deformation of the QRS complex.

5 Assessment of fluid balance: The bladder should be catheterised and continuous drainage allowed so that hourly volumes can be recorded. A central venous pressure (CVP) line should be established, preferrably via the antecubital vein. Where the patient is deeply shocked the subclavian vein may be used, but this route should be avoided when artificial ventilation is likely, because of the danger of pneumothorax. This complication is unlikely to arise using the right internal jugular vein, a route that has the added advantage that the catheter tip invariably enters the right atrium. The right atrial pressure (RAP) serves as an indicator of volume of blood returning to the right side of the heart and the response of the right ventricle to a volume load.

An intravenous therapy line, preferably in a central vein, should also be established. Exact therapy will depend on the biochemical disturbance(s) and CVP or RAP readings.

Administration of large amounts of fluid in acute tubular necrosis is both useless and fraught with danger. Blood loss must be taken into account; it is frequently understimated especially if there has been an antepartum haemorrhage, which is often concealed.

6 Fetal salvage: If this has to be taken into consideration then a decision will have to be taken regarding the timing and route of delivery.

DIAGNOSTIC PITFALLS

It is difficult and often impossible to decide which of the three types of acute renal failure (acute tubular necrosis, acute corticol necrosis, prerenal failure) is present. Total anuria or alternating periods of anuria and polyuria strongly suggests obstruction, but normal urine volumes do not exclude obstruction. Complete anuria and/or evidence of disseminated intravascular coagulation are suggestive of acute cortical necrosis but this diagnosis can only be firmly established by renal biopsy.

The differential diagnosis between functional renal insufficiency caused by dehydration or hypotension (prerenal failure or vasomotor nephropathy) and acute tubular or cortical necrosis is of practical importance as their therapy is diametrically different.

Urine/plasma (U/P) osmolality ratio.   This ratio is the single most valuable indicator of early acute renal failure (Luke *et al* 1965). Prerenal failure is suggested when the ratio is greater than 1.5, whereas in acute tubular or cortical necrosis it is closer to unity.

Urine specific gravity. This is inadequate because misleadingly high values may be caused by sugar or protein admixture and comparison wih plasma is not possible.

Urinary sodium concentration. This index is only useful when oliguria is present because a low sodium concentration can be found in non-oliguric acute renal failure (Vertel and Knochel 1967). In prerenal failure the urine is concentrated with low sodium concentration (less than 20 mmol/l) and in acute tubular necrosis the urine is isotonic to plasma with a relatively high sodium concentration (greater than 60 mmol/l) (Luke *et al* 1965).

Trial i.v. infusion of 100 ml 25% mannitol. Mannitol infusion is a relatively safe therapeutic test and may be helpful in distinguishing between reversible prerenal failure and established acute tubular necrosis provided the period of oliguria does not exceed 48 hours and the U/P osmolality ratio is greater than 1.05 (Luke *et al* 1965).

If a diuresis is established within three hours (more than 50 ml per hour or double the previous urine volume) then urine output should be replaced exactly with intravenous isotonic saline in an attempt to sustain adequate urine flow for at least 24–36 hours, after which the danger of acute tubular necrosis has probably passed. By determining urinary electrolytes the losses can be replaced accordingly. If urine flow subsequently decreases to less than 30 ml then the mannitol infusion can be repeated 6–8 hourly.

If attempts to increase urine flow are unsuccessful, the objective is to support the functionally anephric patient until the kidneys recover (*see* p. 241).

Use of diuretics. Increments in urine flow produced by 'loop diuretics' such as frusemide may represent conversion of oliguric renal failure to a polyuric form, rather than reversal of prerenal failure. Furthermore, there is no evidence of any beneficial effect of frusemide on the period of oliguria, immediate prognosis or mortality (Jørgensen 1981).

Role of renal biopsy. Since acute cortical necrosis is usually irreversible, biopsy is indicated in patients with protracted oliguria or anuria who fail to improve, in order to allow an assessment of prognosis. Diagnosing acute cortical necrosis early, however, is not mandatory, since the management of the acute stage is no different from that of acute tubular necrosis.

GENERAL MANAGEMENT PLAN

Prerenal failure or vasomotor nephropathy

The basic principle is to adequately replace blood and fluid losses and maintain blood pressure at levels that will permit adequate renal perfusion. Evidence of continuing blood loss calls for localisation and control of the bleeding. Volume correction should always precede the use of diuretics, with the exception of mannitol (both a volume expander and an osmotic diuretic) which may usefully reduce endothelial cell swelling and thereby help to restore renal blood flow.

Volume and metabolic control

Fluid intake and output must be determined daily. Insensible fluid losses cannot be measured directly, but weighing the patient every day is helpful in assessing the state of hydration, and haematocrit and total protein determinations are additional evaluators.

Volume balance is achieved by allowing the adult, non-febrile patient an intake of

500 ml of fluid plus the total output of the preceding 24 hours. If the patient is febrile 200 ml of additional intake is needed for each 1°C increment. If fluid volume is in balance then bodyweight should decrease approximately 0.3–0.5 kg per 24 hours because of tissue catabolism. Overhydration must be avoided and if present must be promptly corrected, if necessary by dialysis. Continuous careful supervision and replacement of urinary fluid electrolyte losses is even more important in the polyuric phase, as 50 per cent of deaths occur at this time.

There is a need for oral or parenteral administration of at least 1500 calories of a protein-free fat/carbohydrate combination which is low in potassium and sodium. Carbohydrate calories are important for decreasing gluconeogenesis from protein (protein-sparing effect), thus retarding the development of azotaemia/acidosis. Volume limitations dictate that glucose should be administrated as a hypertonic (up to 50 per cent) solution via a central vein.

Administration of essential L-amino acids improve wound healing, result in reductions of plasma potassium, magnesium and phosphate levels, and generally improve survival and hasten recovery (Abel *et al* 1973).

Acid–base and electrolyte balance

Treatment of metabolic acidosis should be instituted whenever the clinical situation warrants it or when plasma bicarbonate (P_{HCO_3}) drops below 12 mmol/l. A rough estimate of the amount of bicarbonate required can be obtained as follows:

$$\text{Dosage (mmol)} = (25 - P_{HCO_3}) \times \text{Bodyweight (kg)} \times 0.6$$

In severe acidosis only half of the calculated dose should be given initially, with the remaining dosage subsequently adjusted according to frequent pH and P_{CO_2} determinations. Care should be taken not to overload the oliguric patient with sodium and water which are inevitably present in bicarbonate solution. If fluid overload appears likely, then acidosis should be treated by dialysis at the outset.

Correction of blood pH is an important contribution to the prevention or treatment of potentially fatal hyperkalaemia which frequently develops rapidly, especially in the hypercatabolic patient. Prevention requires absolute restriction of potassium intake and sometimes prophylactic use of a cation exchange resin, either by the oral or rectal route.

Bacteriological control

It is neither necessary nor advisable to treat the uninfected uraemic patient with broad spectrum antibiotics. They are potentially toxic in the oliguric patient and may favour overgrowth of resistant pathogens and thus lead to nosocomial infection which is difficult to control. Prophylaxis can be achieved by expert nursing care, aseptic technique during instrumentation and wound care, frequent changing of intravenous therapy sites and impeccable management of indwelling bladder catheters.

If antibiotics are needed their initial use must be empirical until culture and sensititivies specify the appropriate agents. Vigorous treatment is mandatory, if possible guided by antibiotic serum levels (Levy 1977).

DIALYSIS FOR ACUTE RENAL FAILURE

Indications

The indications for dialysis differ slightly from centre to centre but overall the choice should be dictated by the prevailing clinical circumstances rather than the facilities available. The main indications for dialysis are: volume overload and congestive heart failure; severe hyperkalaemia; severe acidosis; and uraemic symptoms (nausea, vomiting and encephalopathy) not treatable by conventional methods.

In such circumstances dialysis should be started regardless of plasma biochemistry, but when creatinine and urea levels rise rapidly because of a hypercatabolic state, dialysis is indicated even if clinical symptoms have not yet appeared. Early 'prophylactic' dialysis, before the onset of uraemic symptoms, allows more liberal intake of protein, salt and water as well as preventing hyperkalaemic emergencies (Lindheimer *et al* 1982). Furthermore, it decreases the incidence of infectious complications, improves wound healing, increases patient comfort and appears to improve patient survival.

Peritoneal dialysis

Peritoneal dialysis has many advantages and can be used in pregnant or recently delivered women (Smith *et al* 1968). It is easily available, simple, inexpensive and has a relatively low complication rate. There are no absolute contraindications and it can be used even in the presence of pelvic peritonitis. Relative contraindications are intraperitoneal adhesions, open wounds or drains in the abdomen and recent retroperitoneal operations (Kleinknecht *et al* 1973). Occasionally peritoneal dialysis may be complicated by peritonitis or trauma to the intra-abdominal viscera.

Haemodialysis

Haemodialysis depends on an adequate shunt blood flow and has limited usefulness in the presence of hypotension. It is contraindicated in the actively bleeding patient, since even well controlled regional heparinisation does not ensure the safety of the procedure.

Acute renal failure and septic shock (*see also* p. 494)

Septicaemia associated with pregnancy is commonly due to septic abortion whereas pyelonephritis, chorioamnionitis and puerperal sepsis occur less frequently (Hawkins *et al* 1975; Chugh *et al* 1976). Only occasionally is the abortion spontaneous, although detailed questioning may be required to elicit evidence that abortifacients have been used. Although this life-threatening condition is now very rare the clinician should not be lulled into false sense of security given the ever present potential of antibiotic-resistant bacterial strains.

PATHOLOGY

There are many reasons why acute renal failure should be associated with septic abortion. The patient is both dehydrated and hypotensive—a combination which leads to considerable renal ischaemia. Haemoglobinuria (due to haemolysis) and dissemi-nated intravascular coagulation (DIC) are often present and soap and lysol (common abortifacients) have specific nephrotoxic effects (Bartlett and Yahia 1969). The severity of the renal dysfunction associated with clostridial infections suggest that clostridia produce a specific nephrotoxin (Richet and Alagille 1975). However, most pregnancy sepsis is due to Gram-negative bacteria (clostridia is responsible for only 0.5 per cent), so that marked haemolysis due to bacteria and/or abortifacients is sufficient by itself to provoke renal shutdown.

DIAGNOSIS AND INVESTIGATION

The presentation can be quite dramatic, especially in cases of *E. coli* and clostridia infection. There is an abrupt rise in temperature (to 40°C) often associated with myalgias, vomiting and diarrhoea, the latter occasionally bloody.

Once symptoms commence, hypotension, tachypnoea and progression to acute shock occur rapidly. The patients are usually jaundiced, with a particular bronze-like colour ascribed to the association of jaundice with cutaneous vasodilatation, cyanosis and pallor. Despite the presence of fever, the extremeties are often cold, with purplish areas which may be precursors of small patches of necroses on the toes, fingers or nose.

There is laboratory evidence of severe anaemia due to haemolysis with hyperbiliru-binaemia of the direct type. There are also alterations in clotting factors which suggest DIC (p. 76). Leucocytosis (25 000 per mm^3) with marked shifts to the left are the rule and thrombocytopenia of less than 50 000 per mm^3 is often observed. Hypocalcaemia, severe enough to provoke tetany, can occur (Hawkins *et al* 1975).

Abdominal X-ray may demonstrate air in the uterus or abdomen—the result of gas-forming organisms and/or perforation. Despite this toxic and septicaemic picture bacterial identification may be difficult and the situation is further confused because clostridia are normally present in the female genital tract (Smith *et al* 1971).

Full initial assessment should be conducted with a nephrologist along the lines discussed for acute renal failure with the following additional important points:

Skin and core temperature differential.   The relationship of skin temperature to central body temperature serves as an indicator of adequacy of peripheral perfusion. Peripheral temperature can be measured from the medial aspect of the big toe and central body temperature by a probe placed in the rectum, in the lumen of the oesophagus or over the sternum. A large difference between the two (more than 2°C) implies poor peripheral perfusion. This is commonly associated with lactic acidosis and occasionally with DIC.

Serum albumin. This should always be assessed in any patient with severe sepsis. Levels less than 25 g/l are commonly found, predisposing the patient to pulmonary oedema. Albumin replacement should be considered.

Blood sugar. Diabetes must be excluded. Blood from a finger prick should not be used if there is poor skin perfusion.

Acid–base status. The patient may be hypoxic, through ventilation-perfusion inequality. The $Paco_2$ is usually low in order to compensate for the increasing metabolic acidosis. An elevated $Paco_2$ is unusual: it may imply deterioration in the level of consciousness with loss of respiratory drive or, occasionally, may precede respiratory failure or depression due to sedative drugs.

Metabolic acidosis is generally related to inadequate peripheral oxygenation, anaeorobic metabolism and the onset of lactic acid acidosis. An increasing and irreversible metabolic acidosis following initial resuscitation is a bad prognostic sign.

Coagulation indices (*see* Chapter 3). Hypercoagulability may be seen early and can alternate with hypocoagulability. Haematological evidence of DIC correlates with the severity of the shock and poor peripheral oxygenation. The potential for blood loss in septic abortion increases the susceptibility to DIC. Thrombocytopenia alone can occur in the presence of significant sepsis.

Cardiovascular investigation. Occasionally routine cardiovascular assessment is insufficient for haemodynamic evaluation. More elaborate investigations may be needed such as right ventricular output assessment or pulmonary capillary wedge pressure (PCWP), and these require skilled personnel as well as specialised equipment. Therefore, should a patient fail to respond to volume replacement, metabolic correction and antibiotics or be severely shocked, treatment must be conducted in an appropriately equipped intensive therapy unit.

DIAGNOSTIC PITFALLS

The clinician may be misled by an asymptomatic patient admitted with an incomplete abortion who rapidly becomes shocked within hours. The generalised muscular pains, often most intense in the thorax and abdomen, may lead to confusion with intra-abdominal inflammatory processes; this is especially true when a history of provoked abortion is denied or not sought for, since heavy vaginal bleeding is often not a prominent feature.

Recent treatment with antibiotics or other drugs must be pursued as it will give pointers to bacterial resistance, suppressed infection and drug-modified physiology.

GENERAL MANAGEMENT PLAN

The initial steps include vigorous supportive therapy and the use of antibiotics in high doses. The use of clostridia antitoxin, steroids and the role of surgical intervention are controversial.

The role of surgery

Three or four decades ago women with septicaemia due to septic abortion were usually considered too ill to undergo surgery. It was later suggested that in such patients the placenta served as a huge culture site for bacterial growth, from which bacteria and toxins could easily pass into the maternal circulation (Studdiford and Douglas 1956). This led to the hypothesis that if this nidus could be contained by securing the ovarian and uterine vessels, the patient's blood pressure would respond favourably and rapidly. In a series of 77 women with soap-provoked septic abortion, 60 per cent of patients who underwent surgery survived compared to 30 per cent of those treated by supportive therapy alone (Janovski *et al* 1963). Bartlett and Yahia (1969) described five successive gravely ill women whose abortion had been induced by soap and/or phenol; each of them survived, and this success rate was attributed to the rapid performance of abdominal hysterectomy.

Such results led many to advocate a radical approach, where abdominal hysterectomy is performed in patients who are responding poorly to volume replacement and vasoactive agents (Cavanaugh and Singh 1970; Emmanouel and Katz 1973). However, this approach was questioned by Hawkins and co-workers (1975) who described 19 patients managed with intensive antibiotic therapy, dialysis as required, and an absolute minimum of surgical intervention; 17 out of 19 of these patients survived while a twentieth patient who had undergone hysterectomy died. These authors state that modern antibiotic therapy alone is usually capable of confining the infection to the pelvis and eventually eradicating it from the uterus. They further noted that many young women with septic abortion may want a pregnancy in the future, and in their series of 11 women who subsequently attempted to conceive, 7 achieved normal pregnancies.

The debate concerning radical versus conservative treatment continues (Lindheimer *et al* 1982). Data supporting the surgical approach have not always been as favourable as the small series of Bartlett and Yahia (1969), and none of the reported studies are controlled. On the other hand, the picture of a necrotic and grossly infected uterus that often accompanies these chemically-produced abortions is sufficient to convince many that hysterectomy is necessary. While the results of Hawkins *et al* (1975) are impressive, it should be noted that most of their patients were transferred from other hospitals, and constituted a group that had already survived for several days with a conservative approach.

Volume and metabolic control

It is essential to restore an adequate circulating volume as soon as possible, and the volume infused must be regulated according to central venous pressure (CVP) or right atrial pressure (RAP) readings. When both the blood pressure and the CVP are low, fluid should be infused until the systolic pressure rises to 100 mmHg or higher and/or the CVP is up to 8 cm H_2O. An increase in urinary output to above 40 ml per hour is an excellent prognostic sign.

The fluid selected for volume replacement will depend upon whether there is an obvious electrolyte deficit, possible albumin depletion, or fluid is merely required to increase the circulating volume. Plasma-protein-fraction (PPF) is the solution of choice for volume replacement. Should the urinary output improve, potassium supplementation is generally necessary.

Sodium chloride (as normal saline) should only be given when there has been obvious sodium loss. A low serum sodium is common in the septic patient but does not necessarily reflect a fall in total body sodium. Blood should not be used for volume replacement, unless the haematocrit is 30 per cent or less, because it increases viscosity and hence may encourage capillary sludging. Dextran-70 should not be used if there is evidence of a bleeding diathesis or a history of skin allergy or bronchospasm.

In an appreciable number of cases anuria may persist for up to three or more weeks (Hamburger *et al* 1968). Often it is just when the patient is thought to have cortical rather than tubular necrosis that the diuretic phase commences. Some women with septic abortion do develop cortical necrosis, however, perhaps due to a severe ischaemic insult or massive DIC.

Digoxin should be used (provided the plasma potassium is normal) when there is evidence of myocardial failure or the patient develops atrial flutter or fibrillation. Other drugs which may improve the haemodynamic state include dopamine, isoprenaline and phentolamine; their use must be based on expert assessment of the haemodynamic situation (Hanson 1978).

Bacteriological control

Appropriate antibiotic therapy is essential but in the shocked patient it is of secondary importance to restoration of adequate perfusion. Before antibiotics are given the appropriate specimens for aerobic and anaerobic cultures must be taken. A bactericidal antibiotic may produce temporary clinical deterioration because of breakdown of bacteria and endotoxin release. This is an additional reason for performing basic resuscitation procedures before starting antibiotic therapy.

In patients without previous antibiotic therapy, it is reasonable to commence with a combination of a cephalosporin and metronidazole. Should the shock be severe and a pseudomonas or proteus infection diagnosed or a resistant klebsiella or coliform suspected, then gentamicin should be included. The dosage of gentamicin must be regulated according to daily blood levels. Once the sensitivities are available, the antibiotic therapy may need to be modified. Antibiotics should be given intravenously at first, changing to the intramuscular and then the oral route once the shock phase is over.

Haematological control

Sequential assessment of the coagulation indices is essential. A steady deterioration may be seen consistent with a diagnosis of DIC, and is commonly associated with overall clinical deterioration. Active treatment is not required where there are minor changes in the coagulation indices without clinical evidence of bleeding and where shock is rapidly corrected.

Should the clotting factors continue to deteriorate, in spite of the preceding resuscitative measures, fresh frozen plasma (FFP) should be given. Heparin may be considered if there is a further fall in the fibrinogen titre, in spite of FFP. A persistent thrombocytopenia (platelet count of less than $40\,000/mm^3$) and capillary oozing in spite of replacement of clotting factors is an indication for an infusion of platelets or platelet-enriched plasma.

Other measures

Hyperbaric oxygen and exchange transfusion have both been used to treat clostridial sepsis, but results are too fragmentary to recommend specific protocols (Eaton and Pearson 1971).

Acute renal failure in pre-eclampsia/eclampsia

When considering hypertension in pregnancy it is difficult to distinguish clinically between the different aetiological categories—pre-eclampsia, hypertension secondary to renal disease, essential hypertension, and combinations of these separate pathological states (Lindheimer and Katz 1981a, 1981b, 1982). Consequently, some cases diagnosed as pre-eclampsia progressing to renal failure are incompletely or improperly classified. In multiparous patients the diagnosis of pure pre-eclampsia is particularly suspect (Fisher *et al* 1980).

Pre-eclampsia is accompanied by a characteristic renal lesion in which the glomeruli enlarge and become ischaemic due to swelling of the intracapillary cells, glomerular endothelioses and mesangioses (Fisher *et al* 1981). Renal failure is usually due to acute tubular necrosis but acute cortical necrosis always results from glomerular cell swelling which can lead to complete obliteration of the capillary lumen. This appears unlikely, as the extent of the morphological lesion correlates poorly with renal functional alterations (Fisher *et al* 1981). As the vasculature of women with pre-eclampsia is exquisitely sensitive to the vasoactive influence of angiotensin II and catecholamines these vasoconstrictors may play a role in the genesis of the acute renal failure.

The pre-eclampsia patient is vasoconstricted and haemoconcentrated and has a reduced intravascular volume (Gallery *et al* 1979). The decrement usually precedes the development of the hypertension and the susceptibility of hypertensive pregnant women to develop prerenal azotaemia when salt-restricted and/or prescribed diuretics is well known. It is therefore possible that these patients (who also have an increased incidence of placental abruption) may be more susceptible than healthy women to the adverse renal effects of antepartum and intrapartum haemorrhage (Tatum and Mulé 1956).

Acute renal failure and pyelonephritis

Acute pyelonephritis is the most common renal complication during pregnancy. In the absence of complicating features such as obstruction, calculi, papillary necrosis and analgesic nephropathy, acute pyelonephritis is an extremely rare cause of acute renal failure in nonpregnant subjects, but this association appears to be more frequent in pregnant women (Ober *et al* 1956). The reason is obscure. It is known that, in pregnant women, acute pyelonephritis is accompanied by marked decrements in GFR as well as significant increments in plasma creatinine levels (Whalley *et al* 1975) and this contrasts with the situation in nonpregnant patients. The vasculature in pregnancy may be more sensitive to the vasoactive effect of bacterial endotoxins.

Acute fatty liver of pregnancy (*see also* Chapter 9)

Acute fatty liver of pregnancy (also called obstetric pseudo-acute yellow atrophy) is characterised by jaundice and severe hepatic dysfunction in late pregnancy or the early postpartum period (Sheehan 1940).

The renal failure appears to be due to haemodynamic factors (as in the 'hepatorenal syndrome') but some cases have been associated with DIC and/or the parenteral administration of tetracyclines (Schiffer 1966). Reversible urea cycle enzyme deficiencies (ornithinine transcarbamylase and carbamyl phosphate synthetase), resembling those seen in Reye's syndrome, have been described (Reye *et al* 1963; Weber *et al* 1979) and it may be an adult form of Reye's syndrome provoked by the metabolic stress of pregnancy.

A typical patient presents with nausea, vomiting and abdominal pain in late pregnancy. She then rapidly develops fever, severe jaundice, and hepatic encephalopathy (Long *et al* 1977) and common misdiagnoses are pre-eclampsia with liver involvement or septicaemia. It has been suggested that acute fatty liver and pre-eclampsia co-exist in approximately 20 per cent of the cases (Hatfield *et al* 1972).

Serum transaminases are only minimally increased (if at all), despite the marked hyperbilirubinaemia and severe hepatic failure. Also, and in contrast to patients with viral hepatitis, the serum glutamic oxaloacetic acid transaminase concentration is higher than the pyruvate transaminase level. Alkaline phosphatase and amylase levels are occasionally elevated and hyperammonaemia has been recorded (Cano *et al* 1975; Long *et al* 1976). As previously mentioned, a substantial number of patients manifest laboratory evidence of DIC. Serum urate levels may be elevated out of proportion to the degree of renal dysfunction: in fact, hyperuricaemia may precede the clinical presentation (Quigley 1974).

Treatment consists of termination of the pregnancy and supportive therapy for hepatic and renal failure. The efficacy of termination, however, has not been proven. The mortality rate is high with death resulting from hepatic rather than renal failure.

Haemolytic uraemic syndrome (Idiopathic postpartum renal failure)

The patient usually has an uncomplicated pregnancy but 3–6 weeks after delivery she develops severe hypertension and uraemia, often accompanied by microangiopathic haemolytic anaemia and platelet consumption. The pathophysiology is unknown and the controversies about management reflect this uncertainty (Sun *et al* 1975; Segonds *et al* 1979).

It has a poor prognosis despite treatment with dialysis, immunosuppression, heparin, streptokinase, dipyridamole, acetylsalicyclic acid or corticosteroids, alone or combined. Other forms of management have evolved in recent years and have been used with some success. A supposed lack of plasma prostacyclin (PGI_2)—a powerful vasodilator and potent endogenous inhibitor of platelet aggregation—can be counteracted by exchange transfusion or even plasma infusion alone (Remuzzi *et al* 1979). Prolonged PGI_2 infusions have been tried with the aim of restoring the deficiency, thus controlling the hypertension and reversing the platelet consumption (Webster *et al* 1980).

Because DIC may be of pathogenic significance, with placental thromboplastin release during labour, antithrombin III (AT-III) may have a protective effect. AT-III can be given as a concentrate and there have been reports of low plasma AT-III concentrations at the onset of the syndrome (Brandt *et al* 1980). Interestingly, heparin increases the turnover rate of AT-III, and giving heparin to patients with potentially decreased plasma AT-III levels may therefore paradoxically increase an existing risk of thrombosis.

References

Abel R.M., Abbott W.M. & Fischer J.E. (1973) Intravenous essential L-amino acids and hypertonic dextrose in patients with acute renal failure. *American Journal of Surgery* **123**, 695–9.

Ackrill P., Goodwin F.J., Marsh F.P., Stratton D. & Wagman H. (1975) Successful pregnancy in patient on regular dialysis. *British Medical Journal* **2**, 172–4.

Andrioli V.T. (1975) Bacterial Infections. In Burrow G.N. and Ferris T.F. (eds) *Medical Complications During Pregnancy*, pp. 382–95. W.B. Saunders & Company, Philadelphia.

Bailey R.R. & Rolleston G.L. (1971) Kidney length and ureteric dilation in the puerperium. *Journal of Obstetrics and Gynaecology of the British Commonwealth* **78**, 55–61.

Bartlett R.H. & Yahia C. (1969) Management of septic abortion with renal failure: Report of five consecutive cases with five survivors. *New England Journal of Medicine* **281**, 747–50.

Bear R.A. (1976) Pregnancy in patients with renal disease: A study of 44 cases. *Obstetrics and Gynecology* **48**, 13–18.

Blumenkrantz M.J., Gallagher N., Bashore R.A. & Teuckhoff M.D. (1981) Retrograde menstruation in women undergoing chronic peritoneal dialysis. *Obstetrics and Gynecology* **57**, 667–70.

Borgeson B.D. (1982) Continuous ambulatory peritoneal dialysis (CAPD): Some psychosocial observations. *Dialysis and Transplantation* **11**, 54–6.

Brandt P., Jesperson, J. & Gregerson G. (1980) Post-partum haemolytic–uraemic syndrome successfully treated with antithrombin III. *British Medical Journal* **i**, 449.

Brenner B.M., Meyer T.W. & Hostetter T.H. (1982) Dietary protein intake and the progressive nature of kidney disease: The role of hemodynamically mediated glomerular injury in the pathogenesis of progressive glomerular sclerosis in ageing, renal ablation and intrinsic renal disease. *New England Journal of Medicine* **307**, 652–9.

British Medical Journal (Editorial) (1976) Pregnancy after renal transplantation. **i**, 733–4.

British Medical Journal (Editorial) (1982) Effect of transplantation on non-renal effects of renal failure. **284**, 221–2.

Briedahl P., Hurst P.E., Martin J.D. & Vivian A.B. (1972) The post-partum investigation of pregnancy bacteriuria. *Medical Journal of Australia* **2**, 1174–7.

Brumfitt W. (1981) The significance of symptomatic and asymptomatic infection in pregnancy. *Contributions to Nephrology* **25**, 23–9.

Calne R.Y., White D.J.J.G., Thiru S., Evans D.B., Dunn D.C., Henderson R.G., Lewis P., Rolles K., McMaster P., Craddock G.N. & Aziz S. (1979) Cyclosporin A initially as the only immunosuppressant in 34 recipients of cadaveric organs: 32 kidneys, 2 pancreases, and 2 livers. *Lancet* **2**, 1033–6.

Cano R.I., Delman M.R., Pitchumoni C.S., Lev R. & Fosenberg W.S. (1975) Acute fatty liver of pregnancy. Complication of disseminated intravascular coagulation. *Journal of the American Medical Association* **231**, 159–61.

Cavanaugh D. & Singh K.B. (1970) Endotoxin shock in abortion. In Schurmer W. and Nyhus L.M. (eds) *Corticosteroids in the Treatment of Shock*, p. 86. University of Illinois Press.

Chamberlain G.V.P., Lewis P.J., de Swiet M. & Bulpitt C.J. (1978) How obstetricians manage hypertension in pregnancy. *British Medical Journal* **i**, 626–9.

Chesley L.C. (1978) *Hypertension in Pregnancy*. Appleton-Century-Crofts, New York.

Chesley L.C. (1980) Hypertension in pregnancy: Definitions, familial factor and remote prognosis. *Kidney International* **18**, 234–40.

Chesley L.C. & Williams L.O. (1945) Renal glomerular and tubular function in relation to the hyperuricaemia of pre-eclampsia and eclampsia. *American Journal of Obstetrics and Gynecology* **50**, 367–75.

Chng P.K. and Hall M.H. (1982) Antenatal prediction of urinary tract infection in pregnancy. *British Journal of Obstetrics and Gynaecology* **89**, 8–11.

Chugh K.S., Singhal P.C., Shamra B.K., Pal Y., Mathew M.T., Dohall K. & Dotta B.N. (1976) Acute renal failure of obstetric origin. *Obstetrics and Gynecology* **48**, 642–6.

Clark H., Ronald A.R., Cutler R.E. & Turck M. (1969) The correlation between site of infection and maximal concentrating ability in bacteriuria. *Journal of Infectious Diseases* **120**, 47–53.

Coe F.C., Parks J.H. & Lindheimer M.D. (1978) Nephrolithiasis during pregnancy. *New England Journal of Medicine* **298**, 324–6.

Cohen S.N. & Kass E.H. (1967) A simple method for quantitative urine culture. *New England Journal of Medicine* **277**, 176–80.

Condie A.P., Brumfitt W., Reeves D.S. & Williams J.D. (1973) The effects of bacteriuria in pregnancy on fetal health. In Brumfitt W. & Asscher A.W. (eds) *Urinary Tract Infection*, pp. 108–16. Oxford University Press, London.

Confortini P., Galanti G., Ancona G., Giongo A., Bruschi E. & Lorenzini E. (1971) Full term pregnancy and successful delivery in a patient on chronic haemodialysis. In Cameron J.S. (ed) *Proceedings of the European Dialysis and Transplant Association*, pp. 74–8. Pitman Medical Limited, London.

Coulam C.B., Moyer T.P., Jiang M.-S. & Zincke H. (1982) Breast-feeding after renal transplantation. *Transplantation Proceedings* **14**, 605–9.

Coulam, C.B. & Zincke, H. (1981) Successful pregnancy in a renal transplant patient with a 75-year-old kidney. *Surgical Forum* **32**, 457–9.

Coulam, C.B., Zincke, H. & Sterioff, S. (1982a) Relationship between donor age and outcome of pregnancy in a renal allograft population. *Transplantation* **33**, 97–9.

Coulam, C.B., Zincke, H. & Sterioff, S. (1982b) Pregnancy after renal transplantation: estrogen secretion. *Transplantation* **33**, 556–8.

Coyne S.S., Walsh J.W., Tisnado J., Brewer W.H., Sharpe A.R., Amendola M.A., Mendez-Picon G. & Lee H.M. (1981) Surgically correctable renal transplant complications: An integrated clinical and radiologic approach. *American Journal of Radiology* **136**, 1113–19.

Crawford J.S. (1977) Epidural analgesia in pregnancy hypertension. *Clinical Obstetrics and Gynecology* **4**, 735–49.

Davison J.M. (1975) Renal nutrient excretion. *Clinics in Obstetrics and Gynaecology* **2**, 365–480.

Davison J.M. (1978) Changes in renal function in early pregnancy in women with one kidney. *Yale Journal of Biological Medicine* **51**, 347–9.

Davison J.M. & Hytten F.E. (1974) Glomerular filtration during and after pregnancy. *Journal of Obstetrics and Gynaecology of the British Commonwealth* **81**, 588–95.

Davison J.M. & Noble M.C.B. (1981) Serial changes in 24-hour creatinine clearance during normal menstrual cycles and the first trimester of pregnancy. *British Journal of Obstetrics and Gynaecology* **88**, 10–17.

Davison J.M. & Dunlop W. (1980) Renal hemodynamics and tubular function in normal human pregnancy. *Kidney International* **18**, 152–61.

Davison J.M. & Lindheimer M.D. (1982a) Gynaecological and obstetrical problems after renal transplantation. *Nieren und Hochdruckkrankheiten* **11**, 258–65.

Davison J.M. & Lindheimer, M.D. (1982b) Pregnancy in renal transplant recipients. *Journal of Reproductive Medicine* **27**, 613–21.

Davison J.M., Lind T. & Uldall P.R. (1976) Planned pregnancy in a renal transplant recipient. *British Journal of Obstetrics and Gynaecology* **83**, 518–27.

Davison J.M., Dunlop W. & Ezimokhai M. (1980) Twenty-four hour creatinine clearance during the third trimester of normal pregnancy. *British Journal of Obstetrics and Gynaecology* **87**, 106–9.

Dunlop W. (1981) Serial changes in renal haemodynamics during normal human pregnancy. *British Journal of Obstetrics and Gynaecology* **88**, 1–9.

Eaton C.J. & Peterson E.P. (1971) Diagnosis and acute management of patients with advanced clostridial sepsis complicating abortion. *American Journal of Obstetrics and Gynecology* **109**, 1162–5.

Elmstedt E. (1981) Avascular bone necrosis in the renal transplant patient. *Clinical Orthopaedics and Related Research* **158**, 149–57.

Emmanouel D.S. & Katz A.I. (1973) Acute renal failure in obstetric shock. Current views on pathogenesis and management. *American Journal of Obstetrics and Gynecology* **117**, 145–9.

Emmanouel D.S., Lindheimer M.D. & Katz A.I. (1980) Pathogenesis of endocrine abnormalities in uremia. *Endocrine Reviews* **1**, 28–44.

European Multicentre Trial (1982) Cyclosporin A as sole immunosuppressive agent in recipients of kidney allografts from cadaver donors. Preliminary results of a European Multicentre trial. *Lancet* **2**, 57–60.

Evans T.J., McCollum J.P.K. & Valdimasson H. (1975) Congenital cytomegalovirus infection after maternal renal transplantation. *Lancet* **1**, 1359–60.

Faber M., Kennison R.D., Jackson H.T., Sbarra A.J. & Widnere B. (1976) Successful pregnancy after renal transplantation. *Obstetrics and Gynecology* **48**, 2–4.

Fagerholm M.I., Coulam C.B. & Moyer T.P. (1980) Breast feeding after renal transplantation: 6-mercaptopurine content of human breast milk. *Surgical Forum* **31**, 447–9.

Fairley K.F., Bond A.G. & Adey F. (1966) The site of infection in pregnancy bacteriuria. *Lancet* **1**, 939–41.

Fairley K.F., Bond A.G., Brown R.B. & Habasberger P. (1967) Simple test to determine the site of urinary-tract infection. *Lancet* **2**, 427–9.

Fairley K.F., Whitworth J.S. & Kincaid-Smith P. (1973) Glomerulonephritis and pregnancy. In Kincaid-Smith P., Mathew T.H. and Becker E.L. (eds) *Glomerulonephritis* (Part II), pp. 997–1011. Wiley, New York.

Felding C.F. (1969) Obstetric aspects in women with histories of renal disease. *Acta Obstetricia et Gynecologica Scandinavica* **48**, 2–43.

Ferris T.F. (1977) Toxaemia of pregnancy: A model of human hypertension. *Cardiovascular Medicine* **2**, 877–86.

First M.R., Ooi B.S., Wellington J. & Pollak V.E. (1978) Pre-eclampsia with the nephrotic syndrome. *Kidney International* **13**, 166–77.

Fisher K.A., Luger A., Spargo B.H. & Lindheimer M.D. (1980) A biopsy study of hypertension in pregnancy. In Bonnar J., MacGillivray I. and Symonds E.M. (eds) *Pregnancy Hypertension*, pp. 333–8. MTP Press, Lancaster.

Fisher K., Luger A., Spargo B.H. & Lindheimer M.D. (1981) Hypertension in pregnancy: Clinical-pathological correlations and remote prognosis. *Medicine* **60**, 267–74.

Folger G.K. (1955) Pain and pregnancy: Treatment of painful states complicating pregnancy, with particular emphasis on urinary calculi. *Obstetrics and Gynecology* **5**, 513–15.

Gallery E.D.M., Delprado W. & Györy A.Z. (1981) Antihypertensive effect of plasma volume expansion in pregnancy-associated hypertension. *Australian and New Zealand Journal of Medicine* **2**, 20–4.

Gallery E.D.M., Hunyor S.M. & Györy A.Z. (1979) Plasma volume contraction: A significant factor in both pregnancy-associated hypertension (pre-eclampsia) and chronic hypertension in pregnancy. *Quarterly Journal of Medicine* **192**, 573–602.

Gant N.F., Worley R.J., Everett R.B. & MacDonald P.C. (1980) Control of vascular responsiveness during human pregnancy. *Kidney International* **18**, 253–8.

Gerety R.J. & Schweitzer I.L. (1977) Viral hepatitis B during pregnancy, the neonatal period and infancy. *Journal of Paediatrics* **90**, 368–74.

Gilstrap L.C., Cunningham F.G. & Whalley P.J. (1981a) Acute pyelonephritis in pregnancy: an anterospective study. *Obstetrics and Gynecology* **57**, 408–13.

Gilstrap L.C., Leveno K.J., Cunningham F.G., Whalley P.J. & Roark M.L. (1981b) Renal infection and pregnancy outcome. *American Journal of Obstetrics and Gynecology* **141**, 709–16.

Godfrey K.A. (1981) Fetal monitoring in pregnancy and labour. *Practitioner* **225**, 1253–9.

Goldby F.S. & Beilin L.J. (1972) Relationship between arterial pressure and the permeability of arterioles to carbon particles in acute hypertension in the rat. *Cardiovascular Research* **6**, 384–90.

Goldsmith J.H., Menzies D.N., De Boer C.H. & Caplan W. (1971) Delivery of healthy infants after five week's dialysis treatment for fulminating toxaemia of pregnancy. *Lancet* **2**, 738–40.

Gower P.E., Haswell B., Sidaway M.E. & de Wardener H.E. (1968) Follow-up of 164 patients with bacteriuria of pregnancy. *Lancet* **1**, 990–4.

Greiss Jr F.C. (1966) Pressure-flow relationship in the gravid uterine vascular bed. *American Journal of Obstetrics and Gynecology* **96**, 41–8.

Gross A., Fein A., Serr D.M. & Nebel L. (1976) The effect of imuran on implantation and early embryonic development in rats. *Obstetrics and Gynecology* **50**, 713–18.

Grünfeld J.P., Boise E.P. & Hinglais N. (1973) Progressive and non-progressive hereditary chronic nephritis. *Kidney International*, **4**, 216–20.

Grünfeld J.P., Ganeval D. & Bournerias F. (1980) Acute renal failure in pregnancy. *Kidney International* **18**, 179–91.

Guttmann R.D. (1979) Renal transplantation (I and II). *New England Journal of Medicine* **301**, 975–81 and 1038–48.

Hall B.M. (1982) Immunosuppression in renal transplantation. *Medical Journal of Australia* **2**, 415–18.

Hamburger J., Richet G., Crosnier J., Funck-Brentano J.L., Mery J.P. & Moutera H.D. (1968) Acute tubular and interstitial nephritis ('acute tubular necrosis'). *Nephrology*, vol. I, Chap. 16, p. 501. W.B. Saunders Co., Philadelphia.

Hanson G.C. (1978) Shock and infection. In Hanson G.C. and Weight P.L. (eds) *The Medical Management of the Critically Ill*, pp. 367–73. Academic Press, London.

Harris R.E. & Dunnihoo D.R. (1967) The incidence and significance of urinary calculi in pregnancy. *American Journal of Obstetrics and Gynecology* **99**, 237–43.

Hatfield A.K., Stein H., Greenberger N.J., Abernathy R.W. & Ferris T.F. (1972) Idiopathic acute fatty liver of pregnancy. *American Journal of Digestive Diseases* **17**, 167–71.

Hauth J.C., Cunningham F.G. & Whalley P.J. (1976) Management of pregnancy-induced hypertension in the nullipara. *Obstetrics and Gynecology* **48**, 253–9.

Hawkins D.F., Sevitt L.H., Fairbrother P.F. & Tothil A.U. (1975) Management of chemical septic abortion with renal failure: use of a conservative regimen. *New England Journal of Medicine* **292**, 722–5.

Hayslett J.P. & Lynn R.I. (1980) Effect of pregnancy in patients with lupus nephropathy. *Kidney International* **18**, 207–20.

Heineman H.S. & Lee J.H. (1973) Bacteriuria in pregnancy. *Obstetrics and Gynecology* **41**, 22–6.

Hogan W.J. & Price J.W. (1967) Proteinuria as a cause of false positive results in pregnancy tests. *Obstetrics and Gynecology* **29**, 585–9.

Hoover R. & Fraumeni J.R. (1973) Risk of cancer in renal transplant recipients. *Lancet* **2**, 55–7.

Horbach J., van Liebergen F., Mastboom J. & Wijdeveld P. (1973) Pregnancy in a patient after cadaveric renal transplantation. *Acta Medica Scandinavica* **194**, 237–40.

Houser M.T., Fish A.J., Tegatz G.E., Williams P.P. & Michael A.F. (1980) Pregnancy and systemic lupus erythematosus. *American Journal of Obstetrics and Gynecology* **138**, 409–13.

Howie P.W., Prentice C.R.M. & Forbes C.D. (1975) Failure of heparin therapy to affect the clinical course of severe pre-eclampsia. *British Journal of Obstetrics and Gynaecology* **82**, 711–17.

Huffer W.E., Kuzela D. & Popovtzer M.M. (1975) Metabolic bone disease in chronic renal failure. II. Renal transplant patients. *American Journal of Pathology* **78**, 385–98.

Hytten F.E. & Thomson A.M. (1976) Weight gain in pregnancy. In Lindheimer M.D., Katz A.I. and Zuspan F.P. (eds) *Hypertension in Pregnancy*, pp. 179–87. John Wiley & Sons, New York.

Ibels L.S., Alfrey A.C. & Huffer W.E. (1978) Aseptic necrosis of bone following renal transplantation: experience in 194 transplant recipients and review of the literature. *Medicine (Baltimore)* **57**, 25–45.

Janovski N.S., Weimer L.E. & Ober W.B. (1963) Soap intoxication following criminal abortion. *New York Medical Journal* **63**, 1463–5.

Jørgensen K.A. (1981) Acute renal failure: diuretic treatment. *Scandinavian Journal of Urology* (Suppl. 57) 31–35.

Joyce III T.H., Debnath K.S. & Baker E.A. (1979) Pre-eclampsia—relationship of CVP and epidural analgesia. *Anesthesiology* **51**, S297.

Kaplan A.L., Smith J.P. & Tillman A.J.B. (1962) Healed acute and chronic nephritis in pregnancy. *American Journal of Obstetrics and Gynecology* **83**, 1519–25.

Karlan J.R. & Cook W.A. (1970) Renal scleroderma and pregnancy. *Obstetrics and Gynecology* **44**, 349–52.

Kass E.H. (1956) Asymptomatic infections of the urinary tract. *Transactions of the Association of American Physicians* **60**, 56–63.

Katz A.I., Davison J.M., Hayslett J.P., Singson E. & Lindheimer M.D. (1980) Pregnancy in women with kidney disease. *Kidney International* **18**, 192–206.

Katz A.I., Davison J.M., Hayslett J.P. & Lindheimer M.D. (1981) Effect of pregnancy on the natural history of kidney disease. *Contributions to Nephrology* **25**, 53–60.

Kaufmann J.J., Dignam W., Goodwin W.E., Martin D.C., Goldman R. & Maxwell M.H. (1967) Successful normal childbirth after kidney homotransplantation. *Journal of the American Medical Association* **200**, 162–5.

Keller A.J., Irvine W.J., Jordan J.J. & London N.B. (1976) Phytohemagglutin-induced lymphocyte transformation in oral contraceptive users. *Obstetrics and Gynecology* **49**, 83–91.

Kerr D.N.S. & Elliott R.W. (1963) Renal disease in pregnancy. *Practitioner* **190** 459–64.

Kincaid-Smith P., Fairley K.F. & Bullen M. (1967) Kidney disease and pregnancy. *Medical Journal of Australia* **2**, 1155–9.

Kincaid-Smith P., Whitworth J.A. & Fairley K.F. (1980) Mesangial IgA nephropathy in pregnancy. *Clinical and Experimental Hypertension* **2**, 821–38.

Kitzmiller J.L., Brown E.R., Philipe M., Stark M.R., Acker D., Kaldany A. & Hare J.W. (1981) Diabetic nephropathy and perinatal outcome. *American Journal of Obstetrics and Gynecology* **141**, 741–51.

Kleinknecht D., Grünfeld J.P., Gomez P.C., Moreau J.F. & Garcia-Torres R. (1973) Diagnostic procedures and long-term prognosis in bilateral renal cortical necrosis. *Kidney International* **4**, 390–400.

Klockars M., Saarikoski S., Ikonen E. & Kuhlback B. (1980) Pregnancy in patients with renal disease. *Acta Medica Scandinavica* **207**, 207–14.

Kobayashi H., Matsumoto Y., Otsubo O., Otsubo K. & Naito T. (1981) Successful pregnancy in a patient undergoing chronic hemodialysis. *Obstetrics and Gynecology* **57**, 382–6.

Kraus G.W. & Marchese J.R. (1966) Prophylactic use of hydrochlorothiazide in pregnancy. *Journal of the American Medical Association* **198**, 1150–4.

Kuhlback B. & Widholm O. (1966) Plasma creatinine in normal pregnancy. *Scandinavian Journal of Clinical and Laboratory Investigation* **18**, 654–8.

Kunin C.M. (1970) The natural history of recurrent bacteriuria in schoolgirls. *New England Journal of Medicine* **282**, 1443–8.

Lattanzy D.R. & Cook W.A. (1980) Urinary calculi in pregnancy. *Obstetrics and Gynecology* **56**, 462–70.

Lawson D.H. & Miller A.W.F. (1971) Screening for bacteriuria in pregnancy. *Lancet* **i**, 9–11.

Lawson D.H. & Miller A.W.F. (1973) Screening for bacteriuria in pregnancy: a critical reappraisal. *Archives of Internal Medicine* **132**, 925–8.

Leppert P., Tisher C.C., Shu-Chung S.C. & Harlan W.R. (1979) Antecedent renal disease and the outcome of pregnancy. *Annals of Internal Medicine* **90**, 747–51.

Leveno K.J., Harris R.E. Gilstrap L.C., Whalley P.J. & Cunningham F.G. (1981) Bladder versus renal bacteriuria during pregnancy: recurrence after treatment. *American Journal of Obstetrics and Gynecology* **139**, 403–406.

Levy G. (1977) Pharmacokinetics in renal disease. *American Journal of Medicine* **62**, 461–5.

Lewis P.J., Bulpitt C.J. & Zuspan F.P. (1982) A comparison of current British and American practice in the management of hypertension in pregnancy. *American Journal of Obstetrics and Gynecology* **1**, 78–82.

Lewis G.J., Lamont C.A.R., Lee H.A. & Slapak M. (1983) Successful pregnancy in a renal transplant recipient taking Cyclosporin A. *British Medical Journal* **286**, 603.

Lim V.S., Henriquez C., Sievertsen G. & Frohman L.A. (1980) Ovarian function in chronic renal failure: Evidence suggesting hypothalaemic anovulation. *Annals of Internal Medicine* **57**, 7–12.

Lim D.T.Y. & Fairweather D.V.I. (1981) The management of preterm labour. In Elder M.G. and Hendricks C.H. (eds) *Preterm Labour*, pp. 231–58. Butterworths, London.

Lindheimer M.D., Fisher K.A., Spargo B.H. & Katz A.I. (1981) Hypertension in pregnancy: a biopsy study with long term follow-up. *Contributions to Nephrology* **25**, 71–7.

Lindheimer M.D. & Katz A.I. (1977) *Kidney Function and Disease in Pregnancy*. New York, Lea and Febiger.

Lindheimer M.D. & Katz A.I. (1981a) Pathophysiology of pre-eclampsia. *Annual Review of Medicine* **32**, 273–89.

Lindheimer M.D., & Katz A.I. (1981b) The renal response to pregnancy. In Brenner B.M. and Rector F.C. Jr. (eds) *The Kidney*, pp. 1762–1815. W.B. Saunders, Philadelphia.

Lindheimer M.D. & Katz A.I. (1984) Hypertension and pregnancy. In Genest J. *et al* (eds.) *Hypertension: Physiopathology and Treatment*. McGraw-Hill, New York.

Lindheimer M.D., Spargo B.H. & Katz A.I. (1975) Renal biopsy in pregnancy-induced hypertension. *Journal of Reproductive Medicine* **15**, 189–94.

Lindheimer M.D. Katz A.I., Ganeval D. & Grünfeld J.P. (1982) Renal failure in pregnancy. In Brenner B.M., Lazarus J.H. and Myers B.D. (eds) *Acute Renal Failure*. W.B. Saunders, Philadelphia. (in Press).

Long R.G., Scheur P.J. & Sherlock S. (1977) Pre-eclampsia presenting with deep jaundice. *Journal of Clinical Pathology* **30**, 212–16.

Luke R.G., Linton A.L., Briggs J.D. & Kennedy A.C. (1965) Mannitol therapy in acute renal failure. *Lancet* **1**, 980–32.

MacGillivray I., Rose G.A. & Rowe B. (1969) Blood pressure survey in pregnancy. *Clinical Science* **37**, 395–401.

McFadyen I.R., Eykryn S.J., Gardner N.H.N., Vanier T.M., Bennett A.E., Mayo M.E. & Lloyd-Davies R.W. (1973) Bacteriuria of pregnancy. *Journal of Obstetrics and Gynaecology of the British Commonwealth* **80**, 385–405.

MacLean A.B., Abbott G.D., Aickin D.R., Bailey R.R., Bashford D.H. & Little P.J. (1977) Successful pregnancy after renal transplantation. *Australian and New Zealand Journal of Obstetrics and Gynaecology* **17**, 224–8.

MacLean A.B., Sharp F., Briggs J.D. & MacPherson S.G. (1980) Successful triplet pregnancy following renal transplantation. *Scottish Medical Journal* **25**, 320–2.

Maresca L. & Koucky C.J. (1981). Spontaneous rupture of the renal pelvis during pregnancy presenting as acute abdomen. *Obstetrics and Gynecology* **58**, 745–7.

Marwood R.P., Ogg C.S., Coltart T.M. & Klopper A.I. (1977) Plasma oestrogens in a pregnancy associated with chronic haemodialysis. *British Journal of Obstetrics and Gynecology* **84**, 613–17.

Mead P.B. & Gump D.W. (1976) Asymptomatic bacteriuria in pregnancy. In de Alvarez R.R. (ed) *The Kidney*, pp. 45–67. John Wiley & Sons, New York.

Meares E.M. (1978) Urologic surgery during pregnancy. *Clinics in Obstetrics and Gynecology*, **21**, 907–15.

Merkatz I.R., Schwartz G.H., David D.S., Stenzel K.H., Riggio R.R. & Whitsell J.C. (1971) Resumption of female reproductive function following renal transplantation. *Journal of the American Medical Association* **216**, 1749–54.

Mitra S., Vertes V., Roza O. & Berman L.B. (1970) Periodic haemodialysis in pregnancy. *American Journal of Medical Science* **259**, 333–9.

Mulley A.G., Silverstein M.D. & Dienstag J.L. (1982) Indications for use of hepatitis B vaccine, based on cost-effectiveness analysis. *New England Journal of Medicine* **307**, 644–52.

Mundt K.A. & Polk B.F. (1979) Identification of urinary tract infections by antibody-coated bacteria assay. *Lancet* **2**, 1172–5.

Myerowitz R.L., Medeiros A.A. & O'Brien T.F. (1972) Bacterial infection in renal homotransplant recipients: a study of fifty-three bacteremic episodes. *American Journal of Medicine* **53**, 308–14.

Nadler N., Salinas-Madrigal L., Charles A.G. & Pollak V.E. (1969) Acute glomerulonephritis during late pregnancy. *Obstetrics and Gynecology* **34**, 277–80.

Naik R.B., Clark A.D. & Warren D.J. (1979) Acute proliferative glomerulonephritis with crescents and renal failure in pregnancy successfully managed by intermittent haemodialysis. *British Journal of Obstetrics and Gynaecology* **86**, 819–22.

Nolan G.H., Sweet R.L., Laros R.K. & Roure C.A. (1974) Renal cadaver transplantation followed by successful pregnancies. *Obstetrics and Gynecology* **43**, 732–9.

Nolten W.E. & Ehrlich E.N. (1980) Sodium and mineralocorticoids in normal pregnancy. *Kidney International* **18**, 162–72.

Norden C.W. & Kass E.H. (1968) Bacteriuria of pregnancy—a critical reappraisal. *Annual Review of Medicine* **19**, 431–70.

Ober W.E., Reid D.E., Romney S.L. & Merrill J.P. (1956) Renal lesions and acute renal failure in pregnancy. *American Journal of Medicine* **21**, 781–810.

Page E.W. & Christianson R. (1976) The impact of mean arterial pressure in the middle trimester upon the outcome of pregnancy. *American Journal of Obstetrics and Gynecology* **125**, 740–6.

Parsons V., Bewick M., Elias J., Snowden S.A., Weston M.J. & Rodeck C.H. (1979) Pregnancy following renal transplantation. *Journal of the Royal Society of Medicine* **72**, 815–17.

Penn I., Makowski E.L. & Harris P. (1980a) Parenthood following renal transplantation. *Kidney International* **18**, 221–33.

Penn I., Makowski E.L. & Harris P. (1980b) Parenthood following renal and hepatic transplantation. *Transplantation* **30**, 397–400.

Porreco R., Penn I., Droegemneller W., Greer B. & Makowski E.L. (1975) Gynecologic malignancies in immunosuppressed organ homograft recipients. *Obstetrics and Gynecology* **45**, 359–64.

Price H.V., Salaman J.R., Laurence K.M. & Langmaid H. (1976) Immunosuppressive drugs and the fetus. *Transplantation* **21**, 294–8.

Pritchard J.A. (1980) Management of pre-eclampsia and eclampsia. *Kidney International* **18**, 259–66.

Quigley M.M. (1974) Acute obstetric yellow atrophy presenting as idiopathic hyperuricemia. *Southern Medical Journal* **67**, 142–6.

Rabau-Friedman E., Mashiach S., Cantor E. & Jacob E.T. (1982) Association of hypoparathyroidism and successful pregnancy in kidney transplant recipient. *Obstetrics and Gynecology* **59**, 126–8.

Rao V.K., Smith E.J. & Alexander J.W. (1976) Thromboembolic disease in renal allograft recipients. *Archives of Surgery* **111**, 1086–92.

Rasmussen P., Fasth A., Ahlmén J., Brynger H., Iwarson S. & Kjellmer I. (1981) Children of female renal transplant recipients. *Acta Paediatrica Scandinavica* **70**, 869–75.

Ready B.L. & Johnson E.S. (1981) Epidural block for treatment of renal colic during pregnancy. *Canadian Anaesthetists Society Journal* **28**, 77–9.

Recommendations of the Immunization Practices Advisory Committee (1982) Immune globulins for protection against viral hepatitis. *Annals of Internal Medicine* **96**, 193–7.

Redman C.W.G. (1980) Treatment of hypertension in pregnancy. *Kidney International* **18**, 267–78.

Registration Committee of the European Dialysis and Transplant Association (1980) Successful pregnancies in women treated by dialysis and kidney transplantation. *British Journal of Obstetrics and Gynaecology* **87**, 839–45.

Reid D.E., Ryan K.J. & Benirschke K. (1972) Medical and surgical diseases in pregnancy. In *Principles and Management of Human Reproduction*, p. 734. W.B. Saunders Co., Philadelphia.

Reimers T.J. & Sluss P.M. (1978) 6-Mercaptopurine treatment of pregnant mice: Effects on second and third generations. *Science* **201**, 65–7.

Remuzzi G., Misiani R., Marchesi D., Livio M., Mecca G., De Gaetano G. & Donati M.B. (1979) Treatment of hemolytic uremic syndrome with plasma. *Clinical Nephrology* **12**, 279–84.

Renal Transplant Registry Advisory Committee (1977) The 13th report of the human renal transplant registry. *Transplant Proceedings* **9**, 9–26.

Reye R.D.K., Morgan G. & Banal J. (1963) Encephalopathy and fatty degeneration of the viscera. A disease entity in childhood. *Lancet* **2**, 749–52.

Richet G. & Alagille D. (1975) La proteolyse precose au course des anurics hemolytiques du postabortum. *Revue française d'études cliniques et biologiques* **2**, 475–9.

Rifle G. & Traeger J. (1975) Pregnancy after renal transplantation: an international review. *Transplant Proceedings* (Suppl. 1) **7**, 723–8.

Rigenbach M., Renger B., Beavais P., Imbs J.F., Eschbach J. & Frey G. (1978) Grossesse et accouchment d'un enfant vivant diez une patiente traitée par hamodialyse interative. *Journal d'urologie et de néphrologie* **84**, 360–6.

Roberts J. (1976) Hydronephrosis of pregnancy. *Urology* **8**, 1–5.

Roberts A.P., Robinson R.E. & Beard R.W. (1967) Some factors affecting bacterial colony counts in urinary infection. *British Medical Journal* **1**, 400–3.

Robertson E.G. & Cheyne G.A. (1972) Plasma biochemistry in relation to oedema of pregnancy. *Journal of Obstetrics and Gynaecology of the British Commonwealth* **79**, 769–76.

Romagnoli A. & Batra M.S. (1973) Continuous epidural block in the treatment of impacted ureteric stones. *Canadian Medical Association Journal* **109**, 968.

Rosenbaum A.L., Churchill J.A., Shakhasashiri Z.A. & Moody R.L. (1969) Neuropsychologic outcome of children whose mothers had proteinuria during pregnancy. *Obstetrics and Gynecology* **33**, 118–23.

Rosenkrantz J.G, Githens J.H., Cox S.M. & Kellum D.L. (1967) Azathioprine (Imuran) and pregnancy. *American Journal of Obstetrics and Gynecology* **97**, 387–94.

Rubin J., Rogers W.A., Taylor H.M., Everett E.D., Prowant B.F., Fruto L.V. & Nolph K.D. (1980) Peritonitis during continuous ambulatory peritoneal dialysis. *Annals of Internal Medicine* **92**, 7–13.

Rudolph J.E., Shwihizir R.T. & Barius S.A. (1979) Pregnancy in renal transplant patients: A review. *Transplantation* **27**, 26–9.

Saarikoski S. & Seppala M. (1973). Immunosuppression during pregnancy: transmission of azathioprine and its metabolites from mother to the fetus. *American Journal of Obstetrics and Gynecology* **115**, 1100–6.

Salant D.J., Marcus R.G. & Milne F.J. (1976) Pregnancy in renal transplant recipients. *South African Medical Journal* **50**, 1288–92.

Salerno L.J., Stone M.L. & Ditchik P. (1959) A clinical evaluation of chlorothiazide in prevention and treatment of toxaemia of pregnancy. *Obstetrics and Gynecology* **14**, 188–91.

Savage W.E., Hajj S.N. & Kass E.H. (1967) Demographic and prognostic characteristics of bacteriuria in pregnancy. *Medicine* (*Baltimore*) **46**, 385–407.

Savdie E., Caterson R.J., Mahony J.F. & Clifton-Bligh P. (1982) Successful pregnancies in women treated by haemodialysis. *Medical Journal of Australia* **2**, 9.

Schewitz L.J., Friedman E.A. & Pollak V.E. (1965) Bleeding after renal biopsy in pregnancy. *Obstetrics and Gynecology* **26**, 295–304.

Schiffer M. (1966) Fatty liver associated with administration of tetracycline in pregnancy and non-pregnant women. *American Journal of Obstetrics and Gynecology* **96**, 326–32.

Sciarra J.J., Toledo-Pereyra L.H., Bendel R.P. & Simmons R.L. (1975) Pregnancy following renal transplantation. *American Journal of Obstetrics and Gynecology* **123**, 411–25.

Schloss W.A. & Solomkin M. (1952) Acute hydronephrosis of pregnancy. *Journal of Urology* **68**, 885–8.

Scott J.R. (1977) Fetal growth retardation associated with maternal administration of immunosuppressive drugs. *American Journal of Obstetrics and Gynecology* **128**, 668–76.

Scott J.R., Cruikshank D.P. & Corry (1978) Ectopic pregnancy in kidney transplant patients. *Obstetrics and Gynecology* **51**, 565–85.

Scott J.R., Cruikshank D.P., Kochenour N.K., Pitkin R.M. & Warenski J.C. (1980) Fetal platelet counts in the obstetric management of immunologic thrombocytopenic purpura. *American Journal of Obstetrics and Gynecology* **136**, 495–9.

Segonds A., Louradour N., Suc J.M. & Orfila C. (1979) Postpartum hemolytic uremic syndrome: A study of three cases with a review of the literature. *Clinical Nephrology* **12**, 229–42.

Seigler A.M. & Spain D.M. (1965) Polyarteritis nodosa and pregnancy. *Clinical Obstetrics and Gynecology* **8**, 322–9.

Sheehan H.L. (1940) The pathology of acute yellow atrophy and delayed chloroform poisoning. *Journal of Obstetrics and Gynaecology of the British Empire* **47**, 49–56.

Sheehan H.L. (1961) Jaundice in pregnancy. *American Journal of Obstetrics and Gynecology* **81**, 427–33.

Sheriff M.H.R., Hardman M., Lamont C.A.R., Shepherd R. & Warrent D.J. (1978) Successful pregnancy in a 44-year-old haemodialysis patient. *British Journal of Obstetrics and Gynaecology* **85**, 386–9.

Sims E.A.H. (1961) Serial studies of renal function in pregnancy complicated by diabetes mellitus. *Diabetes* **10**, 190–5.

Skinhöj P., Cohn J. & Bradburne A.F. (1976) Transmission of hepatitis type B from healthy HBsAg-positive mothers. *British Medical Journal* **1**, 10–11.

Slavin M.J. (1980) Renal function and hypertension associated with pregnancy. *Journal of the American Obstetric Association* **80**, 258–63.

Smith K., Browne J.C.M. Schackman R. & Wrong O.M. (1965) Acute renal failure of obstetric origin. An analysis of 70 patients. *Lancet* **2**, 351–4.

Smith K., Browne J.C.M., Schackman R. & Wrong O.M. (1968) Renal failure of obstetric origin. *British Medical Bulletin* **24**, 49–64.

Smith L.P., McLean A.P.H. & Maughan G.B. (1971) *Clostridium welchii* Septicotexemia: a review and report of three cases. *American Journal of Obstetrics and Gynecology* **110**, 135–40.

Soffer O. (1980) Sexual dysfunction in chronic renal failure. *Southern Medical Journal* **73**, 1599–601.

Spencer E.S. & Anderson H.K. (1979) Viral infections in renal allograft recipients treated with long-term immunosuppression. *British Medical Journal* **2**, 829–30,

Stamey T.A., Goven D.E. & Palmer J.M. (1965) The localisation and treatment of urinary tract infections: The role of bactericidal levels as opposed to serum levels. *Medicine (Baltimore)* **44**, 1–36.

Steinhausen M., Dallenbach F.D., Dussel R. & Nelinski D. (1981) Pathophysiological mechanisms of acute renal failure. *Contributions to Nephrology* **25**, 151–6.

Strauch B.S. & Hayslett J.P. (1974) Kidney disease and pregnancy. *British Medical Journal* **4**, 378–82.

Strong D.W., Murchison R.J. & Lynch D.F. (1978) The management of ureteral calculi during pregnancy. *Surgery, Gynecology and Obstetrics* **146**, 604–8.

Studd J.W.W. & Blainey J.D. (1969) Pregnancy and the nephrotic syndrome *British Medical Journal* **1**, 276–8.

Studdiford W.E. & Douglas G.W. (1956) Placental bacteriuria: a significant finding in septic abortion accompanied by vascular collapse. *American Journal of Obstetrics and Gynecology* **71**, 842–7.

Sun N.C.J., Johnson W.J., Sung D.T.W. & Woods J.E. (1975) Idiopathic postpartum renal failure:

Review and case report of a successful renal transplantation. *Mayo Clinic Proceedings* **50**, 395–401.

Swapp G.H. (1973) Asymptomatic bacteriuria, birthweight and length of gestation in a defined population. In Brumfitt W. and Asscher A.W. (eds) *Urinary Tract Infection*, pp. 92–102. London, Oxford University Press.

Tatum H.J. (1976) Clinical aspects of intrauterine contraception: circumspection. *Fertility and Sterility* **28**, 3–27.

Tatum H.J. & Mulé J.G. (1956) Puerperal vasomotor in patients with toxemia of pregnancy: a new concept of the etiology and a rational plan of treatment. *American Journal of Obstetrics and Gynecology* **71**, 492–98.

Taylor E.S. (1975) Editorial comments. *Obstetrical and Gynaecological Survey* **30**, 739.

Taylor E.S., McMillan J.H., Greer B.E., Droegemueller W. & Thompson H.E. (1975) The intrauterine device and tubo-ovarian abscess. *American Journal of Obstetrics and Gynecology* **123**, 338–48.

Tenney B. & Dandrow R.V. (1961) Clinical study of hypertensive disease in pregnancy. *American Journal of Obstetrics and Gynecology* **81**, 8–15.

Texter J.H., Bellinger M., Kawamoto E. & Koontz W.E. (1980) Persistent haematuria during pregnancy. *Journal of Urology* **123**, 84–7.

Thomson A.M., Billewicz W.Z. & Hytten F.E. (1968) The assessment of fetal growth. *Journal of Obstetrics and Gynaecology of the British Commonwealth* **75**, 903–16.

Thomson N.M., Rigby R.J., Atkins R.C. & Walters W.A.W. (1978) Successful pregnancy in a patient on recurrent haemodialysis. *Australian Society of Nephrology* **8**, 243.

Tillman A.J.B. (1955) The effect of normal and toxemic pregnancy on blood pressure. *American Journal of Obstetrics and Gynecology* **70**, 589–603.

Trebbin W.M. (1979) Hemodialysis and pregnancy. *Journal of the American Medical Association* **241**, 1811–12.

Turck M. (1975) Localisation of the site of recurrent urinary tract infection in women. *Urology Clinics of North America* **2**, 433–4.

Turck M., Ronald A.R. & Petersdorf R.G. (1968) Relapse and reinfection in chronic bacteriuria. II. The correlation between site of infection and pattern of recurrence in chronic bacteriuria. *New England Journal of Medicine* **278**, 422–7.

Unzelman R.F., Alderfer G.R. & Chojnacki R.E. (1973) Pregnancy and chronic hemodialysis. *Transactions of the American Society of Artificial Internal Organs* **19**, 422–7.

UK Transplant Service Annual Report (1981) 26–36.

Vertel R.M. & Knochel J.P. (1967) Non-oliguric acute renal failure. *Journal of the American Medical Association* **200**, 598–604.

Waltzer W.C. (1981) The urinary tract in pregnancy. *Journal of Urology* **125**, 271–6.

Waltzer W.C., Coulam C.B., Zincke H., Sterioff S. & Frohnert P.P. (1980) Pregnancy in renal transplantation. *Transplant Proceedings* **12**, 221–8.

Warren S.E., Mitas J.A. & Evertson L.R. (1981) Pregnancy after renal transplantation: Reversible acidosis and renal dysfunction. *Southern Medical Journal* **74**, 1139–41.

Weber F.L., Snodgrass P.J., Powell D.E., Rao P., Hoffman S.L. & Brady P.G. (1979) Abnormalities of hepatic mitochrondrial urea-cycle enzyme activities and hepatic ultrastructure in acute fatty liver of pregnancy. *Journal of Laboratory and Clinical Medicine* **94**, 27–41.

Webster J., Rees A.J., Lewis P.J. & Hensby C.N. (1980) Prostacyclin deficiency in haemolytic uraemic syndrome. *British Medical Journal* **281**, 271.

Werkö L. & Bucht H. (1956) Glomerular filtration rate and renal blood flow in patients with chronic diffuse glomerulonephritis during pregnancy. *Acta Medica Scandinavica* **153**, 177–86.

Whalley P.J. (1967) Bacteriuria of pregnancy. *American Journal of Obstetrics and Gynecology* **97**, 723–38.

Whalley P.J., Martin F.G. & Peters P.C. (1965) Significance of asymptomatic bacteriuria detected during pregnancy. *Journal of the American Medical Association* **193**, 879–81.

Whalley P.J., Cunningham, F.G. & Martin F.G. (1975) Transient renal dysfunction associated with acute pyelonephritis of pregnancy. *Obstetrics and Gynecology* **46**, 174–9.

Whetam J.C.G., Cardelle C. & Harding M. (1980) Effect of pregnancy on graft function and graft survival in renal cadaver transplant recipients. *American Journal of Obstetrics and Gynecology* **145**, 193–7.

Williams P.F. & Jelen J. (1979) Eclampsia in a patient who had had a renal transplant. *British Medical Journal* **2**, 972.

Williamson R.A. & Karp L.E. (1981) Azathioprine toxicity: review of the literature and case report. *Obstetrics and Gynecology* **58**, 247–50.

Woods J.R. Jr. & Brinkman III C.R. (1975) The treatment of gestational hypertension. *Journal of Reproductive Medicine* **15**, 195–200.

Systemic Lupus Erythematosus and
     Other Connective Tissue Diseases

Michael de Swiet

Systemic lupus erythematosus

Systemic lupus erythematosus (SLE) is a multi-system disease which most frequently presents in young women. It is therefore relatively common in pregnancy, and it is certainly the connective tissue disease that has been studied most intensively. The apparent prevalence has increased as more mild forms of the disease are recognised. In 1974 Fessel found a prevalence of one in 700 women aged 15 to 64 years. In black women the prevalence was one in 245. The diagnosis may be based on the patient having at least four of the features noted by the American Rheumatism Association, either simultaneously or following each other (Table 8.1).

Since the publication of the American Rheumatism Association Criteria, the measurement of antinuclear factor and of anti-DNA antibodies has largely replaced the LE cell test in the diagnosis of SLE. In pregnancy, proteinuria and thrombocytopenia can lead to confusion with pre-eclampsia. The clinical features of pre-eclampsia, which usually run a much more acute course, remit after delivery, and are not associated with other features summarised in Table 8.1, normally distinguish the two conditions. However, proteinuria may occasionally appear early in pregnancy, the process may not be so acute, and in this situation, measurement of antinuclear factor helps to distinguish SLE from other renal conditions and pre-eclampsia.

The disease runs a fluctuating course. In the advanced forms, with severe nephritis or nervous system involvement, the overall prognosis is bad, but as less severe forms are recognised, the prognosis has improved, so that many centres now report a greater than 95 per cent survival at five years. If treatment is required, the drugs most commonly used are aspirin, prednisone, and antimalarials such as hydroxychloroquine and azathioprine. For other reviews of SLE in pregnancy *see* Boelaert *et al* (1980); Devoe and Taylor (1979); and Scott (1979).

EFFECT OF PREGNANCY ON SLE

As in the case with most illnesses which run a fluctuating course, such as asthma or disseminated sclerosis, it is difficult to document any special effect of pregnancy on SLE.

Table 8.1 Criteria for the diagnosis of SLE as suggested by the American Rheumatism Association (Tan *et al* 1982). To substantiate the diagnosis, the patient should have at least four features, either simultaneously, or following each other.

---

1. Facial butterfly rash
2. Discoid lupus
3. Photosensitivity—skin rash as a result of unusual reaction to sunlight
4. Oral or nasopharyngeal ulceration
5. Nonerosive arthritis involving two or more peripheral joints
6. Pleurisy or pericarditis
7. Proteinuria >0.5 g/day or cellular casts
8. Psychosis or convulsions
9. One of: (a) haemolytic anaemia; (b) leucopenia, wcb <4000 mm^{-3} on two or more occasions; (c) lymphopenia <1500 mm^{-3} on two or more occasions; (d) thrombocytopenia 100 000 mm^{-3}
10. Immunological disorder: (a) positive LE cell preparation; (b) antibody to native DNA in abnormal titre, (c) antibody to SM nuclear antigen; (d) chronic false-positive syphillis serology for six months
11. Antinuclear antibody in abnormal titre

The general consesus is that pregnancy does not affect the long-term prognosis of SLE (Garsenstein *et al* 1962), but that pregnancy itself may be associated with more 'flare ups', particularly in the puerperium (Mund *et al* 1963; Fraga *et al* 1974). Since patients are usually observed more closely in pregnancy this is not surprising. Also, patients with SLE are normally advised against conceiving during an active phase of the disease and therefore conceive when they are well (Estes and Larson 1965). If the effect of pregnancy is judged by a comparison of the state of pregnancy with that before conception (*see* for example Zulman *et al* 1980), their condition can only either stay unchanged if they were well before pregnancy or can deteriorate; this is a further cause of bias. However, in a comparison with the prepregnancy period, Garsenstein *et al* (1962) found that the exacerbation rate was three times greater in the first half of pregnancy, one and one-half times greater in the second half, and at least six times greater in the puerperium—the time when the majority of maternal deaths occur (Zulman *et al* 1980). These deaths have been due to pulmonary haemorrhage (Spiera 1980) or lupus pneumonitis (Lulman *et al* 1980; Ainslie *et al* 1979).

It is interesting that successive pregnancies do not necessarily affect an individual in the same way (Estes and Larson 1965). Chorea gravidarium is a rare complication of SLE in pregnancy (Lubbe and Walker 1983; Donaldson and Espiner 1971).

The relationship of pregnancy to renal disease caused by SLE is also considered in Chapter 7.

EFFECT OF SLE ON PREGNANCY

There are three main ways in which SLE affects pregnancy and its outcome. SLE increases the risk of abortion, increases the risks of late pregnancy losses due to hypertension and renal failure, and is an important cause of heart block and other cardiac defects in the newborn. This latter effect may be part of a more general neonatal lupus syndrome.

Abortion

The incidence of abortion in patients with SLE may be as high as 40 per cent (Fraga *et al* 1974). On reviewing previous pregnancies, even those occurring before the onset of SLE, Fraga *et al* (1974) found that the incidence of abortion was 23 per cent—about twice as high as in a group of control patients. Chesley (1978) also analysed the outcome of 630 pregnancies in mothers with SLE and found that there was a 36 per cent failure rate.

The risk of abortion is not clearly related to the severity of the condition. In SLE, abortion often occurs later than the usual 12–14 weeks' gestation and, indeed, may occur at any gestation up to 28 weeks. SLE should always be considered as an important, though rare, cause of recurrent late abortion. Many of these cases have serological evidence of SLE with no other clinical manifestations. The risk of abortion is not shared by other connective tissue diseases such as rheumatoid arthritis (Kaplan and Diamond 1965) or scleroderma (Johnson *et al* 1964). Baesnihan *et al* (1977) showed a high titre of lymphocytotoxic antibodies in 3 of 4 patients with SLE, whose pregnancies ended in abortion. These antibodies can be absorbed by trophoblast which indicates a number of possible mechanisms for the cause of abortion in SLE (Baesnihan *et al* 1977). For example, Abramowsky *et al* (1980) have described necrotising decidual vascular lesions with immunoglobulin deposition in placentas of women whose pregnancies were complicated by SLE.

An alternative approach has been to examine the relationship between the lupus inhibitor and recurrent abortion. Between five and ten per cent of patients with SLE develop an inhibitor of the coagulation pathway which causes prolongation of the partial thromboplastin or prothrombin times (Schlieder *et al* 1976). Firkin *et al* (1980) found the lupus inhibitor in four women with recurrent abortion, only one of whom had established SLE, as judged by antinuclear factor antibodies. Carreras *et al* (1981) suggested that the lupus inhibitor or related antibodies might damage the fetoplacental unit by interfering with prostacyclin release.

Other causes of fetal wastage

As indicated above, patients with trivial SLE, or even no clinical evidence of SLE, have a much higher risk of abortion. The other group of patients at risk of fetal morbidity are those with renal involvement who may also have hypertension. For example, Houser *et al* (1980) studied 18 pregnancies in patients with SLE. Ten occurred in patients with no evidence of renal disease and were uncomplicated. The remaining eight occurred in patients with renal disease. There were four abortions (one elective), three premature deliveries, and only one normal term delivery. It is difficult to be precise as to what level of renal impairment is significant, but a creatinine clearance of less than 65 ml/min/m^3 or proteinuria greater than 2.4 g/24 hours would be ominous (*see* Chapter 7).

The neonatal lupus syndrome

This includes haematological complications, cardiac abnormalities, babies in whom skin lesions are present (Lockshin *et al* 1983) or the only abnormalities, and neonates who develop SLE in the absence of any involvement in the mother (Hardy *et al* 1979). Maternal antibodies have been shown to cross the placenta (Hardy *et al* 1979), and it is likely that SLE is one of the conditions—such as rhesus disease, Graves' disease or myasthenia gravis—where transplacental passage of antibodies harms the fetus. However, in SLE, the precise antibody which affects the fetus has not been identified, and the fetal outcome cannot be correlated with fetal (or maternal) antibody levels. The haematological abnormalities are haemolytic anaemia, leucopenia and thrombocytopenia. They are usually transient and not a major problem (Nathan and Snapper 1958).

The cardiac abnormalities have been best defined by McCue (1977) and Scott (Esscher and Scott 1979). By far the most common abnormality is complete heart block which may be present and detected antenatally (Altenburger *et al* 1977). Although the majority of infants born to mothers with SLE are normal, about one in three mothers (38 per cent) who deliver babies with congenital heart block have, or will have, a connective tissue disease (Esscher and Scott 1979). Most frequently, the disease is SLE, but in 16 per cent of cases the mother had rheumatoid arthritis, and 25 per cent had a less well-defined form of connective tissue disease.

About 60 per cent of mothers who deliver a child with congenital heart block have anti-R_0 antibodies. In one series, these autoantibodies were invariably present in the mothers with SLE that delivered an affected child but they were also present in some of those asymptomatic women who had a child with congenital heart block (Maddison *et al* 1983). There is therefore strong circumstantial evidence to implicate the anti-R_0 system in the pathogenesis of congenital heart block.

The baby usually survives the perinatal period, and often does not require pacing. Fatal cases may be associated with endomyocardial fibrosis (Esscher and Scott 1979) or pericarditis (Doshi *et al* 1980).

Meuiston and Schoch (1954) first described discoid skin lesions in a neonate whose mother subsequently developed SLE. The lesions are usually on the face or the scalp and are present at birth. They have normally disappeared by one year of life, and only rarely are associated with other organ involvement (Vonderheid *et al* 1976).

MANAGEMENT OF SLE IN PREGNANCY

It was originally hoped that the use of corticosteroids would decrease the high abortion rate associated with SLE. In general, this has not been the case (Fraga *et al* 1974). However, occasional successes after habitual abortion have been reported with prednisone alone (Hartkainen-Sorri and Kaila 1980), prednisone and aspirin (Lubbe and Walker 1983) or plasmapheresis (Hubbard and Portnoy 1979).

Minor manifestations of SLE can be treated with paracetamol. Acetylsalicyclic acid has been found to cause abnormalities of platelet function in mothers and their babies which can lead to significant bleeding in both if taken within five days of delivery, and in mothers if taken in the puerperium (Stuart *et al* 1982). High doses of aspirin taken in the last six months of pregnancy have been associated with a higher incidence of postmaturity, prolonged labour and excessive antepartum and postpartum haemorrhage (Collins and Turner 1975), as noted above. In addition, aspirin is a prostaglandin synthetase inhibitor and may cause premature closure of the ductus arteriosus (*see* p. 265).

The mainstay of maternal management is glucocorticoid therapy. As in the nonpregnant state, the smallest dose of steroids that will control the condition should be used. Since the ESR is elevated in normal pregnancy, reduction of C_3 complement can be used as an objective index of disease activity (Zurier *et al* 1978). There is no evidence that corticosteroids, given in the usual clinical dosage, harm the fetus (Chapter 1). Parenteral steroid cover should be given in labour. Our practice is to use hydrocortisone 100 mg i.m. 6-hourly, until the patient is taking oral medication. Because of the risk of dangerous exacerbation of SLE in the puerperium, steroid dosage should only be reduced with great care after delivery. The possible use of azathioprine in pregnancy is considered in Chapter 7.

The timing of delivery in patients with SLE depends on the severity of the condition and whether the patients have renal involvement or hypertension. If there are none of these complications, the patient should be delivered at term. Increasing degrees of renal failure or hypertension will necessitate early delivery, either for these reasons alone or because of evidence of fetal compromise, as judged by poor growth, falling oestriol levels in plasma or urine, or cardiotocography. With the advent of cardiotocography and widespread use of ultrasound to measure fetal growth, there is less emphasis on oestriol levels. These can also be depressed purely by corticosteroid therapy, although usually only in dosages greater than 75 mg of cortisol per day (Oakey 1970).

If the fetus has congenital heart block which is discovered before delivery, it is probably best delivered by Caesarean section. This is because of the difficulty of diagnosing fetal distress when the fetal heart rate is not under autonomic control; also, although most fetuses do not suffer haemodynamic problems from complete heart block, some do, and may not be able to withstand the stress of labour.

Clotting defects are usually not a problem at delivery of patients with SLE, but it is reassuring to perform a clotting screen at the onset of labour and be prepared to treat any major abnormalities.

Rheumatoid arthritis

The finding by Hench (1938) that rheumatoid arthritis improved in 24 of 30 pregnancies, coupled with a belief that cortisol levels were markedly elevated in pregnancy, was so important that it led to the successful use of steroids in patients with rheumatoid arthritis who were not pregnant. These observations have been confirmed by Kaplan and Diamond (1965), and difficulties in the management of rheumatoid arthritis are rare in pregnancy, although exacerbations may occur in the puerperium. Unger *et al* (1983) have correlated the improvement in rheumatoid arthritis with the level of pregnancy-associated α_2-glycoprotein which has immunosuppressive actions. However, pregnancy induces many other changes in the immune system and therefore there may be other reasons why rheumatoid arthritis improves.

In contrast to SLE there is no increased risk of abortion in patients with rheumatoid arthritis (Kaplan and Diamond 1965).

As indicated above, there is a small risk of congenital heart block in the newborn. The other potential problems are in abduction of the hip during vaginal delivery, or extension of the neck and opening of the mouth for intubation in general anaesthesia.

The most common difficulty concerns drug administration. As indicated above, the dangers of steroid therapy have been exaggerated, and paracetamol is a better analgesic for use in pregnancy than aspirin.

Indomethacin and other prostaglandin antagonists are quite extensively used for the treatment of rheumatoid arthritis in nonpregnant patients. However, there are many reports of primary pulmonary hypertension of the newborn associated with the use of indomethacin for the treatment of premature labour (*Lancet* 1980). It is postulated that the pulmonary hypertension is due to premature closure of the ductus arteriosus caused by inhibition of prostaglandin synthetase. In addition, there are case reports of convulsions in a breast-fed infant, after the mother had taken indomethacin for analgesia (Eeg-Olofsson 1978; Fairhead 1978). For these reasons indomethacin should not be used in pregnancy, or in women who are breast feeding.

There is little experience with the use of phenylbutazone in pregnancy. In nonpregnant patients, phenylbutazone can cause sodium retention and bone marrow dyscrasias. It is not known whether these and other abnormalities occur in the fetus exposed to phenylbutazone before delivery. The situation is similar concerning gold therapy. In the adult, gold causes blood dyscrasias, drug rashes and nethropathy. However, gold is very strongly protein-bound and little appears to cross the placenta (Rocker and Henderson 1976).

Antimalarial drugs such as chloroquine are used in the treatment of rheumatoid arthritis. Chloroquine has been reported to cause chromosome damage, but there is no evidence that this results in stable chromosome abnormalities which might be of genetic or neoplastic significance (Gifford 1975). A greater worry is that chloroquine may cause retinopathy in the neonate because it is concentrated in the fetal uveal tract (Ullberg *et al* 1970). Congenital deafness has also been reported (Hart and Naunton 1964). Antimalarial drugs should therefore not be used in the treatment of rheumatoid arthritis in pregnancy, particularly since alternative treatments exist. Nevertheless, the risks of their use have probably been exaggerated. Because there is no alternative women must, and do, take antimalarial drugs for the treatment or prophylaxis of malaria in pregnancy (Lewis *et al* 1973) (*see* p. 294); a high incidence of fetal damage associated with malaria has not been reported.

Immunosuppressive drugs are occasionally used in the treatment of rheumatoid arthritis. Azathioprine is the drug that has been used most frequently and it appears to be relatively safe, although it has still not been extensively tried (Chapter 7). Penicillamine is also used in the treatment of rheumatoid arthritis. There are occasional reports of suspected teratogenesis (Solomon *et al* 1977) and neonatal abnormalities of connective tissue, which may be irreversible (Mjølnerød *et al* 1971) or reversible (Linares *et al* 1979). However, there are two series (totalling 56 pregnancies) in which the only abnormality (which could have occurred by chance) was one child with a small ventricular septal defect (Scheinberg and Sternlieb 1975; Lyle 1978). It would therefore seem that penicillamine is reasonably safe in pregnancy (*see* p. 318).

In summary, if a patient with rheumatoid arthritis requires treatment in pregnancy, she should be given paracetamol. If this does not give adequate relief, corticosteroids should be used. Penicillamine treatment also appears to be safe.

Scleroderma and other connective tissue diseases

Scleroderma is a connective tissue disease affecting skin, gastrointestinal tract (oesophagus) kidneys and lungs. There have been four series of 87 patients (Leinwald *et al* 1954; Johnson *et al* 1964; Slate *et al* 1968; Haynes 1969) and several case reports (*see* Karlen and Cook 1974), describing the interaction of scleroderma and pregnancy. As in SLE, pregnancy does not seem to influence the course of scleroderma unless there is already renal involvement, or unless renal involvement and/or pre-eclamptic toxaemia develops during pregnancy. Under these circumstances, the maternal prognosis is bad and consideration should be given to termination of pregnancy if the renal function is deteriorating (Karlen and Cook 1974). The fetal outcome is also impaired. In a review of 17 pregnancies reported in the literature, Karlen and Cook (1974) documented five perinatal deaths, and five instances of premature delivery. The one patient that we have managed at Queen Charlotte's Maternity Hospital with scleroderma had a growth-retarded infant in each of two pregnancies. She did not have renal involvement but did have a severe reduction of pulmonary transfer factor.

Other connective tissue diseases which rarely complicate pregnancy are polyarteritis nodosa (Debeukelaer *et al* 1973), dermatomyositis (Spiera 1980) and Wegner's granulomatosis (Cooper *et al* 1970).

References

Abramowsky C.R., Vegas M.E., Swinehart G. & Gyves M.T. (1980) Decidual vasculopathy of the placenta in lupus erythematosus. *New England Journal of Medicine* **303**, 668–72.

Ainslie W.H., Britt K. & Moshipur J.A. (1979) Maternal death due to lupus pneumonitis in pregnancy. *The Mount Sinai Journal of Medicine* **46**, 494–9.

Altenburger K.M., Jedziniak M., Roper W.L. & Hernandez J. (1977) Congenital complete heart block with hydrops fetalis. *Journal of Pediatrics* **91**, 618–20.

Baesnihan B., Grigor R.R., Oliver M., Lewkonia R.M., Hughes G.R.V., Lovins R.E. & Faulk W.P. (1977) Immunological mechanism for spontaneous abortion in systemic lupus erythematosus. *Lancet* **2**, 1205–7.

Boelaert J., Ryckaert R., Tser Kezoglou A. & Daneels R. (1980) Systemic lupus erythematosus and pregnancy. *Acta Clinica Belgica* **35**, 183–92.

Carreras L.O., Defreyn G., Machin S.J., Vermylen J., Deman R., Spitz B. & Van Assch A. (1981) Arterial thrombosis, intrauterine death and 'lupus' anticoagulant: detection of immunoglobulin interfering with prostacyclin formation. *Lancet* **1**, 244-6.

Chesley L.C. (1978) *Hypertensive Disorders in Pregnancy*, p. 504. Appleton-Century-Crofts, New York.

Cohen A.S. & Canoso J.J. (1972) Criteria for the classification of systemic lupus erythematosus—status. *Arthritis and Rheumatism* **15**, 540–3.

Collins E. & Turner G. (1975) Maternal effects of regular salicylate ingestion in pregnancy. *Lancet* **2**, 335–8.

Cooper K., Stafford J. & Turner Warwick M. (1970) Wegner's granulomatosis complicating pregnancy. *Journal of Obstetrics and Gynaecology of the British Commonwealth* **77**, 1028–30.

Debeukelaer M.M., Travis L.B. & Roberts D.K. (1973) Polyarteritis and pregnancy: report of a successful outcome. *Southern Medical Journal* **66**, 613–15.

Devoe L.D. & Taylor R.L. (1979) Systemic lupus erythematosus in pregnancy. *American Journal of Obstetrics and Gynecology* **135**, 473–9.

Donaldson I.M. & Espiner E.A. (1971) Disseminated lupus erythematosus presenting as chorea gravidarum. *Archives of Neurology* **25**, 240–4.

Doshi N., Smith B. & Klionsky B. (1980) Congenital pericarditis due to maternal lupus erythematosus. *Journal of Pediatrics* **96**, 699–701.

Eeg-Olofsson O., Malmros I., Elwin C. & Steen B. (1978) Convulsions in a breast-fed infant after maternal indomethacin. *Lancet* **2**, 215.

Esscher E. & Scott J.S. (1979) Congenital heart block and maternal systemic lupus erythematosus. *British Medical Journal* **1**, 1235–8.

Estes D. & Larson D.L. (1965) Systemic lupus erythematosus and pregnancy. *Clinical Obstetrics and Gynecology* **8**, 307–21.

Fessel W.J. (1974) Systemic lupus erythematosus in the Community. Incidence, prevalence, outcome and first symptoms; the high prevalence in black women. *Archives of Internal Medicine* **134**, 1027–35.

Fraga A., Mintz G., Orozco J. & Orozco J.H. (1974) Sterility and fertility rates, fetal wastage and maternal morbidity in systemic lupus erythematosus. *Journal of Rheumatology* **1**, 1293–8.

Fairhead F.W. (1978) Convulsions in a breast-fed infant after maternal administration. *Lancet* **2**, 576.

Firkin B.G., Howard M.A. & Radford N. (1980) Possible relationship between lupus inhibitor and recurrent abortion in young women. *Lancet* **2**, 366.

Garsenstein M., Pollak V.E. & Karik R.M. (1962) Systemic lupus erythematosus and pregnancy. *New England Journal of Medicine* **267**, 165–9.

Gifford R.H. (1975) Rheumatic diseases. In Burrow G.N. and Ferris T.F. (eds) *Medical Complications During Pregnancy*, W. B. Saunders Co., Philadelphia.

Hardy J.D., Solomon S., Banwell G.S., Beach R., Wright V. & Howard F.M. (1979) Congenital complete heart block in the newborn associated with maternal systemic lupus erythematosus and other connective tissue disease. *Archives of Disease of Childhood* **54**, 7–13.

Hart C.W. & Naunton R.F. (1964) The ototoxicity of chloroquine phosphate. *Archives of Otolaryngology* **80**, 407.

Hartikainen-Sorri A. & Kaila J. (1980) Systemic lupus erythematosus and habitual abortion. *British Journal of Obstetrics and Gynaecology* **87**, 729–31.

Haynes D.M. (1969) Collagen diseases in pregnancy. In Haynes D.M. (ed.) *Medical Complications during Pregnancy*. McGraw Hill, New York.

Hench A.B. (1938) The ameliorating effect of pregnancy on chronic atrophic (infectious rheumatoid) arthritis; fibrositis and intermittent hydrothosis. *Proceedings of the Mayo Clinic 1938* **13**, 161.

Heymann M.A., Rudolph A.M. & Silverman N.H. (1976) Closure of the ductus arteriosus in premature infants by inhibition of prostaglandin synthesis. *New England Journal of Medicine* **295**, 530–4.

Houser M.T., Fish A.J., Tagatz G.E., Williams P.P. & Michael A.F. (1980) Pregnancy and systemic lupus erythematosus. *American Journal of Obstetrics and Gynecology* **138**, 409–13.

Hubbard H.C. & Portnoy B. (1979) Systemic lupus erythematosus in pregnancy treated with plasmapheresis. *British Journal of Obstetrics and Gynaecology* **101**, 87–9.

Johnson T.R., Banner E.A. & Winkelmann R.K. (1964) Scleroderma and pregnancy. *Obstetrics and Gynecology* **23**, 467–9.

Kaplan D. & Diamond H. (1965) Rheumatoid arthritis and pregnancy. *Clinical Obstetrics and Gynecology* **8**, 286–303.

Karlen J.G. & Cook W.A. (1974) Renal scleroderma and pregnancy. *Obstetrics and Gynecology* **44**, 349–54.

Lancet (Editorial) (1980) PG-synthetase inhibition in obstetrics and after. *Lancet* **2**, 185–6.

Leinwald I. & Durgee A.W. (1954) Scleroderma. *Annals of Internal Medicine* **41**, 1033–41.

Lewis R., Lauersen N.H. & Birnbaum S. (1973) Malaria associated with pregnancy. *Obstetrics and Gynecology* **42**, 696–700.

Linares A., Zarranz J.J., Rodriguez-Alarcon J. & Diaz-Perez J.L. (1979) Reversible cutis taxa due to maternal d-penicillamine treatment. *Lancet* **2**, 43.

Lockshin M.D., Gibofsky A., Peebles C.L., Gigli I., Fotino M. & Hurwitz S. (1983) Neonatal lupus erythematosus with heart block: family study of a patient with anti-SS-A and SS-B antibodies. *Arthritis and Rheumatism* **26**, 210–13.

Lubbe W.F., Buttler W.S., Palmer S.J. & Liggins G.C. (1983) Fetal survival after prednisone suppression of maternal lupus anticoagulant. *Lancet* **1**, 1361–3.

Lubbe W.F. & Walker E.B. (1983) Chorea gravidarum associated with lupus anticoagulant: successful outcome of pregnancy with prednisone and aspirin therapy. Case report. *British Journal of Obstetrics and Gynaecology* **90**, 487–90.

Lyle W.H. (1978) Penicillamine in pregnancy. *Lancet* **1**, 606–7.

McCue C.M., Matakas M.E., Tinglestad J.B. & Ruddy S. (1977) Congenital heart block in newborns of mothers with connective tissue disease. *Circulation* **56**, 82–90.

McCuiston C.H. & Schoch E.P. (1954) Possible discoid lupus erythematosus in a new born infant; report of case with subsequent development of acute systemic lupus erythematosus in mother. *Archives of Dermatology and Syphilology* **70**, 782–5.

Maddison P.J., Skinner R.P., Esscher E., Taylor P.V., Scott O. & Scott J.S. (1983) Serological studies in congenital heart block. *Annals of the Rheumatic Diseases* **42**, 218–19.

Meurman O., Terho P. & Salmi A. (1978) Actuation of rheumatoid factor during pregnancy. *Lancet* **2**, 685–6.

Mjølnerød I.K., Rasmussen K., Dommerud S.A. & Gjeruldsen S.T. (1971) Congenital connective-tissue defect probably due to d-penicillamine treatment in pregnancy. *Lancet* **1**, 673–5.

Mund A., Simson J. & Rothfield N. (1963) Effect of pregnancy on course of systemic lupus erythematosus. *Journal of the American Medical Association* **183**, 917–20.

Nathan D.J. & Snapper I. (1958) Simultaneous placental transfer of factors responsible for LE cell formation and thrombocytopenia. *American Journal of Medicine* **25**, 647.

Oakey R.E. (1970) The interpretation of urinary oestrogen and pregnanediol excretion in women receiving corticosteroids. *Journal of Obstetrics and Gynaecology of the British Commonwealth* **77**, 922–7.

Rocker I. & Henderson W.J. (1976) Transfer of gold from mother to fetus. *Lancet* **2**, 1246.

Scheinberg I.H. & Sternlieb I. (1975) Pregnancy in penicillamine-treated patients with Wilson's disease. *New England Journal of Medicine* **293**, 1300–2.

Schlieder M.A., Nachman R.L., Jaffe E.A. & Coleman M. (1976) A clinical study of the lupus anticoagulant. *Blood* **48**, 499–509.

Scott J.S. (1979) Systemic lupus erythematosus and allied disorders in pregnancy. *Clinics in Obstetrics and Gynecology* **6**, 461–71.

Solomon L., Abrams G., Dinner M. & Berman L. (1977) Neonatal abnormalities associated with D-penicillamine treatment during pregnancy. *New England Journal of Medicine* **296**, 54–5.

Spiera H. (1980) Connective tissue disease in pregnancy. *The Mount Sinai Journal of Medicine* **47**, 438–41.

Slate W.G. & Graham A.R. (1968) Scleroderma and pregnancy. *American Journal of Obstetrics and Gynecology* **101**, 335–41.

Stuart M.J., Gross S.J., Ellad H. & Graeber J.E. (1982) Effects of acetylsalicyclic-acid ingestion on maternal and neonatal hemostasis. *New England Journal of Medicine* **307**, 909–12.

Tan E.M., Cohan A.S., Aries J.F., Masi A.T., McShane D.J., Rothfield N.F., Schaller J.G., Talal N. & Winchester R.J. (1982) The 1982 revised criteria for the classification of systemic lupus erythematosus. *Arthritis and Rheumatism* **25**, 1271–7.

Ullberg S., Lindquist N.G. & Sjostrand S.E. (1970) Accumulation of retinotoxic drugs in the foetal eye. *Nature* **227**, 1257.

Unger A., Kay A., Griffin A.J. & Panayi G.S. (1983) Disease activity and pregnancy-associated α_2-glycoprotein in rheumatoid arthritis during pregnancy. *British Medical Journal* **286**, 750–2.

Vonderheid E.C., Koblenzer P.J., Ming P., Ming L. & Burgoon C.F. (1976) Neonatal lupus erythematosus, report of four cases with a review of the literature. *Archives of Dermatology* **112**, 698–705.

Zuckerman H., Reis U. & Rubinstein I. (1974) Inhibition of human premature labour by indomethacin *Obstetrics and Gynecology* **44**, 787–92.

Zulman J.I., Talal N., Hoffman G.S. & Epstein W.V. (1980) Problems associated with the management of pregnancies in patients with systemic lupus erythematosus. *The Journal of Rrheumatology* **7**, 37–49.

Zurier R.B., Argyros T.G., Urman J.D., Warren J. & Rothfield N.F. (1978) Systemic lupus erythematosus. Management during pregnancy. *Obstetrics and Gynecology* **51**, 178–80.

9 Disorders of Gastrointestinal Tract, Pancreas and Hepato-biliary System

Elizabeth A. Fagan & Vinton S. Chadwick

INVESTIGATIVE PROBLEMS IN PREGNANCY

The gastroenterologist is naturally reluctant to expose the pregnant woman to X-rays, for example during an investigation of symptoms of abdominal pain, diarrhoea or jaundice. On the other hand it is mandatory to avoid unnecessary delay in diagnosis, especially for problems which may require surgical intervention. In the case of the acute abdomen in pregnancy, erect and supine X-rays of the abdomen and a chest X-ray would be ordered without hesitation, whereas in a patient with less acute upper abdominal pain or diarrhoea, flexible fibreoptic gastroscopy or sigmoidoscopy would be preferred to conventional barium studies.

The advent of ultrasonography has revolutionised the investigation of cholestatic jaundice; finding non-dilated intrahepatic bile ducts makes extrahepatic obstruction unlikely, and suggests liver biopsy as the next appropriate investigation. In contrast, dilated intrahepatic ducts would be a clear indication for conventional cholangiography to delineate the site of obstruction. Ultrasound may show gallstones, tumours or cysts in the liver, pancreas and other sites, and abscess cavities. This powerful and safe technique is often the first line investigation in pregnancy for these reasons. For example, if a pregnant patient presented with a hepatic mass, ultrasound could distinguish a cystic lesion (leading to a hydatid complement fixation test and a conservative approach) from a solid lesion (arteriography and appropriate biopsy procedure). In this way, the potential hazards of X-rays are reserved for those patients for whom radiology is essential. Similarly, flexible sigmoidoscopy and biopsy procedures may confirm inflammatory bowel disease in a pregnant patient without resort to radiology, and permit institution of rational therapy. With this approach, the gastroenterologist is far from diagnostically destitute; routine blood, urine and stool tests complete the spectrum of available diagnostic procedures.

It may, under certain circumstances, be necessary to expose pregnant patients to X-rays. It has been estimated that exposure of up to 2 rads is without apparent harmful effects to the developing fetus. This exposure would permit most conventional X-ray procedures with a very wide margin for safety; of course the minimum number of films should be taken and every available measure adopted to screen the fetus.

MANAGEMENT PROBLEMS IN PREGNANCY

Self-medication for gastroenterological disorders is widespread, and an individual patient may be taking proprietary antacids, anti-emetics, laxatives or antidiarrhoeal medicines before she realises she is pregnant, or because she is unaware that warnings about drug ingestion in pregnancy apply to these readily available agents. Most practitioners are reluctant to prescribe drugs for pregnant patients, but persistent and severe nausea, vomiting or constipation may require medication and the safest agent should then be selected. If patients with pre-existing diseases such as inflammatory bowel disease or chronic active hepatitis are already taking drugs, the decision to continue, modify or discontinue therapy depends on the relative risks to fetus and to the mother, should she suffer a relapse. Suggestions for therapy included in this chapter are given on the understanding that many drugs have not been subjected to extensive clinical trials in pregnancy. In general, drugs should not be used for self-limiting disorders of short duration and only prescribed with some reluctance for other conditions when there is no reasonable alternative, and then only exceptionally in the first trimester.

DIETARY HABITS IN PREGNANCY

Changes in dietary selection are common in pregnancy. Aversion to coffee, alcohol, cigarettes, fried foods, poultry and oregano are common, and are related to exacerbations of nausea, vomiting or gastro-oesophageal reflux. Dietary cravings are also common but their mechanisms are not understood. In a survey of dietary preference in 1000 women, Taggart (1961) found that 50 per cent reported an increase in appetite with particular preference for dairy produce, vegetables, fruit and cereals. Pica is also common, and women admit to cravings for clay, chalk, starch, coal, soap, toothpaste and disinfectants (Harries and Hughes 1957).

Disorders of the oral cavity

Benign disorders of the mouth, gingiva and teeth are common in the general population, and disorders of the gingiva are particularly prevalent in pregnancy.

APHTHOUS STOMATITIS

Benign aphthous stomatitis ulceration may occur in up to 20 per cent of the population and, although often idiopathic, occurs more frequently in women than men and in particular around the time of the menses. There is often a family history. A significant proportion (17 per cent) appear to relate to an underlying nutritional deficiency of folic acid, Vitamin B_{12} and/or iron (Wray *et al* 1975), or may herald the onset of gastrointestinal or systemic diseases such as coeliac disease, inflammatory bowel disease, Behçet's syndrome, Reiter's syndrome or haematological disturbances, such as leucopenia, leukaemia or pernicious anaemia (Antoon and Miller 1980). Important factors in their pathogenesis include exogenous microbes, trauma, nutritional deficiencies, hormonal changes, physiological stress and autoimmune disease.

The innumerable and diverse forms of medication testify to the limited success of treatments for aphthous stomatitis. Management is generally palliative, aiming to relieve pain, reduce the number of ulcer days, extend the remission period, and exclude underlying nutritional deficiency or disease. Treatment regimes include good dental hygiene together with topical steroids (hydrocortisone, betamethasone lozenges, triamcinolone paste). Symptomatic relief is helped by additional application of a topical anaesthetic (lignocaine rinses and orabase barrier cream). Nystatin or amphotericin should be considered for super-added oral candidiasis. Caustic astringents (e.g. silver nitrate) are best avoided since these may cause tissue damage with protracted use.

HYPERPLASTIC GINGIVITIS

Hyperplasia of gingival tissues is sometimes seen at puberty in males and females in association with elevation in gonadotrophins and sex hormones (oestrogens/androgens) (Gorlin and Goldman 1970), and is commonly seen in pregnancy (Löe and Silness 1963). In an extensive study of periodontal disease in pregnancy, Löe and Silness found gingivitis in all women studied between the second and eighth months of pregnancy, with regression in the ninth month and after delivery. The gingival tissue may be lobulated or nodular (pregnancy tumour, pregnancy granuloma) and in extreme cases the colour of the gingival margin and interdental papillae change to deep red or purple, with excessive contact bleeding (Gorlin and Goldman 1970). Histology shows a nodular inflammatory hyperplasia with endothelial proliferation, vascular dilatation and sometimes features similar to pyogenic granuloma. Management is difficult as these conditions are prone to recur, but some improvement occurs with careful oral dental hygiene, removal of dental plaque and debris, and use of soft toothbrushes.

DENTAL CARIES

Deficiency of calcium, once believed to play a dominant role in the development of dental caries in pregnancy, is now considered of secondary importance. The increase in incidence of caries found in pregnancy (1.5–2 times greater than in the nonpregnant) relates to the increased incidence of acidophilic microorganisms (*Str. mutans*, *Lactobacillus acidophilus*) in plaque and subgingiva, compared to normals. Predisposing factors include raised levels of oestradiol and progesterone (Kornman and Loesche 1980).

Gastro-oesophageal disorders

GASTRO-OESOPHAGEAL REFLUX

Pathophysiology

Dyspepsia and heartburn due to gastro-oesophageal reflux (De Paula Castro 1967) are distressing symptoms that often commence in early pregnancy and occur in up to 70 per cent of pregnant women (Van Thiel *et al* 1977; McClure Browne 1978), particularly in the third trimester (Feeney 1982).

Various theories have been put forward to explain the predisposition to reflux in pregnancy including mechanical factors such as changes in lower oesophageal sphincter pressure (LOSP) (Byrne 1972; Dodds *et al* 1978), increased intragastric pressure (Cohen and Harris 1972; Brock-Utne *et al* 1981) and reduced competence of the pyloric sphincter with back wash of alkaline bile (Atlay *et al* 1973). Hormonal changes (Van Thiel and Wald 1981; Feeney 1982), diet (Nebel and Castell 1972; Bassey 1977) and even racial predisposition (Bassey 1977) have also been emphasised.

Hiatus hernia

Hiatus hernia is common in both the nonpregnant and pregnant patient and can be demonstrated in 10–20 per cent of women in late pregnancy (Burrow and Ferris 1975). There is currently considerable controversy concerning the relationships among LOSP, intragastric pressure, symptoms of gastro-oesophageal reflux and the presence of a hiatus hernia (Cohen and Harris 1971; Bassey 1977).

Oesophagitis

Inflammation of the oesophageal mucosa results from contact with acid or alkaline gastric contents. The most common cause is gastro-oesophageal reflux of acid peptic juice, with or without hiatus hernia (Cohen and Harris 1972), although alkaline oesophagitis may also occur (Kaye and Showalter 1974). There is no direct correlation between symptom severity and degree of oesophagitis as seen at endoscopy or on histology. In a retrospective survey of the complications of oesophagitis in pregnancy,

Scott and Deutch (1955) collected 34 cases from the literature of severe, erosive and haemorrhagic oesophagitis often, but not invariably, associated with vomiting during pregnancy.

Management of gastro-oesophageal reflux

Gastro-oesophageal reflux and oesophagitis are distressing symptoms which often require treatment. In late pregnancy, during labour and during obstetrical anaesthesia there is additional concern regarding the increased risk of vomiting and regurgitation with tracheal aspiration of acid gastric contents leading to chemical pneumonitis, hypoxia and pulmonary oedema (Mendelson's syndrome) (*see* p. 24).

In early pregnancy, ingestion of small carbohydrate-rich meals with avoidance of excess fat (Nebel and Castell 1972) and alcohol (Hogan *et al* 1972) and maintenance of upright posture are sufficient to alleviate symptoms in over 50 per cent of cases. The use of antacids may, however, be necessary and in a retrospective study (Nelson and Forfar 1971) up to 34 per cent of women were shown to have taken antacids at some time during pregnancy.

Studies on the teratogenicity of conventional simple antacids, i.e. aluminium or magnesium preparations, suggest that they are probably safe (Nelson and Forfar 1971), although prospective data from controlled trials is lacking. Antacid therapy in doses of 10–15 ml two or three times daily, between meals and at night is usually sufficient. Severe symptoms may benefit from additional use of coating gels. Proprietary antacids are best avoided since many contain anticholinergic agents that are well absorbed, are known to reduce LOSP (Brock-Utne *et al* 1981; Fisher *et al* 1978) and are excreted into breast milk (Wilson *et al* 1980). In patients with coeliac disease and/or milk/lactose intolerance, Nulacin, which contains gluten, milk fats and lactose should be avoided.

NAUSEA AND VOMITING

Nausea and vomiting during uncomplicated pregnancy occurs so frequently in Western countries with reported incidences of 50–80 per cent (Midwinter 1971; Biggs and Vesey 1980) that these symptoms are considered by many women as diagnostic of pregnancy and its normal physiological consequences. Symptoms of nausea and vomiting occur most commonly between the sixth and fourteenth week, but in some 20 per cent of cases can continue through pregnancy into the second and third trimesters (Midwinter 1971).

The commonest variety of nausea and vomiting, the 'morning sickness' syndrome, involves mild symptoms of nausea and vomiting limited to the first trimester and does not influence health. *Hyperemesis gravidarum* is defined as vomiting occurring before the twentieth week and requiring admission to hospital (Fairweather 1968). Vomiting of a persistent nature through pregnancy and particularly occurring in the third trimester suggests intercurrent disease, for example pyelonephritis, hepatitis, pancreatitis, intestinal obstruction, or adrenocortical insufficiency (Midwinter 1971; Biggs and Vesey 1980).

Management

Morning sickness

'Morning sickness' generally improves following reassurance that symptoms eventually resolve with the taking of small carbohydrate-rich meals and avoidance of large volume drinks in the early morning (Biggs and Vesey 1980). Therapy with anti-emetic drugs is rarely necessary. There is some evidence that women who abort in early pregnancy have less nausea and vomiting (Medalie 1957). A smaller number of mothers of infants born with major abnormalities consumed anti-emetics in the first trimester (7.4 per cent) than mothers of normal infants (13.1 per cent), suggesting an inverse relation between nausea and vomiting (anti-emetic therapy) and fetal abnormalities (Nelson and Forfar 1971).

Hyperemesis gravidarum

Hyperemesis gravidarum presents with profound vomiting, dehydration and ketosis and occasionally jaundice with hepatic dysfunction (*see* p. 301) at or before the twentieth week of pregnancy. The cause is unknown. High levels of circulating oestrogens and human choriogonadotrophin (hCG) have been implicated in some but not all studies (Fairweather and Loraine 1962) since the condition may be associated with multiple pregnancy, hydramnios or hydatidiform mole (Guttmacher 1960; Fairweather 1968; Winship 1975). Hyperemesis gravidarum is also associated with a history of a previously unsuccessful pregnancy, and may recur in subsequent pregnancies (Semmens 1957). Various psychological and social factors have also been implicated (Katon *et al* 1980), but the cause is probably multifactorial.

Management of hyperemesis gravidarum involves admission to hospital and removal from a stressful home environment, withdrawal of oral foods and fluids, rehydration with intravenous fluids, replacement of electrolytes, vitamin B therapy and antihistamine anti-emetics or metoclopramide (Winship 1975). Corticosteroids have been used in early studies with some reported success (Wells 1953) but information from controlled trials is lacking.

Anti-emetic drug therapy

The majority of cases of 'morning sickness' can be managed without recourse to drug therapy. Concern about the teratogenic potential and consequent safety of many anti-emetics in humans following the thalidomide tragedy has led to the reappraisal of the use of anti-emetic drugs in human pregnancy.

Retrospective (Nelson and Forfar 1971) and prospective (Kullander and Källén 1976) studies, involving large numbers of women, suggest that a variety of commonly used anti-emetics such as meclozine, cyclizine and dimenhydrinate are safe for use in pregnancy, with the possible exception of an increased risk of congenital hip dislocation in babies born to mothers who have taken promethazine during early pregnancy

(Kullander and Källén 1976; Huff 1980). Data on human teratogenicity studies remain sparse, and in the light of the thalidomide tragedy, animal studies may not be reliable (McBride 1961; Lenz and Knapp 1962). The compound Bendectin (dicyclomine hydrochloride, doxylamine succinate and pyridoxine hydrochloride) is widely used in the treatment of nausea and vomiting in pregnancy (Fagan and Chadwick 1983). Coincidental skeletal and intestinal anomalies have been reported with each of these drugs (Patterson 1969; Donnai and Harris 1978) including individual reports for Debendox (Mellor 1978; Smithells and Sheppard 1978) and Bendectin (Patterson 1977); retrospective (Harron *et al* 1980) and prospective (Nelson and Forfar 1971) studies for Debendox (Smithells and Sheppard 1978) and Bendectin (Shapiro *et al* 1977; FDA 1979) have failed to confirm a clear teratogenic effect. The anticholinergic component dicyclomine has been withdrawn in America. In Great Britain the component doxylamine has been withdrawn because of lack of efficacy. Metoclopramide has been effectively used in the management of hyperemesis gravidarum (Singh and Lean 1970) and may have greater efficacy than prochlorperazine or placebo (Singh and Lean 1970), but less than the antihistamines. This drug is a base which readily crosses the placenta and is also excreted in breast milk (Schulze-Delrieu and Koch-Weser 1981). Metoclopramide is generally considered to be safe for use in idiopathic cases of vomiting of late pregnancy and labour, but information concerning its effects on the fetus or neonate is lacking. Prochlorperazine enjoyed popularity as a safe, general anti-emetic in pregnancy in the 1950s–60s particularly in the treatment of hyperemesis gravidarum, but has been superseded by metoclopramide which causes less side-effects.

Gastrointestinal disorders

PEPTIC ULCERATION

Gastric acid secretion

Despite problems in studying gastric physiology during pregnancy, it is generally accepted that gastric secretion of acid is reduced during pregnancy (Hytten 1980), particularly in the mid trimester (Hunt and Murray 1958). Gastric acid outputs clearly do not correlate with serum gastrin levels which rise to 2–3 times the nonpregnant level by the third trimester (Françavilla *et al* 1978). Despite these findings, several authors feel that the magnitude of the reduction in acid secretions seen during pregnancy is too small to explain the reported reduction in peptic ulcer symptoms (Parbhoo and Johnston 1966; Waldrum *et al* 1980).

Prevalence

Peptic ulceration arising *de novo* in pregnancy is remarkably uncommon. In nearly 23 000 deliveries only six women had documented active ulceration (Baird 1966). In a study of 118 women with already documented peptic ulceration prior to pregnancy, 89 per cent either improved or became symptom-free (Clark 1953). There are, however, scattered reports of increased severity of peptic ulcer symptoms and complications during pregnancy (Langmade 1956; Crisp 1960; Baird 1966; Peden *et al* 1981), particularly in association with toxaemia (Langmade 1956; Jones *et al* 1969). Furthermore, quiescent ulcers may suddenly erupt (Crisp 1960), particularly in the puerperium (Clark 1953; Langmade 1956; Jones *et al* 1969). Presentation may then be acute with massive haemorrhage (Sandweiss *et al* 1943; Carangelo and Efstation 1948) or perforation (Anderson 1942; Sandweiss *et al* 1943).

The reduction in symptoms of peptic ulceration during pregnancy has been attributed to good diet, close medical supervision and increased intake of food, e.g. milk (Crisp 1960). Hormonal factors may also play a role.

Management

Management of the pregnant patient should be similar in most respects to that of the nonpregnant (Jones *et al* 1969). Conservative management includes prohibition of smoking, bedrest and regular antacids (Ippolilti *et al* 1978) with endoscopic monitoring of ulcer healing.

The H_2-receptor antagonists, cimetidine and ranitidine, are of proven value in promoting the healing of duodenal and gastric ulcers (Finkelstein and Isselbacher 1978; Langman *et al* 1980), but only cimetidine has been assessed in pregnancy. Cimetidine, when used in late pregnancy, appeared safe (McGowan 1979) despite reports of hepatic dysfunction in two newborn infants (Glade *et al* 1980). It may have a place in elective obstetrical anaesthesia (Howe *et al* 1980), in particular in prophylaxis against Mendelson's syndrome (*see* p. 25). Carbenoxolone (Taylor *et al* 1977) and De-Nol (Boyes *et al* 1975; Connor 1977; Poulantzas *et al* 1978) have been shown to be of equal efficacy to cimetidine in controlled clinical trials in nonpregnant patients, but the recognised side-effects of the former (fluid retention, electrolyte imbalance, etc.) and lack of experience with either drug in pregnancy prohibit their use.

Indications for surgery, and the outcome (mortality), are the same as in the nonpregnant patient (Baird 1966; Jones *et al* 1969). Haemorrhage and/or perforation are fortunately uncommon in late pregnancy, but the associated high maternal and fetal loss should underline the need for awareness of this possibility. Prompt resuscitation of the mother may be followed by surgery and, if necessary, delivery by Caesarean section (Jones *et al* 1969).

COELIAC DISEASE

Coeliac disease (gluten-sensitive enteropathy) may be defined as an abnormality of the small intestinal mucosa caused by the ingestion of gluten-containing substances in susceptible individuals. In most cases, histology from a jejunal biopsy shows sub-total villous atrophy, and withdrawal of gluten from the diet results in marked clinical and histological improvement, although return to normal histological appearances may take many months and is often incomplete in adult coeliac disease.

Epidemiology

The prevalence of the disease in the general Western population has been estimated at 0.03 per cent (Carter *et al* 1959), but the incidence varies considerably from 1 in 6500 of the general population in Sweden (Borgfors and Selander 1968) and 1 in 890 in Switzerland (Shmerling *et al* 1972) to between 1 in 2000 and 1 in 8000 in the UK (British Medical Journal 1970). The highest recorded incidence is 1 in 300 for Western Ireland (McCarthy *et al* 1974). These values may underestimate the true incidence, since they tend to reflect early studies of patients with 'classical' more florid presentations (*see below*). Coeliac disease was originally considered to occur predominantly in temperate climates, but probably occurs world-wide since it is now documented in natives of tropical regions (Misra *et al* 1966). Several reports suggest a preponderance of females (Green and Wollaeger 1960; Benson *et al* 1964; Visakorpi *et al* 1970) but others suggest an equal male to female ratio (Cooke *et al* 1953; Mann *et al* 1970).

Clinical features

Coeliac disease is not the only cause of a flat jejunal biopsy; other causes include Crohn's disease, cows' milk protein intolerance (Walker-Smith *et al* 1978), soy protein intolerance (Ament and Ruben 1972) and tropical sprue, but it remains the commonest cause in Western Europe.

There is evidence that coeliac disease can present at any age (Green and Wollaeger 1960; British Medical Journal 1970) with either an abrupt or insidious presentation in children (Ebbs 1956) or adults (Ebbs *et al* 1950; Green and Wollaeger 1960). In adult life, although the classical presentation of diarrhoea, anorexia and weight loss with evidence of malabsorption is well recognised, this mode is not invariable and probably only occurs in a minority of older patients (Cooke *et al* 1953; Brooks *et al* 1966; Mann *et al* 1970; Visakorpi *et al* 1970). Clinical symptoms may disappear around the time of puberty despite persistently abnormal biopsies (Mortimer *et al* 1968; Sheldon 1969) and symptoms may reappear following gastric surgery (Hedberg *et al* 1966; Ek 1967, 1969; Binder 1970), stress, intercurrent infection (Ebbs *et al* 1950; Brooks *et al* 1966), or during pregnancy (Ek 1967, 1969; Sheldon 1969; Mann *et al* 1970).

Adult patients frequently present with extra-gastrointestinal manifestations to non-gastroenterological departments, e.g. with megaloblastic or iron deficiency anaemias, particularly in pregnancy (Cooke *et al* 1953; Green and Wollaeger 1960; Ek 1967, 1969), or a variety of other haematological problems which may occur in the absence of diarrhoea and steatorrhoea (McGrugan and Volwiler 1964; Kowlessar and Phillips 1970; Mann *et al* 1970; Croese 1979) or symptoms attributable to anaemia (Benson *et al* 1964; Ek 1967, 1969). Other presentations include bone pain from bony complications, e.g. osteoporosis, and osteomalacia and rarely tetany (Cooke *et al* 1953; Green and Wollaeger 1960), secondary to malabsorption of calcium and vitamin D (Juergens *et al* 1956). Neurological manifestations range from generalised muscle weakness to peripheral neuropathies, encephalopathy and other syndromes associated with deficiencies of vitamins B_6 or B_{12} and even frank psychiatric illnesses and psychoses (Cooke and Smith 1966; Pallis and Lewis 1974). Changes in the skin and mucous membranes are not uncommon, and patients may present with glossitis, cheilitis, stomatitis, aphthous ulceration (Cooke *et al* 1953), skin pigmentation, dermatitis herpetiformis and oedema (Cooke *et al* 1953; Green and Wollaeger 1960; Benson *et al* 1964; Mann *et al* 1970). These extra-intestinal features are generally more common when coeliac disease first presents in adult life rather than in childhood (Cooke *et al* 1953; Green and Wollaeger 1960; Visakorpi *et al* 1967). To direct questioning, however, many adult patients will declare symptoms dating from childhood (Cooke *et al* 1953; Benson *et al* 1964; Steward *et al* 1967; Mortimer *et al* 1968).

Effects on fertility

Early studies considered the effects of coeliac disease on fertility and menstrual function. In a study of 41 female patients with coeliac disease the average age at menarche was 14.8 years (range 12–19 years) (Cooke *et al* 1953), and in a similar study of 25 coeliac patients the average age at menarche was 15 years (range 13–17 years) compared with an average of 13.4 years for the general population (Linsay *et al* 1956). In a larger series of 73 women with coeliac disease, covering the years 1945–54, menarche and menstruation were considered normal in 50 but scanty flow or amenorrhoea was recorded in 14 patients (Green and Wollaeger 1960).

Female or male patients with untreated coeliac disease may have an increased risk of infertility and this may return to normal during treatment with a gluten-free diet (*see* below) (Morris *et al* 1970; Ogborn 1975; Baker and Read 1975). Early data on fertility have been indirectly assessed from records of the number of children produced. In the series of Cooke *et al* (1953) of 32 married women, there were seven women without children but an average of two children for each of the remaining 25 patients. They also studied 38 males with coeliac disease and found eleven childless, but information on results of fertility screening was lacking. In recent studies of male patients with untreated coeliac disease, Farthing *et al* (1982, 1983) found an incidence of impotence in 18%, sperm motility was reduced in 75%, and 46% had abnormal sperm morphology. Only the latter improved on gluten withdrawal. Dysfunction of the hypothalamic-pituitary axis with subsequent elevations in levels of plasma testosterone and luteinizing hormone (Farthing *et al* 1983) or serum prolactin (Stevens and Craig 1981) found in some male coeliacs may play a role but these findings require further confirmation.

Effects in pregnancy

In Ogborn's study (1975), 26 women with coeliac disease were followed through pregnancy and symptoms documented. Although four women claimed that their symptoms improved during pregnancy, 14 noted exacerbation of symptoms during pregnancy and the puerperium, and a further 8 experienced symptoms in the puerperium alone. Information on factors such as histological status of the gut and dietary management is lacking and this issue is unresolved.

There are several reports of an association between untreated coeliac disease and both recurrent abortion (Martin and Davis 1964; Joske and Martin 1971; Ogborn 1975) and megaloblastic anaemia (Ek 1967, 1969; Mann *et al* 1970) secondary to folic acid deficiency (Hibbard and Hibbard 1963; Martin *et al* 1965; Hibbard and Smithells 1965; Ek 1967, 1969; Croese 1979). Ek (1967) collected records in Sweden over the period 1952–61 of 39 women with coeliac disease and found five with a previous documented history of megaloblastic anaemia in former pregnancies. In a later follow-up study of 32 women previously diagnosed (over 10 years before) as having megaloblastic anaemia in pregnancy, Ek found low serum folates in 41 per cent compared with 11 per cent of normal matched controls and raised faecal fats in 27 per cent of patients suggesting malabsorption (Ek 1969). Problems in the assessment of folic acid status in pregnancy are considered in Chapter 2.

In a study at the Hammersmith Hospital of 25 women (60 pregnancies) over the period 1965–73, diagnosed on jejunal biopsy as having coeliac disease and supplemented in pregnancy with carbohydrate and vitamin supplements, Ogborn (1975) found eight first trimester abortions in 38 pregnancies (21 per cent) in previously untreated coeliacs compared with only one spontaneous abortion in 22 pregnancies in women strictly adherent to a gluten-free diet. In both the untreated and treated (gluten-free) groups there was an increased incidence of small-for-dates (16 per cent v. 19 per cent) infants and similar (7 per cent v. 10 per cent) high perinatal mortalities. Two abnormal babies were born to mothers in the treated group. Ogborn concluded that successful pregnancy could occur both before and after diagnosis and treatment of coeliac disease but that abortion and intrauterine growth retardation were the main associated obstetric problems and these occurred on or off gluten-containing foods. Folic acid deficiency was common in the untreated group but the association between congenital abnormalities and folate deficiency has only been seen in rats (Hibbard and Smithells 1965) and has not been confirmed for humans (Pritchard *et al* 1971). Ogborn also reported frequently low serum vitamin B_{12} levels. Further information on levels of serum vitamin B_{12} is lacking but there have been reports of infertility in patients with pernicious anaemia (Varadi 1967; Jackson *et al* 1967; Hall & Davidson 1968).

Management in pregnancy

Women with a past medical history of infertility or recurrent abortion, low levels of serum folate, red blood cell folate or serum vitamin B_{12} warrant further investigation, including a barium series and jejunal biopsy, rather than immediate administration of vitamin supplements.

Women presenting for the first time during pregnancy with diarrhoea, weight loss, anaemia, malabsorption or other features suggesting coeliac disease should be thoroughly investigated, and although radiological investigation and jejunal biopsy with a standard capsule are not recommended, coeliac disease can be diagnosed (or excluded) on a duodenal biopsy obtained during fibreoptic gastroduodenoscopy.

Those women already known to have coeliac disease should be encouraged to adhere strictly to a gluten-free diet if a pregnancy is planned (Morris *et al* 1970; Ogborn 1975) and careful attention should be paid to deficiencies of vitamin B_{12}, folic acid, iron and trace metals, e.g. zinc, with supplements given throughout pregnancy, the puerperium and during lactation as necessary. Severe zinc deficiency which may occur in acrodermatitis enteropathica is an established cause of congenital malformation, particularly neural tube defect (Hambedge *et al* 1975). Babies, particularly those breast fed and born to mothers with low serum B_{12} levels, will also have low serum and liver stores, and should receive supplements (Srikantia and Reddy 1967).

Failure to respond to a gluten-free diet or clinical relapse should be investigated in the same way as in the nonpregnant patient with attention to dietary indiscretion, possible inadvertent ingestion gluten-containing drugs (Booth 1970), intercurrent infection or infestation or associated diseases. Dyspepsia and dysphagia occurring in coeliac disease should be taken seriously and endoscopy performed in view of the association of oesophageal malignancy and coeliac disease.

Follow-up of patients with coeliac disease should be lifelong. In the majority of adults in whom the disease is neglected (McCrae *et al* 1975) or who reintroduce gluten into the diet (Kumar 1979), histological evidence of relapse occurs, frequently within seven weeks, but symptoms and histological severity do not necessarily correlate (McCrae *et al* 1975; Kumar 1979), and haematological and nutritional abnormalities are common even in 'asymptomatic' patients (Croese 1979). Genetic studies show a familial incidence of coeliac disease (MacDonald *et al* 1965; Mylotte *et al* 1972). Relatives may have biochemical abnormalities suggesting malabsorption (low serum folate, low xylose excretion, increased faecal fat) making coeliac disease a likely diagnosis (Ek 1969). A further genetic link has been shown with HLA typing where up to 80 per cent of coeliacs have been shown to be positive for the histocompatibility antigen HLA B8 (Falchuk *et al* 1972).

INFLAMMATORY BOWEL DISEASE

The incidence and prevalence of the various conditions (e.g. ulcerative colitis, Crohn's disease and non-specific colitis) collectively grouped as the non-specific inflammatory bowel diseases (IBD), have risen in the last 40 years (Kyle 1971; Kewenter *et al* 1974; Miller *et al* 1974; Brahme *et al* 1975; Mayberry *et al* 1979; Gilat and Rozen 1979; Rozen *et al* 1979; Kyle and Stark 1980; Sedlack *et al* 1980; Sinclair *et al* 1980). Ulcerative colitis and Crohn's disease are more common in certain countries, e.g. North America, England and Scandinavia, with a prevalence rate of 40–100 per 100 000 and incidence of 4–6 per 100 000 per year (Kirsner and Shorter 1982b). The incidence of Crohn's disease in particular has increased fourfold (1.9–6.6 per 100 000) between 1935 and 1979 in the USA (Sedlack *et al* 1980) and increases have been reported in Wales (Mayberry *et al* 1979) and Israel (Gilat and Rozen 1979; Rozen *et al* 1979). The trend suggesting a rise in incidence of Crohn's disease for Scotland and Sweden (Kyle and Clark 1980) has not been sustained. Inflammatory bowel disease is apparently rare in certain areas, e.g. Morocco and Saudi Arabia (Kirsner and Shorter 1982b), and is much less common in blacks than whites (Segal *et al* 1980) and in the non-Jewish than the Jewish population (Brahme *et al* 1975).

IBD can occur in any age group although in general there is a bimodal peak in incidence. The disease often becomes manifest before the age of 30 with peaks between 15–20 (Rogers *et al* 1971) and 55–60 years (Kirsner and Shorter 1982b); it has an almost equal ratio of females to males (Kirsner and Shorter 1982b). Thus, the prevalence of IBD in the childbearing years has led to awareness of the impact of IBD and therapies on pregnancy and maternal and fetal outcomes. Opinions on fertility, the clinical course during pregnancy and fetal outcome have recently changed with the advent of earlier diagnosis and instigation of therapies, and improved control of inflammation prior to and during pregnancy and the puerperium.

Effects on fertility

Female

Some studies have suggested that women with IBD may have a higher rate of involuntary infertility than the normal population, but details of relevant factors, such as the spouse's fertility and nutritional status, were often unavailable (Fielding and Cooke 1970; De Dombal *et al* 1972; Homan and Thorbjarnarson 1976). Two groups found that conception was less frequent in women with Crohn's colitis (67 per cent) compared with small bowel disease alone (Fielding and Cooke 1970) or ileitis and ileocolitis (De Dombal *et al* 1972). In contrast, in Homan and Thorbjarnarson's study (1976), only women with small intestinal disease had fertility rates below the normal population (0.053 v. 0.088 pregnancy/woman/year). Results on fertility rates in women with ulcerative colitis are also conflicting. Crohn *et al* (1956a) found no impairment in fertility in ulcerative colitis, providing the disease was well controlled. De Dombal *et al* (1965), however, in a study of 107 pregnancies of women with ulcerative colitis, had only three women in their subgroup with active disease at the time of conception, compared with 63 who had clinically quiescent disease, and suggested that active disease may impair the chance of conception. In a later report, however (Willoughby and Truelove 1980), of 147 women with ulcerative colitis of variable disease activity, only ten (6.8 per cent) were involuntarily infertile and this proportion is comparable to the figure of 10 per cent for the general population (Harrison 1977). Studies on women with Crohn's disease suggest that amenorrhoea and subsequent involuntary infertility correlates with disease activity, but that normal fertility can be anticipated in well controlled disease.

Details of disease activity and drug therapy are often lacking in the above studies. No data are currently available on the effects of drug treatment, namely salazopyrine, on *female* fertility. There is no evidence that corticosteroids cause infertility. The safety of azathioprine, which is occasionally used in IBD, is discussed in p. 226.

Infertility following surgery (colectomy and ileostomy) has not been directly considered although obstructive complications which may follow surgery or arise *de novo*, such as pyosalpinx, ureteric obstruction, adhesions, fistulae and infections must add to the general morbidity (Fielding and Cooke 1970; Hudson 1972; Barwin *et al* 1974; Homan and Thorbjarnarson 1976). Psychological problems with sexual dysfunction, particularly after resective surgery (Gruner *et al* 1977) or with chronic disease, may also be relevant (Gazzard *et al* 1978; Meyers *et al* 1980).

In summary, the present literature suggests that a woman with Crohn's disease may have a significant risk (32–55 per cent) of being infertile (Vender and Spiro 1982), but that this may grossly overestimate the true risk because many factors, e.g. unrelated obstruction to Fallopian tubes or infertility of the spouse, have only recently been considered (Willoughby and Truelove 1980; Vender and Spiro 1982). The possible influence of the site of disease on fertility in women with Crohn's disease, and the whole issue of infertility in women with ulcerative colitis, remains open.

Male

Salazopyrine (sulphasalazine) is an important cause of male infertility (Levi *et al* 1979).

Deficiencies of trace metals may also contribute to infertility. Low serum levels of zinc or chromium have been found in IBD, and in isolated studies have been associated with hypogonadism in Crohn's disease (McClain *et al* 1980).

Effects of disease on pregnancy

Several early reports stressed the detrimental effect of IBD on pregnancy and fetal outcome (Barnes and Hayes 1931; Bauman 1931; Feder 1938; Bargen *et al* 1939; Babson 1946; Kirsner *et al* 1948; Raffensperger 1948). Barnes and Hayes (1931) in a case study recorded two out of three fetal deaths in three women who subsequently developed ulcerative colitis postpartum. Babson (1946) reported a single case of a woman with Crohn's disease requiring a colostomy for small bowel obstruction during pregnancy, with subsequent premature labour and death of the fetus. A similar case was reported by Raffensperger (1948) of a woman with a colostomy for Crohn's disease, who subsequently had a twin pregnancy resulting in premature labour and fetal loss. Despite these and later reports for ulcerative colitis (Bauman 1931; Feder 1938; Bargen *et al* 1939; Kirsner *et al* 1948) and Crohn's disease (Schofield *et al* 1970; Martinbeau *et al* 1975) indicating that IBD may have a detrimental effect on pregnancy and fetal outcome, there have been many later reports of larger numbers of pregnancies that counteract these earlier pessimistic impressions and present a more optimistic viewpoint.

In the first large series of 50 pregnancies in 34 women with ulcerative colitis, there were 43 (86 per cent) normal births and 5 (10 per cent) spontaneous abortions (Felsen and Wolarsky 1948). The first large series by Crohn and colleagues of 84 pregnancies in 53 women with terminal ileitis (regional enteritis) reported a normal delivery and outcome in 81 per cent, premature labour in 5 per cent; 4 per cent went to Caesarean section and 6 per cent had spontaneous abortions (Crohn *et al* 1956b). These authorities and other studies involving patients with ulcerative colitis (Abramson *et al*

1951; Crohn *et al* 1956a; Banks *et al* 1957) have reported normal deliveries and good fetal outcome in 70–90 per cent of cases if the IBD pre-dated the pregnancy and was firstly quiescent at the time of conception and throughout pregnancy, and secondly was quiescent at the time of conception but relapsed during pregnancy, or first became manifest in the puerperium (Abramson *et al* 1951; Crohn *et al* 1956a; Banks *et al* 1957).

These and other workers (Martinbeau *et al* 1975) have shown a deleterious effect on fetal outcome in those patients where IBD first became manifest during pregnancy. Abramson *et al* (1951) reported fetal loss in three out of five pregnancies in women in this subgroup with ulcerative colitis, and Crohn *et al* (1956b) in two out of three pregnancies in women with terminal ileitis. In a later study (Martinbeau *et al* 1975) of eleven pregnancies in ten women, where Crohn's disease commenced during pregnancy, there was a 55 per cent fetal loss, and in the six women who required surgery for severe disease, there were four fetal deaths. In the earlier study by Crohn and co-workers (Crohn *et al* 1956a) there was only one fetal death among 19 pregnancies where ulcerative colitis first developed during the course of pregnancy, but there was an increase in rate of spontaneous abortion if quiescent ulcerative colitis became reactivated during pregnancy. Many authorities feel, however, that the rates of spontaneous abortion reported in women with pre-existing IBD for ulcerative colitis (7–16 per cent) (Machella 1952; Zetzel 1975; MacDougall 1956; Krawitt 1959; Maddix 1962; De Dombal *et al* 1965; McEwan 1972; Willoughby and Truelove 1980) or Crohn's disease (6–18 per cent) (Crohn *et al* 1956b; Fielding and Cooke 1970; De Dombal *et al* 1972; Norton and Patterson 1972; Homan and Thorbjarnarson 1976) are not significantly different from figures drawn from the healthy pregnant population (Harlap *et al* 1979).

The overall consensus for the impact of pre-existing IBD on subsequent pregnancy is that a woman can anticipate a full-term normal delivery of a healthy infant, as can her healthy counterpart (Zetzel 1975; Willoughby and Truelove 1980) but the physician should anticipate frequent relapses during the pregnancy (Abramson *et al* 1951). The prospects of having a full-term, normal birth are improved (84 compared to 73 per cent) if the IBD is quiescent rather than active at the time of conception (Willoughby and Truelove 1980) and these figures are comparable if remission is maintained (83 per cent) or relapse occurs (73 per cent) during pregnancy (Webb and Sedlack 1974). That the rate of spontaneous abortion may be increased if quiescent disease becomes reactivated was only seen in Crohn's study in patients with ulcerative colitis (Crohn *et al* 1956a) and has not been confirmed by later studies for either ulcerative colitis (De Dombal *et al* 1965) or Crohn's disease (De Dombal *et al* 1972; Norton and Patterson 1972).

Where the disease becomes severe (Schofield *et al* 1970) or should surgery (e.g. colectomy) be required during pregnancy (Babson 1946; Martinbeau *et al* 1975) for obviously severe disease (McEwan 1972) then the outlook for the fetus is less good; rates of spontaneous abortion or stillbirth being 44–66 per cent (McEwan 1972; Martinbeau *et al* 1975). Women who have, however, previously undergone colectomy or ileostomy, and who later embark on a pregnancy, have (from one rather limited study of nine such patients) a 66 per cent chance of reaching term with a normal birth and healthy infant (Banks *et al* 1957) (*see* p. 295).

Women who present for the first time with IBD in pregnancy, according to some authors, appear to run a particularly severe course (Abramson *et al* 1951; Crohn *et al* 1956b) but this is by no means generally accepted (Crohn *et al* 1956a and b; Banks *et al* 1957), and so remains an unresolved issue. There appears to be no overall increase in risk of congenital defects (De Dombal *et al* 1965; Fielding and Cooke 1970; Homan and Thorbjarnarson 1976) and the rate of Caesarean section or elective termination of pregnancy is not increased in later studies (Krawitt 1959; De Dombal *et al* 1965; Crohn *et al* 1956a and b; Fielding and Cooke 1970; Homan and Thorbjarnarson 1976).

There is little doubt that this more optimistic viewpoint has emerged with the advent of early therapeutic intervention with salazopyrine and corticosteroids (*see below*). Those early studies where pregnancy was commenced during active IBD and where relapses remain frequent during the pregnancy (Abramson *et al* 1951) occurred before the advent of conventional treatment with salazopyrine and corticosteroids (Willoughby and Truelove 1980; Vender and Spiro 1982) and concern over the frequency of low birthweight in mothers on corticosteroids during relapse has not been substantiated (Willoughby and Truelove 1980).

Information on anatomical site and severity of disease and quantitative correlations of disease activity, drug therapy and pregnancy outcome is lacking.

Effects of pregnancy on disease

The effects of pregnancy on the course of IBD are controversial, and studies have yielded conflicting results. These findings arise partly because the studies extend over a 50 year period (1931–82), and more recent cases have been influenced by earlier diagnosis, better control of inflammation with drug treatments and resective surgery for fulminant, uncontrolled disease.

The early report by Barnes and Hayes (1931) of two maternal and fetal deaths in three women who subsequently developed ulcerative colitis postpartum led to the initial pessimistic conclusion that women with *already known* ulcerative colitis should avoid pregnancy. During 1950–56 there were several reports of women with pre-existent ulcerative colitis who *subsequently* became pregnant and these indicated an increase in numbers of relapses during pregnancy and particularly postpartum (Tumen and Cohn 1950; Abramson *et al* 1951; Crohn *et al* 1956a). The course was also stormy and maternal prognosis poor, with several maternal deaths, where ulcerative colitis first became manifest during pregnancy or in the postpartum period.

However, several follow-up studies have now shown a high relapse rate (about 40 per cent per annum) for both pregnant and nonpregnant women with either ulcerative colitis (De Dombal *et al* 1965; Willoughby and Truelove 1980) or Crohn's disease (Crohn *et al* 1956b; Fielding and Cooke 1970; De Dombal *et al* 1972; Norton and Patterson 1972; Homan and Thorbjarnarson 1976). De Dombal *et al* (1965) conducted a one year follow-up study (through pregnancy and three months postpartum) of 80 women with ulcerative colitis, clinically quiescent at the time of conception, and found that 27 out of 80 (34 per cent) had recurrences within the year, but that this was not statistically different from a rate of 47 per cent in their comparable control (nonpregnant) group. Clinical relapse from IBD may occur at any time during pregnancy but tends to occur particularly in the first trimester and early postpartum (Crohn *et al* 1956b; Fielding and Cooke 1970).

In addition, although studies have yielded conflicting results, there is general agreement that patients with Crohn's disease limited to the ileum, fare better in pregnancy and postpartum than those with colonic Crohn's disease or ulcerative colitis. However, studies with more precise data on disease site, extent and activity, and assessment of inflammation (rather than just relying on clinical scores) are lacking.

In summary, women with quiescent ulcerative colitis or Crohn's disease at the time of conception have approximately a 40–50 per cent clinical relapse rate but this is probably not significantly different from a comparable control, nonpregnant population (age 15–45 years). Also relapses occur most often in the first trimester and postpartum; and women in whom IBD becomes manifest for the first time in pregnancy or early postpartum generally tend to run a severe course, although these can now often be managed by medical therapy.

Management

Patients with already documented ulcerative colitis or Crohn's disease should be encouraged to embark on a pregnancy when their disease is clinically quiescent (Willoughby and Truelove 1980) (*see above*) and when taking a minimum number of medications (Seymour and Chadwick 1979). Investigation is limited and radiological investigations are not recommended in early pregnancy, but flexible fibreoptic endoscopy is safe and should be gently performed if the diagnosis is in doubt. Medical treatment and management is the same as for the nonpregnant patient (Seymour and Chadwick 1979; Willoughby and Truelove 1980; Vender and Spiro 1982).

Acute severe disease

In acute severe IBD, the pregnant patient should be admitted to hospital and stools taken for routine cultures for *E. coli*, Salmonella and Shigella, and also for Campylobacter spp. jejuni (Blaser *et al* 1979; Gribble *et al* 1981; Vesikari *et al* 1981) and *Clostridium difficile* toxin, since these organisms can also cause bloody diarrhoea, abdominal pain and fever. Stools should also be screened for parasites, including *Entamoeba histolytica* and *Strongyloides stercoralis*, prior to treatment, particularly with corticosteroids, since the latter may cause disseminated parasitosis. Treatment in general consists of bed rest, nil by mouth, oral corticosteroids, e.g. prednisolone 20–60 mg/day, rectal corticosteroids, oral salazopyrine (3–4 g/day) and intravenous fluids. The adrenal corticosteroids (hydrocortisone, prednisone, prednisolone, methyl prednisolone) remain the single most effective group of drugs for active IBD (Summers *et al* 1979; Kirsner 1980a). In patients who have not been previously treated with corticosteroids, intravenous ACTH may be superior to intravenous hydrocortisone, but intramuscular administration appears to have no additional advantage (Kirsner and Shorter 1982a). This regime is usually effective in lessening symptoms, using clinical disease activity scores, e.g. the Crohn's disease activity index (CDAI), and reducing inflammation as measured by laboratory indices, including serum albumin, erythrocyte sedimentation rate (ESR) and the C-reactive protein (Fagan *et al* 1982). Oral feeding may usually be resumed within 48 hours. The daily dose of prednisolone may be reduced from 30 to 20 mg by the end of seven days' treatment and below 20 mg by reducing 2 mg weekly (Fagan and Chadwick 1983). Therapy with corticosteroids should be withdrawn completely since there is no evidence that they prevent relapse in either Crohn's disease or ulcerative colitis (Singleton *et al* 1979a; Summers *et al* 1979). In a moderately severe attack, treatment with topical corticosteroid (Lee *et al* 1980), enemata (Ruddell *et al* 1980) and oral salazopyrine (1.0 g twice daily) or salazopyrine enemata should suffice, together with additional oral prednisolone up to 20 mg daily.

There have been no reports before 1980 of women given steroids for IBD during pregnancy but reassuring information is now available from some studies (Willoughby and Truelove 1980) of ulcerative colitis during pregnancy. The overall safety of steroids in pregnancy is discussed in Chapter 1.

The general consensus of opinion suggests that when corticosteroids are indicated for the treatment of an underlying disorder, they are not associated with an increased risk of abortion or congenital abnormality (Vender and Spiro 1982). The indications for their use in IBD are essentially the same as in the nonpregnant patient (Crohn *et al* 1956a and b; De Dombal *et al* 1965; De Dombal *et al* 1972; Willoughby and Truelove 1980) but doses should be kept to a minimum, i.e. below 20 mg/day, if possible, particularly in early pregnancy.

Salazopyrine (sulphasalazine) has been found to be a valuable drug in the treatment of colonic IBD in the nonpregnant (Singleton *et al* 1979b; Summers *et al* 1979) and pregnant patient (McEwan 1972; Holtermüller and Weis 1979; Mogadam *et al* 1981). This drug has been extensively studied, and shown to be superior to placebo in both ulcerative colitis and Crohn's disease when subjected to several controlled, randomised, double-blind, clinical studies, using either the oral (Singleton *et al* 1979b; Summers *et al* 1979) or rectal form (Möller *et al* 1978; Palmer *et al* 1981). Salazopyrine is split by colonic bacteria into the components sulphapyridine and 5-aminosalicylic acid, and general toxicity appears to relate to the sulphapyridine and acetylator status. Sulphapyridine has been show to be the major component responsible for many of the common side-effects, including headaches and skin rashes (Klotz *et al* 1980). The component 5-aminosalacyclic acid is unstable but believed to be the major active principle in IBD (Klotz *et al* 1980). Results of preliminary studies of a new oral preparation of 5-aminosalicylic acid (Dew *et al* 1982) are promising.

Salazopyrine is generally considered safe for use throughout pregnancy and the puerperium (McEwan 1972; Mogadam *et al* 1981) and also in breast-feeding mothers (Järnerot and Into-Malmberg 1979; Willoughby and Truelove 1980). The sulphapyridine component is a sulphonamide, but despite its well-documented potential to cause cleft palate and skeletal abnormalities in rats, and reports of similar findings in women taking a variety of other sulphonamides, reports of toxicity of salazopyrine in obstetric practice are few. Salazopyrine and its components cross the placenta, and fetal blood levels rapidly approach maternal levels (Hensleigh and Kauffman 1977). In late pregnancy sulphapyridine may displace bilirubin and impair its transport; kernicterus has been reported (Hensleigh and Kauffman 1977). Salazopyrine is excreted into breast milk, and although sulphapyridine levels may reach 40 per cent of maternal blood levels, these are not considered toxic in breast-fed infants (Järnerot and Into-Malmberg 1979). Salazopyrine impairs absorption of folic acid, necessitating additional supplements during pregnancy (Franklin and Rosenberg 1973; Lederer and Kump 1979). In view of the low but obvious potential side-effects of oral salazopyrine, and the important implications as a cause of infertility in males with IBD in oral or rectal form (Toovey *et al* 1981), the results of recent trials of rectal and oral preparations of the active component 5-aminosalicylic acid are awaited with interest.

Other treatments for acute IBD include administration of antibiotics, such as ampicillin; since the penicillin derivatives are generally considered safe in pregnancy, there appears no contraindication to its use. Metronidazole has been widely used in the non-pregnant population in the treatment of trichomoniasis (Rodin and Hass 1966), giardiasis (Jokipii and Jokippi 1979), amoebiasis (Peterson *et al* 1966; Prakash *et al* 1974), and Crohn's disease (Bernstein *et al* 1980; Finegold 1980; Sachar 1980). Its adverse effects include chromosome breakage (Vender and Spiro 1982), association with peripheral neuropathy after extended use and production of tumours in some (Howard and Hill 1979) but not all (Peterson *et al* 1966) animals after administration in large doses. Metronidazole crosses the placenta and is excreted in breast milk (Gray *et al* 1961; Finegold 1980). Its safety in pregnancy and during breast feeding is questionable.

Azathioprine and its component 6-mercaptopurine (6-MP) has been used in nonpregnant patients with severe Crohn's disease generally unresponsive to corticosteroids and salazopyrine (Lennard-Jones and Powell-Tuck 1979; Summers *et al* 1979, Korelitz 1980; Present *et al* 1980; Sleisenger 1980). Although azathioprine was considered *not* to be superior to placebo in the short-term in the National Co-operative Crohn's Disease Study (Singleton *et al* 1979a; Summers *et al* 1979), this trial has been criticised. Long-term studies with azathioprine or 6-MP have shown benefit and minimal toxicity in the nonpregnant population (Korelitz *et al* 1973; O'Donoghue *et al* 1978; Present *et al* 1980). Although there are limited data confirming the safety of azathioprine in pregnancy, particularly in patients with renal transplants (*see* p. 226), more studies are necessary before the use of azathioprine can be freely advocated.

Numerous other therapies have been used to treat acute relapse of IBD in the nonpregnant patient, including parenteral intravenous feeding for small bowel Crohn's disease (Dickinson *et al* 1980; Elson *et al* 1980; Fleming *et al* 1980) or IBD in general (Driscoll and Rosenberg 1978). Hyperalimentation has not been well studied in pregnancy (Webb 1980) but Tresadern *et al* (1983) have recently reported one successful pregnancy in a patient with Crohn's disease maintained on parenteral home nutrition. No data are available on the use of elemental diets (Kirsner and Shorter 1982a; Logan *et al* 1981) for acute IBD in pregnancy or on the drugs disodium cromoglycate (Bernstein *et al* 1978) or levamisole (Lennard-Jones and Powell-Tuck 1979; Vendor and Spiro 1982).

Chronic disease

Assessment of nutritional status is important in any patient with chronic IBD. Supplementation with folic acid (5–10 mg/day) is advisable in all pregnant patients and Vitamin B_{12} is essential in patients with ileal Crohn's disease or after ileal resection (*see* p. 49). Ideally measurement and assessment of trace metals including chromium, zinc and copper should be performed in pregnancy and also in cases of suspected infertility (*see* p. 283). Osteomalacia and Vitamin D deficiency syndromes are well recognised in Crohn's disease and require early therapeutic intervention (*see* p. 441). Patients with chronic IBD and blood loss may require iron supplements in pregnancy (*see* p. 41). Many oral iron preparations cause diarrhoea and this may be a problem, particularly in the ileostomy patient.

Since colonic function often improves and diarrhoea lessens in pregnancy, the use of anti-motility agents and stool thickeners, viz. codeine phosphate and diphenoxylate with atropine (Lomotil), should be kept to a minimum.

Lomotil and codeine phosphate are excreted into breast milk (Wilson *et al* 1980) and should, like other opiate/anticholinergic agents, be avoided (Anderson 1977). Severe diarrhoea should be investigated with the emphasis on treating underlying inflammation and/or infection rather than prescribing symptomatic measures.

Constipation should be avoided in patients with IBD, particularly with strictures, and also because it may impair the efficiency of action of oral salazopyrine on the left colon ('constipated colitis'). The pregnant patient should be encouraged to take adequate fluids and, in the absence of strictures, a high fibre diet, processed hydrophilic agents that are poorly absorbed (Godding 1976b) or magnesium hydroxide. Salazopyrine has been shown to be superior to placebo (2–4 g/day) in maintenance of remission in chronic ulcerative colitis but not apparently in Crohn's disease. There is no evidence that corticosteroids are useful in maintaining a remission in IBD.

The effects of surgical therapy

In the non-pregnant population, current surgical trends for IBD resistant to medical therapy are influenced by the site and extent of involvement of disease. Surgery may be required for up to 25 per cent of patients with fulminant ulcerative colitis (Kirsner and Shorter 1982a) or up to 40–50 per cent of patients with small bowel or ileocolonic Crohn's disease with complications such as obstruction, fistulae or abdominal suppuration (Kirsner and Shorter 1982a). The usual operation for fulminant or complicated colonic IBD involves a single-stage colectomy and ileostomy without/with preservation of the rectal stump (Kirsner and Shorter 1982a). In Crohn's disease limited gut resection and end-to-end anastomosis is preferred to previously performed bypass procedures or extensive resections with healthy tissue margins for anastomosis. The rate of clinical relapse and obvious disease recurrence at or near the site of previous resective surgery for Crohn's disease is over 90 per cent and does not appear to relate to the disease site, severity of inflammation or extent of resection (Kirsner and Shorter 1982a).

In pregnancy surgery has in the past been reserved for severe fulminant IBD. Early studies generally concluded that the subsequent outlook for both mother and fetus was poor. The early individual case reports by Babson (1946) and Raffensperger (1948) respectively of two women with Crohn's disease who required colostomy for obstructive symptoms during or prior to pregnancy, show that both resulted in fetal death.

Fetal and maternal mortalities following surgery for Crohn's disease that developed during pregnancy were high (Martinbeau *et al* 1975) and similar results were found for ulcerative colitis (McEwan 1972). There is no doubt that with improved medical therapy the outlook for mother and child has considerably improved (Willoughby and Truelove 1980; Vender and Spiro 1982).

The effect of prior surgery and possible outcome in a subsequent pregnancy was considered by Crohn and co-workers in their original series (Crohn *et al* 1956b). This group evaluated the rate of clinical relapse in women with known ileitis who had undergone ileocolic resection and bypass prior to pregnancy. They concluded that an operation prior to pregnancy might lessen the chances of clinical relapse. These results are difficult however to evaluate, since they arose before the advent of modern medical therapy, and also patients with ileal Crohn's disease alone may have a better overall prognosis and less severe course than those with colonic or ileocolonic IBD. Bypass procedures are discouraged today because of the residual inflammation, potential problems with blind loop (bacterial overgrowth) and increased risk of carcinoma (Kirsner and Shorter 1982a).

Ileostomy and colostomy

Ileostomy (or colostomy) performed for urinary or alimentary diversion is no contraindication to subsequent pregnancy. The majority of women (70–75 per cent) will have fullterm, normal vaginal deliveries (Crohn *et al* 1956a; Scudamore *et al* 1957; Banks *et al* 1957; Krawitt 1959; De Dombal *et al* 1965; Hudson 1972; McEwan 1972; Barwin *et al* 1974) but data on patients with Crohn's disease is lacking. In one large review using questionnaires from the Ileostomy Society, Hudson in 1972 reviewed 75 women, through 89 pregnancies, who had had a previous ileostomy performed at some time before pregnancy, for vesicovaginal fistula following previous obstetric trauma or colectomy for IBD. Pregnancy was uneventful to term in 84 of the 89 instances and normal vaginal delivery achieved in 71 per cent of cases. The increase in use of forceps occurred from impaired ability to push. Caesarean section was performed in 16 cases for obstetrical reasons, and in only one for ileal prolapse. Intestinal obstruction occurred in 10 per cent of cases, leading to one maternal death following a Caesarean section, and also one case of spontaneous abortion. Details of disease activity and anatomical site were not available.

In general, loss of up to 50 per cent of small bowel and/or colon is well tolerated in the nonpregnant subject and adaptation in the ileostomy occurs with time (Urban & Weser 1980). More extensive small and large bowel resection is attended by complex metabolic and neuroendocrine dysfunction (Filipsson *et al* 1978; Bryant and Bloom 1979; Mitchell *et al* 1980; Cosnes *et al* 1981; Griffin *et al* 1982). The pregnant woman with an ileostomy or massive gut resection may develop from problems such as malabsorption of fat, fat soluble vitamins, Vitamin B_{12}, water and electrolyte imbalance, hyperoxaluria and cholelithiasis. Complications such as obstruction of ureters or Fallopian tubes, and effects of surgery on subsequent fertility and sexual function, should also be anticipated.

INFECTIONS AND INFESTATIONS

Infections and infestations affecting the gastrointestinal system cause significant morbidity worldwide (*see* Table 9.1), but studies of their effects and management in pregnancy are few. Information on some of the following infections and infestations affecting the gastrointestinal system in pregnancy is available.

Bacterial infections

Travellers' diarrhoea

Acute diarrhoea, particularly in travellers, is commonly due to gastrointestinal infection with *Escherichia coli* (40–70 per cent of cases). Other organisms, e.g. Shigella, may be isolated from stools in 5–20 per cent of cases. Less commonly isolated organisms include the genus Campylobacter and also *Clostridium difficile*.

Table 9.1   Gastrointestinal infections and infestations.

Bacterial—specific	*Protozoa*
E. coli	Malaria
Salmonella	Toxoplasmosis
Shigella	Amoebiasis
Campylobacter sp.	Giardiasis
Cholera	
Clostridium difficile	*Nematodes*
	Enterobiasis
Bacterial—miscellaneous	Ascariasis
Bacterial overgrowth	Ancylostomiasis
Tropical sprue	Strongyloidiasis
Whipple's disease	
	Trematodes
Viral Infections	Shistosomiasis
Polio	
Cytomegalovirus	*Cestodes*
Listeriosis	Taeniasis
Herpes hominis	Hydatid

Campylobacter and Listeria

Gastrointestinal infection with the genus Campylobacter in pregnancy can cause a gastroenteritis (*C. fetus* spp. jejuni) characterised by abdominal pain, prolonged fever and often but not always bloody diarrhoea (Gribble *et al* 1981). The organisms can be grown from blood cultures, stool and placenta but require prolonged incubation under microaerophilic conditions using selective media (Blaser *et al* 1979; Karmali and Tan 1980; Gilbert *et al* 1981; Gribble *et al* 1981; Vesikari *et al* 1981).

In a review of seven women with systemic *C. fetus* infection documented in late pregnancy, there were three cases of premature labour and stillbirth, and a further baby died of neonatal sepsis. The mothers had a febrile illness with respiratory symptoms, but although one woman had a fulminant course with septic shock, in two cases the mothers were asymptomatic (Gribble *et al* 1981). *C. fetus* was isolated from blood cultures, fetal spleen and brain and placenta. The latter was abnormal with necrosis, infarction or abscess formation. The source of infection was not identified. In cases of neonatal meningitis or enteritis, the source of infection is probably by the faecal-oral route, from mothers with Campylobacter diarrhoea at delivery (Karmali and Tan 1980).

Treatment consists of four weeks of oral erythromycin stearate or erythromycin base (but not erythromycin estolate which is hepatotoxic) for maternal gastroenteritis, and in addition, gentamicin if systemic campylobacteriosis is suspected (Gribble *et al* 1981). Relapses are common with shorter courses. Erythromycin has been used in pregnancy in the treatment of genital mycoplasmal infections, and may cause elevations in serum aspartate aminotransferase; it crosses the placenta, but fetal blood levels remain low (McCormack *et al* 1977).

Listeria monocytogenes has been isolated from the faeces of many pregnant women. In some, infection is associated with febrile illness and after entering via the gut, the organism may cross the placenta resulting in abortion or preterm labour. The ratio of clinical infection to carriage is low. Treatment of Listeria infections is with ampicillin (Tobin *et al* 1977) (*see* p. 494).

Miscellaneous

The treatment of bacterial overgrowth, tropical sprue and Whipple's syndrome traditionally involve the use of tetracyclines but these are contraindicated in pregnancy. There is no informed experience on the management of these diseases in pregnancy.

Management principles

In the non-pregnant and pregnant population, acute diarrhoea lasting 24–96 hours can often be managed conservatively, with clear liquids and rehydration, without recourse to drugs. Common remedies, e.g. kaolin, pectin and hydrated aluminium silicate, act by absorbing water and hence reduce stool frequency but there is no evidence that these agents reduce water loss from the gut (Gorbach 1982). Controlled prospective trials in nonpregnant subjects using charcoal, kaolin/pectin preparations or diphenoxylate showed no influence on outcome or speed of resolution of symptoms (72 hours) compared to controls receiving simple fluid replacements (Alestig *et al* 1979), and these agents may even exacerbate symptoms and delay excretion of certain organisms, e.g. Shigella (Gorbach 1982).

Every patient with acute diarrhoea lasting more than 96 hours should have stools sent directly for microscopic examination for ova, cysts and parasites, and culture for bacterial organisms (*see* Table 9.1), and if diarrhoea is more prolonged, then there should be careful sigmoidoscopic or gastroduodenoscopic examination to exclude other causes of diarrhoea, such as inflammatory bowel disease or coeliac disease (*see above*). In pregnancy, as in the nonpregnant state, all cases of persistent diarrhoea should be investigated.

Amoxycillin 1 g every six hours remains the safest antibiotic to use in cases of typhoid, paratyphoid and their carriers (Scioli *et al* 1972; Pillay *et al* 1975; Scragg and Rubidge 1975) or Shigellosis in pregnancy, although it may reduce the activity of hepatic glucuronyl transferase in preterm infants. These infections run a similar course to that in the nonpregnant patient, but in pregnancy transplacental infection with congenital disease has been recorded (Diddle and Stevens 1939; Freedman *et al* 1970).

The widespread use of antibiotics, in particular clindamycin (Tedesco *et al* 1974) and lincomycin, and tetracyclines, erythromycin and ampicillin, has led to awareness of the association of diarrhoea and/or colitis (pseudomembraneous colitis) with their administration (Larson and Price 1977). The diagnosis of antibiotic-associated colitis should be considered in any pregnant patient with diarrhoea complicating recent or previous antimicrobial therapy, and sigmoidoscopy may reveal the characteristic yellow-white plaques, copious mucus and erythematous mucosa. Stools should be positive for *Clostridium difficile* toxin (Larson and Price 1977). Withdrawal of all antibiotics and administration of vancomycin in an oral dose of 125 mg every six hours remains the treatment of choice (Keighley *et al* 1978). Although vancomycin is a poorly absorbed antibiotic, its use in pregnancy can result in damage to the fetal eighth cranial nerve (Stirrat and Beard 1973).

Viral infections

These are also considered in Chapter 15.

Polio virus

In a study of 310 women, to whom oral polio vaccine was administered, the immune response was similar to that measured in the nonpregnant population. This study included 69 women in the first eleven weeks of pregnancy, and there were five abortions and three babies with congenital deformities (Prem *et al* 1961) which agrees with a previous study of natural infection (Weinstein and Meade 1955). Infection acquired in the third trimester has been associated with neonatal paralysis and stillbirth.

Cytomegalovirus

This has been recorded as causing gastroenteritis (Weller 1971) and jaundice with hepatitis (Stern 1972). The fetus may be mentally retarded or deaf (*Lancet* 1983b).

Herpes virus

Hepatitis in mothers and their newborn infants has also been reported due to Herpes hominis virus (Hamory *et al* 1981).

Protozoal infections and infestations

Malaria

Plasmodium infection should be considered in any patient with fever and/or jaundice who has recently travelled through India, South-East Asia, Africa or South America. Patients with acute falciparium malaria may develop jaundice from haemolytic anaemia or hepatic congestion and deposition of haemosiderin.

Pregnant women have an increased prevalence of infection, and parasitaemia may be great (Bray and Anderson 1979) probably due to impaired host defences (Gilles *et al* 1969). Haemolytic anaemia with jaundice may be severe in pregnancy, and hepatorenal syndrome is often the cause of death. It has recently been recognised that patients with falciparum malaria may have severe hypoglycaemia. The risk of this complication is markedly increased by pregnancy (White *et al* 1983). Malaria may infect the placenta leading to spontaneous abortion, stillbirth and low birth weight. Malarial parasites may cross the placenta, particularly in non-immune mothers (Jelliffe 1967). Immune primagravidae are prone to relapse in the second trimester (Trussell and Beeley 1981).

Prophylaxis and treatment depend on the local area, the dominant plasmodium type and pattern of drug resistance. Chloroquine is the treatment of choice for severe infestation with *P. falciparium* in chloroquine-sensitive areas (Lancet 1983c), even though this drug has been suspected of causing neonatal deafness if used in the first trimester (Trussell and Beeley 1981). Quinine is less safe in pregnancy, although in a collaborative perinatal study of 106 women exposed to quinine in early pregnancy there was no increase in frequency of congenital malformation (Heinonen *et al* 1977). The metabolism of quinine may be impaired and should be avoided if hepatic dysfunction is severe. In choroquine-resistant areas, the combination, pyrimethamine and dapsone (Malaprim) has been used in pregnancy and is probably safe providing extra folate (10 mg per day) is given (Bruce-Chwatt 1983) (pyrimethamine and proguanil are folate antagonists). Pyrimethamine is excreted in breast milk but appears harmless to the breast-fed infant. The sulphone drug dapsone, and various sulphona-mides, are often used in combination with trimethoprim or pyrimethamine or primaquine, but haemolysis may occur in neonates, and adults with glucose-6-phosphate dehydrogenase deficiency.

Malaria prophylaxis with chloroquine or proguanil should be continued through pregnancy and visitors to high risk (holoendemic areas) should continue with their prophylaxis for at least the last trimester and preferably until after delivery (Lawson and Stewart 1967; Bruce-Chwatt 1980).

Amoebiasis

Infestation with *Entamoeba histolytica* may result in dysenteric or non-dysenteric colitis, amoebic appendicitis, amoeboma or hepatic abscess. *E. histolytica* is endemic in the tropics and subtropics but also occurs in Great Britain, Europe and North America. Amoebiasis may mimic or coexist with other diarrhoeal illnesses, e.g. bacillary dysentery, schistosomiasis or ulcerative colitis (inflammatory bowel disease), and should be considered in their differential diagnosis by regular examination of stools and careful sigmoidoscopy in all patients with dysenteric illnesses. Amoebiasis in pregnancy is reported to follow a severe course (Lawson & Stewart 1967; Steven 1981).

In the general population, metronidazole (800 mg three times daily) for five days has been used to treat intestinal and hepatic amoebiasis. Studies of metronidazole have shown it to be free from teratogenic effects in the rat, rabbit, mouse and guinea-pig, but large doses may produce tumours in certain species (Howard and Hill 1979) although it does not appear to be teratogenic in man (Beard *et al* 1979). Although metronidazole crosses the placenta and is also excreted in breast milk (Gray *et al* 1961), and its safety in pregnancy and the puerperium remains questionable, many pregnant patients have been given metronidazole without adverse effects. Tinidazole may be more effective than metronidazole in the treatment of amoebiasis (Prakash *et al* 1974) but has not been evaluated in pregnancy. Diloxanide (500 mg three times daily) for 14 days has been used to increase elimination of parasites from the bowel (Trussell and Beeley 1981).

Giardiasis

Infestations with *Giardia lamblia* (*Giardia intestinalis*) is a common cause of travellers' diarrhoea and malabsorption but is also endemic in Great Britain and Europe. This infestation may occur de novo, but susceptibility to infection is increased in patients with achlorhydria, hypogammaglobulinaemia, coeliac disease, chronic pancreatitis and protein malnutrition. Clinical features include abdominal discomfort, dyspepsia, diarrhoea with steatorrhoea and malabsorption. Diagnosis is confirmed by isolation of parasites or cysts from stools but duodenal aspirates and small intestinal biopsy may improve diagnostic yields. Treatment is with metronidazole and a lactose-free diet for secondary lactose intolerance. Prophylaxis involves filtering and boiling water, since cysts are resistant to simple chlorination.

Helminthic infestations

Nematodes and cestodes

Infestation with worms, e.g. hookworm (*Ankylostoma duodenale* or *Necator americanus*), threadworm (*Enterobius vermicularis*), roundworm (*Ascaris lumbricoides*) or the tapeworms (*Taenia saginata* or *Taenia solium*) can generally be managed conservatively. Anaemia from hookworm may require additional supplementation with iron. Abdominal discomfort, dyspepsia and diarrhoea from taeniasis is usually tolerated in pregnancy.

In severe infestation with hookworm, bephenium has been used (single dose 5 g) safely in pregnancy, but relapses are common particularly in the puerperium. The treatment of whipworm or mixed helminth infestations involves the use of mebendazole, but in view of its teratogenic effects in rats it should be avoided in early pregnancy. Piperazine has been used in pregnancy for the treatment of roundworm and threadworm but should only be used for large worm burdens (Lee 1975). Purgation using laxatives, e.g. senna or liquid paraffin, are often used to supplement the treatment of worm infestations but severe purgation and liquid paraffin should be avoided if possible in pregnancy (*see below*) (Trussell and Beeley 1981).

Trematodes

Shistosomiasis affects over 200 million individuals worldwide with a particularly high prevalence in Africa, Egypt and South America. *Shistosoma mansoni* and *S. japonicum* affect predominently the gastrointestinal tract (acute phase) and liver (chronic phase), whereas infestation with *S. haematobium* affects the urinogenital system. The course of the disease is not generally affected by pregnancy and so therapy can often be withheld until the puerperium. All drugs used in the treatment of shistosomiasis, such as niridazole, hycanthone, oxamniquine, and praziquantel, are effective but very toxic. Facilities for Caesarean section should be available since vaginal delivery may be impossible because of scarring of the cervix and vagina in chronic disease. Acute schistosomiasis should be considered in the differential diagnosis of bloody diarrhoea, and chronic disease in most cases of hepatosplenomegaly and portal hypertension. Diagnosis is by microscopic examination of stools and rectal biopsy material for eggs, and sigmoidoscopic examination should be performed to exclude the possible association of carcinoma of the colon.

CONSTIPATION IN PREGNANCY

Constipation is difficult to define but is said to occur when there is a reduction in stool frequency (3–5 stools/week) and/or weight (35 g/day), with a variable reduction in stool size and change in consistency (Martelli *et al* 1978). Constipation is often considered a common consequence of pregnancy although difficulties in definition and lack of objective data may be misleading. Evaluation of patterns of bowel habit in one study of 1000 healthy Israeli women during pregnancy showed that a reduction in stool frequency occurred only in 11 per cent; 1.5 per cent requiring laxatives. In 55 per cent there was no change, and 34 per cent in fact had increased frequency of stool evacuation (Levy *et al* 1971). Studies on motility of the intestine during pregnancy have been few and limited to the small bowel (Parry *et al* 1970a and b). Parry and co-workers assessed transit time in the small bowel (stomach to caecum) using mercury-loaded capsules in 22 healthy pregnant women between the 12th and 20th week and in 12 nonpregnant female controls. Mean stomach to caecum transit times were 57.9 hours compared with 51.7 hours in the nonpregnant group; over a third of the pregnant group exceeded 60 hours. Direct studies on colonic motility have not been performed. One study (Parry *et al* 1970b) showed increased water and sodium absorption in the colon during pregnancy and, although they attributed this to reduced colonic activity, other hormonal mechanisms could be involved. Although progesterone is known to cause relaxation of smooth muscle and has been implicated in the general hypotonia of smooth muscle in pregnancy (Kumar *et al* 1962) direct proof for this action on the gut in pregnancy is lacking. One study of small bowel transit time in nonpregnant women showed an association between increased transit time (stomach to caecum) and elevation in serum progesterone seen during the luteal phase of the menstrual cycle (Wald *et al* 1981). Recently, plasma motilin levels have been shown to be significantly reduced during the second and third trimester and these rapidly return to normal postpartum (Christofides *et al* 1982). Motilin has been shown to improve gastric emptying, increase the LOS pressure, promote activity of smooth muscle and hasten gall bladder emptying. The inhibitory action of progesterone on motilin may therefore explain these effects in pregnancy (Christofides *et al* 1982).

Management

The management of every patient with 'constipation' requires a careful inquiry into the patient's definition, dietary and laxative habits and drug therapy as well as a general history and investigation. Poor dietary habits, ignoring the call to stool and chronic drug or laxative ingestion are all important causes. General measures include education of the patient on the normal (variable) pattern of bowel function and instruction on the need to include a high intake of fibre-containing foodstuffs and adequate fluids (Burgess 1972). Unprocessed (Miller's) bran (1–2 tablespoons daily) may be added as a fibre supplement or alternatively processed hydrophilic stool bulking agents such as methyl cellulose, ispaghula, sterculia etc. with a high fluid intake (Godding 1976b).

Laxative therapy

The laxative therapies of choice in pregnancy include hydrophilic stool bulking agents, magnesium hydroxide tablets (4–6 tablets daily) or Senokot, if these fail. Magnesium hydroxide causes increased osmotic retention of fluid in the colon, and although up to 20 per cent of magnesium salts may be absorbed (Fingl 1975), no adverse effects have been reported in pregnancy. Senokot, an anthraquinone, is widely used in pregnancy and the puerperium (Sichel 1961; Shelton 1980; Fagan and Chadwick 1983). Senna glycosides, the active principles, are released into the colon after undergoing an enterohepatic circulation. Senna metabolites have been reported by some to pass into breast milk but have not been detected by others, and in controlled studies have had no effect on infants (Baldwin 1963; Werthmann and Krees 1973; Shelton 1980). Senokot is of particular value in prevention of constipation in the puerperium. In one study, two Senokot tablets daily during the first four days postpartum reduced the requirement for an enema from 83 per cent to 1 per cent without adverse effects (Shelton 1980). Senna may colour the urine and lead to erroneous estimation of urinary oestrogens.

Liquid paraffin is contraindicated in pregnancy since it impairs absorption of fat-soluble vitamins, namely vitamins D and K, and aspiration and lipoid pneumonia may occur during vomiting. Seepage through the anal sphincter may cause anal pruritus (Goodman and Gilman 1970). Soap enemata are outdated and should not be used in obstetric practice (Smith 1967; Young *et al* 1968).

The polyphenolic laxatives include phenolphthalein, oxyphenacetin and bisacodyl (Dulcolax). Phenolphthalein is excreted in breast milk and should not be used in pregnancy or the puerperium. In one study 1 gram given to breast-feeding mothers resulted in infant colic (Tyson *et al* 1937). Bisacodyl is effective and has been safely used in pregnancy in enema form (Goosen 1962), or as suppositories (Baydoun 1953), without adverse effects on the fetus. In the puerperium it is more effective than glycerine suppositories (Sweeney 1963). Lactulose, a synthetic disaccharide (fructose and galactose) has not been evaluated in pregnancy (Avery *et al* 1972). Castor oil containing tri-ricinolein is hydrolysed by pancreatic lipase to a hydroxy fatty acid ricinoleate, the active principle (Gaginella *et al* 1977). Although generally considered safe in pregnancy its use has been superseded by other, less violent drugs.

IRRITABLE BOWEL SYNDROME

The irritable bowel syndrome is a heterogeneous group of conditions characterised by intermittent abdominal pain ('spastic colon'), constipation and/or painless diarrhoea. Studies in the nonpregnant have shown abnormalities of fasting myoelectrical activity, not only in the colon (Snape *et al* 1976) but throughout the gut.

There are no specific studies of this syndrome in pregnancy. In the nonpregnant, the combinations of psychotropic agents (e.g. lorazepam), anticholinergic smooth muscle relaxants (e.g. hyoscine, merbeverine, loperamide or lomotil) and stool bulking agents (e.g. ispaghula or bran) have been found beneficial (Ritchie and Truelove 1980). In pregnancy the syndrome should be treated with high-fibre diets with, if necessary, hygroscopic stool bulking agents; the value of anticholinergic antispasmodic agents remains controversial (Ivey 1975) and they are contraindicated in pregnancy. Psychotropic drugs, in particular the tricyclic antidepressants (e.g. amitryptiline) are best avoided in pregnancy in view of their possible teratogenic effects (Beeley 1981).

Ano-rectal disorders

EPIDEMIOLOGY AND CLINICAL FEATURES

Minor ano-rectal disorders are commonly seen during pregnancy in the antenatal clinic and also postpartum. Haemorrhoids are most common with or without fissure-*in-ano* (Simmons 1964; Atkinson and Hudson 1970). In a study of 40 patients with ano-rectal disorders studied in the puerperium, 95 per cent had external haemorrhoids and 37.5 per cent in addition internal haemorrhoids. Prolapse or thrombosis of haemorrhoids was found in 20 per cent. Fissure-*in-ano* was only present in 5 per cent (Atkinson and Hudson 1970). Women who are prone to develop haemorrhoids commonly present for the first time in pregnancy and there is an increased incidence in multiparous patients (Atkinson and Hudson 1970). These conditions are aggravated by constipation (*see* p. 296) and during labour, where rectal prolapse, thromboses or strangulation of haemorrhoids are common. Perineal problems may be further aggravated following episiotomy and later infection.

Mechanisms for the development of haemorrhoids remain unclear. Mechanical factors, such as high pressure in pelvic veins, were once considered, but haemorrhoids often appear in pregnancy before significant enlargement of the uterus. Hormonal effects on the unique anatomy of the haemorrhoidal plexus may predispose to haemorrhoids (Thulesius and Gjöres 1973; Thomson 1975).

Common presentations of ano-rectal disorders in pregnancy include pruritus, rectal bleeding or perineal pain. Mucoid or purulent discharge may occur with secondary inflammation or infection. Uncomplicated haemorrhoids are said not to cause pruritus ani (Gallagher 1971) and the presence of this symptom warrants investigation for underlying causes (*see below*).

MANAGEMENT

Prophylactic measures for most ano-rectal conditions include a high residue diet, early response to the urge to defaecate and avoidance of straining at stool. Persistent constipation should be treated promptly by dietary measures, and, if necessary, with hygroscopic (stool bulking) agents and increased fluid intake.

In most ano-rectal and perineal disorders associated with pruritus a careful history and appropriate tests to exclude fungal or parasitic diseases, recent antibiotic therapy and topical applications of soaps, deodorants and alkaline irritants, etc. and systemic diseases such as diabetes mellitus, should be performed. A thorough physical examination, including proctosigmoidoscopy, is mandatory in all patients presenting with ano-rectal disorders or 'bleeding piles', to exclude underlying causes, e.g. inflammatory bowel disease, venereal disorders, tuberculosis or colorectal carcinoma. Therapeutic measures include frequent warm baths for all conditions, hydrocortisone cream/foam 1 per cent with local anaesthetic, e.g. proctofoam, for severe cases of idiopathic pruritus ani or uncomplicated internal haemorrhoids (Atkinson and Hudson 1970) and anal fissures. Ointments, suppositories and other local therapies containing emollients, astringents or local anaesthetics are of limited value in the management of haemorrhoids or anal fissure, but may be useful in pregnancy in preference to surgical treatment. The treatment of choice for prolapsed haemorrhoids that remain refractory to gentle manual manipulation is prompt surgical management including sclero-therapy. Acute thrombosis, prolapse or inflammation of haemorrhoids in pregnancy should be treated initially with bed rest, analgesia, cold compresses and stool-bulking laxatives. Manual dilatation of the anus, and emergency haemorrhoidectomy may be required to relieve severe symptoms and prevent complications (Schrock 1978).

Hepatic disorders

PHYSIOLOGY, ANATOMY AND HISTOLOGY

In a normal pregnancy, with adequate nutrition, the metabolic changes that occur appear to be without significant effect on liver metabolism or function. Table 9.2 summarises the changes in standard liver function tests which are observed in pregnancy. When due allowance is given for these 'physiological changes', it is clear that hepatic function is not significantly impaired. Abnormalities on liver function testing therefore suggest either coincidental liver disease or an effect of complications of pregnancy, e.g. hyperemesis or toxaemia on the liver. The liver in pregnancy shows no

Table 9.2   Liver function tests in pregnancy.

Serum tests		Change in pregnancy	
General			
Bilirubin	2–14 μmol/l	No change	
Transaminase	7–40 IU/l	No change	
γGT	< 30 IU/l	No change	Alteration signifies hepatic dysfunction
5-nucleotidase	2–17 IU/l	No change	
Prothrombin time	12–14 sec	No change	
Proteins			
Total protein	65–80 g/l	Fall	By 10 g/l by 16th–20th week
Albumin	35–55 g/l	Fall	By 10 g/l mostly in first trimester
Globulin	30–50 g/l	Rise	Progressive increase to term
Fibrinogen	2–4 g/l	Rise	Progressive increase to term
Lipids			
Cholesterol	4–6.5 mmol/l	Rise	Progressive increase to term
Triglyceride	< 1.5 mmol/l	Rise	Progressive increase to term
Enzymes			
Alkaline Phosphatase	30–130 IU/l	Rise	Progressive increase after 5th week to term (1.5 × normal) —placental component skeletal component

undue susceptibility to drugs or toxins. Hepatic blood flow is not increased in pregnancy and therefore a smaller proportion of the increase in cardiac output passes through the liver (Steven 1981).

Hypercholesterolaemia in pregnancy is well documented in both animal and human studies (Richman 1965). Carbohydrate metabolism in the liver during normal pregnancy has been studied in humans and remains undisturbed.

Anatomical relations of the liver are not altered in the first or second trimester. In the third trimester the liver may occupy a more posterio-superior position with displacement to the right, and subsequent reduction in dullness to percussion (Haemmerli 1975); therefore a palpable liver suggests underlying liver disease.

In early studies, the liver in normal pregnancy was considered to show specific histological features with central stasis of bile, dilatation of bile ducts and central vein, and centrilobular steatosis (Hofbauer 1908). Later studies, however, showed no specific changes apart from mild steatosis (Richman 1965).

Certain disorders of the liver are peculiar to pregnancy, others occur in both non-pregnant and pregnant individuals and it is helpful to consider these separately.

LIVER DISEASES PECULIAR TO PREGNANCY

Hyperemesis gravidarum

Haemmerli (1966), in an extensive review of 456 cases of jaundice in pregnancy, found only 27 cases of jaundice due to hyperemesis gravidarum; one resulted in premature labour and perinatal death (Richard *et al* 1970). Sheehan (1940) in a study of 19 cases of fatal hyperemesis, six of whom were jaundiced, reported that liver histology at postmortem was non-specific and included fatty infiltration with centrilobular necrosis. These features are, however, common to severe vitamin and protein malnutrition and may, for example, be found in Wernicke's encephalopathy (Richman 1965).

The aetiology of hyperemesis gravidarum is unknown. Its incidence is greatest in prima gravidae, but there is no relation to maternal age.

In an early clinical study, Thorling (1955) described six cases: five had hyperbilirubinaemia and three raised serum alkaline phosphatase. In a later study of 103 patients, liver function was abnormal in 46 patients: a third had hypoalbuminaemia, 25 per cent had elevated serum transaminases and 60 per cent had increased retention of bromosulphthalein (reduced dye excretion). Liver biopsy performed in four patients was normal, in contrast to findings in viral hepatitis (Adams *et al* 1968).

Pre-eclampsia and eclampsia (*see* p. 163)

The liver is not primarily involved in pre-eclampsia or eclampsia, although in Sherlock's study in 1968 of 17 cases of jaundice in pregnancy, four were attributed to pre-eclampsia and among these were one maternal death and three stillbirths. Haemmerli (1966) attributed 21 of 456 cases of jaundice occurring in pregnancy to eclampsia, and this occasionally may include a haemolytic component (Sheehan 1939).

Histological changes in the liver include multiple petechial haemorrhages, particularly in periportal areas, with confluent necrosis and deposition of fibrin, but no inflammatory infiltrate. These features resemble those of disseminated intravascular coagulation (Antia *et al* 1958; Haemmerli 1966). A vascular theory for the aetiology of the hepatic lesions seems likely, in view of the associated hypertension and renal damage, the extensive haemorrhages and venous congestion (Sheehan 1950), and central and midzonal necrosis of the liver with thrombosis of portal venules and hepatic arterial radicles (Ingerslev and Teilum 1945; Govan and Mukherjee 1950). Hormonal factors may also play a role since the clinical features are similar to those seen after administration of massive doses of oestrogens (Glyn 1950).

Necrosis of the liver may occur rarely in severe cases of eclampsia and management should be similar to that of fulminant hepatic failure (p. 314). Another serious complication of eclampsia is liver rupture (Steven 1981).

Hepatic rupture

Subcapsular haemorrhages in the liver are found in 80 per cent of cases of pre-eclampsia or eclampsia (Margolis and Naidoo 1974). These result from disseminated intravascular coagulation, with deposition of fibrin and thrombosis of hepatic sinusoids, and may lead to tears in the liver (Sommer *et al* 1979). Liver rupture may be precipitated by trauma, uterine contractions, vomiting or convulsions (Bis and Waxman 1976). Vascular malformations, amoebic abscess or tumour account for a minority of cases (Steven 1981). The majority of cases, particularly in association with pre-eclamptic toxaemia, occur in the final trimester, but spontaneous rupture may occur at any time through pregnancy or in the puerperium (Steven 1981). The patient is typically multiparous, hypertensive and approaching term. Onset is sudden with epigastric or right upper quadrant pain, nausea, and/or vomiting. In severe cases rupture may be heralded by shock, hypotension and haemoperitoneum. Laparotomy for suspected perforated viscus reveals the subcapsular tear of haematoma, most commonly in the right lobe.

Management remains difficult with resulting high maternal and fetal mortality (Browne *et al* 1975; Steven 1981). In one study of 60 cases, maternal mortality was 59 per cent, and fetal mortality 62 per cent (Bis and Waxman 1976), although in a later study of four patients, there were no maternal deaths and only one fetal death (Herbert and Brenner 1982). Following hepatic rupture, hepatic failure, renal failure, sepsis, abscess formation and pleural effusion may occur (Steven 1981; Herbert and Brenner 1982).

Diagnosis of intra-abdominal haemorrhage and maternal prognosis have improved with the use of paracentesis (Perry and Strate 1972), radionuclide technetium sulphur colloid scanning to detect hepatic haematoma (Castaneda *et al* 1970) and ultrasonography (Herbert and Brenner 1982). Identification of the site and arrest of bleeding are the primary aims. Bleeding may be arrested by direct ligation of the hepatic artery or selective arterial embolisation (Herbert & Brenner 1982). Lobectomy is performed only when these procedures fail, while some authors favour immediate delivery by Caesarean section (Browne *et al* 1975).

Intrahepatic cholestasis of pregnancy (ICP)

Idiopathic intrahepatic cholestasis (ICP) has been reported to occur in between 1 in 40 (Rannevik *et al* 1972) and 1 in 7000 (Haemmerli 1966) pregnancies, but geographical variation is wide. There appears to be a predilection for this disease in Scandinavian and Mediterranean countries (Bennett *et al* 1979), Chile (Rannevik *et al* 1972), Poland (Roszkowski and Wojcicka 1968) and Australia (Steel and Parker 1973).

The original description of intrahepatic cholestasis of pregnancy as a clinical syndrome of generalised pruritus, mild jaundice and intrahepatic cholestasis occurring predominantly in the third trimester was attributed to Thorling (1955), although this condition was originally described 100 years ago (Eliakim *et al* 1966). Svanborg (1954) described seven women with similar features, but in addition included fatigue and mild abdominal pain. He noted that this condition subsided after delivery but had a tendency to recur in subsequent pregnancies.

Today the classical description of ICP is one of generalised pruritus as the dominant symptom presenting in the third trimester, although the onset may be as early as the sixth week (Fallon 1975; Seymour and Chadwick 1979). Jaundice may develop 7–14 days later, right upper quadrant pain is present in a minority of patients, but hepatomegaly and splenomegaly do not occur. The syndrome persists from 1 to 33 weeks, but promptly clears (often within 48 hours) following delivery (Fallon 1975). The general health of the patient is preserved and fetal prognosis is generally good but ICP commonly recurs in subsequent pregnancies (Fallon 1975; Bennett *et al* 1979; Seymour and Chadwick 1979). Typically the serum bilirubin is elevated to about 70 μmol/l (normal <17) and the alkaline phosphatase to about 40 KA units (normal <15) (Bennett *et al* 1979). The other liver enzymes are only marginally elevated.

Histology of the liver in ICP is normal excepting non-specific centrilobular cholestasis; hepatocellular necrosis and inflammatory infiltration are absent (Seymour and Chadwick 1979).

Intrahepatic cholestasis could result from exaggeration of the normal physiological mechanisms of pregnancy. Measurement of oestrogenic components have shown a reduction in urinary oestriol glucuronide, elevated levels of the sulphated conjugate and impaired biliary excretion of oestriol (Tikkanen and Adlercreutz 1973; Adlercreutz *et al* 1974). Progestins may play a synergistic role (Perez and Gorodisch 1974). Serum biliary lipids are elevated in normal pregnancy and levels are not significantly altered in ICP. Retention of maternal bile acids has been suggested as important, both in fetal distress and intrauterine death (Laatikainen 1983).

The aetiology of this condition is uncertain. There is a positive family history of ICP in 18–44 per cent of cases (Sherlock 1968; Furhoff and Hellstrom 1973; Reyes *et al*

1976). Similar features have been described in nonpregnant patients (Summerskill and Walshe 1959; De Pagter *et al* 1976) recurring with menstruation (Kreek *et al* 1967), in women taking the contraceptive pill, and at the time of the menopause (Orellana-Alcade and Dominguez 1966; Kreek *et al* 1967; Ockner and Davidson 1967; Urban *et al* 1968; Drill 1974; Jeppsson and Rannevik 1976).

The outcome and prognosis for both mother and child are excellent (Seymour and Chadwick 1979). The mother should be reassured that the itching and jaundice will resolve postpartum and that ICP is not always recurrent. She should be warned, however, that pruritus and/or jaundice may recur in subsequent pregnancies. In one study of 27 multiparous women with ICP, 15 had pruritus or jaundice in one subsequent pregnancy, three in more than one pregnancy but the remaining nine were not affected in later pregnancies (Furhoff and Hellstrom 1973).

Pruritus can sometimes be relieved by treatment with cholestyramine, a non-absorbable anion-exchange resin. This drug binds bile acids and has to be used in high dose (16–20 g daily) for effect. Cholestyramine should be gradually introduced and gastrointestinal side-effects are common. This drug also binds anionic drugs and interferes with absorption of fat-soluble vitamins, such as vitamin K. Enzyme-inducing agents, e.g. barbiturates, have been used, with variable results; their prime effect probably acts via sedation (Seymour and Chadwick 1979). Women with a history of ICP should be advised to avoid the contraceptive pill. Screening for viral hepatitis (cholestatic phase) should be performed and serum analysed for mitochondrial antibodies. Hepatic ultrasonography should be performed in all cases to exclude extrahepatic cholestasis, such as large bile duct obstruction from associated gall-stones (Samsioe *et al* 1975) or even cholangio-carcinoma (*see* p. 321). Liver biopsy may be indicated in obscure cases to exclude other causes of intrahepatic cholestasis, e.g. drug toxicity, or in the rare case of ICP where pruritus and/or jaundice occur before the twentieth week, or where serum bilirubin levels remain high even eight weeks after delivery (Misra *et al* 1980).

Management of the fetus is more difficult. In one report of 56 pregnancies in women with ICP, there were five stillbirths and five infants with intrapartum asphyxia (Reid *et al* 1976), but this was not found in a later study (Johnston and Baskett 1979). An increase in incidence of preterm labour and also postpartum haemorrhage was reported by both groups (Reid *et al* 1976; Johnston and Baskett 1979). Measurement of oestriol levels (*see* p. 303) as an index of fetal wellbeing was unsatisfactory. Fetal distress should be anticipated. Vitamin K therapy should be given to the mother during labour and the puerperium and to the child to prevent haemorrhage.

Acute fatty liver

This condition was first recognised as an entity in 1934 by Stander and Cadder, but the differentiation from fulminant viral hepatitis is attributed to Sheehan (1940). Acute fatty liver of pregnancy (AFLP) is rare and, together with pre-eclampsia and hyperemesis gravidarum, accounts for less than 10 per cent of cases of jaundice in pregnancy. However, it is a serious disorder, usually occurring in obese primiparous women often with pre-eclampsia in the last trimester. But occasionally it presents before thirty weeks (Haemmerli 1966) or even in the puerperium (Stander and Cadder 1934; Sheehan 1940; Breen *et al* 1970; Hatfield *et al* 1972; Holtzbach 1974; Cano *et al* 1975; Moldin and Johansson 1978; Varner and Rinderknecht 1980; Burroughs *et al* 1982; Hague *et al* 1983). Interestingly in mothers with AFLP, the incidence of male fetuses is about three times greater than that of females (Hague 1982).

Symptoms develop acutely with abdominal pain (58 per cent), vomiting and headache (35 per cent), jaundice (93 per cent) and impaired conscious level (83 per cent), and may rapidly progress to fulminant hepatic failure, renal failure, bleeding diatheses, coma and death (Kunelis *et al* 1965; Hatfield *et al* 1972; Cano *et al* 1975; Varner and Rinderknecht 1980). The diagnosis of AFLP should always be considered in any patient presenting with vomiting or abdominal pain which are serious symptoms in late pregnancy. Other complications include pancreatitis (Kunelis *et al* 1965; Mackenna *et al* 1972) and necrotising enteritis (colitis) (Varner and Rinderknecht 1980).

Maternal (80 per cent) and fetal (70 per cent) mortalities are exceptionally high, but in the minority of women who survive, fetal loss is around 40 per cent, and maternal recovery is complete. AFLP is said not to recur in subsequent pregnancies (Breen *et al* 1972), and surviving infants are not affected. Fig. 9.1 illustrates the liver function tests through two pregnancies in a woman who had typical acute fatty liver of pregnancy in the first, and remained perfectly well throughout the second pregnancy.

Laboratory findings include a gross neutrophil leucocytosis, the blood urea, creatinine and uric acid levels are also raised, and there is a severe metabolic acidosis.

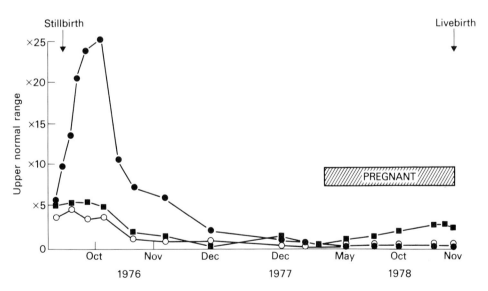

Fig. 9.1   Acute fatty liver of pregnancy: liver function tests during first (abnormal) and second (normal) pregnancies, showing the normal rise in placental alkaline phosphatase in the second pregnancy. ● Bilirubin, ■ Alkaline phosphatase, ○ AST.

Serum urate levels may be elevated out of proportion to the degree of renal dysfunction; hyperuricaemia may even precede the clinical presentation. Abnormalities in liver function tests are not marked. The serum bilirubin is only mildly raised, rarely above 170 μmol/l (10 mg/decilitre) and serum aspartate aminotransferase (AST), alanine (AAT) aminotransferase and serum alkaline phosphatase show small elevations only in contrast to acute viral hepatitis (*see* p. 308). Measurements of clotting parameters are commonly grossly deranged, with elevations in prothrombin (PT) and partial thromboplastin (PTT) times, and fibrin degradation products together with low platelet counts suggesting disseminated intravascular coagulation (Moldin and Johansson 1978; Varner and Rinderknecht 1980).

Morphological changes described at postmortem examination are widespread with fatty infiltration and haemorrhages in many organs including the gut, pancreas, kidney, brain and bone marrow (Kunelis *et al* 1965; Hatfield *et al* 1972). Characteristic features have been described in the liver, which is often small. Hepatic steatosis is marked with microdroplets of fat within hepatocytes. The distribution is panlobular with sparing of periportal areas (Figs 9.2 and 9.3). Centrilobular cholestasis may be prominent but infiltration by inflammatory cells is often mild (Kunelis *et al* 1965; Breen

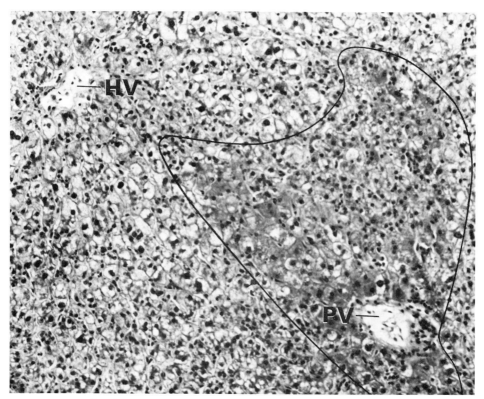

Fig. 9.2   Acute fatty liver of pregnancy (× 150, H&E) showing typical sparing of periportal area (ringed).

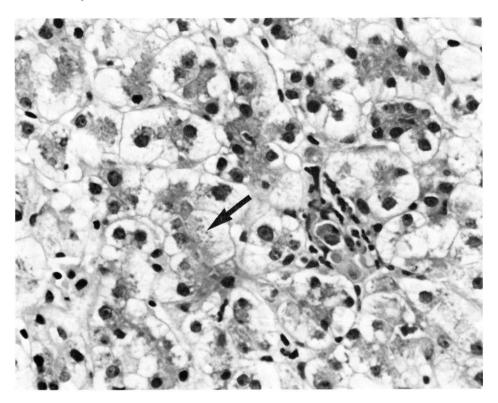

Fig. 9.3   Acute fatty liver of pregnancy (× 600, H&E) showing perinuclear microvesicular steatosis (arrowed) without liver cell necrosis.

et al 1970; Mackenna *et al* 1972). The intrahepatic lipids are free fatty acids in contrast to the triglycerides seen in steatosis associated with obesity, diabetes mellitus or alcoholic liver disease (Eisele *et al* 1975).

The aetiology of this condition remains unknown. Possible predisposing factors have included toxins, viruses, pre-eclampsia, protein and vitamin malnutrition and depression of protein synthesis by tetracyclines (Kunelis *et al* 1965; Hatfield *et al* 1972; Varner and Rinderknecht 1980; Wenk *et al* 1981; Harpey and Charpentier 1983), or less specifically with hypertension. The association with pre-eclampsia, which can also produce changes in the liver and coagulopathy in pregnancy, is important. There may be a common pathophysiological pathway; also some of the 29 maternal deaths ascribed to hypertensive disease in the Confidential Maternal Mortality Census 1976–78 and associated with cerebral haemorrhage, coagulopathy and hepatorenal failure, may have been due to AFLP rather than pre-eclampsia (*Lancet* 1983a).

The chemical syndrome and liver histology of AFLP is very similar to that of Reye's syndrome, a fulminating liver disorder which occurs in children. Transient deficiency of ornithine transcarbamylose and carbamyl synthetase have been described in both conditions (Weber *et al* 1979).

Kunelis and co-workers (1965) reviewed 54 cases of acute fatty liver including ten survivors. There was a history of pyelonephritis in twelve patients and eleven of these had received intravenous tetracyclines, but in four, therapy with tetracyclines had not been recorded, so tetracycline therapy is unlikely to be the only causative factor.

Management involves supportive treatment for fulminant hepatic failure (*see* p. 314), with fresh blood transfusions and clotting factors (Cano *et al* 1975). Hypoglycaemia may be profound, large quantities of glucose may be required (Breen *et al* 1970), and renal dialysis may be necessary. Early delivery by Caesarean section has been advocated (Haemmerli 1966; Conaster and Harris 1975) to improve maternal and fetal prognosis. Epidural anaesthesia should not be used because of the risk of epidural haematoma associated with the coagulopathy.

LIVER DISEASES INCIDENTAL TO PREGNANCY

Acute viral hepatitis

Types and serology

It is now possible to distinguish the common types of acute viral hepatitis using serological tests (Burrell 1980). The presence of the surface antigen, HBsAg, in association with clinical and biochemical features of hepatitis suggest acute infection with type B virus. Subsequent disappearance of HBsAg and appearance of the antibody, anti-HBs, confirms recent infection and signals the development of immunity. For type A hepatitis the infective agent cannot be detected in blood, though virus may be demonstrated by immune electron microscopy in faeces. A rising titre of IgM class antibody to hepatitis A virus (anti-HAV) is the conventional means of confirming recent infection. The absence of the above markers suggests non-A, non-B hepatitis providing other hepatitic viruses such as EB virus, cytomegalovirus and in some geographical areas yellow fever virus are excluded.

Diagnosis in type B virus infection is complicated by the occurrence of a carrier state which may be asymptomatic. Furthermore, it is not inconceivable that type A or non-A, non-B hepatitis could occur in a patient already positive for HBsAg, thus causing confusion. In practice such diagnostic difficulties are unusual. In infections or carrier states due to type B virus, other immunological markers may help to define the type of infection and assess the risk of infectivity, and in particular the risk of materno-fetal vertical transmission (*see* p. 311). Serological studies indicate that all three types of viral hepatitis can occur in pregnancy; the incidence varying with geographical location and ethnic factors.

Clinical features

Clinical features of viral hepatitis are identical in the pregnant and nonpregnant populations. The onset of hepatitis A is usually abrupt, while that of type B and non-A, non-B is more prolonged. Anorexia, nausea, vomiting, upper abdominal pain and malaise usually precede the development of jaundice. Arthralgias and skin rashes are occasional prodromal features, especially in type B infection. Anicteric illnesses are not uncommon. Physical signs are usually limited to jaundice and tender hepatomegaly. The main biochemical features are elevations in serum transaminases with or without elevation of the serum bilirubin. The serum alkaline phosphatase usually shows modest elevations only. The leucocyte count is normal or low, a useful differential point in distinguishing viral hepatitis from acute fatty liver of pregnancy which is associated with leucocytosis (*see* p. 305). Abnormalities of blood clotting are not unusual, but the presence of marked prolongation in the prothrombin time or appearance of thrombocytopenia and fibrin degradation products indicative of disseminated intravascular coagulation suggest fulminant viral hepatitis or acute fatty liver of pregnancy. Renal function is usually preserved in viral hepatitis, but is characteristically impaired in acute fatty liver of pregnancy or in eclampsia.

Clinical and biochemical features together with serological tests usually permit a clear diagnosis. Figs 9.4 and 9.5 illustrate the course of uncomplicated type A and type B hepatitis in pregnancy, with the timing of appearance of the serological markers of infection. Hepatitis A resolves usually within 2–3 weeks after the onset of symptoms, but in the other types recovery may take up to six months. The differential diagnosis of infectious hepatitis in pregnancy is illustrated in Table 9.3. Liver biopsy is not indicated in the majority of patients but when diagnostic difficulties arise, biopsy is safe in pregnancy providing blood clotting parameters are satisfactory.

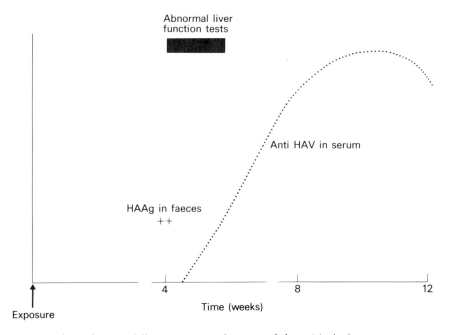

Fig. 9.4   Serological events following acute infection with hepatitis A virus.

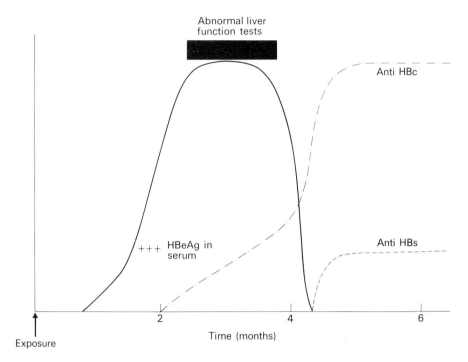

Fig. 9.5   Serological events following acute infection with hepatitis B virus.

Outcome

The effects of viral hepatitis on the course and outcome of pregnancy vary markedly with geographical area and ethnic group. Reviews of the European literature (Haemmerli 1966) reported a maternal mortality of 1.8 per cent similar to that in nonpregnant patients. Furthermore, apart from a possible increase in preterm birth (about 20 per cent), obstetrical complications and congenital malformations were not increased (Siegel 1973; Hieber *et al* 1977). Hepatitis running a non-fulminant course may have little influence on the course of pregnancy, even in areas where the incidence of fulminant hepatitis during pregnancy is much increased, e.g. in Kashmir (Khuroo *et*

Table 9.3   Differential diagnosis of infective hepatitis in pregnancy.

First trimester	Second trimester	Third trimester
Hyperemesis gravidarum Drug reaction	Gallstones Cirrhosis Pyelonephritis	Intrahepatic cholestasis (ICP) Gallstones Cirrhosis Acute fatty liver Eclampsia Pyelonephritis

al 1981). The strikingly high incidence of fulminant hepatitis in pregnancy in some areas, e.g. Kashmir and Iran (22–50 per cent), and appallingly high maternal (greater than 80 per cent) and fetal (100 per cent) mortalities remain unexplained. Of the factors which appear to be relevant, hepatitis in the third trimester and maternal malnutrition have been suggested. A high incidence of hepatitis B is probably not responsible for the high incidence of fulminant hepatitis in certain regions since, in Kashmir, non-A, non-B hepatitis was established as the cause of an outbreak (Khuroo *et al* 1981), and an outbreak in Libya was also not associated with hepatitis B (Christie *et al* 1976). Whether non-A, non-B, hepatitis A or hepatitis B infections differ in their propensity to cause fulminant hepatitis in susceptible ethnic groups remains unresolved.

Fulminant hepatitis

The key features are deterioration in conscious level (encephalopathy), marked abnormalities in blood clotting with development of haemorrhagic manifestations, and hypoglycaemia. Initially jaundice may be absent but it becomes marked in those who survive more than 48 hours. Most cases are due to hepatitis B (Chiaramonte *et al* 1974) but type A and non-A, non-B can cause fulminant hepatitis (Rakela *et al* 1978). Management is intensive (*see* p. 313) involving careful monitoring of vital functions, maintenance of normoglycaemia, correction of coagulopathies and anticipation of infection.

Materno-fetal transmission

The risk of transmission of hepatitis B virus (HBV) from HBsAg positive mothers is much less in Europeans (Boxall *et al* 1980) than in certain other ethnic groups, e.g. the Chinese (up to 64 per cent). In general, there is a high incidence of neonatal HBV infection when maternal hepatitis occurs near term, estimated at 78 per cent for the third trimester (Schweitzer *et al* 1973) and particularly in the presence of maternal 'e' antigen. There is a much lower incidence (approximately 10 per cent) of transmission when maternal infection occurs within the first trimester. This implies that transplacental passage of anti-HBs antibody may prevent transmission of infection occurring early in pregnancy, and that transmission is maximal at or near birth (Woo *et al* 1979). In endemic areas such as Nigeria (Tabor and Gerety 1979) most HBsAg-positive babies (age range 0.5–2 years) were infected very early in life. Furthermore, 85–90 per cent of newborns infected with HBV become chronic carriers for HBsAg (Tong *et al* 1981). These findings support the prevailing view that passive immunization is of prime importance, and that any successful schedule must be carried out very early, probably at birth or within 48 hours, for maximum efficacy.

Passive immunisation with hepatitis B immunoglobulin (anti HBs titre of 1 : 100 000) is currently advised for infants of HBsAg-positive mothers, with repeated doses monthly for six months (Zuckerman 1980). Active immunisation with inactivated hepatitis B virus is effective in chimpanzees (Hilleman *et al* 1978; Purcell and Gerin 1978) and has been evaluated with promising results in adult males

(Hilleman *et al* 1978). These vaccines are currently being evaluated in paediatric practice, and the newborn appears to mount a vigorous immune response following paediatric vaccination (Barin *et al* 1982). Current policy is to recommend vaccination with the triple inactivated hepatitis B vaccine in the neonates of all HBe antigen-positive mothers at birth.

Although vertical transmission of hepatitis B is well accepted there is no consensus view as to whether there is materno-fetal transmission of hepatitis A or non-A, non-B hepatitis. Perinatal transmission of non-A, non-B hepatitis agents has been suggested by the observation of elevated liver enzymes in infants whose mothers had acute liver disease in late pregnancy (Tong *et al* 1981), but in the absence of specific markers, this issue remains open.

Chronic hepatitis

Types

Acute hepatitis may be followed by complete clinical remission with restoration of normal liver function tests and histology. However, in some individuals a period of mild, non-specific ill-health associated with persistently abnormal liver function tests and mild periportal inflammation on biopsy ('chronic persistent hepatitis') occurs. In a further group, a chronic relapsing disorder with more severe constitutional disturbances, disordered liver function and more extensive inflammatory change in the liver occurs ('chronic active hepatitis').

Chronic persistent hepatitis

This disorder is usually thought to be benign and not to progress to cirrhosis. It may persist for several months following acute viral hepatitis. Pregnancy documented in individuals with chronic persistent hepatitis was not associated with any maternal or fetal morbidity and spontaneous labour and normal delivery occurred (Infield *et al* 1979).

Chronic active hepatitis

Little information is available about HBsAg positive chronic active hepatitis. However, in Western countries, most cases of chronic active hepatitis are not HBsAg-positive but have autoimmune features with hypergammaglobulinaemia and anti-smooth muscle antibodies. Histologically, the characteristic features include a chronic inflammatory cell infiltrate in the portal tracts with extension beyond the 'limiting plate' to surround islands of hepatocytes ('piecemeal necrosis') or with extension of inflammation and necrosis towards central veins ('bridging necrosis'). Untreated, the disorder is associated with amenorrhoea and infertility, progression to cirrhosis and even liver failure. Introduction of corticosteroids and azathioprine has led to increased fertility (Steven *et al* 1979) and a marked improvement in the pregnant and nonpregnant patient. Liver function is preserved during pregnancy but an increased incidence of fetal prematurity and low birthweight has been recorded (Steven *et al* 1979). Obstetrical complications (urinary infections, toxaemia) are also frequent and in some series fetal loss was high reaching from 33 per cent to 55 per cent but with no increased incidence of congenital malformation (Steven *et al* 1979; Whelton and Sherlock 1968).

Prednisolone therapy for chronic active hepatitis should be continued throughout pregnancy and the conventional dose (10–20 mg daily) increased with any sign of relapse (Whelton and Sherlock 1968) although this is unusual (10–15 per cent) (Steven *et al* 1979). Azathioprine has an established role in the treatment of chronic active hepatitis per se as maintenance therapy (50–100 mg per day) in combination with prednisolone (10 mg daily) but during pregnancy disease activity should be controlled with corticosteroids alone and azathioprine re-introduced only if control is inadequate (Fallon 1975) (*see* p. 226 for a discussion of azathioprine in pregnancy). Corticosteroids are less effective in HBsAg positive chronic active hepatitis, and in one report (Schweitzer and Peters 1976) two maternal deaths occurred during pregnancy.

Fulminant hepatic failure

Definition and aetiology

Fulminant hepatic failure (FHF) is a rare disorder that follows massive necrosis of presumably previously normal hepatocytes and should be differentiated from acute hepatic failure superimposed on a background of chronic liver disease (Braude *et al* 1981). In the nonpregnant population, fulminant hepatic failure may occur following paracetamol overdose or viral hepatitis. Uncommon causes include idiosyncratic drug reactions, halothane anaesthesia or Wilson's disease. In pregnancy this clinical syndrome typically occurs in acute fatty liver of pregnancy (*see* p. 304) and may also be a complication of viral hepatitis (*see* above).

Clinical features and management

Fulminant hepatic failure is heralded by restlessness, confusion, hallucinations, drowsiness, convulsions and vomiting, and these rapidly progress to stupor, coma and death. Onset may be so acute that these neurological features precede the development of jaundice although deep jaundice usually occurs within a few days. Clinical features in addition include fetor hepaticus, asterixis and constructional apraxia (grade I encephalopathy) progressing to deep coma with hypertonia and decerebrate and decorticate posturing (Grade IV). Haemorrhage from the gastrointestinal tract (both haematemesis and melaena) and other sites secondary to disseminated intravascular coagulation is well recognised, and there may be renal failure due to hypovolaemia, acute tubular necrosis or infections (Wilkinson *et al* 1974). The liver may be very small; there may be no stigmata of chronic liver disease. Laboratory findings initially include a very high serum transaminase and prolonged prothrombin time, leucocytosis (in contrast to the leucopaenia typically seen in uncomplicated acute viral hepatitis) and occasional thrombocytopenia when associated with disseminated intravascular coagulation. The serum albumin remains normal and serum alkaline phosphatase is only modestly elevated. The serum transaminases may fall early in the course of illness, when there is limited regeneration of hepatocytes, and correspondingly signifies a poor prognosis.

The management of any patient with fulminant hepatic failure requires meticulous intensive care in a specialist centre where facilities for full medical, surgical and obstetric support are available, and where complications can be anticipated. Although the mortality rate from FHF remains alarmingly high, the regenerative capacity of the liver in those few survivors (approximately 15 per cent) is high, and full functional recovery is possible.

A low protein (20 g), high carbohydrate (3000 Cal) and low salt (22 mMol) diet should be prescribed. Hypoglycaemia is frequent and should be anticipated with regular estimations of blood sugar and infusions of 10 per cent dextrose. Concomitant drug therapy, in particular sedative agents, should be completely withdrawn and intercurrent infections treated. Cardiovascular problems include hypotension and dysrhythmias. Monitoring of potassium levels is essential since both hypo- and hyperkalaemia occur. Regular estimations of prothrombin time are essential and rapidly rising values indicate a poor prognosis. Common modes of death are via:

1   Gastrointestinal haemorrhage from gastric erosions; mortality rates are less with cimetidine prophylaxis (MacDougall *et al* 1977).
2   Cerebral oedema from raised intracranial pressure; direct measurement may be required to effect early treatment with osmotic agents, e.g. mannitol, since the classical sign of raised intracranial pressure—papilloedema—is often absent.
3   Renal failure (functional or secondary to acute tubular necrosis) with severe acid-base imbalance, lactic acidosis and hyponatraemia are common and sinister.
4   Respiratory arrest is common from raised intracranial pressure, but hyperventilation and a respiratory alkalosis may also occur.
5   Acute haemorrhagic pancreatitis.

Corticosteroids are not of proven benefit. Charcoal or membrane haemoperfusion provide the best hope of artificial liver support (Jenkins and Williams 1980). In those who recover, chronic liver disease and cirrhosis are said not to occur.

Fulminant viral hepatitis may be difficult to differentiate clinically from acute fatty liver in pregnancy. Laboratory features in acute fatty liver show serum bilirubin and transaminase levels lower than in fulminant viral hepatitis and the liver histology (where possible) is diagnostic. In fulminant hepatic failure from viral hepatitis the serum transaminases are usually very high, e.g. 2000 IU/litre. In the UK, only 25 per cent show the surface antigen HBsAg (Trewby and Williams 1977), and although a marker for hepatitis A is now available (*see* p. 308) this remains a rare cause (Redeker 1978).

Cirrhosis

Pregnancy in patients with advanced cirrhosis remains uncommon and, until 1965, there were only eighteen reported cases with five maternal deaths (including four from hepatic causes), and two fetal deaths (Richman 1965). Recent surveys have clarified the prognosis for mother and fetus and the effects of the pregnancy on co-existing liver disease (Cheng 1977; Britton 1982).

Effects on fertility and pregnancy

Irregular menses (oligomenorrhoea and amenorrhoea) are common in cirrhotic women and relate to the degree of hepatic dysfunction (Britton 1982). Compensated cirrhosis secondary to extrahepatic obstruction generally has a good prognosis in pregnancy (Fallon 1975; Cheng 1977; Britton 1982). Studies of the effects of existing maternal cirrhosis on fetal survival show that, overall, there is a high perinatal mortality of 11–18 per cent, predominantly from stillbirths (7–13 per cent) (Huchzermeyer 1971; Cheng 1977; Britton 1982) and this may relate to maternal nutritional status (Cheng 1977). In early pregnancy there is increased risk of spontaneous abortion. The rate in cirrhotic women was 10–11 per cent (Huchzermeyer 1971; Britton 1982) and appeared further increased (17 per cent) in patients without prior porto-systemic shunt surgery (Cheng 1977). The cause of the increased abortion rate in advanced cirrhosis remains unknown; it does not correlate directly with the level of hepatic dysfunction on testing (Cheng 1977).

Maternal prognosis depends on the degree of decompensation of cirrhosis (Fallon 1975; Cheng 1977). The incidence of toxaemia and anaemia do not appear to be increased. There is an increased risk (25 per cent) of postpartum haemorrhage in cirrhotic patients, particularly in patients who have previously undergone porto-systemic shunt surgery (Cheng 1977).

In general, maternal prognosis depends on the degree of hepatic dysfunction during the pregnancy, and not necessarily on the type (aetiology) of the cirrhosis, although bilary and postnecrotic cirrhosis, if compensated, carry the best prognosis. The presence of a portacaval shunt is not necessarily a contraindication to future pregnancy, and the latter does not add to the risk of chronic liver disease (Cheng 1977).

Effects of pregnancy on disease

The gloomy prognosis of mother and child once associated with co-existing maternal cirrhosis has now been modified. In general, if hepatic function is well compensated without portal hypertension, and if the liver histology is bilary, postnecrotic in type or consistent with Wilson's disease, the prognosis for the mother is good (Richman 1965; Britton 1982). In one study of 16 pregnancies there was only one maternal death and one variceal bleed, although overall hepatic function deteriorated (Whelton and Sherlock 1968). In Cheng's literature survey (1977) 54 per cent of women with documented severe cirrhosis had successful term pregnancies without maternal complications. In a study of oesophageal varices in a total of 160 pregnancies, variceal bleeds occurred on 38 occasions with associated maternal mortalities from variceal bleeds of 18 per cent in the cirrhotic, and 2 per cent in the non-cirrhotic group respectively. These figures compared with a 38 per cent mortality in nonpregnant cirrhotic patients and suggests that there is no increased risk of fatal haemorrhage from oesophageal varices in pregnancy (Britton 1982). The spontaneous abortion rate was also only 10 per cent.

In some studies, liver function during pregnancy has been shown to improve for primary biliary cirrhosis (Ahrens *et al* 1950), Wilson's disease (Bihl 1959; Sherwin *et al* 1960; Dreifuss and McKinney 1966) and other diseases (Bennett *et al* 1963; Slaughter and Kranz 1963; Borhanmanesh and Haghighi 1970).

In contrast, adverse effects of the pregnancy on the mother and fetus are common in cirrhotic women with decompensated liver disease (Fallon 1975; Cheng 1977). Liver dysfunction is further impaired (Whelton and Sherlock 1968; Huchzermeyer 1971) in at least one-third of cases (Huchzermeyer 1971; Britton 1982). The increased incidence of hepatic failure and coma has been linked with toxic effects of oestrogens on the liver (Johnston *et al* 1965). There is increased risk of bleeding from varices reported in many (Moore and Hughes 1960; Gordon and Johnston 1963; Johnston *et al* 1965; Huchzermeyer 1971) but not all studies (Whelton and Sherlock 1968; Britton 1982).

Management

The management of cirrhosis in pregnancy requires a rational programme. When pregnancy occurs in a patient with compensated cirrhosis, without jaundice or previously impaired liver function, the pregnancy should be allowed to proceed to term with attendance to rest, vitamin supplements and diet (high carbohydrate and low protein in advanced cirrhosis) (Richman 1965). Although vaginal delivery is safely achieved in the majority of cases (Britton 1982) a protracted second stage of labour should be anticipated and interrupted by early forceps delivery to avoid excess straining with subsequent rise in portal pressure. Excess blood loss should also be anticipated and facilities to deal with bleeding oesophageal varices made available (Cheng 1977). In patients with chronic liver disease, care with sedation is required, particularly with opiates. Other agents such as halothane, general anaesthesia and chlorothiazide diuretics should be used with caution since these and other factors, including excess blood loss, occult infection, hypoglycaemia, hypotension and constipation can all precipitate hepatic encephalopathy. Tetracyclines are contraindicated in pregnancy (p. 18) and particularly in patients with liver disease (p. 308).

Surgical intervention by Caesarean section should be reserved for urgent situations to save the infant in the presence of rapidly deteriorating liver function, but the prognosis for mother and child in these circumstances remains poor (Cheng 1977). Elective termination of pregnancy should only be considered in advanced, decompensated cirrhosis, and then, only in the first trimester (Richman 1965).

Portal hypertension and varices

Many, although not all (Britton 1982), authors agree that there is an increased risk of bleeding from oesophageal varices if they are present in pregnancy. Haematemesis can occur at any time, but most frequently in the second trimester (Britton 1982). The risk appears to be independent of variceal size. The prognosis for mother and child is very poor. Cheng (1977) found a 60 per cent maternal mortality, although in Britton's later survey (1982) overall maternal and fetal mortality was approximately 10 per cent.

Porto-systemic shunt surgery

In Cheng's retrospective survey (1977) of 117 pregnant women with cirrhosis, there was a lower rate of spontaneous abortion and lower incidence of toxaemia and anaemia in women who had undergone previous shunt surgery before pregnancy. Maternal mortality was also lower in the group with previous shunt surgery. There were twelve maternal deaths; nine in women without and three with prior shunt surgery. Porto-systemic shunt surgery can be safely performed during pregnancy; seven women with cirrhosis and one with extrahepatic dysfunction proceeded to surgery during pregnancy for acute variceal bleeds with no maternal loss and relatively good fetal outcome (one death). Bleeds from oesophageal varices occurred on 24 occasions in 117 cirrhotic women, and on 14 occasions in 32 women with portal hypertension and varices secondary to extrahepatic obstruction. There were 17 deaths in the first group and one death in the second group, suggesting a better maternal prognosis in the group with extrahepatic obstruction.

Postpartum haemorrhage is a particular hazard to the pregnant woman with intrahepatic portal hypertension and the risk appears increased in patients with prior shunt surgery (Whelton and Sherlock 1968).

Primary biliary cirrhosis

Until recently, pregnancy in primary biliary cirrhosis (PBC) had been rarely reported (Ahrens *et al* 1950; Sherlock 1981). In an early study (Whelton and Sherlock 1968) fetal mortality was high and prognosis poor. In Cheng's retrospective survey (1977) covering the years 1923–77, there were 124 recorded cases of PBC, all without prior shunt surgery; three patients had spontaneous abortions, but there were no maternal deaths. Early studies on PBC concentrated on the disease in its advanced stage at presentation. Today PBC may present in less advanced stages or indeed be asymptomatic (Long *et al* 1977); reappraisal of this disease is therefore necessary in pregnancy. Early studies on intrahepatic cholestasis of pregnancy (*see* p. 303) have undoubtedly included cases of PBC, and the latter has previously been underdiagnosed. These two conditions are very similar in presentation, although the finding of mitochondrial antibodies in more than 95 per cent of patients with PBC (Munzoz *et al* 1981) should help to differentiate PBC from intrahepatic cholestasis in a patient with intractable pruritus during pregnancy. Also ICP usually resolves in the puerperium. The effects of pregnancy on the disease, in its newly recognised milder form, are difficult to assess. Results of liver function are variable, with reports of deterioration (Whelton and Sherlock 1968) or even improvement (Ahrens *et al* 1950) during pregnancy. There are no prospective studies on later maternal prognosis in women with early PBC first diagnosed in pregnancy. Therapy for this disease is generally disappointing. Trials of penicillamine in PBC in the nonpregnant have concentrated on advanced forms of the disease, and although liver function tests may improve, this drug does not appear to significantly arrest the progression of liver histology. There are no trials relating to pregnancy (*see* Wilson's disease below).

Wilson's disease

Pregnancy, although uncommon in untreated Wilson's disease, has been reported (Bihl 1959; Toaff *et al* 1977; Walshe 1977). Subfertility, spontaneous abortions and amenorrhoea are frequent, but successful treatment with chelating agents appears to correct the subfertility. The neurological state appears to improve during pregnancy and this is thought to be due to the extraction of copper by the fetus (Toaff *et al* 1977). Liver function has also been shown to improve (Bihl 1959; Sherwin *et al* 1960; Dreifuss and McKinney 1966). Pregnancy is very uncommon in patients with advanced cirrhosis and portal hypertension from Wilson's disease, with resulting high maternal and fetal morbidities and mortalities.

Penicillamine therapy is generally considered safe and should be continued throughout pregnancy (Walshe 1977). Continuous treatment is associated with a lower risk of miscarriage and clinical relapse of disease (Walshe 1977). D-penicillamine crosses the placenta (Crawhall *et al* 1967) but fetal abnormalities are very uncommon (Walshe 1977). In 87 patients with Wilson's desease taking penicillamine there were only two fetal abnormalities (Endres 1981) (*see* p. 266).

Treatment therefore consists of D-penicillamine throughout pregnancy with possible reduction in dose, i.e. 0.25–0.5 g daily (Marecek and Graf 1976). Pyridoxine supplements are also recommended since D-penicillamine may deplete maternal stores (Steven 1981).

Budd–Chiari syndrome

The Budd–Chiari syndrome is defined as obstruction to the hepatic venous outflow tract, extending from the sublobular veins to any site up to entry of the inferior vena cava into the right atrium (Sherlock 1974). The first case described by Chiari in 1899 followed childbirth and between then and 1980 there have been over 28 cases occurring during pregnancy or postpartum (Krass 1957; Hancock 1968; Datta *et al* 1972; Dentsch *et al* 1972; Khuroo and Datta 1980). The aetiology of this condition is unclear. In the nonpregnant Western population, polycythaemia rubra vera remains a major association (Tavill *et al* 1975).

There is an increased incidence of Budd–Chiari syndrome in women taking the contraceptive pill (Khuroo and Datta 1980; Steven 1981). Clotting factor activities are increased in pregnancy (Nilsson and Kullanders 1967) although no increase was found in studies of Budd–Chiari syndrome following pregnancy (Khuroo and Datta 1980).

Clinical symptoms and signs commonly include acute abdominal pain, rapidly developing ascites and abdominal distension. In one study of 105 patients with Budd–Chiari syndrome occurring between 1963 and 1968, 16 patients presented in association with pregnancy (Khuroo and Datta 1980). In 15, presentation occurred four days to four weeks postpartum, and in only one patient did presentation occur during pregnancy. The prognosis for Budd–Chiari associated with pregnancy is uniformly bad (Steven 1981). Only two of 16 patients gained relief of symptoms despite various treatments, including anticoagulation, reinfusion of ascites or surgery involving porta-caval, splenorenal or mesocaval shunts. The maternal mortality following surgical intervention was 50 per cent (Khuroo and Datta 1980).

Diagnosis is best achieved by a combination of percutaneous liver biopsy and percutaneous hepatic venous catheterisation. Liver histology, although not entirely specific for Budd–Chiari, commonly shows centrizonal venous congestion, haemorrhage, necrosis and dilatation of sinusoids and central veins (Krass 1957; Datta *et al* 1972; Tavill *et al* 1975). Hepatic venography is diagnostic.

Inflammatory bowel disease and the liver

Abnormalities of the liver detected by liver function testing occur in a significant proportion (8 per cent) of patients with inflammatory bowel disease (Perrett *et al* 1971a and b; BMJ 1979). Clinically overt liver disease may occur in up to 5 per cent of patients with inflammatory bowel disease (Greenstein *et al* 1976). Liver biopsies taken at surgery or postmortem from patients with inflammatory bowel disease show hepatic abnormalities in at least 50–95 per cent of specimens (Palmer *et al* 1964; Eade 1970). Sclerosing cholangitis and bile duct carcinoma occur more commonly in ulcerative colitis than in Crohn's colitis. Hepatic involvement in small bowel Crohn's disease is unusual. These abnormalities bear no constant relation to length of symptoms or mode of therapy and the aetiology of these extraintestinal manifestations remains unknown. There are no specific reports of the significance in pregnancy of liver abnormalities in IBD.

Oral contraceptive steroids and the liver

Various benign and malignant hepatic lesions have been found more commonly in users than non-users of oral contraceptive steroids (*see* p. 320). Hepatic adenoma and follicular nodular hyperplasia, although rare, are well-recognised associations in women taking mestranol, or occasionally with ethynyl oestradiol, and the validity of classifying them as totally benign is uncertain. Other histological diagnoses of benign lesions have been variously reported including cholestasis, haemartomata, solitary hyperplastic nodule, focal cirrhosis (Huggins 1981) peliosis hepatitis and periportal sinusoidal dilatation, the latter possibly in association with inflammatory bowel disease (Camilleri *et al* 1981).

Liver transplantation

Two normal, consecutive pregnancies have been reported occurring 27 and 56 months respectively following orthotopic liver transplantation for Budd–Chiari syndrome in a patient taking azathioprine and prednisolone (Schmid and Newton 1980).

Gastrointestinal and hepatic malignancies

GASTRIC AND COLONIC CANCERS

Malignancy of the gastrointestinal tract, discovered during a normal pregnancy, is a considerable problem both for the patient and her physician. Less than 20 often single case reports of primary adenocarcinoma of the stomach (Sims *et al* 1980), primary (Banner *et al* 1945; Swartley *et al* 1947; Der Brucke 1949; Putzki *et al* 1949; Waters and Fenimore 1954; Green *et al* 1975) and metastatic (Watson and Kennedy 1980) carcinoma of the large intestine have been reported, but the true incidence of gastrointestinal malignancy complicating pregnancy is unknown. Although malignancies in general occurring in normal pregnancy are rare, they formed a significant proportion (21 of 387) of maternal deaths in England and Wales during 1973–5 (DHSS 1979), and excluding the five deaths from cerebral tumours, deaths from colorectal malignancy (three cases) were second commonest. The single case reports suggest that colorectal carcinoma may be diagnosed late in pregnancy after metastatic spread and possibly because of delay in initiating investigations (Girard *et al* 1981). These reports highlight the need to consider gastrointestinal malignancy in cases of protracted vomiting (Sims *et al* 1980), abdominal pain, constipation and rectal bleeding (Green *et al* 1975), and to proceed to fibreoptic endoscopic and even radiological investigation if necessary (Sims *et al* 1980; Girard *et al* 1981). Pregnancy appears to have no adverse effect on the carcinoma or vice versa. The maternal prognosis in reported cases is, however, extremely poor, with no survivors beyond five years (Girard *et al* 1981).

Reports are too limited to speculate on possible aetiological factors. In a controlled survey of 143 women in the general population with colorectal cancer there was an association between lower parity (compared with controls) and future incidence of colonic (but not rectal) cancer and these findings were consistent with those from a previous report (Weiss *et al* 1981) but the possible interrelation between endometrial cancer, colonic cancer and exogenous or endogenous oestrogens remains an open issue (Schottenfeld *et al* 1969; Weiss 1978; Weiss *et al* 1981).

HEPATIC TUMOURS

Hepatic adenomata, and the related lesion focal nodular hyperplasia (FNH), although generally uncommon, are found most frequently in young women, with a high proportion aged 26–30 years and taking the contraceptive pill (Grabowski *et al* 1975; Mays *et al* 1976; Fechner 1977; Klatskin 1977; Knowles *et al* 1978; Rooks *et al* 1979; Goldman 1980) and an increased occurrence in patients using mestranol rather than ethynyl oestradiol compounds (Vana *et al* 1977). Some of these lesions show features of both adenoma and FNH. Carcinomatous changes have been documented in hepatic adenomata suggesting an interrelationship between hepatic adenoma, focal nodular hyperplasia and carcinoma (Klatskin 1977) and casting doubt on their 'benign' classification. Cases of hepatic adenoma (Kent *et al* 1977; Check *et al* 1978; Kent *et al*

1978) and focal nodular hyperplasia (Whelan *et al* 1973; Knowles *et al* 1978) becoming manifest in pregnancy have been reported.

These lesions often present acutely with rupture of the tumour (Davies *et al* 1973; Mays *et al* 1976; Kent *et al* 1978; Rooks *et al* 1979) or liver (Hibbard 1976). The patient at highest risk from spontaneous rupture is a woman with a large hepatic adenoma taking a high dose combined contraceptive pill preparation for more than four years (Huggins 1981), and rupture is more frequent during pregnancy or menstruation (Keifer and Scott 1977). Clinical features include the finding of an asymptomatic mass, but the majority of patients complain of epigastric or right upper quadrant pain, and may present in shock. Routine blood tests do not help in differential diagnosis and liver function tests remain unimpaired. Diagnosis is best made by hepatic ultrasound and selective coeliac axis arteriography. These tumours are very vascular, and percutaneous needle biopsy is hazardous and should be performed under direct vision. Surgical resection still carries a significant mortality (Whelan *et al* 1973). Spontaneous regression may occur following delivery or withdrawal of exogenous oestrogens, so that a conservative approach in benign lesions may be contemplated (Steven 1981).

Primary hepatocellular carcinoma and cholangiocarcinoma (Haemmerli 1966) occurring in pregnancy have been rarely reported (less than ten cases), and this is surprising considering the high incidence of both diseases in certain countries such as Africa, their prevalence in younger persons of childbearing age and their known associations and markers—HBsAg and alpha-fetoprotein—both widely measured in antenatal screening (Purtilo *et al* 1975; Egwnatu 1980; Haddow *et al* 1980). In the six cases (two cholangiocarcinoma, four hepatocellular carcinoma) collected up to 1980, cirrhosis was only found in the hepatocellular group (Egwuatu 1980). The clinical features of abdominal pain and a mass are similar to findings in the nonpregnant population (Salih *et al* 1978) and regardless of pregnancy the maternal and fetal outlook remains poor (Egwuatu 1980; Steven 1981).

CHORIO-CARCINOMA

The persistence of elevated or rising titres of urinary human chorionic gonadotrophin (hCG) after evacuation of a hydatidiform mole indicates residual functional trophoblastic tissue, and possibly the malignant transformation to chorio-carcinoma (gestational trophoblastic neoplasia) (Grumbine *et al* 1980; Huggins 1981). Those patients with metastases to the liver are often classified as high risk from life-threatening hepatic haemorrhage. Rarely hepatic metastases in the infant have been reported (Aozaga *et al* 1981). Combined treatment with selective hepatic arterial embolisation and multiagent chemotherapy is perhaps the approach offering the least morbidity and best chance of survival (Grumbine *et al* 1980).

Biliary disorders

CHOLESTEROL CHOLELITHIASIS

Epidemiology and pathophysiology

Cholesterol gallstones are common in Europe and Western countries and are found in women more often than in men (Bennion and Grundy 1978). This sex difference commences during puberty and remains during reproductive life. Other established risk factors for the development of cholesterol cholelithiasis include obesity, endogenous or exogenous female sex hormones, gastrointestinal disorders with bile salt malabsorption, such as ileal disease, e.g. Crohn's disease or small bowel resection. Parity and/or pregnancy may also be risk factors (Samsioe *et al* 1975; Bennion and Grundy 1978; Braverman *et al* 1980).

In the pathogenic sequence of cholesterol cholelithiasis, a prerequisite for stone formation includes the hepatic secretion of lithogenic bile (Everson *et al* 1982). In the nonpregnant female (compared to the male) there is a reduction in total bile acid pool, in particular the chenodeoxycholic acid (CDCA) pool. Studies on the composition of bile in pregnancy yield conflicting results although in general there appears to be an additional increase in bile saturation (and reduction in CDCA pool). These findings mimic those found during oestrogen therapy (Bennion and Grundy 1978).

Other factors that may play an important role in cholesterol cholelithiasis involve impaired gallbladder function (emptying). In pregnancy, cholycystographic and ultrasonographic studies have shown impaired rates of gallbladder emptying (decreased by 30 per cent) and increased gallbladder residual volumes, following a liquid meal after the first trimester (Braverman *et al* 1980) or through pregnancy (Everson *et al* 1982). Gallbladder emptying was shown to be impaired in the luteal phase of the ovulatory cycle in one study (Nilsson and Stattin 1967) but was considered normal in a recent study (Everson *et al* 1982). Conversely, women taking oral contraceptive steroids were found to have either normal gallbladder volumes and emptying (Braverman *et al* 1980) or increased fasting volumes (Everson *et al* 1982) on ultrasonographic analysis after a liquid meal. These effects may result from the relaxant action of progestogens on smooth muscle, although the progressive rise seen in serum progestogens after the eleventh week of pregnancy does not directly correlate with gallbladder dysfunction, which can be seen before the twelfth week. Oestrogens may impair water absorption by the gallbladder by inhibiting the action of the sodium-potassium ATP-ase pump (Braverman *et al* 1980). In America, the Food & Drugs Administration require that information on the increased risks of gallbladder disease be included with instructions to users of oral contraceptive steroids (FDA 1978).

Management

Jaundice and biliary obstruction by gallstones occurring in pregnancy is considered rare (less that 5 per cent of cases of jaundice in pregnancy) by some (Haemmerli 1966), but not others (Richards *et al* 1970; Steel and Parker 1973). The management of acute cholecystitis or biliary obstruction occurring in pregnancy is the same as in the non-pregnant patient and includes bed rest, withdrawal of oral feeding, rehydration with intravenous fluids and antibiotics such as ampicillin. Diagnosis can often be made by ultrasound, which is safe in pregnancy. For simple biliary colic and/or cholecystitis, a conservative approach is reasonable with consideration for cholecystectomy postpartum. Surgical intervention is obligatory in the presence of large duct obstruction to avoid recurrent attacks and other complications: cholangitis, pancreatitis (p. 324) and empyema of the gallbladder. Rarely, biliary obstruction may be due to cholangiocarcinoma (Haemmerli 1966) or even *Clonorchis silensis* (in the Far East), and management is similar to that in the nonpregnant.

The use of bile acid therapy, chenodeoxycholic (Schoenfield *et al* 1981; Maton *et al* 1982) or ursodeoxycholic acids to dissolve cholesterol gallstones is not indicated in pregnancy. Although no adverse effects on the mother or fetus have been recorded in isolated reports, the Committee on the Safety of Medicines has not approved their use in pregnancy and, should pregnancy occur on therapy, they should be withdrawn.

Pancreatic disorders

Exocrine pancreatic function tests have not been performed in the human during pregnancy.

ENDOCRINE PANCREATIC FUNCTION (*see also* Chapter 10)

In pregnancy there is a reduced level of fasting blood glucose but increased postprandial response. Plasma levels of pancreatic polypeptide (PP) are reduced in pregnancy and the response to a glucose tolerance test is reduced compared to that in the nonpregnant (Kitzmiller *et al* 1980; Hornnes and Kühl 1981). In pregnancy, there appears to be a reduction in cholinergic tone, and this is consistent with a reduced signal to PP secretion in the pancreas via cholinergic nerves rather than a direct effect of glucose on the PP-containing cell (Glaser *et al* 1980; Hornnes and Kühl 1981). Other factors, e.g. delay in gastric emptying, may affect the PP response but this is not invariably found in pregnancy (Hornnes and Kühl 1981). Limited studies of other hormones, i.e. glucagon and insulin have been performed in humans during pregnancy and the puerperium. The responses of plasma glucagon and insulin to an oral alanine load were measured in seven normal pregnant females in the third trimester and during the puerperium (Kitzmiller *et al* 1980). Increased levels of basal plasma glucagon and insulin, together with an elevated response to oral alanine were seen at 34 weeks compared to postpartum levels. In the late puerperium there was both a reduction in basal levels of glucagon and insulin, and a reduced response to the oral load compared to levels taken during pregnancy. The comparison of levels of pancreatic hormones measured in the puerperium, with those measured during pregnancy, may not, however, be strictly valid (Kitzmiller *et al* 1980).

ACUTE PANCREATITIS

Epidemiology and clinical features

Acute pancreatitis is an uncommon cause of abdominal pain in pregnancy, occurring in one in 1066–3800 pregnancies (Joupilla *et al* 1974) or one in 1100–11 000 live births (Corlett and Mishell 1972; Wilinson 1973).

The morbidity and mortality from severe acute pancreatitis remains high in both nonpregnant and pregnant populations. Deaths from acute pancreatitis were 11.4 per million in the general population, according to the Registrar General's Statistical Review for England & Wales (1969). In early surveys of acute pancreatitis in pregnancy, maternal deaths were as high as 20 per cent (Langmade and Edmondson 1951; Montgomery and Miller 1970) with neonatal losses between 35 and 50 per cent (Montgomery and Miller 1970; Wilinson 1973).

In a study of 590 cases of acute pancreatitis in the general population between 1950 and 1969 that included four pregnant patients and 13 postpartum, Trapnell and Duncan (1975) found biliary tract disease present in 53.6 per cent of cases. Alcoholism was present in 4.4 per cent of cases, whereas drugs (steroids), hyperparathyroidism and infection, e.g. mumps, accounted for 1 per cent each respectively. In a similar study in pregnancy (Berk *et al* 1971) biliary tract disease was present in 36 per cent of cases, alcoholism 1 per cent, whereas drugs (chlorothiazides) accounted for 8 per cent, infections 25 per cent and significantly, toxaemia in 9 per cent of patients.

The aetiological mechanisms of acute pancreatitis in pregnancy are poorly understood. There is no specific association between pregnancy and pancreatitis per se but a definite association between pancreatitis and gallstones (McKay *et al* 1980). Gallstones are found in many patients who present with acute pancreatitis in pregnancy (Berk *et al* 1971). One suggested mechanism proposed is that atony of the biliary tract and bile stasis in the duodenum secondary to the actions of progesterone, promote reflux of bile into the pancreatic duct (Peters *et al* 1951; Richman 1956; Joupilla *et al* 1974). In toxaemia, pancreatitis has been suggested to result from extreme elevations in abdominal pressure from vomiting, leading to raised intrapancreatic pressure, rupture of pancreatic ducts and release of enzymes (Berk *et al* 1971).

Primary hyperparathyroidism remains a rare cause of pancreatitis during pregnancy, although over 50 cases have been now reported (Thomason *et al* 1981). The first reported case in 1968 of acute hyperparathyroidism in pregnancy presented with hyperemesis gravidarum in the sixteenth week of pregnancy, with subsequent maternal and fetal death (Soyannwo and McGowan 1968). Other rare associations with pancreatitis in pregnancy include a hyperfunctioning parathyroid carcinoma (Hess *et al* 1980) and familial hypertriglyceridaemia (Glueck *et al* 1980).

The common symptoms and signs of acute pancreatitis are similar in nonpregnant and pregnant patients. Acute pancreatitis most commonly occurs in the third trimester or early puerperium (Montgomery and Miller 1970) but can occur at any time and there appears to be no influence from maternal parity or age on its incidence (Langmade and Edmondson 1951; Corlett and Mishell 1972).

Diagnosis in pregnancy may be difficult. Acute pancreatitis remains an uncommon cause of abdominal pain in pregnancy (Fischer and Dudley 1971). Furthermore, the serum amylase, the serum ratio of amylase to creatinine (S.am/S.creat per cent) and serum lipases may be misleadingly low in the first trimester (Fitzgerald 1955). The renal clearances of amylase and creatinine are correspondingly elevated in pregnancy and the ratio of renal clearances of amylase to creatinine (C.am/C.creat per cent) is diagnostically superior to ratios of these in serum since the latter may remain in the normal (nonpregnant) range despite severe acute pancreatitis (De Vore *et al* 1980).

Management

The aims of treatment are twofold—first to induce a state of pancreas and bowel rest, and second, to prevent complications. The use of nasogastric suction, although traditional, lacks evidence for its efficacy and may even promote elevation in serum amylase and delay the return of bowel sounds.

Various therapeutic agents have been used as inhibitors of pancreatic secretion including anti-cholinergic agents, glucagon, steroids, prostaglandins, vasopressin and ε-amino-caproic acid but controlled clinical trials are lacking. Cimetidine inhibits the acid stimulus to pancreatic secretion but has no demonstrable effect on biliary or pancreatic secretion. Trypsin inhibitors, e.g. aprotinin (Trasylol), have been subjected to various double blind studies but are without benefit (Dreiling *et al* 1976).

A major consideration in the management of severe acute pancreatitis includes the prevention/management of complications. These may include hypovolaemia, respiratory complications such as infection or pulmonary oedema, electrolyte (calcium and magnesium) imbalance, carbohydrate intolerance, renal failure, fat necrosis, haemorrhage, thrombosis, intestinal damage, pancreatic cysts, ascites, jaundice and hepatic and/or metabolic encephalopathy.

The management of severe acute pancreatitis in pregnancy poses additional problems. Therapeutic agents are without proven benefit in the nonpregnant (Ettien and Webster 1980) and therefore their benefit versus safety ratio is even more controversial in pregnancy. Elective induction of labour in the third trimester has been recommended but it remains controversial (Wilinson 1973; Joupilla *et al* 1974). Furthermore, termination of pregnancy offers no guarantee of cessation of the pathological state since the acute process may continue after delivery (spontaneous or induced) and into the puerperium (Langmade and Edmondson 1951; Montgomery and Miller 1970). Acute pancreatitis is less common in either the first or second trimester, and termination of pregnancy has no effect on maternal survival (Wilinson 1973).

The majority of pregnant patients with acute pancreatitis have gallstones (Berk *et al* 1971; Corlett and Mishell 1972; McKay *et al* 1980). In general, treatment is conservative in the first or second trimester although surgery is feasible. The latter requires a balanced decision in the third trimester (Thomason *et al* 1981).

CYSTIC FIBROSIS

This condition, which can affect the pancreas in pregnancy (Siegel and Siegel 1960), is described in Chapter 1.

References

Abramson D., Jankelson I.R. *et al* (1951) Pregnancy in idopathic ulcerative colitis. *American Journal of Obstetrics and Gynecology* **61**, 121–9.

Adams R.H., Gordon J. *et al* (1968) Hyperemesis gravidarum. I. Evidence of hepatic dysfunction. *Obstetrics and Gynecology* **31**, 659–64.

Adlercreutz H., Tikkanen M.J. *et al* (1974) Recurrent jaundice in pregnancy. IV. Quantitative determination of urinary and biliary estrogens, including studies in pruritus gravidarum. *Journal of Clinical Endocrinology and Metabolism* **38**, 51–7.

Ahrens E.H., Payne M.A. *et al* (1950) Primary biliary cirrhosis. *Medicine (Baltimore)* **29**, 299–364.

Alestig K., Trollfors B. *et al* (1979) Acute non-specific diarrhoea studies on the use of charcoal, kaolin-pectin and diphenoxylate. *Practitioner* **222**, 859–62.

Ament M.E. & Ruben C.E. (1972) Soy protein—another cause of a flat intestinal lesion. *Gastroenterology* **62**, 227–34.

Anderson G.W. (1942) Pregnancy complicated by acute perforated peptic ulcer. *American Journal of Obstetrics and Gynecology* **43**, 883–7.

Anderson P.O. (1977) Drugs and breast feeding—a review. *Drug Intelligence and Clinical Pharmacy* 208–23.

Antia F.P., Bharadiwaj T.P. *et al* (1958) Liver in normal pregnancy, pre-eclampsia and eclampsia. *Lancet* **2**, 776–8.

Antoon J.W. & Miller R.L. (1980) Aphthous ulcers—a review of the literature on etiology, pathogenesis, diagnosis and treatment. *Journal of the American Dental Association* **101**, 803–8.

Aozaga K., Ito H. *et al* (1981) Choriocarcinoma in infant and mother. *Acta Pathologica Japonica* **31**, 317–22.

Atkinson R.E. & Hudson C.H. (1970) Ano-rectal and perineal disorders of pregnancy and the puerperum. *Practitioner* **205**, 789–90.

Atlay R.D., Gillison E.W. *et al* (1973) A fresh look at pregnancy heartburn. *Journal of Obstetrics and Gynaecology of the British Commonwealth* **80**, 63–6.

Avery G.S., Davies E.F. *et al* (1972) Lactulose—a review of its properties with reference to metabolism and action in portal systemic encephalopathy. *Drugs* **4**, 7–12.

Babson W.W. (1946) Terminal ileitis with obstruction and abscess complicating pregnancy. *New England Journal of Medicine* **235**, 544–7.

Baird R.M. (1966) Peptic ulceration in pregnancy: report of a case with perforation. *Canadian Medical Association Journal* **94**, 861–2.

Baker P.G. & Read A.E. (1975) Reversible infertility in male coeliac patients. *British Medical Journal* **ii**, 316–17.

Baldwin W.F. (1963) Drugs in pregnancy. Senna—clinical study of senna administered to nursing mothers: assessment of effects on infant bowel habits. *Canadian Medical Association Journal* **89**, 566–8.

Banks B.M., Korelitz B.I. *et al* (1957) The course of non-specific ulcerative colitis: Review of twenty years' experience and late results. *Gastroenterology* **32**, 983–1012.

Banner E.A., Hunt A.B. *et al* (1945) Pregnancy associated with carcinoma of the large bowel. *Surgery, Gynecology and Obstetrics* **80**, 211–16.

Bargen J.A., Nunez C.J. *et al* (1939) Pregnancy associated with chronic ulcerative colitis. *American Journal of Obstetrics and Gynecology* **38**, 146–8.

Barin F., Goudeau A. *et al* (1982) Immune response in neonates to hepatitis B vaccine. *Lancet* **i**, 251–3.

Barnes C.S. & Hayes H.M. (1921) Ulcerative colitis complicating pregnancy and the puerperum. *American Journal of Obstetrics and Gynecology* **22**, 907–12.

Barwin B.N., Hartley J.M.G. *et al* (1974) Ileostomy and pregnancy. *British Journal of Clinical Practice* **28**, 256–8.

Bassey O.O. (1977) Pregnancy heartburn in Nigerians and Caucasians with theories about aetiology based on manometric recordings from the oesophagus and stomach. *British Journal of Obstetrics and Gynaecology* **84**, 439–43.

Bauman F. (1931) Ulcerative colitis complicated by pregnancy. *American Journal of Obstetrics and Gynecology* **22**, 944–5.

Baydoun A.B. (1953) Bisacodyl suppositories: a practical means of securing bowel evacuation during labour. *American Journal of Obstetrics and Gynecology* **85**, 905–7.

Beard C.M., Noller K.L. *et al* (1979) Lack of evidence for cancer due to use of metronidazole. *New England Journal of Medicine* **301**, 519–22.

Beeley L. (1981) Adverse effects of drugs in later pregnancy. In Wood S.M. and Beeley L. (eds) *Prescribing in Pregnancy Clinics in Obstetrics and Gynaecology*, p. 281. W. B. Saunders Co. Ltd., London.

Bennett A.G., Kunin A.S. *et al* (1963) Liver disease in pregnancy. Report of a case complicated by jaundice and cirrhosis with a review of the literature. *Obstetrical and Gynecological Survey* **18**, 919–34.

Bennett N. McK., Lehmann N.I. *et al* (1979) Viral hepatitis and intrahepatic cholestasis of pregnancy. *Australian and New Zealand Journal of Medicine* **9**, 54–7.

Bennion L.J. & Grundy S.M. (1978) Risk factors for the development of cholelithiasis in man (second of two parts). *New England Journal of Medicine* **299**, 1221–27.

Benson G.D., Kowlessar O.D. *et al* (1964) Adult celiac disease with emphasis upon response to the gluten-free diet. *Medicine (Baltimore)* **43**, 1–40.

Berk J.E., Smith B.H. *et al* (1971) Pregnancy pancreatitis. *American Journal of Gastroenterology* **56**, 216–26.

Bernstein I.L., Johnson C.L. *et al* (1978) Therapy with cromolyn sodium. *Annals of Internal Medicine* **89**, 228–33.

Bernstein L.H., Frank M.S. *et al* (1980) Healing of perineal Crohn's disease with metronidazole. *Gastroenterology* **79**, 357–65.

Biggs J.S.G. & Vesey E.J. (1980) Treatment of gastrointestinal disorders of pregnancy. *Drugs* **19**, 70–6.

Bihl J.H. (1959) The effect of pregnancy on hepatolenticular degeneration (Wilson's disease). *American Journal of Obstetrics and Gynecology* **78**, 1182–88.

Binder H.J. (1970) Celiac sprue—'unmasking' after vagotomy and hiatal-hernia repair. *New England Journal of Medicine* **283**, 520–1.

Bis K.A. & Waxman B. (1976) Rupture of the liver associated with pregnancy: A review of the literature and report of two cases. *Obstetrical and Gynecological Survey* **31**, 763–73.

Blaser M.J., Berkowtiz I.D. *et al* (1979) Campylobacter enteritis: Clinical and epidemiologic features. *Annals of Internal Medicine* **91**, 179–85.

Booth C.C. (1970) The enterocyte in coeliac disease. *British Medical Journal* **4**, 14–17.

Borgfors N. & Selander P. (1968) The incidence of coeliac disease in Sweden. *Acta Paediatrica Scandinavica* **57**, 260.

Borhanmanesh F. & Haghighi P. (1970) Pregnancy in patients with cirrhosis of the liver. *Obstetrics and Gynecology* **36**, 315–24.

Boxall E.H., Flewett T.H. *et al* (1980) Specific immunoglobulin for babies born to HBsAg carriers. *Lancet* **i**, 419–20.

Boyes B.E., Woolf I.L. *et al* (1975) Treatment of gastric ulceration with a bismuth preparation. *Postgraduate Medical Journal* **51** (Suppl. 5), 29–33.

Brahme F., Lindstrom C. *et al* (1975) Crohn's disease in a defined population. An epidemiological study of incidence, prevalence, mortality and secular trends in the city of Malmo, Sweden. *Gastroenterology* **69**, 342–51.

Braude S., Gimson A.E.S. *et al* (1981) Progress in the management of fulminant hepatic failure. *Intensive Care Medicine* **7**, 101–3.

Braverman D.Z., Johnson M.L. *et al* (1980) Effects of pregnancy and contraceptive steroids on gallbladder function. *New England Journal of Medicine* **302**, 362–4.

Bray R.S. & Anderson M.J. (1979) Falciparum malaria and pregnancy. *Transactions of the Royal Society of Tropical Medicine and Hygiene* **73**, 427–31.

Breen K.J., Perkins K.W. *et al* (1970) Idiopathic acute fatty liver of pregnancy. *Gut* **11**, 822–5.

Breen K.J., Perkins K.W. *et al* (1972) Uncomplicated subsequent pregnancy after idiopathic fatty liver of pregnancy. *Obstetrics and Gynecology* **40**, 813–15.

British Medical Journal editorial (1970) Coeliac disease. *British Medical Journal* **4**, 1–2.

British Medical Journal editorial (1979) Liver dysfunction in inflammatory bowel disease. *British Medical Journal* **2**, 688–9.

Britton R.C. (1982) Pregnancy and esophageal varices. *American Journal of Surgery* **4**, 421–5.

Brock-Utne J.G., Dow T.G.B. *et al* (1981) Gastric and lower oesophageal sphincter (LOS) pressures in early pregnancy. *British Journal of Anaesthesia* **53**, 381–4.

Brooks F.P., Powell K.C. *et al* (1966) Variable clinical course of adult celiac disease. *Archives of Internal Medicine* **117**, 789–94.

Browne C.H., Hanson G.C. *et al* (1975) Rupture of subcapsular haematoma of the liver in a case of eclampsia. *British Journal of Surgery* **62**, 237–8.

Bruce-Chwatt L.J. (1980) *Essential Malariology.* Heinemann Medical, London.

Bruce-Chwatt L.J. (1983) Malaria and pregnancy. *British Medical Journal* **286**, 1457–8.

Bryant M.G. & Bloom S.R. (1979) Distribution of the gut hormones in the primate intestinal tract. *Gut* **20**, 653–9.

Burgess D.E. (1972) Constipation in obstetrics. In Avery Jones, Sir Francis and Godding E.W. (eds) *Management of Constipation,* pp. 176–88. Blackwell Scientific Publications, Oxford.

Burrell C.J. (1980) Serological markers of hepatitis B infection. *Clinical Gastroenterology* **9**, 47–63.

Burroughs A.K., Seong N.G. *et al* (1982) Idiopathic acute fatty liver of pregnancy in 12 patients. *Quarterly Journal of Medicine* **41**, 481–97.

Burrow G.N. & Ferris T.F. (eds) (1975) *Medical Complications During Pregnancy.* W. B. Saunders Co., Philadelphia.

Byrne J.J. (1972) Diagnostic evaluation of patients with intestinal problems. *Clinical Obstetrics and Gynecology* **15**, 473–83.

Camilleri M., Schafler K. *et al* (1981) Periportal sinusoidal dilatation, inflammatory bowel disease and the contraceptive pill. *Gastroenterology* **80**, 810–15.

Cano R.I., Delman M.R. *et al* (1975) Acute fatty liver of pregnancy. Complication by disseminated intravascular coagulation. *Journal of the American Medical Association* **231**, 159–61.

Carangelo J. & Efstation T.D. (1948) Massive gastric hemorrhage in pregnancy. *American Journal of Obstetrics and Gynecology* **56**, 191–4.

Carter C.O., Sheldon W. *et al* (1959) Coeliac disease. *Annals of Human Genetics* **23**, 266.

Castaneda H., García-Romèro H. *et al* (1970) Hepatic haemorrhage in toxaemia of pregnancy. *American Journal of Obstetrics and Gynecology* **107**, 578–84.

Check J.H., King L.C. *et al* (1978) Uncomplicated pregnancy following oral contraceptive-induced liver hepatoma. *Obstetrics and Gynecology (Suppl. 1)* **52**, 28S–9S.

Cheng Y.S. (1977) Pregnancy in liver cirrhosis and/or portal hypertension. *American Journal of Obstetrics and Gynecology* **128**, 812–22.

Chiaramonte M., Dardanoni L. *et al* (1974) Observations on acute phase and follow-up of similar series of cases of HB-Ag positive and HB-Ag negative hepatitis. *Rendicorti di Gastro-enterologica* **6**, 1–5.

Chiari H. (1899) Über die Selbständinge Endo-phlebitis obiterans der Haupstamme der Venae Hepaticae als Todesurache. *Beiträge zur Pathologischen Anatomie* **26**, 1–18.

Christie A.B., Allam A.A. *et al* (1976) Pregnancy hepatitis in Libya. *Lancet* **2**, 827–9.

Christofides N.D., Ghatei M.A. *et al* (1982) Decreased plasma motilin concentration in pregnancy. *British Medical Journal* **285**, 1453–4.

Clarke D.H. (1953) Peptic ulcer in women. *British Medical Journal* **1**, 1254–7.

Cohen S. & Harris L.D. (1971) Does hiatus hernia effect competence of the gastroesophageal sphincter? *New England Journal of Medicine* **284**, 1053–6.

Cohen S. & Harris L.D. (1972) The lower esophageal sphincter. *Gastroenterology* **63**, 1066–73.

Conaster D.G. & Harris R.E. (1975) Fatty liver of pregnancy. *Journal of the American Medical Association* **232**, 1125.

Connon J.J. (1977) De Nol, an effective drug in the therapy of duodenal ulceration. *Journal of the Irish Medical Association* **70**, 206–7.

Cooke W.T., Peeney A.L.P. *et al* (1953) Symptoms, signs and diagnostic features of idiopathic steatorrhoea. *Quarterly Journal of Medicine* **22**, 59–77.

Cooke W.T. & Smith W.T. (1966) Neurological disorders associated with adult coeliac disease. *Brain* **89**, 683–722.

Corlett R.C. & Mishell D.R. (1972) Pancreatitis in pregnancy. *American Journal of Obstetrics and Gynecology* **113**, 281–90.

Cosnes J., Hecketsweiler P. *et al* (1981) Consequences of extensive bowel resection in Crohn's disease: a study of 53 cases. *Gastroenterologie Clinique et Biologique* **5**, 198–206.

Crawhall J.C., Scowen E.F. *et al* (1967) Dissolution of cystine stones during D-penicillamine treatment of a pregnant patient with cystinuria. *British Medical Journal* **2**, 216–18.

Crisp W.E. (1960) Pregnancy complicating peptic ulcer. *Postgraduate Medicine* **27**, 445–7.

Croese J. (1979) Coeliac disease. Haematological features and delay in diagnosis. *Medical Journal of Australia*. **2**, 335–8.

Crohn B.B., Yarnis H. *et al* (1956a) Ulcerative colitis and pregnancy. *Gastroenterology* **30**, 391–403.

Crohn B.B., Yarnis H. *et al* (1956b) Regional ileitis complicating pregnancy. *Gastroenterology* **31**, 615–28.

Datta D.V., Chhuttani P.N. *et al* (1972) Clinical spectrum of Budd–Chiari syndrome in Chandigarh with particular reference to obstruction of intrahepatic portion of the inferior vena cava. *Gut* **13**, 372–8.

Davies J.B., Shenken J.R. *et al* (1973) Massive haemoperitoneum from rupture of benign hepatocellular adenoma. *Surgery* **73**, 181–4.

De Dombal F.T., Burton I.L. *et al* (1972) Crohn's disease and pregnancy. *British Medical Journal* **3**, 550–3.

De Dombal F.T., Watts J.M. *et al* (1965) Ulcerative colitis and pregnancy. *Lancet* **2**, 599–602.

Dentsch V., Rosenthal T. *et al* (1972) Budd–Chiari syndrome. Study of angiographic findings and remarks of etiology. *American Journal of Roentgenology* **116**, 430–9.

De Pagter A.G.F., Van Berge Henegouwen G.P. *et al* (1976) Familial benign recurrent intrahepatic cholestasis. Interrelation with intrahepatic cholestasis of pregnancy and from oral contraceptives? *Gastroenterology* **71**, 202–7.

Department of Health and Social Security (1979) *Report on Confidential Enquiries into Maternal Deaths in England and Wales, 1973–1975*. HMSO, London.

De Paula Castro L. (1967) Reflux esophagitis as the cause of heartburn in pregnancy. *American Journal of Obstetrics and Gynecology* **98**, 1–10.

Der Brucke M.G. (1949) Intestinal obstruction due to malignancy complicating pregnancy. *American Journal of Obstetrics and Gynecology* **40**, 307–11.

De Vore G.R., Bracken M. & Berkowitz R.L. (1980) The amylase/creatinine ratio in normal pregnancy and pregnancies complicated by pancreatitis, hyperemesis gravidarium and toxaemia. *American Journal of Obstetrics and Gynecology* **138**, 747–54.

Dew M.J., Hughes P.H. *et al* (1982) Maintenance of remission in ulcerative colitis with oral preparation of 5-aminosalicylic acid. *British Medical Journal* **285** 1012–13.

Dickinson R.J., Ashton M.G. *et al* (1980) Controlled trial of intravenous hyperalimentation and total bowel rest as an adjunct to the routine therapy of acute colitis. *Gastroenterology* **79**, 1199–1204.

Diddle A.W. & Stevens R.L. (1939) Typhoid fever in pregnancy: probable intrauterine transmission of the disease. *American Journal of Obstetrics and Gynecology* **38**, 300–5.

Dodds W.J., Dent J. *et al* (1978) Pregnancy and the lower esophageal sphincter. *Gastroenterology* **74**, 1334–6.

Donnai D. & Harris R. (1978) Unusual fetal malformations after antiemetics in early pregnancy. *British Medical Journal* **1**, 691–2.

Dreifuss F.E. & McKinney W.M. (1966) Wilson's disease (hepatolenticular degeneration) and pregnancy. *Journal of American Medical Association* **195**, 960–2.

Dreiling D.A., Leichtling J.J. *et al* (1976) Trasylol revisited: the value of proteolytic inhibitors in the therapy of pancreatitis. *Mount Sinai Journal of Medicine, New York* **43**, 409–14.

Drill V.A. (1974) Benign cholestatic jaundice of pregnancy and the benign cholestatic jaundice from oral contraceptives. *American Journal of Obstetrics and Gynecology* **119**, 165–74.

Driscoll R.H. & Rosenberg I.H. (1978) Total parenteral nutrition in inflammatory bowel disease. *Medical Clinics of North America* **62**, 185–201.

Eade M.N. (1970) Liver disease in ulcerative colitis. 1. Analysis of operative liver biopsy in 138 consecutive patients having colectomy. *Annals of Internal Medicine* **72**, 475–87.

Ebbs J.H. (1956) Coeliac disease. *Canadian Medical Association Journal* **75**, 885–93.

Ebbs J.H., Thompson M. *et al* (1950) Etiologic factors in celiac disease. *American Journal of Diseases of Children* **79**, 936–7.

Egwuatu V.E. (1980) Primary hepatocarcinoma in pregnancy. *Transactions of the Royal Society of Tropical Medicine and Hygiene* **74**, 793–4.

Eisele J.W., Barber E.A. *et al* (1975) Lipid content in the liver of fatty metamorphosis of pregnancy. *American Journal of Pathology* **81**, 545–60.

Ek B. (1967) On the familial incidence of idiopathic sprue and the significance of pregnancy and partial gastrectomy for the manifestation of the symptoms. *Acta Medica Scandinavica Supplement* **181**, 125–6.

Ek B. (1969) Studies on idiopathic sprue. Familial incidence and relation to pregnancy and partial gastrectomy. *Acta Medica Scandinavica Supplement* **185**, 463–4.

Eliakim M., Sadovsky E. *et al* (1966) Recurrent cholestatic jaundice of pregnancy. Report of five cases and electron microscopic observations. *Archives of Internal Medicine* **117**, 696–705.

Elson C.O., Layden T.J. *et al* (1980) An evaluation of total parenteral nutrition in the management of inflammatory bowel disease. *Digestive Diseases and Science* **25**, 42–8.

Endres W. (1981) D-Penicillamine in pregnancy—to ban or not to ban? *Klinische Wochenschrift* **59**, 535–7.

Ettien J.T. & Webster P.D. (1980) The management of acute pancreatitis. *Advances in Internal Medicine* **25**, 169–98.

Everson G.T., McKinley C. *et al* (1982) Gallbladder function in the human female: effect of the ovulatory cycle, pregnancy and contraceptive steroids. *Gastroenterology* **82**, 711–19.

Fagan E.A., Dyck R.F. *et al* (1982) Serum levels of C-reactive protein in Crohn's disease and ulcerative colitis. *European Journal of Clinical Investigation* **12**, 351–9.

Fagan E.A. & Chadwick V.S. (1983) Drug treatment of gastrointestinal disorders in pregnancy. In Lewis P.J. (ed.) *Clinical Pharmacology in Obstetrics*, Chapter 10, 114–37. John Wright & Sons Ltd., Bristol.

Fairweather D.V.I. (1968) Nausea and vomiting in pregnancy. *American Journal of Obstetrics and Gynecology* **102**, 135–75.

Fairweather D.V.I. & Loraine J.A. (1962) Urinary excretion of human chorionic gonadotrophin in patients with hyperemesis gravidarium. *British Medical Journal* **1**, 666–9.

Falchuk Z.M., Rogentine G.N. *et al* (1972) Predominance of histocompatibility antigen HLA B8 in patients with gluten-sensitive enteropathy. *Journal of Clinical Investigation* **51**, 1602–5.

Fallon H.J. (1975) Liver disease. In Burrow G.N. and Ferris T.F. (eds) *Medical Complications During Pregnancy*, p. 357. W. B. Saunders Co., Philadelphia.

Farthing M.J.C., Edwards C.R.W., Rees L.H. & Dawson A.M. (1982) Male gonadal function in coeliac disease. I. Sexual dysfunction, infertility, and semen quality. *Gut* **23**, 608–14.

Farthing M.J.C., Rees L.H., Edwards C.R.W. & Dawson A.M. (1983) Male gonadal function in coeliac disease. II Sex hormones. *Gut* **24**, 127–35.

Fechner R.E. (1977) Benign hepatic lesions and orally administered contraceptives. A report of seven cases and a critical analysis of the literature. *Human Pathology* **8**, 255–68.

Feder I.A. (1938) Chronic ulcerative colitis: An analysis of 88 cases. *American Journal of Digestive Diseases* **5**, 239–45.

Feeney J.G. (1982) Heartburn in pregnancy. *British Medical Journal* **284**, 1138–9.

Felson J. & Wolarsky W. (1948) Chronic ulcerative colitis and pregnancy. *American Journal of Obstetrics and Gynecology* **56**, 751–5.

Fielding J.F. & Cooke W.T. (1970) Pregnancy and Crohn's disease. *British Medical Journal* **2**, 76–7.

Filipsson S., Hulten L. *et al* (1978) The metabolic consequences of surgery in Crohn's disease. *Scandinavian Journal of Gastroenterology* **13**, 471–9.

Finegold S.M. (1980) Metronidazole. *Annals of Internal Medicine* **93**, 585–7.

Fingl E. (1975) Laxatives and cathartics. In Goodman L.S. and Gilman A. (eds) *The Pharmacological Basis of Therapeutics*, pp. 976–86. Macmillan, New York.

Finkelstein W. & Isselbacher K.J. (1978) Medical intelligence: Drug therapy: cimetidine. *New England Journal of Medicine* **299**, 992–6.

Fischer E.P. & Dudley A.G. (1971) Acute pancreatitis in pregnancy. A review and case report. *Military Medicine* **136**, 578–81.

Fisher R.S., Roberts G.S. *et al* (1978) Altered bowel esophageal sphincter function during early pregnancy. *Gastroenterology* **74**, 1233–7.

Fitzgerald O. (1955) Pancreatitis following pregnancy. *British Medical Journal* **1**, 349.

Fleming C.R., Beart R.W. *et al* (1980) Home parenteral nutrition for management of the severely malnourished adult patient. *Gastroenterology* **79**, 11–18.

Food Drug Administration, Department of Health, Education and Welfare (1978) Oral contraceptive labelling. *FDA Drug Bulletin* **8**, 12–13.

Food and Safety Administration (1979) Bendectin. *Federal Register* **44**, 41068.

Françavilla A., Panella C. *et al* (1978) Serum gastrin levels during normal pregnancy. *VI World Congress in Gastroenterology*, p. 216.

Franklin J.L. & Rosenberg I.H. (1973) Impaired folic acid absorption in inflammatory bowel disease: effects of salicylazosulfapyridine/Azulfidine. *Gastroenterology* **64**, 517–25.

Freedman M.L., Christopher P. *et al* (1970) Typhoid carriage in pregnancy with infection of neonate. *Lancet* **i**, 310–11.

Furhoff A.K. & Hellstrom K. (1973) Jaundice in pregnancy. A follow-up study of the sera of women originally reported by L. Thorling. I. The pregnancies. *Acta Medica Scandinavica* **193**, 259–66.

Gaginella T.S., Chadwick V.S. *et al* (1977) Perfusion of rabbit colon with ricinoleic acid: dose-related mucosal injury, fluid secretion and increased permeability. *Gastroenterology* **73**, 95–101.

Gallagher D.M. (1971) Pruritus ani. *Modern Treatment.* **8**, 963–70.

Gazzard B.G., Price H.L. *et al* (1978) The social toll of Crohn's disease. *British Medical Journal* **2**, 1117–19.

Gilat T. & Rozen P. (1979) Epidemiology of Crohn's disease and ulcerative colitis: etiologic implications. *Israel Journal of Medical Science* **15**, 305–8.

Gilbert G.L., Davoren R.A. *et al* (1981) Midtrimester abortion associated with septicaemia caused by Campylobacter jejuni. *Medical Journal of Australia* **1**, 585–6.

Gilles H.M., Lawson J.B. *et al* (1969) Malaria, anaemia and pregnancy. *Annals of Tropical Medicine and Parasitology* **63**, 245–63.

Girard R.M., Lamarche J. *et al* (1981) Carcinoma of the colon associated with pregnancy: report of a case. *Diseases of the Colon and Rectum* **24**, 473–5.

Glade G., Saccar C.L. *et al* (1980) Cimetidine. Transient liver impairment in the newborn. Case report. *American Journal of Diseases of Children* **134**, 87–8.

Glaser B., Vinik A.I. *et al* (1980) Plasma human pancreatic polypeptide responses to administered secretin: effects of surgical vagotomy, cholinergic blockade and chronic pancreatitis. *Journal of Clinical Endocrinology and Metabolism* **50**, 1094–9.

Glueck C.J., Christopher C. *et al* (1980) Pancreatitis, familial hypertriglyceridemia and pregnancy. *American Journal of Obstetrics and Gynecology* **136**, 755–61.

Glyn L.E. (1950) Relation of nutrition of hepatic disease and toxemias of pregnancy. In *Toxemias of Pregnancy, Human and Veterinary*, p. 19 et seq. (Ciba Foundation Symposium) Blakiston Co., Philadelphia.

Godding E.W. (1976a) Constipation and allied disorders. *Pharmaceutical Journal* **2**, 8.

Godding E.W. (1976b) Constipation and allied disorders. *Pharmaceutical Journal* **2**, 17.

Goldman R.L. (1980) Liver cancer and oral contraceptives (letter). *American Journal of Surgical Pathology* **4**, 208.

Goodman L.S. & Gilman A. (1970) *The Pharmacological Basis of Therapeutics* 4th edn, p. 1027. Macmillan, London.

Goosen C.J. (1962) The use of Bisacodyl in place of an enema in obstetrics. *Mediese Bydraes* **8**, 107–8.

Gorbach S.L. (1982) Travelers' diarrhea. *New England Journal of Medicine* **307**, 881–3.

Gordon A.G. & Johnston G.W. (1963) Portal hypertension in pregnancy. *Journal of Obstetrics and Gynaecology of the British Commonwealth* **70**, 1056–9.

Gorlin R.J. & Goldman H.M. (eds) (1970) Hyperplastic gingivitis. In *Thoma's Oral Pathology* 6th edition, Vol. 1, pp. 400–2. C.V.Mosby Company, St Louis.

Govan A.D.T. & Mukherjee C.L. (1950) Vascular supply to the liver and anatomy of eclampsia. *British Journal of Experimental Pathology* **31**, 485–94.

Grabowski G.M., Stenram V. *et al* (1975) Focal nodular hyperplasia of the liver, benign hepatomas, oral contraceptives and other drugs affecting the liver. *Acta Pathologica et Microbiologica Scandinavica; Section A: Pathology* **83**, 615–22.

Gray M.S., Kane P.O. *et al* (1961) Further observations on Metronidazole (Flagyl). *British Journal of Venereal Diseases* **37**, 278–9.

Green L.K., Harris R.E. *et al* (1975) Cancer of the colon during pregnancy. A review of the literature and report of a case associated with ulcerative colitis. *Obstetrics and Gynecology* **46**, 480–3.

Green P.A. & Wollaeger E.E. (1960) The clinical behavior of sprue in the United States. *Gastroenterology* **38**, 399–418.

Greenstein A.J., Janowitz H.D. *et al* (1976) The extra-intestinal complications of Crohn's disease and ulcerative colitis: A study of 700 patients. *Medicine (Baltimore)* **55**, 401–12.

Gribble M.J., Salit I.E. *et al* (1981) Campylobacter infections in pregnancy. Case report and literature review. *American Journal of Obstetrics and Gynecology* **140**, 423–6.

Griffin G.E., Fagan E.A. *et al* (1982) Enteral therapy in the management of massive gut resection complicated by chronic fluid and electrolyte depletion. *Digestive Diseases and Science* **27**, 902–8.

Grumbine F.C., Rosenshein N.B. *et al* (1980) Management of liver metastasis from gestational neoplasia. *American Journal of Obstetrics and Gynecology* **137**, 959–61.

Gruner O.-P.N., Naas R. *et al* (1977) Marital status and sexual adjustment after colectomy. *Scandinavian Journal of Gastroenterology* **12**, 193–7.

Guttmacher A.F. (1960) Hyperemesis. In Guttmacher A.F. and Rovinsky J.J. (eds) *Medical, Surgical and Gynecological Complications of Pregnancy*, pp. 166–9. Williams & Wilkins, Baltimore.

Haddow J.E., Thompson D.K. *et al* (1980) Maternal hepatoma detected during serum AFP screening. *Lancet* **2**, 806–7.

Haemmerli U.P. (1966) Jaundice during pregnancy with special reference on recurrent jaundice during pregnancy and its differential diagnosis. *Acta Medica Scandinavica Supplement* **444**, 1–111.

Haemmerli U.P. (1975) Jaundice during pregnancy. In Schiff L. (ed.) *Disease of the Liver*, pp. 1336–8. J.B. Lippincott Co., Philadelphia.

Hague W.M. (1982) Impact of sex ratio on onset and management of labour. *British Medical Journal* **285**, 1577.

Hague W.M., Fenton, D.W. *et al* (1983) Acute fatty liver of pregnancy. *Journal of the Royal Society of Medicine* **76**, 652–61.

Hall M. & Davidson R.J.L. (1968) Prophylactic folic acid in women with pernicious anaemia pregnant after periods of infertility. *Journal of Clinical Pathology* **21**, 599–602.

Hambidge K.M., Neldner K.H. & Walravens P.A. (1975) Zinc, acrodermatitis enternopathica and congenital malformations. *Lancet* **i**, 577–8.

Hamory B.H., Luger A. *et al* (1981) Herpes virus hominis hepatitis of mother and newborn infant. *Southern Medical Journal* **74**, 992–5.

Hancock K.W. (1968) The Budd–Chiari syndrome in pregnancy. *Journal of Obstetrics and Gynaecology of the British Commonwealth* **75**, 746–8.

Harlap S., Shiono P.H. *et al* (1979) A prospective study of spontaneous fetal losses after induced abortions. *New England Journal of Medicine* **301**, 677–681.

Harpey J. & Charpentier C. (1983) Acute fatty liver of pregnancy. *Lancet* **i**, 586–7.

Harries J.M. & Hughes T.F. (1957) An enumeration of the 'cravings' of some pregnant women. *Proceedings of the Nutrition Society (Abstract)* **16**, xx–xxi.

Harris O.D., Cooke W.T. *et al* (1967) Malignancy in adult coeliac disease and idiopathic steatorrhoea. *American Journal of Medicine* **42**, 899–912.

Harrison R.F. (1977) Infertility in women. *British Journal of Hospital Medicine* **17**, 45–6, 50–4.

Harron D.W.G., Griffiths K. *et al* (1980) Debendox and congenital malformations in Northern Ireland. *British Medical Journal* **281**, 1379–81.

Hatfield A.K., Stein J.H. *et al* (1972) Idiopathic acute fatty liver of pregnancy. Death from extrahepatic manifestations. *American Journal of Digestive Diseases* **17**, 167–78.

Hedberg L.A., Melnyk L.S. *et al* (1966) Gluten enteropathy appearing after gastric surgery. *Gastroenterology* **50**, 796–804.

Heinonen O.P., Slone D. *et al* (eds) (1977) Birth defects and drugs in pregnancy. Publishing Sci. Gp. Inc., Littleton, Massachusetts.

Hensleigh P.A. & Kauffman R.E. (1977) Maternal absorption and placental transfer of sulfasalazine. *American Journal of Obstetrics and Gynecology* **127**, 443–4.

Herbert W.N. & Brenner W.E. (1982) Improving survival with liver rupture complicating pregnancy. *American Journal of Obstetrics and Gynecology* **142**, 530–4.

Hess J.M., Dickson J. *et al* (1980) Hyperfunctioning parathyroid carcinoma presenting as acute pancreatitis in pregnancy. *Journal of Reproductive Medicine* **25**, 83–7.

Hibbard B.M. & Hibbard E.D. (1963) Aetiological factors in abruptio placentae. *British Medical Journal* **ii**, 1430–6.

Hibbard E.D. & Smithells R.W. (1965) Folic acid metabolism and human embryopathy. *Lancet* **i**, 1254.

Hibbard L.T. (1976) Spontaneous rupture of the liver in pregnancy: a report of eight cases. *American Journal of Obstetrics and Gynecology* **126**, 334–8.

Hieber J.P., Doeton D. *et al* (1977) Hepatitis and pregnancy. *Journal of Pediatrics* **91**, 545–9.

Hilleman M.R., Bertland A.U. *et al* (1978) Clinical laboratory studies of HBsAg vaccine. In Vyas G., Cohen S.N. and Schmid R. (eds) *Viral Hepatitis*, pp. 525–37. Franklin Institute Press, Philadelphia.

Hofbauer J. (1908) Beitrage zur Aetiologie und zur Klinik der Graviditatstoikosen. *Zeitschrift für Geburtshilge und Gynäkologie* **61**, 200–74.

Hogan W.J., de Andrade S.R.V. & Winship D.H. (1972) Ethanol-induced acute esophageal motor dysfunction. *Journal of Applied Physiology* **32**, 755–60.

Holmes G.K.T., Stokes P.L. *et al* (1974) Coeliac disease, malignancy, and gluten-free diet. *Gut* **15**, 339.

Holtermüller K.H. & Weis H.J. (1979) Gastroenterologishe Erkrankungen in der Schwangershaft. *Gynäkologe* **12**, 35–51.

Holtzbach R.T. (1974) Acute fatty liver of pregnancy with disseminated intravascular coagulation. *Obstetrics and Gynecology* **43**, 740–4.

Homan W.P. & Thorbjarnarson N.B. (1976) Crohn's disease and pregnancy. *Archives of Surgery* **111**, 545–7.

Hornnes P.J. & Kühl C. (1981) Decreased plasma pancreatic polypeptide levels in pregnancy. *Journal of Clinical Endocrinology and Metabolism* **52**, 605–7.

Howard F.M. & Hill J.M. (1979) Drugs in pregnancy. *Obstetrical and Gynecological Survey* **34**, 643–53.

Howe J.P., Moore J. *et al* (1980) Effect of cimetidine in reducing intragastric acidity on patients undergoing elective Caesarian section. Further experience with histamine H_2 receptor antagonists and peptic ulcer disease and progress in histamine research. In Torsoli A., Lucchell P.E. and Brimblecombe R.W. (eds) *European Symposium on H_2 Antagonists*, pp. 174–84. Excerpta Medica, Amsterdam.

Huchzermeyer H. (1971) Schwangershaft bei Leberzirrhose und chronischer Hepatitis (Pregnancy in patients with liver cirrhosis and chronic hepatitis). *Acta Hepatogastroenterologica (Stuttgart)* **18**, 294–305.

Hudson C.N. (1972) Ileostomy in pregnancy. *Proceedings of the Royal Society of Medicine* **62**, 281–3.

Huff P.S. (1980) Safety of drug therapy for nausea and vomiting of pregnancy. *Journal of Family Practice* **11**, 969–70.

Huggins G.R. (1981) Neoplasia and hormonal contraception. *Clinical Obstetrics and Gynecology* **24**, 903–25.

Hunt J.N. & Murray F.A. (1958) Gastric function in pregnancy. *Journal of Obstetrics and Gynaecology of the British Empire* **65**, 78–83.

Hytten F.E. (1980) The alimentary system. In Hytten F.E. and Chamberlain G. (eds) *Clinical Physiology in Obstetrics*, pp. 147–58. Blackwell Scientific Publications, Oxford.

Infield D.S., Sorkowf H.I. *et al* (1979) Chronic persistent hepatitis and pregnancy. *Gastroenterology* **77**, 524–7.

Ingerslev M. & Teilum G. (1945) Biopsy studies on the liver in pregnancy. III. Liver biopsy in albuminuria of pregnancy, eclampsism and eclampsia. *Acta Obstetricia et Gynecologica Scandinavica Supplement* **25**, 361–76.

Ippolilti A.F., Sturdevant R.A.L. *et al* (1978) Cimetidine versus intensive antacid therapy for duodenal ulcer. *Gastroenterology* **74**, 393–5.

Ivey K.J. (1975) Are anticholinergics of use in the irritable colon syndrome? *Gastroenterology* **68**, 1300–7.

Jackson I.M.D., Doig W.B. *et al* (1967) Pernicious anaemia as a cause of infertility. *Lancet* **ii**, 1159–60.

Järnerot G. & Into-Malmberg M.B. (1979) Sulphasalazine treatment during breast feeding. *Scandinavian Journal of Gastroenterology* **14**, 869–71.

Jelliffe E.F.P. (1967) Placental malaria and foetal growth failure. In Aysen R.N. (ed.) *Nutrition and Infection*. CIBA Foundation Study Group 31, Churchill, London.

Jenkins P.J. & Williams R. (1980) Fulminant viral hepatitis. *Clinics in Gastroenterology* **9**, 171–89.

Jeppsson S. & Rannevik G. (1976) Effect of oral 17-beta-oestradiol on the liver in women with intrahepatic cholestasis (hepatosis) during previous pregnancy. *British Journal of Obstetrics and Gynaecology* **83**, 567–71.

Johnston G.W., Gordon A.G. *et al* (1965) Porta-caval shunt performed during pregnancy. *Journal of Obstetrics and Gynaecology of the British Commonwealth* **72**, 292–5.

Johnston W.C. & Baskett T.F. (1979) Obstetric cholestasis. *American Journal of Obstetrics and Gynecology* **133**, 299–301.

Jokipii L. & Jokippi A.M.M. (1979) Single-dose metronidazole and tinidazole as therapy for giardiasis: success rates, side effects and drug absorption and elimination. *Journal of Infectious Diseases* **140**, 984–8.

Jones P.F., McEwan A.B. *et al* (1969) Haemorrhage and perforation complicating peptic ulcer in pregnancy. *Lancet* **iii**, 350–1.

Joske R.A. & Martin J.D. (1971) Coeliac disease presenting as recurrent abortion. *Journal of Obstetrics and Gynaecology of the British Commonwealth* **78**, 754–8.

Joupila P., Mokka R. *et al* (1974) Acute pancreatitis in pregnancy. *Surgery, Gynecology and Obstetrics* **139**, 879–82.

Juergens J.L., Scholz D.A. *et al* (1956) Severe osteomalacia associated with occult steatorrhoea due to nontropical sprue. *Archives of Internal Medicine* **98**, 774–82.

Karmali M.A. & Tan Y.C. (1980) Neonatal campylobacter enteritis. *Canadian Medical Association Journal* **122**, 192–7.

Katon W.J., Ries R.K. *et al* (1980) Hyperemesis gravidarum: A biopsychosocial perspective. *International Journal of Psychiatry in Medicine* **10**, 151–62.

Kaye M.D. & Showalter J.P. (1974) Pyloric incompetence in patients with symptomatic gastroesophageal reflux. *Journal of Laboratory and Clinical Medicine* **83**, 198–206.

Keifer W.S. & Scott J.C. (1977) Liver neoplasms and the oral contraceptives. *American Journal of Obstetrics and Gynecology* **128**, 448–54.

Keighley M.R.B., Burdon D.W.B. *et al* (1978) Randomised controlled trial of vancomycin for pseudomembranous colitis and post operative diarrhoea. *British Medical Journal* **2**, 1667–9.

Kent D.R., Nissen E.D. *et al* (1977) Liver tumors and oral contraceptives. *International Journal of Gynaecology and Obstetrics* **15**, 137–42.

Kent D.R., Nissen E.D. *et al* (1978) Effect of pregnancy on liver tumor associated with oral contraceptives. *Obstetrics and Gynecology* **51**, 148–51.

Kewenter J., Hulten L. *et al* (1974) The relationship and epidemiology of acute terminal ileitis and Crohn's disease. *Gut* **15**, 801–4.

Khuroo M.S. & Datta D.V. (1980) Budd–Chiari syndrome following pregnancy. Report of 16 cases with roentgenologic, hemodynamic and histologic studies of the hepatic outflow tract. *American Journal of Medicine* **68**, 113–21.

Khuroo M.S., Teli M.R. *et al* (1981) Incidence and severity of viral hepatitis in pregnancy *American Journal of Medicine* **70**, 252–5.

Kirsner J.B. (1980) Observation on the medical treatment of inflammatory bowel disease. *Journal of the American Medical Association* **243**, 557–64.

Kirsner J.B., Palmer W.L. *et al* (1948) Clinical course of chronic nonspecific ulcerative colitis. *Journal of the American Medical Association* **137**, 922–8.

Kirsner J.B. & Shorter R.G. (1982a) Recent developments in 'nonspecific' inflammatory bowel disease (first of two parts). *New England Journal of Medicine* **306**, 775–85.

Kirsner J.B. & Shorter R.G. (1982b) Recent developments in 'nonspecific' inflammatory bowel disease (second of two parts). *New England Journal of Medicine* **306**, 837–48.

Kitzmiller J.L., Tanenberg R.J. *et al* (1980) Pancreatic alpha cell response to alanine during and after normal and diabetic pregnancies. *Obstetrics and Gynecology* **56**, 440–5.

Klatskin G. (1977) Hepatic tumours: possible relationship to the use of oral contraceptives. *Gastroenterology* **73**, 386–94.

Klotz U., Maier K. *et al* (1980) Therapeutic efficacy of sulphasalazine and its metabolites in patients with ulcerative colitis and Crohn's disease. *New England Journal of Medicine* **26**, 1499–1502.

Knowles D.M., Casarella W.J. *et al* (1978) The clinical radiologic and pathologic characterisation of benign hepatic neoplasms. Alleged associations with oral contraceptives. *Medicine (Baltimore)* **57**, 223–37.

Korelitz B.I., Glass J.L. *et al* (1973) Long-term immunosuppressive therapy of ulcerative colitis: continuation of a personal series. *American Journal of Digestive Diseases* **18**, 317–22.

Kornman K.S. & Loesche W.J. (1980) The subgingival microbial flora during pregnancy. *Journal of Periodontal Research* **15**, 111–22.

Kowlessar O.D. & Phillips L.D. (1970) Celiac disease. *Medical Clinics of North America* **54**, 647–56.

Krass I.M. (1957) Chiari's syndrome: Report of a case following pregnancy. *Journal of Obstetrics and Gynaecology of the British Commonwealth* **64**, 715–19.

Krawitt E.L. (1959) Ulcerative colitis and pregnancy. *Obstetrics and Gynecology* **14**, 354–61.

Kreek M.J., Sleisenger M.H. *et al* (1967) Recurrent cholestatic jaundice of pregnancy with demonstrated estrogen sensitivity. *American Journal of Medicine* **43**, 795–813.

Kullander S. & Källén B. (1976) A prospective study of drugs and pregnancy. II. Antiemetics. *Acta Obstetricia et Gynecologica Scandinavica Supplement* **55**(2), 105–11.

Kumar D., Goodno J.A. *et al* (1962) Isolation of progesterone from human pregnant myometrium. *Nature* **195**, 1204.

Kumar P.J. (1979) Re-introduction of gluten in adults and children with treated coeliac disease. *Gut* **20**, 743–9.

Kunelis C.T., Peters J.L. *et al* (1965) Fatty liver of pregnancy and its relationship to tetracycline therapy. *American Journal of Medicine* **38**, 359–77.

Kyle J. (1971) An epidemiological study of Crohn's disease in northeast Scotland. *Gastroenterology* **61**, 826–33.

Kyle J. & Stark G. (1980) Fall in the incidence of Crohn's disease. *Gut* **21**, 340–3.

Laatikainen T.J. (1983) Intrauterine fetal death in cholestasis of pregnancy: a case report showing high fetal bile salt levels. *Journal of Obstetrics and Gynecology* **4**, 22.

Lancet editorial (1983a) Acute fatty liver of pregnancy. *Lancet* **i**, 339.

Lancet editorial (1983b) Congenital cytomegalovirus infection. *Lancet* **i**, 801–2.

Lancet editorial (1983c) Malaria in pregnancy. *Lancet* **ii**, 84–5.

Langmade C.F. (1956) Epigastric pain in pregnancy toxaemias *Western Journal of Surgery, Obstetrics & Gynecology* **64**, 540–4.

Langmade C.F. & Edmondson H.A. (1951) Acute pancreatitis during pregnancy and the postpartum period: report of 9 cases. *Surgery, Gynecology and Obstetrics* **92**, 43–52.

Langman M.J., Henry D.A. *et al* (1980) Cimetidine and ranitidine in duodenal ulcer. *British Medical Journal* **281**, 473–4.

Larson H.E. & Price A.B. (1977) Pseudomembranous colitis: Presence of clostridial toxin. *Lancet* **2**, 1312–14.

Lawson J.B. & Stewart D.B. (1967) *Obstetrics and Gynaecology in the Tropics*, pp. 52–9. Edward Arnold, London.

Lederer J. & Kump J. (1979) Mecanisme d'action de la salicylazosulfapyridine sur l'activité de l'acide folique dans la recto colite ulcero-hémorragique. *Gastro-Enterologica Belgica* **42**, 73–81.

Lee D.A.H., Taylor M. *et al* (1980) Rectally administered prednisolone—evidence for a predominantly local action. *Gut* **21**, 215–8.

Lee R.V. (1975) Parasitic infestation. In Burrow G.N. and Ferris T.F. (eds) *Medical Complications During Pregnancy*. W.B. Saunders & Co., London.

Lennard-Jones J.E. & Powell-Tuck J. (1979) Drug treatment of inflammatory bowel disease. *Clinics in Gastroenterology* **8**, 187–217.

Lenz W. & Knapp K. (1962) Thalidomide embryopathy. *Deutsche Medizinische Wochenschrift* **87**, 1232–42.

Levi A.J., Fisher A.M. *et al* (1979) Male infertility due to sulphasalazine. *Lancet* **2**, 276–8.

Levy N., Lemberg E. *et al* (1971) Bowel habit in pregnancy. *Digestion* **4**, 216–22.

Lindsay M.K.M., Nordin B.E.C. *et al* (1956) Late prognosis in coeliac disease. *British Medical Journal* **1**, 14–18.

Löe H. & Silness J. (1963) Periodontal disease in pregnancy. *Acta Odontologica Scandinavica* **21**, 533–51.

Logan R.F.A., Gillon J. *et al* (1981) Reduction of gastrointestinal protein loss by elemental diet in Crohn's disease of the small bowel. *Gut* **22**, 383–7.

Long R.G., Scheuer P.J. *et al* (1977) Presentation and course of asymptomatic primary biliary cirrhosis. *Gastroenteroloty* **72**, 1204–7.

MacDonald W.C., Dobbins W.O. *et al* (1965) Studies of the familial nature of celiac sprue using biopsy of the small intestine. *New England Journal of Medicine* **272**, 448–56.

MacDougall B.R.D., Bailey R.J. *et al* (1977) H_2 receptor antagonists and antacids in the prevention of acute upper gastrointestinal haemorrhage in fulminant hepatic failure. *Lancet* **i**, 617–19.

MacDougall I. (1956) Ulcerative colitis and pregnancy. *Lancet* **271**, 641–3.

Machella T.E. (1952) Problems in ulcerative colitis. *American Journal of Medicine* **13**, 760–76.

Mackenna J., Pupkin M. *et al* (1972) Acute fatty metamorphosis of the liver: a report of two patients who survived. *American Journal of Obstetrics and Gynecology* **40**, 813–15.

Maddix B.L. (1962) Ulcerative colitis and pregnancy. *Minnesota Medicine* **45**, 1097–2011.

Mann J.G., Brown W.R. *et al* (1970) The subtle and variable clinical expressions of gluten-induced enteropathy (adult coeliac disease, non-tropical sprue). An analysis of twenty-one consecutive cases. *American Journal of Medicine* **48**, 357–66.

Marecek Z. & Graf M. (1976) Pregnancy in penicillamine-treated patients with Wilson's disease. *New England Journal of Medicine* **295**, 841–2.

Margolis K. & Naidoo B.N. (1974) Spontaneous postpartum subcapsular haematoma of the liver. *South African Medical Journal* **48**, 1997–8.

Martelli H., Duguay C. *et al* (1978) Some parameters of large bowel motility in normal man. *Gastroenterology* **75**, 612–18.

Martin J.D. & Davis R.E. (1964) Serum folic acid activity and vaginal bleeding in early pregnancy. *Journal of Obstetrics and Gynaecology of the British Commonwealth* **71**, 400–3.

Martin R.H., Harper T.A. *et al* (1965) Serum-folic-acid in recurrent abortions. *Lancet* **i**, 670–2.

Martinbeau P.N., Welch J.S. *et al* (1975) Crohn's disease and pregnancy. *American Journal of Obstetrics and Gynecology* **122**, 746–9.

Maton P.N., Iser J.H. *et al* (1982) The final outcome of chenodeoxycholic acid treatment in 125 patients with radiolucent gallstones, factors influencing efficacy, withdrawal, symptoms and side effects of post dissolution recurrence. *Medicine (Baltimore)* **61**, 86–97.

Mayberry J., Rhodes J. *et al* (1979) Incidence of Crohn's disease in Cardiff between 1934 and 1977. *Gut* **20**, 602–8.

Mays E.T., Christopherson W.M. *et al* (1976) Hepatic changes in young women ingesting contraceptive steroids. Hepatic hemorrhage and primary hepatic tumours. *Journal of the American Medical Association* **235**, 730–2.

McBride W.G. (1961) Thalidomide and congenital abnormalities. *Lancet* **ii**, 1358.

McCarthy C.F., Mylotte M. *et al* (1974) Family studies on coeliac disease in Ireland. In *Proceedings of the Second International Coeliac Symposium, Coeliac Disease*. Stenfert Kroese, Leiden.

McClain C., Soutor C. *et al* (1980) Zinc deficiency: A complication of Crohn's disease. *Gastroenterology* **78**, 272–9.

McClure Browne J.C. (1978) The alimentary system. In McClure Browne J.C. and Dixon G. (eds) *Anti-natal Care*, 11e. Churchill Livingstone, London.

McCormack W.M., George H. *et al* (1977) Hepatotoxicity of erythromycin estolate during pregnancy. *Antimicrobial Agents and Chemotherapy* **12**, 630–5.

McCrae W.M., Eastwood M.A. *et al* (1975) Neglected coeliac disease. *Lancet* **1**, 187–90.

McEwen H.P. (1972) Ulcerative colitis in pregnancy. *Proceedings of the Royal Society of Medicine* **65**, 279–81.

McGowan W.A.W. (1979) Safety of cimetidine in obstetric patients. *Journal of the Royal Society of Medicine* **72**, 902–7.

McGrugan J.E. & Volwiler W. (1964) Celiac-sprue: Malabsorption of iron in the absence of steatorrhoea. *Gastroenterology* **47**, 636–41.

McKay A.J., O'Neill J. *et al* (1980) Pancreatitis, pregnancy and gallstones. *British Journal of Obstetrics and Gynaecology* **87**, 47–50.

Medalie J.H. (1957) Relationship between nausea and/or vomiting in early pregnancy and abortion. *Lancet* **2**, 117–19.

Mellor S. (1978) Fetal malformation after Debendox in early pregnancy. *British Medical Journal* **1**, 1055.

Meyers S., Walfish J.S. *et al* (1980) Quality of life after surgery for Crohn's disease: a psychosocial survey. *Gastroenterology* **78**, 1–6.

Midwinter A. (1971) Causes of vomiting in pregnancy. *Practitioner* **206**, 743–50.

Miller D.S., Keighley A.C. *et al* (1974) Changing patterns in epidemiology of Crohn's disease. *Lancet* **2**, 691–3.

Misra P.S., Evanov F.A. *et al* (1980) Idiopathic intrahepatic cholestasis of pregnancy. Report of an unusual case and review of the recent literature. *American Journal of Gastroenterology* **73**, 54–9.

Misra R.C., Kasthuri S. *et al* (1966) Adult coeliac disease in tropics. *British Medical Journal* **2**, 1230–2.

Mitchell J.E., Breuer R.I. *et al* (1980) The colon influences ileal resection diarrhoea. *Digestive Diseases and Science* **25**, 33–41.

Mogadam M., Dobbins W.O. *et al* (1981) Pregnancy in inflammatory bowel disease: effect of sulfasalazine and corticosteroids on fetal outcome. *Gastroenterology* **80**, 72–6.

Moldin P. & Johansson O. (1978) Acute fatty liver of pregnancy with disseminated intravascular coagulation. *Acta Obstetricia et Gynecologica Scandinavica Supplement* **57**, 179–81.

Möller C., Kiviluoto O. *et al* (1978) Local treatment of ulcerative proctitis with salicylazosulpha-pyridine (salazopyrin) enema. *Clinical Trials Journal (London)* **15**, 199–203.

Montgomery W.H. & Miller F.C. (1970) Views and reviews: Pancreatitis and pregnancy. *Obstetrics and Gynecology* **35**, 658–65.

Moore R.M. & Hughes P.K. (1960) Cirrhosis of the liver in pregnancy. A review of the literature and report of three cases. *Obstetrics and Gynecology* **15**, 753–6.

Morris J.S., Ajdukiewicz A.B. & Read A.E. (1970) Coeliac infertility: an indication for dietary gluten restrictions? *Lancet* **1**, 213–14.

Mortimer P.E., Stewart J.S. *et al* (1968) Follow-up study of coeliac disease. *British Medical Journal* III, 7–9.

Munzoz L.E., Thomas H.C. *et al* (1981) Is mitochondrial antibody diagnostic of primary biliary cirrhosis? *Gut* **22**, 136–40.

Mylotte M.J., Egan-Mitchell B. *et al* (1972) Familial coeliac disease. *Quarterly Journal of Medicine* **41**, 527–8.

Nebel O.T. & Castell D.O. (1972) Lower esophageal sphincter pressure changes after food ingestion. *Gastroenterology* **63**, 778–83.

Nelson M.M. & Forfar J.O. (1971) Associations between drugs administered during pregnancy and congenital abnormalities of the foetus. *British Medical Journal* i, 523–7.

Nillsson I.M. & Kullanders S. (1967) Coagulation and fibrinolytic studies during pregnancy. *Acta Obstetricia et Gynecologica Scandinavica Supplement* **46**, 273–85.

Nilsson S. & Stattin S. (1967) Gallbladder emptying during the normal menstrual cycle. *Acta Chirurgica Scandinavica* **133**, 648–52.

Norton R.A. & Patterson J.F. (1972) Pregnancy and regional enteritis. *Obstetrics and Gynecology* **40**, 711–12.

Ockner R.K. & Davidson C.S. (1967) Hepatic effects of oral contraceptives. *New England Journal of Medicine* **276**, 331–4.

O'Donoghue D.P., Dawson A.M. *et al* (1978) Double blind withdrawal trial of azathioprine as maintenance treatment for Crohn's disease. *Lancet* **2**, 955–7.

Ogborn A.D.R. (1975) Pregnancy in patients with coeliac disease. *British Journal of Obstetrics and Gynaecology* **82**, 293–6.

Orellana-Alcade J.M. & Dominguez J.P. (1966) Jaundice and oral contraceptive drugs. *Lancet* **1**, 1278–80.

Pallis C.A. & Lewis P.D. (1974) Coeliac disease. In *Neurology of Gastrointestinal Diseases*. W.B. Saunders and Co, London.

Palmer K.R., Goepel J.R. *et al* (1981) Sulphasalazine retention enemas in ulcerative colitis: a double-blind trial. *British Medical Journal* **282**, 1571–3.

Palmer W.L., Kirsner J.B. *et al* (1964) Disease of the liver in chronic ulcerative colitis. *American Journal of Medicine* **36**, 856–66.

Parbhoo S.P. & Johnston I.D.A. (1966) Effect of oestrogen and progestogens on gastric secretion in patients with duodenal ulcer. *Gut* **7**, 612–18.

Parry E., Shields R. *et al* (1970a) Transit time in the small intestine in pregnancy. *Journal of Obstetrics and Gynaecology of the British Commonwealth* **77**, 900–1.

Parry E., Shields R. *et al* (1970b) The effect of pregnancy on the colonic absorption of sodium, potassium and water. *Journal of Obstetrics and Gynaecology of the British Commonwealth* **77**, 616–19.

Patterson D. (1969) Congenital deformities (letter). *Canadian Medical Association Journal* **101**, 175–6.

Patterson D. (1977) Congenital deformities associated with Bendectin. *Canadian Medical Association Journal* **116**, 1348.

Peden N.R., Boyd E.J.S. *et al* (1981) Women and duodenal ulcer. *British Medical Journal* **282**, 866.

Perez V. & Gorodisch S. (1974) Female sex hormones and the liver. In Schaffner F., Sherlock S. and Leevy C.M. (eds) *The Liver and its Diseases*, p. 179. Georg Thieme, Stuttgart.

Perrett A.D., Higgins G. *et al* (1971a) The liver in Crohn's disease. *Quarterly Journal of Medicine* **40**, 187–209.

Perrett A.D., Higgins G. *et al* (1971b) The liver in ulcerative colitis. *Quarterly Journal of Medicine* **40**, 211–38.

Perry J.F. & Strate R.G. (1972) Diagnostic peritoneal lavage in blunt abdominal trauma: indications and results. *Surgery* **71**, 898–901.

Peters J.P., Heinemann M. *et al* (1951) Lipids of serum in pregnancy. *Journal of Clinical Investigation* **30**, 388–94.

Peterson W.F., Stauch J.F. *et al* (1966) Metronidazole in pregnancy. *American Journal of Obstetrics and Gynecology* **94**, 243–9.

Pillay N., Adams E.B. *et al* (1975) Comparative trial of amoxycillin and chloramphenicol in treatment of typhoid fever in adults. *Lancet* **2**, 333–4.

Poulantzas J., Polymeropoulos P.S. *et al* (1978) Double-blind evaluation of the effect of tripotassium di-citrato bismuthate in peptic ulcer. *British Journal of Clinical Practice* **32**, 147–8.

Prakash C., Bansal B.C. *et al* (1974) A comparative study of tinidazole and metronidazole in symptomatic intestinal amoebiasis. *Journal of the Association of Physicians of India* **22**, 527–9.

Prem K.A., Fergus J.W. *et al* (1961) Vaccination by oral route of pregnant women and young children with trivalent antipoliomyelitis vaccine of living attenuated virus. *Boletin de la Oficina Sanitaria Panamericana* **50**, 525–49.

Present D.H., Korelitz B.I. *et al* (1980) Treatment of Crohn's disease with 6-Mercaptopurine: A long-term randomised, double-blind trial. *New England Journal of Medicine* **302**, 981–7.

Pritchard J.A., Scott D.E. *et al* (1971) Maternal folate deficiency and pregnancy wastage. IV. Effects of folic acid supplements, anticonvulsants, and oral contraceptives. *American Journal of Obstetrics and Gynecology* **109**, 341–6.

Purcell R.H. & Gerin J.L. (1978) Hepatitis B vaccines: A status report. In Vyas G.N., Cohen S.N. and Schmid R. (eds) *Viral Hepatitis*. Franklin Institute Press, Philadelphia.

Purtilo D.T., Clark J.V. *et al* (1975) Primary hepatic malignancy in pregnant women. *American Journal of Obstetrics and Gynecology* **121**, 41–4.

Putzki P.S., Scully J.H. *et al* (1949) Carcinoma of the colon producing acute intestinal obstruction during pregnancy. *American Journal of Surgery* **77**, 749–54.

Raffensperger E.C. (1948) Recurrence of regional terminal ileitis associated with pregnancy. *Gastroenterology* **10**, 1010–17.

Rakela J., Redeker A.G. *et al* (1978) Hepatitis A virus infection in fulminant hepatitis and chronic active hepatitis. *Gastroenterology* **74**, 879–82.

Rannevik G., Jeppsson S. *et al* (1972) Effect of oral contraceptives on the liver in women with recurrent cholestasis (hepatosis) during previous pregnancies. *Journal of Obstetrics and Gynaecology of the British Commonwealth* **79**, 1128–36.

Redeker A.G. (1978) Advances in clinical aspects of acute and chronic liver disease of viral origin. In Vyas G.N., Cohen S.N. and Schmid R. (eds) *Viral Hepatitis*, pp. 425–9. Franklin Institute Press, Philadelphia.

Reid R., Ivey K.J. *et al* (1976) Fetal complications of obstetric cholestasis. *British Medical Journal* **1**, 870–2.

Reyes H., Ribalta J. *et al* (1976) Idiopathic cholestasis of pregnancy in large kindred. *Gut* **17**, 709–13.

Richards R.L., Willcocks J. *et al* (1970) Jaundice in pregnancy. *Scottish Medical Journal* **15**, 52–7.

Richman A. (1956) Acute pancreatitis. *American Journal of Medicine* **21**, 246–74.

Richman A. (1965) Medical, surgical and gynecologic complications of pregnancy. In Rovinsky

J.J. and Guttmacher A.F. (eds) *The Liver*, Chapter 11, p. 200. E. & S. Livingstone Ltd, Edinburgh.

Ritchie J.A. & Truelove S.C. (1980) Comparison of various treatments for irritable bowel syndrome. *British Medical Journal* **281**, 1317–19.

Rodin P. & Hass G. (1966) Metronidazole and pregnancy. *British Journal of Venereal Diseases* **42**, 210–12.

Rogers B.H.G., Clark L.M. *et al* (1971) The epidemiologic and demographic characteristics of inflammatory bowel disease: An analysis of a computerized file of 1400 patients. *Journal of Chronic Diseases* **24**, 743–73.

Rooks J.B., Ory H.W. *et al* (1979) Epidemiology of hepatocellular carcinoma. The role of oral contraceptive use. *Journal of the American Medical Association* **242**, 644–8.

Roszkowski I. & Wojcicka J. (1968) Jaundice in pregnancy. I. Biochemical assays. *American Journal of Obstetrics and Gynecology* **102**, 839–46.

Rowe A.W. & Boyd W.C. (1932) Metabolism in pregnancy; foetal influence on basal rate. *Journal of Nutrition* **5**, 551–69.

Rozen P., Zonis J. *et al* (1979) Crohn's disease in the Jewish population of Tel-Aviv-Yafo: epidemiologic and clinical aspects. *Gastroenterology* **76**, 25–30.

Ruddell W.S.J., Dickinson R.J. *et al* (1980) Treatment of distal ulcerative colitis (proctosigmoiditis) in relapse: comparison of hydrocortisone enemas and rectal hydrocortisone foam. *Gut* **21**, 885–9.

Sachar D.B. (1980) Metronidazole for Crohn's disease: Breakthrough or ballyhoo? (Editorial). *Gastroenterology* **79**, 393–4.

Salih S.Y., Satir Abdel A. *et al* (1978) Observations on hepatocellular carcinoma in the Sudan. *Journal of Tropical Medicine and Hygiene* **81**, 60–2.

Samsioe G., Svendsen P. *et al* (1975) Studies in cholestasis of pregnancy. V. Gallbladder disease, liver function tests, serum lipids and fatty acid composition of serum lecithin in the non-pregnant state. *Acta Obstetricia et Gynecologica Scandinavica Supplement* **54**, 417–23.

Sandweiss D.J., Podolsky H.M. *et al* (1943) Deaths from perforation and hemorrhage of gastroduodenal ulcer during pregnancy and the puerperium. *American Journal of Obstetrics and Gynecology* **45**, 131–6.

Schoenfield L.J., Lachin J.M. *et al* (1981) Chenodiol (chenodeoxycholic acid) for dissolution of gallstones—the National Cooperative Gallstone Study—a controlled trial of efficacy and safety. *Annals of Internal Medicine* **95**, 257–83.

Schofield P.F., Turnbull R.B. *et al* (1970) Crohn's disease and pregnancy. *British Medical Journal* **2**, 364.

Schottenfeld D., Berg J.W. *et al* (1969) Incidence of multiple primary cancers. II. Index cancers arising in the stomach or digestive system. *Journal of the National Cancer Institute* **43**, 77–86.

Schrock T.R. (1978) Diseases of the anorectum. In Sleisenger M.H. and Fordtran J.S. (eds) *Gastrointestinal Disease*, 2e, pp. 1875–89. W.B. Saunders & Co, London.

Schulze-Delrieu K. & Koch-Weser J. (1981) Drug therapy: Metoclopramide. *New England Journal of Medicine* **305**, 28–33.

Schweitzer I.L., Mosley J.W. *et al* (1973) Factors influencing neonatal infection by hepatitis B virus. *Gastroenterology* **65**, 277–83.

Schweitzer I.L. & Peters R.L. (1976) Pregnancy in hepatitis B antigen positive cirrhosis. *Obstetrics and Gynecology* (Suppl.) **48**, 535–65.

Scioli C., Fiorentino F. *et al* (1972) Treatment of salmonella typhi carriers with intravenous ampicillin. *Journal of Infectious Diseases* **125**, 170–3.

Scott N.M. & Deutsch D.L. (1955) The esophagus during pregnancy. *American Journal of Gastroenterology* **24**, 305–13.

Scragg J.N. & Rubidge C.J. (1975) Amoxycillin in the treatment of typhoid fever in children. *American Journal of Tropical Medicine and Hygiene* **24**, 860–5.

Scudamore H.H., Rogers A.G. *et al* (1957) Pregnancy after ileostomy for ulcerative colitis. *Gastroenterology* **32**, 295–303.

Sedlack R.E., Whisnant J. *et al* (1980) Incidence of Crohn's disease in Olmsted County, Minnesota 1935–75. *American Journal of Epidemiology* **112**, 759–63.

Segal I., Tim L.O. *et al* (1980) The rarity of ulcerative colitis in South African blacks. *American Journal of Gastroenterology* **74**, 332–6.

Semmens J.P. (1957) Hyperemesis gravidarum: evaluation and treatment. *Obstetrics and Gynecology* **9**, 586–94.

Seymour C.A. & Chadwick V.S. (1979) Liver and gastrointestinal function in pregnancy. *Postgraduate Medical Journal* **55**, 343–52.

Shapiro S., Neinonen O.P. *et al* (1977) Antenatal exposure to doxylamine succinate and dicyclomine hydrochloride (Bendectin) in relation to congenital malformations, perinatal mortality rate, birth weight and intelligence quotient score. *American Journal of Obstetrics and Gynecology* **128**, 480–5.

Sheehan H.L. (1939) The pathology of hyperemesis and vomiting of late pregnancy. *Journal of Obstetrics and Gynaecology of the British Commonwealth* **46**, 685–99.

Sheehan H.L. (1940) The pathology of acute yellow atrophy and delayed chloroform poisoning. *Journal of Obstetrics and Gynaecology of the British Commonwealth* **47**, 49–62.

Sheehan H.L. (1950) Pathological lesions in the hypertensive toxemias of pregnancy. In Ciba Foundation: Symposium: *Toxemias of Pregnancy, Human and Veterinary*, p. 19. Blakiston Co, Philadelphia.

Sheldon W. (1969) Prognosis in early adult life of coeliac children treated with gluten-free diet. *British Medical Journal* **2**, 401–4.

Shelton M.G. (1980) Standardized senna in the management of constipation in the puerperum: a clinical trial. *South African Medical Journal* **57**, 78–80.

Sherlock S. (1968) Jaundice in pregnancy. *British Medical Bulletin* **24**, 39–43.

Sherlock S. (1974) Classification of functional aspects of portal hypertension. *American Journal of Surgery* **127**, 121–8.

Sherlock S. (1981) *Diseases of the Liver and Biliary System*, 6th edn. p. 227 et seq. Blackwell Scientific Publications, Oxford.

Sherwin A.L., Beck I.T. *et al* (1960) The course of Wilson's disease (hepatolenticular degeneration) during pregnancy and after delivery. *Canadian Medical Association Journal* **83**, 160–3.

Shmerling D.H., Leisinger P. *et al* (1972) On the familial occurrence of coeliac disease. *Acta Paediatrica Scandinavica* **61**, 501.

Sichel M.S. (1961) Postpartum and postoperative bowel function. *Northwest Medicine* **60**, 708–9.

Siegel B. & Siegel S. (1960) Pregnancy and delivery in a patient with cystic fibrosis of the pancreas. *Obstetrics and Gynecology* **16**, 438–40.

Siegel M. (1973) Congenital malformations following chicken pox, measles, mumps and hepatitis. *Journal of the American Medical Association* **226**, 1521–4.

Simmons S.C. (1964) Ano-rectal disorders in pregnancy *Journal of Obstetrics and Gynaecology of the British Commonwealth* **71**, 960–2.

Sims E.H., Schlater T.L. *et al* (1980) Obstructing gastric carcinoma complicating pregnancy. *Journal of the National Medical Association* **72**, 21–3.

Sinclair T.S., Brunt P.W. *et al* (1980) Natural history of proctocolitis in the North-east of Scotland: a community study. *Gut* **2**, A924 abstract.

Singh M.S. & Lean T.H. (1970) The use of metoclopramide (Maxolon) in hyperemesis gravidarum. *Proceedings of the Obstetrical and Gynaecological Society of Singapore* **1**, 43.

Singleton J.W., Law D.H. *et al* (1979a) National Cooperative Crohn's Disease Study: adverse reactions to study drugs. *Gastroenterology* **77**, 870–82.

Singleton J.W., Summer R.W. *et al* (1979b) A trial of sulfasalazine as adjunctive therapy in Crohn's disease. *Gastroenterology* **77**, 887–97.

Slaughter C.R. & Krantz K.E. (1963) Cirrhosis of the liver complicating pregnancy. A presentation of 2 cases and a review of the literature. *American Journal of Obstetrics and Gynecology* **86**, 1060–7.

Smith D. (1967) Severe anaphylactic reaction after a soap enema. *British Medical Journal* **IV**, 215.

Smithells R.W. & Sheppard S. (1978) Fetal malformation after Debendox in early pregnancy (letter). *British Medical Journal* **1**, 1055–6.

Snape W.J., Carlson G.M. *et al* (1976) Colonic myoelectric activity in the irritable bowel syndrome. *Gastroenterology* **70**, 326–30.

Sommer D.G., Greenway G.D. *et al* (1979) Hepatic rupture with toxaemia of pregnancy: angiographic diagnosis. *American Journal of Roentgenology* **132**, 455–6.

Soyanno M.A.O., McGeown M.G. *et al* (1968) A case of acute hyperparathyroidism with thyrotoxicosis and pancreatitis presenting as hyperemesis gravidarum. *Postgraduate Medical Journal* **44**, 861–78.

Srikantia S.G. & Reddy V. (1967) Megaloblastic anaemia of infancy and Vitamin B_{12}. *British Journal of Haematology* **13**, 949–53.

Stander H.J. & Cadder J.F. (1934) Acute yellow atrophy of the liver in pregnancy. *American Journal of Obstetrics and Gynecology* **28**, 61–9.

Steel R. & Parker M.L. (1973) Jaundice in pregnancy. *Medical Journal of Australia* **1**, 461.

Steven M.M. (1981) Pregnancy and liver disease. *Gut* **22**, 592–614.

Steven M.M., Buckley J.D. *et al* (1979) Pregnancy in chronic active hepatitis. *Quarterly Journal of Medicine* **48**, 519–33.

Stevens C.E. (1982) Viral hepatitis in pregnancy: the obstetrician's role. *Clinical Obstetrics and Gynecology* **25**, 577–84.

Stevens F.M. & Craig A. (1981) Prolactin and coeliac disease. *Irish Journal of Medical Science* **150**, 329–31.

Stewart J.S., Pollock D.J. *et al* (1967) A study of proximal and distal intestinal structure and absorptive function in idiopathic steatorrhoea. *Quarterly Journal of Medicine* **36**, 425–44.

Stirrat G.M. & Beard R.W. (1973) Drugs to be avoided or given with caution in the second or third trimesters of pregnancy. *Prescribers Journal* **13**, 135–40.

Summers R.W., Switz D.M. *et al* (1979) National Cooperative Crohn's Disease Study: results of drug treatment. *Gastroenterology* **77**, 847–69.

Summerskill W.H.J. & Walshe J.M. (1959) Benign recurrent intrahepatic 'obstructive' jaundice. *Lancet* **ii**, 686–90.

Svanborg A. (1954) A study of recurrent jaundice in pregnancy. *Acta Obstetricia et Gynecologica Scandinavica Supplement* **33**, 434–44.

Swartley W.B., Newton Z.B. *et al* (1947) Perforated carcinoma of large intestine complicating pregnancy: Successful operative management. *Annals of Surgery* **125**, 251–6.

Sweeney W.J. (1963) Use of bisacodyl suppositories as a routine laxative in postpartum patients. *American Journal of Obstetrics and Gynecology* **85**, 908–11.

Tabor E. & Gerety R.J. (1979) Hepatitis B virus infection in infants and toddlers in Nigeria: the need for early interaction. *Journal of Pediatrics* **95**, 647–50.

Taggart N. (1961) Food habits in pregnancy. *Proceedings of the Nutrition Society* **20**, 35–40.

Tavill A.S., Wood E.J. *et al* (1975) The Budd–Chiari syndrome. Correlation between hepatic scintigraphy and clinical radiological and pathological findings in 19 cases of hepatic venous outflow obstruction. *Gastroenterology* **68**, 509–18.

Taylor R.H., Laidlow J.M. *et al* (1977) Double-blind trial comparing cimetidine with carbenoxolone in the treatment of benign gastric ulcer. *Gut* **18**, 420A.

Tedesco F.J., Stanley R.J. *et al* (1974) Diagnostic features of clindamycin-associated pseudomembranous colitis. *New England Journal of Medicine* **290**, 841.

Thomason J.L., Sampson M.B. *et al* (1981) Pregnancy complicated by concurrent primary hyperparathyroidism and pancreatitis. *Obstetrics and Gynecology* **57** (Suppl. 6), 34S–36S.

Thomson H. (1975) Piles: their nature and management. *Lancet* **2**, 494–5.

Thorling L. (1955) Jaundice in pregnancy: A clinical study. *Acta Medica Scandinavica Supplement* **302**, 1–123.

Thulesius O. & Gjöres J.E. (1973) Arterio-venous anastomoses in the anal region with reference to the pathogenesis and treatment of haemorrhoids. *Acta Chirurgica Scandinavica* **139**, 476–8.

Tikkanen M.J. & Adlercreutz H. (1973) Recurrent jaundice in pregnancy. III. Quantitative determination of urinary estriol conjugates, including studies in pruritus gravidarum. *American Journal of Medicine* **54**, 600–4.

Toaff R., Toaff M.E. *et al* (1977) Hepatolenticular degeneration (Wilson's disease) and pregnancy. A review and report of a case. *Obstetrical and Gynecological Survey* **32**, 497–507.

Tobin J. O'H., Jones D.M. *et al* (1977) Aetiology, diagnosis, prevention and control of infections affecting pregnancy in humans. In Coid C.R. (ed.) *Infections and Pregnancy*, pp. 1–45. Academic Press, London.

Tong M.J., Thursby M. *et al* (1981) Studies on the maternal-infant transmission of viruses which cause acute hepatitis. *Gastroenterology* **80**, 999–1004.

Toovey S., Hudson E. *et al* (1981) Sulphasalazine and male infertility: reversibility and possible mechanism. *Gut* **22**, 445–51.

Toth A. (1979a) Male infertility due to sulphasalazine. *Lancet* **2**, 904.

Toth A. (1979b) Reversible toxic effect of salicylazosulfapyridine on semen quality. *Fertility and Sterility* **31**, 538–40.

Trapnell J.E. & Duncan E.H.L. (1975) Patterns of incidence in acute pancreatitis. *British Medical Journal* **2**, 179–83.

Traub A.I., Thompson W. *et al* (1979) Male infertility due to sulphasalazine. *Lancet* **ii**, 639–40.

Tresadern J.C., Falconer G.F. *et al* (1983) Successful completed pregnancy in a patient maintained on home parenteral nutrition. *British Medical Journal* **286**, 602–3.

Trewby P.N. & Williams R. (1977) Pathophysiology of hypotension in patients with fulminant hepatic failure. *Gut* **18**, 1021–6.

Trussell R.R. & Beeley L. (1981) Infestations. In *Clinics in Obstetrics and Gynaecology: Prescribing in Pregnancy*, Vol. 8, Chap. 7, pp. 333–40. W.B. Saunders Co. Ltd, London.

Tumen H.J. & Cohn E.M. (1950) Pregnancy and chronic ulcerative colitis. *Gastroenterology* **16**, 1–11.

Turner E.S., Greenberger P.A. & Patterson R. (1980) Management of the pregnant asthmatic patient. *Annals of Internal Medicine* **93**, 905–18.

Tyson R.M., Shrader E.A. *et al* (1937) Drugs transmitted through breast milk. Part I: Laxatives. *Journal of Pediatrics* **2**, 824–32.

Urban E., Frank B.W. *et al* (1968) Liver dysfunction with mestranol but not with norethynodrel in a patient with Enovid-induced jaundice. *Annals of Internal Medicine* **68**, 598–602.

Urban E. & Weser E. (1980) Intestinal adaptation to bowel resection. *Advances in Internal Medicine* **26**, 265–91.

Vana J., Murphy G.P. *et al* (1977) Primary liver tumors and oral contraceptives. Results of a survey. *Journal of the American Medical Association* **238**, 2154–8.

Van Thiel D.H., Gavaler J.S. *et al* (1977) Heartburn of pregnancy. *Gastroenterology* **72**, 666–8.

Van Thiel D.H. & Wald A. (1981) Evidence refuting a role for increased abdominal pressure in the pathogenesis of the heartburn associated with pregnancy. *American Journal of Obstetrics and Gynecology* **140**, 420–2.

Varadi S. (1967) Pernicious anaemia and infertility. *Lancet* **ii**, 1305.

Varner M. & Rinderknecht N.K. (1980) Acute fatty metamorphosis of pregnancy. A maternal mortality and literature review. *Journal of Reproductive Medicine* **24**, 177–80.

Vender R.J. & Spiro H.M. (1982) Inflammatory bowel disease and pregnancy. *Journal of Clinical Gastroenterology* **4**, 231–49.

Vesikari T., Huffunen L. *et al* (1981) Perinatal campylobacter fetus species jejuni enteritis. *Acta Paediatrica Scandinavica* **70**, 261–3.

Visakorpi J.K.V., Immonen P. *et al* (1967) Malabsorption syndrome in childhood. The occurrence of absorption defects and their clinical significance. *Acta Paediatrica Scandinavica* **56**, 1–9.

Visakorpi J.K., Kuitunen P. *et al* (1970) Intestinal malabsorption: a clinical study of 22 children over 2 years of age. *Acta Paediatrica Scandinavica* **59**, 273.

Wald A., Van Thiel D.H. *et al* (1981) Gastrointestinal transit: the effect of the menstrual cycle. *Gastroenterology* **80**, 1497–1500.

Waldrum H.L., Straume B.K. & Lundgren R. (1980) Serum group I pepsinogens during pregnancy. *Scandinavian Journal of Gastroenterology* **15**, 61–3.

Walker-Smith J.A., Harrison M. *et al* (1978) Cows' milk-sensitive enteropathy. *Archives of Disease in Childhood* **53**, 375–80.

Walshe J.M. (1977) Pregnancy in Wilson's disease. *Quarterly Journal of Medicine* **46**, 73–83.

Waters E.G. & Fenimore E.D. (1954) Perforated carcinoma of cecum in pregnancy. *Obstetrics and Gynecology* **3**, 263–7.

Watson R. & Kennedy J.H. (1980) An unusual case of maternal death. *Scottish Medical Journal* **25**, 241–2.

Webb G.A. (1980) The use of hyperalimentation and chemotherapy in pregnancy: A case report. *American Journal of Obstetrics and Gynecology* **137**, 263–5.

Webb M.J. & Sedlack R.E. (1974) Ulcerative colitis in pregnancy. *Medical Clinics of North America* **58**, 823–37.

Weber F.L., Snodgrass P.J. *et al* (1979) Abnormalities of hepatic mitochondrial urea-cycle enzyme activities and hepatic ultra structure in acute fatty liver of pregnancy. *Journal of Laboratory and Clinical Medicine* **94**, 27–41.

Weinstein L. & Meade R.H. (1955) The effect of the stage of gestation and number of pregnancies on susceptibility to poliomyelitis. *American Journal of Obstetrics and Gynecology* **70**, 1026–30.

Weiss N.S. (1978) Non-contraceptive estrogens and abnormalities of endometrial proliferation. *Annals of Internal Medicine* **88**, 410–12.

Weiss N.S., Daling J.R. *et al* (1981) Incidence of cancer of the large bowel in women in relation to reproductive and hormonal factors. *Journal of the National Cancer Institute* **67**, 57–60.

Weller T.H. (1971) The cytomegaloviruses: ubiquitous agents with protean clinical manifestations. I. *New England Journal of Medicine* **285**, 203–14.

Wells C.N. (1953) Treatment of hyperemesis gravidarum with cortisone. *American Journal of Obstetrics and Gynecology* **66**, 598–601.

Wenk R.E., Gebhardt F.C. *et al* (1981) Tetracycline-associated fatty liver of pregnancy, including possible pregnancy risk after chronic dermatologic use of tetracycline. *Journal of Reproductive Medicine* **26**, 135–41.

Werthmann M.W. & Krees S.V. (1973) Quantitative excretion of Senokot in human breast milk. *Medical Annals of the District of Columbia* **42**, 4–5.

Whelan T.J., Baugh G.H. *et al* (1973) Focal nodular hyperplasia of the liver. *Annals of Surgery* **177**, 150–8.

Whelton M.J. & Sherlock S. (1968) Pregnancy in patients with hepatic cirrhosis. Management and outcome. *Lancet* **2**, 995–9.

White N.J., Warrell D.A. *et al* (1983) Severe hypoglycaemia and hyperinsulinemia in falciparum malaria. *New England Journal of Medicine* **309**, 61–6.

Wilinson E.J. (1973) Acute pancreatitis in pregnancy: A review of 98 cases and a report of 8 new cases. *Obstetrical and Gynecological Survey* **28**, 281–303.

Wilkinson S.P., Blendis L.M. *et al* (1974) Frequency and type of renal and electrolyte disorders in fulminant hepatic failure. *British Medical Journal* **1**, 186–9.

Willoughby C.P. & Truelove S.C. (1980) Ulcerative colitis and pregnancy. *Gut* **21**, 469–74.

Wilson J.T., Brown R.D. *et al* (1980) Drug excretion in human breast milk: principles, pharmakokinetics and projected consequences. *Clinical Pharmacokinetics* **5**, 1–66.

Winship D.H. (1975) Gastrointestinal diseases. In Burrow G.N. and Ferris T.F. (eds) *Medical Complications During Pregnancy*, pp. 275–350. W.B. Saunders Co. Ltd, Philadelphia.

Woo D., Cummins M. *et al* (1979) Vertical transmission of hepatitis B surface antigen in carrier mothers in two west London Hospitals. *Archives of Disease in Childhood* **54**, 670–5.

Wray D., Ferguson M.M. *et al* (1975) Recurrent Aphthae: treatment with Vitamin B_{12} folic acid and iron. *British Medical Journal* **2**, 490–3.

Young J.F., Cave D. *et al* (1968) Enema shock in Hirschsprung's disease. *Diseases of the Colon and Rectum* **11**, 391–5.

Zuckerman A.J. (1980) Prophylaxis of hepatitis type B: Immunoglobulins and vaccines. *Clinics in Gastroenterology* **9**, 65–83.

10 Diabetes

Richard Beard

Management of the pregnant woman with diabetes continues to present a challenge to the physician, obstetrician and paediatrician. Before the availability of insulin, those women with juvenile diabetes who survived to the age of reproduction and were able to become pregnant had less than a 50 per cent chance of having a living child. The problems now are different but nonetheless taxing. The recognition that diabetes results in a disturbance of the environment of the fetus that may seriously interfere with organogenesis and development has led to an acknowledgement that normoglycaemia (*see* Fig. 10.1) is an important objective in diabetic control. Until that can be achieved throughout the early part of pregnancy, there seems little likelihood that it will be possible to reduce the risk of congenital malformation that threatens every diabetic pregnancy. The persistence of an increased incidence of neonatal morbidity from conditions such as hypoglycaemia, respiratory distress and severe jaundice suggests that, even though the baby survives, all was not well with the intrauterine environment. Perhaps, in future, we should be using these complications rather than perinatal mortality as our indices of whether management was successful or not.

The importance of diabetes which is detected for the first time in pregnancy (gestational diabetes) remains disputed. The evidence that diabetes in the mother may lead to permanent damage to the β-cells of the pancreas of her fetus (Hultquist and Olding 1975) raises the possibility of transmission of a tendency to diabetes in later life, if the condition in the mother is not recognised and treated. Equally this is now support for the view that pregnant women with gestational diabetes have a much greater possibility of eventually developing maturity-onset diabetes (O'Sullivan and Mahan 1980).

For these reasons, it is not surprising that so much time and effort is invested in the care of a group of pregnant women who, at most, comprise less than 3 per cent of the obstetric population. A lot has changed in recent years that has dramatically improved the prognosis for the pregnancy of a diabetic. In the past, much of the evidence upon which management was based was speculative, but it is now clear that with better control of diabetes, new systems for monitoring the fetus in late pregnancy, and the outstanding achievements in the care of the newborn, management policies need to be reviewed. This chapter is devoted to a description and rationale of modern management of the pregnant diabetic and her baby.

Terminology

Over the years a variety of descriptive terms have entered the literature of diabetes in pregnancy and it is important that the reader should have a clear idea of their meaning.

PREDIABETES

The term was first used when it was recognised that parous women, who were found to have diabetes in a later pregnancy, had a history of macrosomic babies and perinatal deaths in previous pregnancies. By implication, it was suggested that there was some factor other than the metabolic disturbance of diabetes that affected the fetus adversely. There is no evidence to support this concept and it seems more likely that, if these women had had a glucose tolerance test (GTT) in the 'prediabetic' pregnancy, it would have proved to have been abnormal.

POTENTIAL DIABETES

The term is applied to pregnant women who have certain features in their family or medical or obstetric history which predispose them to increased possibility of developing diabetes in pregnancy. This group is characterised by a number of features, the most important of which are: **1.** diabetes in a close relative, **2.** a bad obstetric history particularly a perinatal death or traumatic delivery of a macrosomic baby, **3.** age of more than 25 and/or obesity. About 30 per cent of most obstetric populations have one or more features of potential diabetes.

GESTATIONAL AND ESTABLISHED DIABETES

In Britain it is customary to classify women with diabetes in pregnancy as having either gestational or established diabetes. *Gestational diabetes*, strictly speaking, is carbohydrate intolerance that arises in pregnancy and disappears after delivery, but this definition is of little practical value because it is rarely possible to be certain that these women did not have subclinical diabetes before they became pregnant, nor is testing carbohydrate tolerance after delivery a widespread practice. The term gestational diabetes is best applied to those women who, for whatever reason, had a GTT in pregnancy which was found to be abnormal. *Established diabetes* on the other hand refers to the condition which is known to have been present for a variable time before pregnancy.

The 'White' classification (*see* Table 10.1) was devised by Dr Priscilla White from Boston, USA, and has widespread acceptance in Europe and the USA (White 1965). Diabetes is graded from A to F according to the severity as judged by the age of onset, duration, and the presence or absence of complications of the disease. In general, the more severe the disease the greater the perinatal mortality and incidence of congenital malformations (Table 10.1). This classification, which is not in general use in Britain, provides a useful system for comparison of results from different centres and has the advantage that the outcome of this pregnancy can be related to the severity of the disease. The interim results of the UK Survey of Diabetes in Pregnancy indicated that, amongst women with established diabetes, 12 per cent were Class A, 24 per cent Class B, 39 per cent Class C, 22 per cent Class D and 3 per cent Class F (Lowy and Beard 1982).

There is a problem in fitting women with gestational diabetes into the White classification because some of them become worse during pregnancy, requiring insulin treatment. Metzger *et al* (1980) has suggested subdividing gestational diabetes into those with and without fasting hyperglycaemia (plasma glucose of more than 5.8 mmol/l); however, until the significance of this subdivision is understood, it is probably wise simply to specify the level of fasting glycaemia and whether the individual was treated with insulin or diet.

Table 10.1   Characteristics of groups according to the White classification.

Group	Characteristic
A	Asymptomatic diabetes shown by glucose tolerance test
B	Diabetes with onset after age 20, duration 0–9 years and no vascular complication
C	Diabetes with onset between ages 10 and 19, duration 10–19 years and no vascular disease
D	Diabetes with onset before age 10, duration 20+ years and vascular disease evidenced by calcification of leg arteries and retinopathy
F	Diabetes with nephropathy
R	Diabetes with retinopathy

Physiology and pathophysiology

Pregnancy by itself induces profound metabolic alterations in the mother which tend to become more marked with advancing gestational age. It seems likely that these changes are adaptive, ensuring an optimal environment for fetal growth and development. A knowledge of some of these changes is essential if an understanding of the principles of care of the diabetic mother and her baby is to be achieved. A full review of this subject is given in the Ciba Foundation Symposium publication, *Pregnancy Metabolism Diabetes and the Fetus* (1979).

MATERNAL GLUCOSE HOMEOSTASIS

Fig. 10.1 shows the remarkably stable concentration of plasma glucose that is maintained by the mother over a 24-hour period. The feature that is noteworthy is the

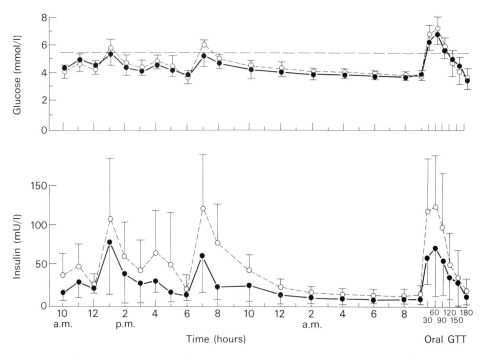

Fig. 10.1 Plasma glucose and insulin concentrations over a 24-hour period and during an oral GTT in nine normal women studied in early and late pregnancy (Gillmer *et al* 1975a). Figures are mean ± SD. ● early pregnancy (12–22 weeks); ○ late pregnancy (32–5 weeks).

small fluctuation around a concentration of 4.0–4.5 mmol/l, except after meals, both in early and late pregnancy. This degree of homeostasis is only maintained by a doubling in the secretion of insulin from the end of the first to the third trimester of pregnancy. In general, the relative normality or otherwise of a diurnal profile is reflected by the GTT. Although there has been some disagreement as to whether glucose tolerance decreases in normal pregnancy, it does appear from this longitudinal study that, if care is exercised in choosing mothers for a complete absence of diabetogenic factors, there is no deterioration of glucose tolerance in late pregnancy.

The precise reasons for the increased demand for insulin during pregnancy are not clear. It seems likely that the placental hormones, in particular oestrogen, progesterone and human placental lactogen (hPL) play an important role. Studies by Kalkhoff and Kim (1979) have suggested that progesterone alone is without effect on carbohydrate tolerance, oestrogen appears to improve it, and, in combination, the effect is enhanced. This could explain the increased secretion of insulin by the β-cells of the pancreas and it seems likely that other hormones such as hPL and glucagon, which are known insulin antagonists, play an important role in this respect. The metabolic picture is further complicated by the 'accelerated starvation of pregnancy', a concept originally proposed by Freinkel *et al* (1972), who observed that withholding food from a pregnant woman resulted in a more rapid fall in plasma glucose, insulin and glucogenic amino acids and an exaggerated rise in free fatty acids and ketone bodies, as compared with nonpregnant controls. It seems likely that this is partly a result of competition by the fetus for glucose and amino acids.

Fig. 10.2 is a striking demonstration of the development of chemical diabetes during pregnancy. The mean diurnal plasma glucose has increased over the 15 weeks between the measurements by about 3 mmol/l, whereas the insulin secretion has increased very little. This failure of insulin to rise is evidence of pancreatic β-cell insufficiency. The established diabetic who has had diabetes for some years before pregnancy often has complete loss of endogenous insulin secretion.

FETAL GLUCOSE HOMEOSTASIS

Glucose crosses the placenta freely in both directions by facilitated diffusion and it is the mother who is responsible for regulating the concentration. In diabetes, wide fluctuations in blood glucose concentration are reflected in the fetus. The normal maternal–fetal difference in glucose concentration is about 0.4–0.5 mmol/l in favour of the mother. With an increase in glucose concentration in the mother, the maternal–fetal difference increases until—around 11–13 mmol/l—the system of 'facilitated

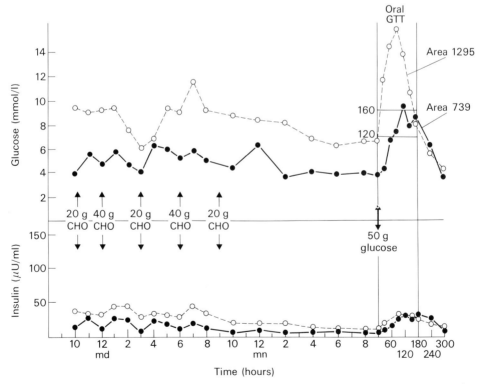

Fig. 10.2 Development of gestational diabetes during the second trimester. ● 12 weeks pregnant; ○ 27 weeks pregnant (Oakley 1976).

diffusion' by which glucose crosses the placenta appears to be saturated, and it is not possible to increase the concentration in the fetus any further. This phenomenon is present in diabetic as well as nondiabetic mothers (Oakley *et al* 1972) and may well be a protective mechanism for the fetus to avoid the damaging effects of severe hyperglycaemia.

Insulin appears in the fetal circulation as early as 10–12 weeks' gestational age when its role is not fully understood. There is general agreement that insulin does not cross the placenta. It used to be said that the β-cells of the fetal pancreas were insensitive to a glucose stimulus until the third day after birth but this has since been disproved by measurement of the response to a maternal glucose infusion in umbilical cord blood and fetal capillary plasma insulin before birth (Milner and Hales 1965; Oakley *et al* 1972). What does seem to be the case is that the response is sluggish and that, in the fetus of the nondiabetic mother, it plays no part in the regulation of glucose homeostasis, its role more likely being as a growth-promoting hormone.

Fig. 10.3 compares the difference between the maternal and fetal glucose and insulin responses to a glucose load in a nondiabetic and in a diabetic woman. The difference in the maternal–fetal glucose concentration increases as the mother becomes more hyperglycaemic. This effect is the same for diabetic as for nondiabetic women. The brisk fetal insulin response in the diabetic is in marked contrast to the sluggish response in the fetus of the nondiabetic mother.

Observations such as these have led to an increasing acceptance of the 'hyperglycaemia–hyperinsulinism' theory (Pedersen 1977). Stated simply, this proposes that the fetal hyperglycaemia resulting from maternal hyperglycaemia stimulates fetal pancreatic β-cell hypertrophy resulting in 'in utero' and inappropriate hyperinsulinism. This theory has gained wide acceptance because it convincingly explains the aetiology of much of the fetal pathology found in diabetic pregnancy. These observations are of particular clinical significance because they point clearly to the possibility that normalisation of the glucose environment of the fetus of the diabetic mother will diminish the tendency to hyperinsulinaemia and hence lead to a diminution of many perinatal problems.

GLYCOSYLATED HAEMOGLOBIN ($A_{1\,a+b+c}$)

HbA_1 is a normally occurring haemoglobin linked to glucose which, in the nonpregnant normoglycaemic woman, represents a fairly constant 5–6 per cent fraction of the total haemoglobin mass. This concentration of HbA_1 correlates well with the level of blood glucose tending to be higher in pregnancy than in the nonpregnant state, though falling slightly as pregnancy advances. It is elevated in diabetics, particularly those individuals whose blood glucose is poorly controlled. Reduced arterial oxygen saturation and Pao_2 in pregnant women who are diabetic, associated with an impaired 2,3-DPG-induced change in haemoglobin oxygen affinity, has been reported recently (Madsen and Ditzel 1982). Table 10.2 shows the mean values described by Schwartz *et al* (1976) for pregnancy, although it must be recognised that values for diabetics are dependent on the metabolic control achieved.

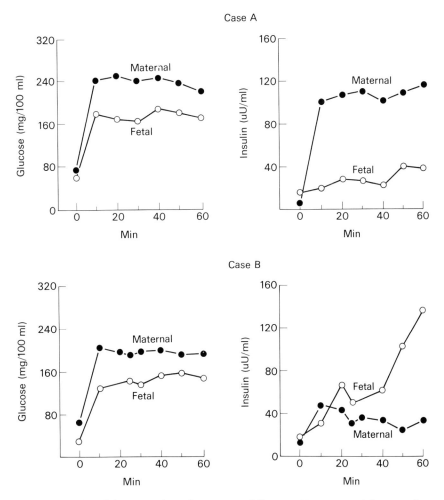

Fig. 10.3   Examples of glucose and insulin response following 60 minutes of glucose infusion in a nondiabetic (case A) and a gestational diabetic (case B) (for conversion to mmol/l divide by 18) (Oakley *et al* 1972).

Table 10.2   Mean HbA$_1$(A–C) values in diabetic and nondiabetic pregnancy (Schwartz *et al* 1976).

Normal nonpregnant females	5.7%
Normal pregnancy	7.0%
Gestational diabetes	8.8%
Pregnant established diabetes	8.5%

The contribution of HbA$_1$ estimations to the management of the pregnant diabetic is that they provide a retrospective measurement of blood glucose concentration. An elevated HbA$_1$ value has been shown to be associated with a number of fetal and neonatal complications which are listed in Table 10.3. In general, a HbA$_1$ value above 8 per cent in the second half of pregnancy suggests an increased possibility of perinatal morbidity (Ylinen *et al* 1981). More specifically the association between a high HbA$_1$ concentration (>10 per cent) and congenital malformations is of value as an indication that a full investigation needs to be initiated at 16 weeks in the form of serum α-fetoprotein and skilled ultrasound scanning of gestational age (Table 10.3). A comparison of HbA$_1$ values with mean blood glucose levels obtained by home

Table 10.3   Recognised associations between elevated HbA$_1$ concentration and fetal and neonatal complications of diabetic pregnancy (Ylinen *et al* 1981; Steel *et al* 1981).

> Congenital malformations
> Perinatal mortality, asphyxia neonatorum
> Excessive size of the baby (macrosomia), birth injury
>
> *Neonatal*
>   hyaline membrane disease, transient tachypnoea
>   hypoglycaemia
>   hyperbilirubinaemia
>   hypocalcaemia and hypomagnesaemia
>   polycythaemia, renal vein thrombosis
>   hypertrophic cardiomyopathy

monitoring over a three-month period showed a highly significant correlation (Paisey *al* 1980). However, in practice, the measurement of HbA$_1$ is only of limited use in the week-by-week control of diabetes because it does not provide the sensitivity required when adjusting insulin treatment which frequent estimations of blood glucose do. In general, if blood glucose values are below 7.0 mmol/l, HbA$_1$ values will be within normal limits. In certain situations HbA$_1$ values can be a valuable guide to management, particularly in the diabetic woman attending for the first time late in pregnancy or when the blood glucose shows marked fluctuations. It has also been proposed as an index of whether a woman who had given birth to a large-for-dates baby is diabetic or not (Steel *et al* 1981).

Burke *et al* (1981) stated '. . . poor fetal outcome in terms of macrosomia, hypoglycaemia and high cord C-peptide concentration, reflecting β-cell hyperplasia was sufficiently well associated with an abnormal HbA$_1$ concentration to conclude that its measurement is a useful test for monitoring diabetic pregnancy.' It seems reasonable to conclude that the estimation of HbA$_1$ is a useful adjunct to serial blood glucose measurement in the management of the pregnant woman with diabetes. In practice, HbA$_1$ estimations are best done at about monthly intervals throughout pregnancy.

Effect of diabetes on the fetus

CONGENITAL MALFORMATIONS

There is now general acceptance of an increased incidence of congenital malformations amongst the offspring of mothers with established diabetes. Malformation rates vary widely ranging from 4.3 per cent (Jervell *et al* 1979) to 11.9 per cent (Schneider *et al* 1980), which can probably be explained by methodological differences between studies and differing susceptibility of populations to malformations. The recent interim results from the UK Survey of Diabetic Pregnancy reported an incidence of 5.7 per cent among 664 mothers with established diabetes. The malformations were about equally divided between major and minor with a predominance of multiple malformations (14 out of the 22 major malformations) (Beard and Lowy 1982).

To date, attention has been directed mainly at malformations that are apparent at or shortly after birth. This means that there is likely to be quite a considerable underestimate because many malformations are overlooked in the neonatal period, only becoming apparent in childhood. In addition, little is known about the 'malformation' rate in organ systems such as the brain where a relatively minor disruption of organogenesis might cause significant behavioural abnormalities in later life. A study from Denmark of 740 children of diabetic mothers (Yssing 1975) showed that 36 per cent had some form of cerebral dysfunction. Although this study was uncontrolled, it serves as a reminder of how seriously one should regard the damaging effects of uncontrolled diabetes in early pregnancy.

The persistence of an increased malformation rate, despite a progressive fall in all other complications associated with diabetic pregnancy, is one of the most consistent features of reports appearing in the world literature in recent years. What is it about diabetes that so unpredictably disrupts fetal organogenesis? Recently, Miller *et al* (1981) have confirmed an earlier suggestion by Leslie *et al* (1978) that the malformation rate was higher amongst the offspring of mothers with established diabetes in whom an abnormally high percentage of glycosylated haemoglobin (HbA_1) had been detected in early pregnancy. This would suggest that there may be a critical concentration of blood glucose above which fetal malformations are much more likely to develop. However, the relationship is not so simple as it might first appear, since there is a considerable overlap between HbA_1 values of women bearing abnormal babies and those with unaffected babies. It has been known for a long time that malformations can be induced in animals by exposing the fetus at the time of organogenesis to insulin (Duraiswami 1952) and high concentrations of glucose (Deuchar 1979), but it has not proved possible to determine which of these is the responsible agent. Recent work in rats (Baker *et al* 1981) has shown that lumbosacral defects in the fetus could only be induced if the mother was diabetic in the first seven days of pregnancy, which corresponds with the period when organogenesis is occurring in the rat. If the mothers were made diabetic after the first week of pregnancy then the defects did not appear.

There is still some debate as to whether the malformation rate is increased in the mother with gestational diabetes but it seems this is more a matter of definition than a rejection of the evidence that hyperglycaemia induces fetal malformations. Pedersen

(1979) reported that the malformation rate was increased by 60 per cent in a large group of White Class A diabetics compared with controls, whereas Malins (1979) found no increase in a similar group. The White Class A of Malins was defined as an abnormal GTT detected in pregnancy for the first time, so that many women in whom hyperglycaemia did not appear until well after the critical period of organogenesis would not have been at risk of malformation. Pedersen on the other hand has defined Class A as mild *pre-existing* diabetes so that his group were all likely to have some degree of hyperglycaemia at this critical time of development in the first trimester.

Logically, efforts to reduce the malformation rate in pregnancy should be directed to normalising the blood glucose of the mother throughout the first trimester of pregnancy. Indirect support for this concept has come from Pedersen and Molsted-Pedersen (1979a) in Copenhagen who reported that the malformation rate amongst 363 White Class B–F diabetics whose diabetes had been well controlled before pregnancy was 7.0 per cent, whilst amongst 284 women with diabetes of similar severity which had been poorly controlled the malformation rate was 14.0 per cent. The recent report of the experience from a prepregnancy clinic for diabetics (Steel *et al* 1982) which showed that the incidence of malformations was significantly lower amongst women who had attempted to improve their diabetic control before pregnancy, adds further support to this concept.

How can good diabetic control in early pregnancy be achieved? At present diabetics are rarely seen before the 10th–12th week of pregnancy. Often control of their diabetes is poor by standards required in pregnancy and sometimes pregnancy may be first detected at the time of a hypo- or hyperglycaemic crisis. Some will be taking oral hypoglycaemic agents, and it is usual for these women to have little understanding of the effect pregnancy will have on their diabetes or of their diabetes on the developing fetus. The remedy must be that the doctors who look after young women with diabetes should be responsible for including an explanation of the harmful effects of diabetes on the fetus as part of routine education. Patients should be told how essential it is to ensure that their diabetes is well controlled before embarking on a pregnancy, by physicians who run diabetic clinics and general practitioners. Further mention is made of this under the sections on Medical management (p. 365) and Contraception (p. 377).

PERINATAL MORTALITY (PNM)

Perinatal mortality rates amongst women with established diabetes have always been higher than those for the population as a whole by a factor of 4–5. However, they have been falling consistently as can be seen from the figures from King's College Hospital, London, shown in Table 10.4. Gillmer *et al* (1984) quoting the Swedish figures for 1973–78, point out that PNM has been falling in the whole obstetric population over this period, and that it is unwise to attribute all of the improvements in diabetic pregnancy to better care of diabetes. The Swedish figures suggest that the major improvement can be ascribed to both diabetic and obstetric care before delivery since the stillbirth rate has fallen more steeply amongst diabetics than nondiabetics. Another factor that has to be taken into account when considering perinatal mortality figures

Table 10.4 Perinatal mortality rates and causes of deaths among 1059 diabetic babies born to diabetic mothers over a 30 year period at King's College Hospital, London. (Personal Communication from Dr D. A. Pyke.)

	n	Perinatal deaths (per 1000)	Causes of death				
			Obstetric	Diabetic	Congenital malformations	Respiratory distress	Unknown
1951–60	318	72 (226)	26	5	6	17	18
1961–70	389	39 (100)	9	2	5	8	15
1971–80	352	13 (37)	3	1	6	1	2

such as those in Table 10.4 is that most reports emanate from centres with a special interest in diabetic pregnancy. In reality the PNM rate for the whole country is higher, as shown by a figure of 61 per 1000 for mothers with established diabetes in Britain in 1979–80 as compared with 37 per 1000 for 1971–80 at King's College Hospital.

Table 10.4 shows the changes in PNM relative to the cause of death. It can be seen that deaths due to obstetric disaster, complications of diabetes, respiratory distress and 'unknown' have all fallen, whereas congenital malformation remains unaltered. The fact that, if malformations are removed from the figures, PNM would be essentially the same as for a nondiabetic population must point towards the effect of improved obstetric and diabetic care. Death from an 'unknown' cause still occurs occasionally and unexpectedly. A number of theories have been advanced to explain these deaths.

1 *Fetal hypoglycaemia* (Beard and Oakley 1976). These authors suggested that, near term, profound fetal hypoglycaemia may develop as a result of excessive endogenous hyperinsulinism and failure of the fetus to mobilise hepatic glycogen. Death from this cause is confined to macrosomic babies.

2 *Fetal hyperglycaemia* (Shelley *et al* 1975). These authors have shown that hyperglycaemia in fetal lambs results in the formation of excess lactic acid which may produce such a profound acidosis that the fetus dies. In theory this could occur at any time during pregnancy, whereas the most usual time for a stillbirth to occur is at the end of pregnancy.

3 *Fetal hypoxia.* Recently the finding of reduced oxygen tension and saturation in diabetic women with elevated concentrations of glycosylated haemoglobin has revived a longstanding hypothesis that unexplained stillbirth of diabetic pregnancy may be due to hypoxia (Madsen and Ditzel 1982).

Hypoxia as a cause of perinatal death in diabetic pregnancy is also proposed by Björk from Stockholm (personal communication). Morphologic studies of the placenta revealed increased branching of villi, and syncytial 'knots' which he interpreted as compensatory in response to hypoxia.

Perinatal mortality in gestational diabetes.

There is still some discussion as to whether PNM is raised in pregnancy complicated by gestational diabetes (Beard and Hoet 1982). There is, however, general acceptance that

PNM is closely related to the severity of the diabetes, whether this is judged by the concentration of plasma glucose (Karlsson and Kjellmer 1972) or by the White Class (Molsted-Pedersen 1976). Gestational diabetes varies in severity from the individual with a mild disturbance of carbohydrate metabolism to the mother whose diabetes deteriorates markedly until she requires treatment with insulin. It is therefore not unreasonable to assume that, in this latter group, the PNM will be higher. Retrospective studies of mothers who develop gestational diabetes in a second or subsequent pregnancy have revealed a PNM as high as 97 per 1000 in previous pregnancies when the diabetes was unsuspected (Merkatz *et al* 1980). In a small prospective study of mothers with untreated gestational diabetes, O'Sullivan *et al* (1973) found a fourfold increase in PNM amongst those mothers as compared with a control group with normal carbohydrate tolerance. On balance, it seems likely that the PNM rate is increased in women with untreated gestational diabetes.

NEONATAL MORBIDITY

Respiratory distress, hypoglycaemia, polycythaemia and jaundice of the newborn are recognised as common sequelae of diabetic pregnancy, yet, because of the concern over perinatal mortality, little attention has been paid to reducing their incidence. Guthberlet and Cornblath (1973) reported an incidence of 30–50 per cent amongst babies of mothers with established diabetes. The appearance of some of these complications during the neonatal period is shown in Fig. 10.4 (Oh 1982).

   The large-for-dates baby is usually defined as a baby whose birthweight for gestational age exceeds the 90th centile (Thomson *et al* 1968). Typically the

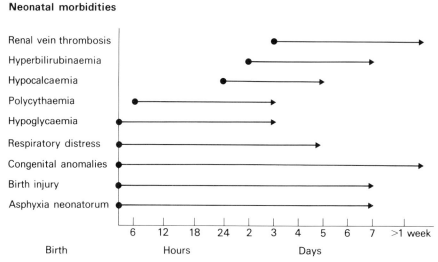

Fig. 10.4   Time of appearance during the neonatal period and duration of complications which can affect infants of diabetic mothers (Oh 1982). ● Usual age of onset of detection; → usual duration of morbidity.

macrosomic baby of the diabetic mother is fat and plethoric. All organs, with the exception of the brain, are enlarged due to an increase in cytoplasmic mass. Subcutaneous fat is markedly increased, the amount being directly related to the maternal blood sugar concentration in the third trimester of pregnancy (Stubbs *et al* 1981). In fact excessive fetal growth does not become apparent before the third trimester of pregnancy. In general morphologic studies of the fetus of the diabetic mother have shown that the greater the percentage area of total pancreatic tissue occupied by the insulin-secreting islet cells, the bigger the baby (Cardell 1953).

The clinical importance of fetal macrosomia which is often accompanied by hydramnios, is that it is a valuable sign of poor diabetic control of the mother and of risk to the fetus. In addition, excessive growth increases the risk of trauma during vaginal delivery. The presence of a large baby may be unrecognised until delivery when the dangerous complication of shoulder impaction may arise. A long-term follow-up study of the Pima Indians also suggests that the prenatal environment of the child of a diabetic mother results in the development of obesity in early adulthood (Pettit *et al* 1983).

Respiratory distress used to be a common complication of diabetic pregnancy from which the baby often died, its aetiology was poorly understood. Recently it has been suggested that excessive amounts of fetal insulin interfere with pulmonary phospholipid production, specifically phosphotidylglycerol, thereby leading to surfactant deficiency (Stubbs and Stubbs 1978). The prevalence of the condition has fallen quite dramatically in recent years and there seem to be a number of reasons for this. Preterm delivery, particularly before 37 weeks of gestation, is less common. There is also an increasing tendency to deliver diabetic mothers per vaginum and nearer term, thereby overcoming the adverse effects in the past of prematurity combined with delivery by Caesarean section, noted by Usher *et al* (1971). Finally, control of maternal diabetes and neonatal care has improved a lot in recent years. In place of hyaline membrane disease, transient tachypnoea, which is characterised by a rapid respiratory rate and transient cyanosis usually disappearing within 24–36 hours of birth, is seen quite commonly. This condition is thought to be due to delayed removal of fetal lung liquid.

Hypoglycaemia is usually asymptomatic in the newborn of the diabetic, and plasma glucose levels of less than 2.0 mmol/l (without evidence of systemic disturbance) are quite common. Kalhan *et al* (1977) have suggested that the combination of decreased hepatic phosphorylase activity, and diminished glucagon and catecholamine release results in decreased output of glucose from the liver of these babies. The symptomatic variety is fortunately less common because it carries an increased likelihood of cerebral damage for the baby, and is heralded by jitteriness and convulsions, or simply by limpness or an abnormal cry (Gentz *et al* 1969). The concentration of plasma glucose in the newborn correlates with the degree of carbohydrate intolerance of the mother in the third trimester of pregnancy (Gillmer *et al* 1975b). It can be attributed to the endogenous hyperinsulinism developing in fetal life that becomes clinically apparent only when the fetus is separated from its supply of glucose from the mother. The condition is usually avoidable by encouraging early feeding and by performing hourly 'Dextrostix' estimations on the newborn after birth. A value below 1.0 mmol/l is an indication for the intravenous administration of glucose.

Polycythaemia and jaundice

Extramedullary haematopoiesis and polycythaemia characterise the infant of the diabetic mother. Animal work suggests that fetal hyperinsulinism results in elevated levels of erythropoietin, leading to increased haematopoiesis. The clinical consequence of this is an increase in blood viscosity leading to increased cardiac work and microcirculatory disturbances. Hyperviscosity within the pulmonary bed may be a contributory factor in the appearance of respiratory distress. The destruction of many red cells and the relative immaturity of the liver of the newborn predispose to the high prevalence of jaundice in these babies. These complications led Persson *et al* (1978) to recommend early clamping of the umbilical cord and of exchange transfusion if the haematocrit exceeds 70 per cent.

Hypertrophic cardiomyopathy

Some 30% of infants of mothers with insulin-dependant diabetes have cardiomegaly and 10% have evidence of cardiac dysfunction (Leslie *et al* 1982). The characteristic abnormality which is best demonstrated by echocardiography (Gutgesell *et al* 1976) is asymetric septal hypertrophy. This is similar to that seen in familial obstructive cardiomyopathy or hypertrophic obstructive cardiomyopathy, except that it is reversible over a period of weeks if the infant survives (Halliday 1981) and that fibre disarray is not a prominent feature (Halliday 1981; Leslie *et al* 1982). The cause is unknown, and the prognosis is good.

The role of fetal hyperinsulinism

It seems likely that fetal hyperinsulinism is an important factor underlying some or all of these complications and that anything which can reduce this is likely to diminish the neonatal complication rate in diabetic pregnancy. Guthberlet and Cornblath (1973) showed that the incidence of neonatal complications after birth was lower amongst mothers with mild diabetes. This fact, and the demonstrable relationship between the maternal glucose tolerance test in the last trimester of pregnancy and the neonatal plasma glucose concentration, strongly suggest that normalisation of maternal plasma glucose in the latter part of pregnancy is likely to reduce the frequency of neonatal complications. Added weight is given to this view by the results of the four surveys of neonatal morbidity following pregnancy in women with established diabetes shown in Table 10.5. The figures of Larsson and Ludvigsson (1974) were obtained from Swedish hospitals where diabetic control was known to be poor with a correspondingly high morbidity rate. The UK Survey (Lowy and Beard 1982) was carried out ten years later when diabetic control was probably better and morbidity rate of associated neonatal complications—except for respiratory distress—much less. The last two surveys are characterised by the provision of diabetic care by a single individual with much greater attention being paid to obtaining good diabetic control throughout pregnancy. This is particularly so in that of Jovanovic *et al* (1981), in which normoglycaemia in the

Table 10.5   Comparison of perinatal morbidity and mortality amongst mothers with diabetic pregnancy.

	A (*n* 157)	B (*n* 664)	C (*n* 113)	D (*n* 55)
Respiratory distress (%)	10	12	4	0
Jaundice (%)	30	20	12	0
Hypoglycaemia (%)	48	15	16	<2
Macrosomia (%)	43	29	—	0
PNM (per 1000)	220	61	26	0

A Larsson and Ludvigsson 1974; B Interim results from the UK National Survey of Diabetic Pregnancy, 1979–80 (Lowry and Beard 1982); C Results from National Maternity Hospital, Dublin (reported by Drury 1982); D Jovanovic *et al* 1981.

mother was maintained for the greater part of pregnancy. The result was the virtual disappearance of neonatal morbidity.

Diagnosis

In considering diagnostic criteria for diabetes, it is important to recognise that the implications of the disease in pregnancy are quite different from those in the nonpregnant condition. Whereas, in the nonpregnant state, minor degrees of carbohydrate intolerance are often not treated because they cause little systemic disturbance, in pregnancy there is a fetus whose development is apparently exquisitely sensitive to small deviations of blood glucose outside the normal range (Beard and Hoet 1982). For this reason, diagnostic criteria and therapeutic goals must be more demanding in pregnancy.

Pregnancy increases the requirement for insulin but this can be accommodated by the pancreas of the nondiabetic woman so that the diurnal plasma glucose remains unaltered. On the other hand, if insulin secretion is insufficient to meet the demand, then relative hyperglycaemia or 'gestational' diabetes appears which may be symptomatic or, if less severe, may simply present as an abnormality of glucose tolerance.

The classical approach to defining abnormal glucose tolerance is to take the limit of two standard deviations above the mean for a group of nondiabetic pregnant women (O'Sullivan and Mahan 1964). The issue of defining 'abnormality' is complicated by whether an oral or intravenous test is performed, the amount of glucose that is given, and the wide variety of methods used for glucose assay, so that there are no agreed diagnostic criteria. The criteria of O'Sullivan *et al* (1973) are generally regarded as being most acceptable because of the careful long-term follow-up of the women following the pregnancy when they had their initial GTT. They used 100 g load of glucose administered orally following prior dietary preparation and collected venous blood half-hourly over three hours. They defined an abnormal result as two or more blood glucose values exceeding the following limits: fasting 5.0 mmol/l, one hour 9.2 mmol/l, two hours 8.1 mmol/l, and three hours 6.9 mmol/l.

An alternative approach has been adopted by Gillmer *et al* (1975a, 1975b) using a three hour GTT and a 50 g oral load. They utilised the known tendency in diabetic pregnancy for the newborn to become hypoglycaemic after birth. By defining neonatal hypoglycaemia two hours after birth as being a plasma glucose value of 1.7 mmol/l or less, they have determined the upper limit of normal glucose tolerance. They found that critical values differed little from those of O'Sullivan *et al* (1973). The best predictor of neonatal hypoglycaemia proved to be the total area of the curve (Fig. 10.5). A value of less than 43 SI area units is used as the upper limit of normal in pregnancy. Although it seems unlikely that diagnostic criteria for diabetes in pregnancy will be agreed in the forseeable future, it should never be forgotten that, because the fetus requires a normoglycaemic environment for normal development, diagnostic criteria must be stricter for pregnant than nonpregnant women. In practice, it is essential that GTT methodology and diagnostic criteria should be agreed by all obstetricians with their physician colleagues in individual hospitals.

Screening for diabetes in pregnancy

Attempts to detect unrecognised diabetes in pregnancy are a part of established practice in every antenatal clinic in this country. The justification for this is the known increased risk of perinatal death amongst women who develop an abnormal GTT in pregnancy. The success of these efforts varies widely because of the generalised lack of any consistent and systematic approach to the problem.

If screening is to be effective it must be comprehensive. The accepted practice in antenatal clinics, of only doing a GTT on a mother if she has one of the features of

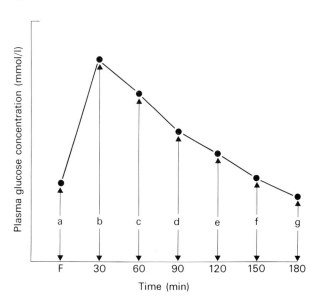

Fig. 10.5   Calculation of the total area under the curve: Area $=\frac{1}{2}$a$+$b$+$c$+$ d$+$e$+$f$+\frac{1}{2}$g units.

potential diabetes, is both time-consuming and imprecise. Screening studies of entire obstetric populations have shown that only 45 per cent of women found to have carbohydrate intolerance have defined features of potential diabetes (O'Sullivan *et al* 1973). The traditional method of waiting for glycosuria to appear is also of little value. Sutherland *et al* (1970) found that 11 per cent of an unselected obstetric population of 1418 women had random glycosuria but less than 1 per cent of the glycosurics had an abnormal GTT. Equally many women with gestational diabetes may never have glycosuria detected when they visit the antenatal clinic. Many screening systems have been advocated but few are worthy of consideration for the reasons given. The most advanced, practical and effective is the 50 g glucose load advocated by O'Sullivan *et al* (1973).

When a mother first attends the antenatal clinic, she is given a fruit-flavoured drink containing 50 g glucose. One hour later blood is taken for glucose assay. If the value is equal to or more than 7.8 mmol/l (> 2 SD of the mean), a full GTT is done. If the GTT is negative or the patient has one of the features of potential diabetes, the screening procedure is repeated at 28 weeks' gestation because of the diabetogenic effect of pregnancy which will unmask incipient diabetes as pregnancy advances. The screening system, and the incidence of abnormal values, is shown in the flow diagram in Fig. 10.6 (Beard *et al* 1980).

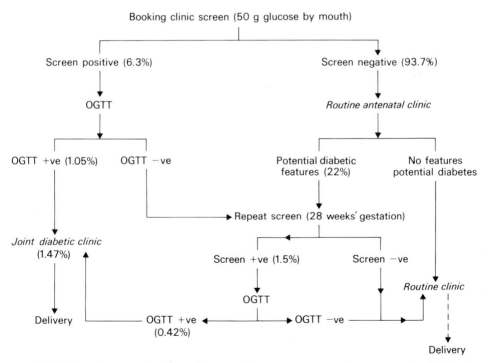

Fig. 10.6 Flow diagram depicting the screening programme and management of patients screened at St Mary's Hospital, London. All percentages are expressed as a proportion of the original booking clinic population screened (Beard *et al* 1980).

Of all the pregnant women tested at their first visit, 6.3 per cent had a positive screening value, of whom 17 per cent had an abnormal GTT. Overall, the incidence of mothers with abnormal GTT values by the beginning of the third trimester was 1.5 per cent, two-thirds of whom had been picked up in the booking clinic and one-third by repeating the screen at 24 weeks' gestation.

Fig. 10.7 shows the distribution of plasma glucose values, in unselected pregnant women who had not been fasted, one hour after a 50 g glucose load.

The Copenhagen group have proposed a different screening system which depends on the presence of glycosuria and certain features of potential diabetes (Guttorm 1975). They showed that the incidence of abnormal OGTT in a group of 514 pregnant women was 5 per cent amongst the glycosuric women and 1 per cent in those without glycosuria. The subdivision of the glycosuric women into those with and without potential diabetic features doubled the detection rate. However, the numbers were small and neither glycosuria nor potential diabetic features showed a degree of diagnostic specificity comparable to that of the O'Sullivan system.

The justification for any screening system is that it should be cost-effective and also acceptable to the patient. A comparison of specificity rates and the relative costs of materials used for the tests is shown in Table 10.6. A full OGTT is clearly time-consuming and disagreeable to pregnant women, apart from being expensive; equally, limiting the test to potential diabetics only is not justified because of the relatively lower pick-up rate. The system proposed by O'Sullivan *et al* (1973) and in the

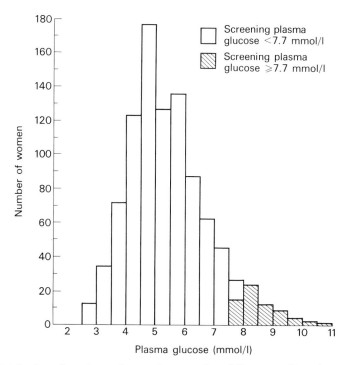

Fig. 10.7   Distribution of one-hour plasma glucose values following a 50 g glucose load.

Table 10.6   Estimate of specificity and cost of various screening systems based on data from 752 women.

	Sensitivity (%)	Relative cost (%)		
		Screen	OGTT	Total
OGTT for whole population	100	—	100	100
OGTT on potential diabetics only[1]	64	—	49	49
O'Sullivan screen on whole population[2]	79	14	16	30
O'Sullivan screen on women aged 25 years	74	7	7	14

1 Beard *et al* 1980; 2 O'Sullivan *et al* 1973.

St Mary's Hospital study (Beard *et al* 1980)—whereby an OGTT is done only on women with a blood glucose above a certain critical level one hour after a 50 g glucose load—has the advantage that it is easy to administer after the first visit to the clinic as part of the overall haematological screening procedure. It is also reasonably specific (79 per cent) and inexpensive. The cost can be halved by confining the screening test to women aged 25 or over, with only a small reduction in diagnostic sensitivity from 79 to 74 per cent. The saving in time, patient and staff involvement, and cost, would seem to justify this modification and it seems likely that it will become the screening method of choice for the future.

Medical management

PROPHYLAXIS

The likelihood that the increased incidence of congenital malformations found in diabetic pregnancy is due to an abnormal metabolic environment for the fetus at the time of organogenesis, suggests that any diabetic woman who is planning to become pregnant should ask her physician to control her diabetes before she does so. Control in these women means a stable diurnal blood glucose which is as near normoglycaemic as possible. This approach has been adopted with some success in Edinburgh where a prepregnancy clinic for diabetics has been established (Steel *et al* 1982). Not only were the HbA$_1$ values lower in those who attended the clinic as compared with those who did not, but the malformation rate was lower. These authors also commented on the importance of the advisory role of such a clinic, particularly amongst women with severe nephropathy, some of whom were dissuaded from becoming pregnant. In general, the establishment of such a clinic in centres with a large diabetic population makes sense. In addition to improving diabetic control, the opportunity can be taken to give general advice regarding the importance of being as healthy as possible at the start of pregnancy—stopping smoking and reducing alcohol intake being obvious examples.

CHOICE OF TREATMENT

There is no consensus view on the choice of treatment, which lies between diet alone or a combination of diet and insulin. In general, gestational diabetics are treated with diet alone, until there is evidence that this is failing to control maternal blood glucose. Equally, established diabetics are changed to insulin in early pregnancy if they have previously been on diet or oral hypoglycaemics. The known effects of oral hypoglycaemic agents on the fetus preclude their use when there are satisfactory alternatives. Drugs such as chlorpropamide cross the placenta and induce fetal hyperinsulinism (Sutherland *et al* 1974) which prevents their use in pregnancy unless there is no satisfactory alternative. The final determinant of which treatment is best will depend on how effective it is in controlling blood glucose at or near normoglycaemia.

Treatment by diet alone

This can be a most effective way of reducing blood sugar as can be seen in Fig. 10.8. In principle, carbohydrates which are the major component of the total calorie intake are reduced. A simple regimen used by the author is to limit the daily carbohydrate intake to 120 g in obese women ($\geqslant 120$ per cent of ideal bodyweight), 140 g in women whose weight is within the normal range (80–119 per cent of ideal bodyweight), and 160 g in thin women (<80 per cent of ideal bodyweight). These figures should not be followed slavishly, the final determinant of the severity of dietary restriction is the plasma glucose. In obese women the restriction may need to be greater, whereas in the woman who has only a mild degree of carbohydrate intolerance, it may be less. Using this system, thin women put on between 4 and 6 kg in a pregnancy whereas the weight of

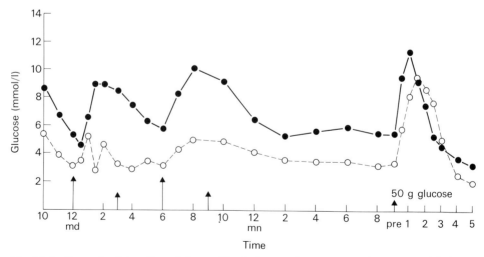

Fig. 10.8 Example of the effect of diet on blood glucose of a woman with gestational diabetes detected at 36 weeks. ● Pre-diet profile, GTT area = 48.5 units; ○ during treatment with diet, 2 weeks later, GTT area = 43.2 units (Oakley 1976).

obese women remains static or may actually fall. Ketonaemia is an unavoidable product of treatment by diet alone which, following the studies in the USA (Berendes 1975), has given rise to some anxiety that it may be a cause of neurological damage to the fetus. However, further work has refuted this view (Naeye 1979) and in Europe the mild ketoacidosis, often found in diabetic women being treated by dieting, is not regarded as harmful. The major problem in obtaining successful control of the blood glucose by this method is to persuade the mother to keep to her diet. A static weight from the time of starting treatment is good evidence that the diet is being strictly observed.

Treatment by insulin

It is now generally accepted that if insulin is to be used to regulate blood glucose in pregnancy, it should be given at least twice a day. Good control can be achieved by combining a medium-acting insulin such as Isophane or Monotard with a short-acting such as Soluble or Actrapid. A convenient mixture of medium- and short-acting insulin is Rapitard, which is suitable for most women in pregnancy; however, if efforts are being made to achieve 24-hour normoglycaemia, it is often more satisfactory to use the insulins separately.

Three approaches to diabetic control are in use at present.

1   The most common method in this country is that advocated by King's College Hospital, London (Essex *et al* 1973). Blood glucose values obtained randomly in the antenatal clinic are maintained below 8.3 mmol/l. After 32 weeks of pregnancy inpatient care begins and efforts are made to keep the blood sugar below 5.5 mmol/l. It has been argued that admission to hospital reduces physical activity thereby making control of blood sugar more difficult. The study by Cassar *et al* (1978) showed that, although nearly half of his diabetic mothers spent more than three weeks in hospital for a variety of reasons—often not connected with diabetic control—routine admission was unnecessary.

2   Home monitoring of blood glucose by the patient has been advocated by Sönksen *et al* (1978), on the grounds that better control can be obtained by involving the mother more in the care of her diabetes. Postprandial peaks and attacks of hypoglycaemia were generally eliminated and blood sugar values at home tended to be lower than those obtained in the clinic. Using this approach Jovanovic *et al* (1981) were able to achieve a mean blood glucose value of between 4.4 and 4.8 mmol/l throughout pregnancy in their group of 53 established diabetics, by giving a standard regimen of three injections of insulin per day; in the morning, before dinner, and before going to bed; the total dose being calculated from the formula 0.7 u/kg. The benefit of providing all young diabetic women with glucose meters, and persuading them to use these reliably, still has to be proven, but the potential for improving the management of these women by this method is attractive. For the woman who is planning to become pregnant, home monitoring offers the possibility of reducing the risk of congenital malformation by careful regulation of blood glucose immediately before conception. For the woman who is already pregnant there is a likelihood that, with good diabetic control at home, the

amount of time she has to spend in hospital before delivery will be reduced. This approach is preferred for the woman who is able to master the home-monitoring procedure.

3 The third approach to diabetic control in pregnancy is that described by Roversi *et al* (1977). In essence, they advocate that as much insulin should be given as the patient will tolerate without developing persistent troublesome symptoms of hypoglycaemia. They describe a series of 479 patients (237 White Class A and 242 Class AB-R). The uncorrected perinatal mortality was 29 per 1000 births and the incidence of total malformations was 1.6 per cent, which is well below that commonly reported in association with diabetic pregnancy (Beard and Oakley 1976). The mean diurnal values reported ranged between 3.0 and 4.2 mmol/l with the exception of a peak of 5.3–5.5 mmol/l at 20.00 hours. The excellence of their results indicates that this approach to diabetic control, which is popular throughout Europe, should be given careful consideration. The disadvantage is that the maternal blood glucose will often be below the physiological norm, and this may reduce the availability to the developing fetus of essential energy-producing substrates which, in theory, could result in fetal growth retardation with a selective effect on organs such as the liver and the brain. In addition, there is the practical disadvantage of the unpleasant side-effects of hypoglycaemia which most patients experience when they first start on the regimen. In practice, most clinics tailor the control of blood glucose to the individual needs of the patient.

ANTENATAL CONTROL OF DIABETES

The joint diabetic clinic

Management of the pregnant diabetic is greatly facilitated by an antenatal clinic which is held weekly and at which all pregnant diabetics are seen. The clinic consists of a physician and an obstetrician with a special interest in diabetes. It is also valuable to have a midwife who is responsible for the organisation of the clinic and the education of the patients about diabetes. The presence of a dietician is also helpful. Diabetic mothers are seen every one or two weeks and a random plasma glucose is measured by a reflectance meter at each visit. It is important to remember that the blood glucose is frequently elevated between 09.00 and 11.00 hours which may be misleading. Regular antenatal examinations and, in the last six weeks of pregnancy, cardiotocography, are done at each visit. By this means it is usually possible to control the diabetes satisfactorily and monitor the condition of the fetus in such a manner that it is not necessary to admit the mother with gestational or established diabetes to hospital until she goes into spontaneous labour. It is only by the 'joint' involvement of physician and obstetrician that it is possible to ensure the correct overall management of the pregnancy. For example, the detection of hydramnios by the obstetrician may well be an indication for tighter control of blood sugar. Equally, difficulty in achieving good control of the diabetes may be a reason for inpatient admission to the antenatal wards.

Control of blood glucose

Satisfactory control of blood glucose—which can be defined as a mean 24-hour profile glucose value of 7.0 mmol/l or less—should be secured as soon as possible after the diabetic mother reports that she is pregnant. This entails admission to hospital so that a 24-hour glucose profile (*see* Figs. 10.1, 10.2 and 10.8) can be done before starting treatment. The profile is a good baseline from which to judge the effect of treatment. A past history of symptomatic hypo- or hyperglycaemia and/or wide fluctuations in the profile values suggests that control of the diabetes may prove troublesome. In general pregnant diabetic mothers are resistant to the effects of injected insulin so that, as pregnancy advances, relatively large doses can be given without risk of inducing profound hypoglycaemia. After starting treatment, the blood glucose profile should be repeated so that if necessary treatment can be readjusted. Attention must be paid to providing an adequate diet and the formula used by Jovanovic *et al* (1981) of 30 Kcal/kg/day is useful in this respect. Nocturnal hypoglycaemia can be treated by reducing the evening insulin or more simply by increasing the dietary intake just before going to bed.

During the course of pregnancy, insulin requirements increase. Providing the mother is seen about every two weeks in pregnancy, insulin dosage can be adjusted to meet requirements. If control becomes difficult it is best to admit her for a further glucose profile. The problem is that the diminished physical activity, which is an inevitable consequence of hospital admission, increases insulin requirements and it is advisable to keep the mother as mobile as possible so that the insulin dosage prescribed in hospital is appropriate for life at home. It goes without saying that diabetic ketoacidosis in pregnancy must be avoided at all costs since it carries a high degree of fetal mortality, in addition to the danger to the mother, and requires immediate admission to hospital.

Other factors affecting control of blood glucose

If blood glucose is to be well regulated, thought must be given to the effect of daily events on insulin requirements. Emotional lability is a potent factor in inducing hyperglycaemia and marked diurnal fluctuations in blood glucose. Many diabetic women continue to work after they are pregnant and this may significantly affect control of the diabetes. An example of this was a nurse whose diabetes failed to respond to a number of changes in insulin regime until it was found that she was working an 8-hour shift in an intensive care unit, often missing meals and getting home exhausted. Transfer to less arduous nursing duties resulted in a significant improvement in her diabetic control.

Control of diabetes during labour

Maintenance of a steady maternal blood glucose near normoglycaemia is essential if the fetus is to withstand the stress of labour. This is best achieved in the established diabetic and the insulin-requiring gestational diabetic by regulating the blood glucose by the simultaneous administration of glucose and insulin intravenously. It is helpful to have a chart on which regular recordings of blood glucose measurements are placed alongside the amount of glucose and insulin being administered and the dilatation of the cervix.

The following regimes are outlined as a guide to the practical management of the diabetic mother before and during labour.

Induction of labour. On the morning of the induction, an intravenous infusion of 7.5 per cent dextrose solution should be commenced about an hour prior to the procedure. (This is prepared by adding 50 ml of 50 per cent dextrose to one litre of 5 per cent dextrose solution BP.) The infusion rate should be adjusted to provide one litre of fluid every eight hours. Twenty units of soluble insulin (0.2 ml of 100 units/ml or 0.5 ml of 40 units/ml strength) should be mixed in 19.5 ml of normal saline BP in a 20 ml syringe which is then administered intravenously by infusion pump.

Before and during labour. The plasma glucose concentration should be estimated prior to deciding whether to start an insulin infusion. It is useful to have a glucose reflectance meter on the labour ward for this purpose. In a woman with established diabetes, if the initial blood glucose is less than 7 mmol/l, then the infusion should be given at a rate of 1 unit/hour; if it exceeds 7 mmol/l, then the infusion should commence at 2 units/hour. Glucose estimations should be repeated at hourly intervals and the insulin infusion rate increased by 1 unit/hour until a stable blood glucose of between 4.5 and 5.5 mmol/l has been achieved. If the concentration falls below 3.5 mmol/l the glucose infusion rate should be increased. After a rise in early labour the glucose concentration tends to fall as labour progresses so that eventually it may be necessary to turn off the insulin and even to administer extra glucose intravenously. The gestational diabetic who is being treated by diet alone may require intravenous insulin if she becomes hyperglycaemic during labour, a level of 7 mmol/l or more being a convenient concentration when this treatment is indicated. Should any additional intravenous fluids be necessary during labour (e.g. prior to commencing epidural analgesia) then solutions which do not contain glucose, such as normal saline, should be used. The insulin and glucose infusions should both be discontinued immediately after delivery to avoid the risk of hypoglycaemia that arises as a result of the increase in insulin sensitivity following the delivery of the placenta. An insulin regime similar to that used before pregnancy should be prescribed for established diabetics; gestational diabetics treated with insulin should discontinue treatment until further blood sugar estimations have been performed a few days after delivery.

MANAGEMENT OF DIABETIC NEPHROPATHY AND/OR RETINOPATHY (WHITE CLASSES F AND/OR R)

These women fortunately represent a small proportion of diabetics who become pregnant. They deserve separate mention because their problems require special consideration.

Diabetic nephropathy is a complication of juvenile-onset diabetes and may get worse during pregnancy. This may be manifested by increasing proteinuria, hypertension, increasing fluid retention—all with or without evidence of diminishing renal function. These women also have a tendency to produce growth-retarded babies. Management must be determined by risk to the mother and fetus. If renal function is seriously impaired before pregnancy, then termination must be considered in early pregnancy, particularly if hypertension is an associated complication. Renal function must be closely monitored throughout pregnancy as it may deteriorate at any time and may require interruption of the pregnancy. Fetal growth retardation is a common accompaniment of the condition, presumably due to the impaired ability of the uteroplacental blood vessels to accommodate the increasing blood flow required to support the growing fetus. Frequent serial measurements by ultrasound of fetal growth, and by cardiotocography of fetal condition are required (*see also* p. 212).

Diabetic retinopathy. The incidence of this condition is not certain but it should be looked for routinely in all diabetic women as soon as they report their pregnancy. A recent study of 55 pregnant women with insulin-requiring diabetes, revealed that the severity of proliferative retinopathy correlates positively with the duration of the diabetes (Dibble *et al* 1982). Regardless of severity, pregnancy often exacerbates retinopathy. Dibble *et al* (1982) noted that photocoagulation of the retinal lesions arrested the progression of the disease.

These are serious complications of diabetes and women with them must accept that pregnancy may shorten still further their reduced life expectancy. It is incumbent on physicians caring for young women with such complications to advise them against pregnancy and, if they become pregnant inadvertently, to consider termination and sterilization.

Obstetric management

There is a certain artificiality in attempting to distinguish between obstetric and medical management of diabetic pregnancy when there are so many problems that require a joint approach. The distinction is further blurred by the interests of the individuals undertaking care of diabetic mothers. In some centres the obstetrician may be responsible for the total management of these women, whereas in others it may be the physician or even a paediatrician who decides on how and when the diabetic mother should be delivered. Nevertheless, although, as has been repeatedly emphasised in this chapter, the most important contribution to management is good control of maternal blood glucose, there are numerous issues which only the obstetrician can decide upon. As the guardian of the fetus he has the responsibility to ensure that fetal development is proceeding satisfactorily from the time of conception until delivery. In early pregnancy congenital malformations have to be excluded; in later pregnancy excessive fetal growth must be detected early as evidence of diabetic control that can be improved and as indicating a fetus at additional risk.

The management decisions with which the obstetrician is faced can be considered sequentially according to the duration of pregnancy.

FIRST TRIMESTER

As soon as pregnancy is confirmed, the diabetic mother should attend the hospital and preferably a joint clinic for antenatal care. An ultrasound examination at this time is essential for dating the pregnancy, although Pedersen and Molsted-Pedersen (1979b, 1981) have suggested that the finding of delayed growth from measurement of the crown–rump length is peculiar to diabetic pregnancy and they claim that it is evidence of future growth retardation and likely congenital malformation. Other authors have been unable to substantiate this observation.

The first admission to hospital provides a good opportunity to educate the mother. The established diabetic needs to be advised on nutrition and to be convinced of the importance of achieving normoglycaemia in the interests of her baby. The admission is also an appropriate time to teach the mother how to measure her own blood glucose at home. The mother who is found to have gestational diabetes needs particularly careful counselling so that she understands that the condition is likely to be confined to pregnancy. At the same time many of these women will be treated by dietary restriction and will need to be motivated to accept the discipline this requires in the interests of their babies.

SECOND TRIMESTER

From the little that is known of intrauterine life in diabetic pregnancy, it appears that the second trimester is a time of relative security for the fetus of the woman with well controlled diabetes. Organogenesis is virtually complete and the problems of fetal hyperinsulinism do not start until later. Diagnosis of fetal abnormality by ultrasound is best done between 16 and 18 weeks of gestational age. Hydrocephaly can be excluded by obtaining a good view of the cerebral ventricles, and spina bifida by scanning the spine. Bony defects, and occasionally major malformations such as exomphalos and renal abnormalities, can also be detected. It seems likely that before long it will be possible to detect other major defects, in particular cardiac anomalies. This is also a satisfactory time for estimating gestational age.

THIRD TRIMESTER

The last twelve weeks of pregnancy is the time when the combination of good medical and obstetric care is likely to have the greatest impact on fetal health. Complications such as pregnancy-induced hypertension, hydramnios and macrosomia, preterm labour and intrauterine death are increased, particularly in the poorly controlled diabetic. The physician has to maintain the good control achieved in the earlier months of pregnancy, often in the presence of increasing insulin requirements, while the obstetrician must be constantly on the lookout for any deterioration in fetal wellbeing, including the development of macrosomia.

PRETERM LABOUR

The incidence of preterm labour (less than 38 weeks' gestation) in diabetic pregnancy is increased. Molsted-Pedersen (1979) reported a threefold increase in women with mild diabetes. There are two major reasons for this. In the UK Survey of Diabetic Pregnancy (1979–80) (Beard and Lowy 1982), 50 per cent of women with established diabetes were delivered before 38 weeks of gestation. Approximately two-thirds of these women were induced or were delivered by elective Caesarean section, either because of suspected fetal compromise or because of established routine management. The remaining third went into spontaneous premature labour for reasons that are not known. All that can be said is that the effect of preterm delivery on the baby of the diabetic mother is likely to be more serious than on that of the nondiabetic because of their known predisposition to complications such as respiratory distress. Tocolytic drugs, which prevent preterm labour by suppressing uterine contractions, and steroids administered to the mother to achieve premature maturation of the fetal lungs, induce hyperglycaemia and cause diabetes to become uncontrolled (*see also* pp. 132 and 133). Beta-sympathomimetic drugs have a glucogenic effect whilst steroids have a similar effect by antagonising insulin. Individual case reports (Borberg *et al* 1978) have suggested that steroids and tocolytics can safely be used in women with diabetes providing blood glucose is well controlled with intravenous insulin (Fig. 10.9). It has been recommended that an initial infusion of 16 units of insulin an hour should be used routinely when tocolytics and steroids are given in combination, in addition to 100–120 mmol of potassium every 24 hours to overcome the hypokalaemia induced by steroids (Barnett *et al* 1980).

This form of treatment is obviously only suitable for a short period, usually 24 hours, while the simultaneously administered steroids are having their effect. There is little place for delaying delivery more than 24 hours with the objective of increasing the maturity of the fetus if phosphatidylglycerol levels in the amniotic fluid show pulmonary maturity.

PREGNANCY COMPLICATIONS

In the past, the incidence of complications such as pregnancy-induced hypertension, antepartum haemorrhage and urinary tract infection were thought to be increased in diabetic pregnancy. In fact there is little evidence that this is so nowadays. Very rarely a woman with insulin-dependent diabetes may suffer antepartum pituitary infarction (*see* p. 415) (Dorfman *et al* 1979). In the UK Survey of Diabetic Pregnancy (1979–80) the incidence of toxaemia—at twelve per cent amongst the established diabetic mothers—was the same as that for the gestational diabetics (Lowy and Beard 1982). However, what is of significance is the increased risk to the fetus of any one of these complications of pregnancy in association with diabetes. Toxaemia and pyelonephritis have a prominent place in Pedersen's classification (Pedersen and Molsted-Pedersen 1965) of prognostically bad signs of pregnancy in diabetics. The appearance of a potentially life-threatening complication of pregnancy to the fetus is an indication for hospital admission and possibly delivery within a short time.

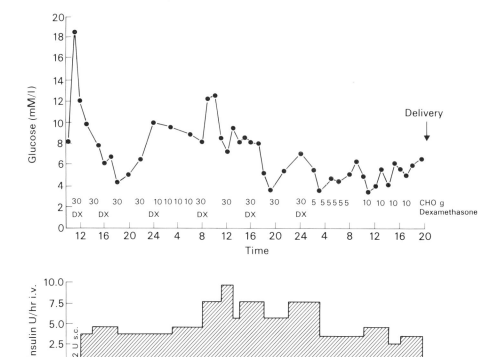

Fig. 10.9   Example of the amount of insulin required to control the blood glucose of a diabetic woman with preterm rupture of membranes who was being treated with dexamethasone. ● Amount of insulin being administered intravenously (milliunits/ml/min) (Borberg *et al* 1978).

INDICES OF FETAL WELLBEING

There is no reliable information on the efficacy of tests of fetal wellbeing in diabetic pregnancy. However, equally there is no evidence that any of the tests of proven value in nondiabetic pregnancy are of less value in diabetic pregnancy.

ULTRASOUND MEASUREMENT OF GROWTH

A majority of studies have shown that the biparietal diameter in diabetic pregnancy remains within normal limits (Szalay *et al* 1975; Stowers and Beard 1982), although one study has shown that growth continues after the 36th week of gestation without the expected slowing found in nondiabetic pregnancy (Murata and Martin 1973). One can only conclude from these observations that the biparietal diameter is an insensitive indicator of excessive fetal growth, for there is no doubt that fetal macrosomia is a common event in all reported series of diabetic pregnancy. It seems possible that a measurement of abdominal circumference of the fetus will prove to be a better index of fetal growth, but until this is confirmed ultrasound has only a limited place in the monitoring of the fetus in late pregnancy.

ANTENATAL FETAL HEART RATE (FHR) MONITORING

Fetal heart rate monitoring is a useful means of assessing fetal health irrespective of whether it is used in mothers with or without diabetes. Curet and Olson (1980), in a study of a heterogeneous population, found that perinatal death was six times higher amongst those with an abnormal contraction stress test than if the test was normal. The non-stress test is a useful means of assisting efforts to prolong pregnancy. If the test is performed two or three times a week (Gillmer and Beard 1975) from 36 weeks' gestation onwards, many diabetics who would be delivered before 38 weeks of gestation because of the obstetrician's anxiety about the possibility of intrauterine death, can be allowed to progress to nearer term.

TOTAL OESTROGEN MEASUREMENTS

There is much disagreement about the value of oestriol or total oestrogen measurement. Most of the large studies have shown an increase in perinatal mortality if oestrogen values are falling (Kitzmiller *et al* 1978; Gillmer and Beard 1975). As in nondiabetic pregnancies, measurements of any particular hormone derived from the placenta are useful, if the concentration is within normal limits and rising, since they help to defer induction or premature Caesarean section (Kitzmiller *et al* 1978).

At present the best indices of fetal health are: 1. the clinical assessment of fetal size with or without hydramnios, by palpation; 2. antenatal fetal heart rate monitoring at regular intervals; and 3. serial urinary or plasma oestrogen measurements.

TIMING AND ROUTE OF DELIVERY

In the past, sudden stillbirth near term was a relatively common event and led to a policy of delivery when the fetus was considered to have a reasonable chance of extrauterine survival (Titus 1937), usually between 36 and 38 weeks of gestation. This policy led to a greater incidence of hyaline membrane disease, which Usher *et al* (1971) ascribed to preterm delivery and to the increased use of Caesarean section. Delayed pulmonary maturation of the fetus is a feature of diabetic pregnancy (Gluck and Kulovich 1973). This is thought by Cunningham *et al* (1978) to be primarily due to a deficiency of one of the important constituents of pulmonary surfactant—phosphatidylglycerol (*see also* p. 359). Measurement of phosphatidylglycerol in the amniotic fluid is a useful index of whether the baby is likely to develop respiratory distress but it involves an amniocentesis near term which most mothers dislike. Fortunately, improved diabetic control and the tendency to allow an increasing number of women to go into spontaneous labour in recent times seems to have diminished the need for phophatidylglycerol measurement and thereby for amniocentesis. It should be measured in cases of preterm labour or prior to induction of labour or elective Caesarean section if there is any doubt about the fetal maturity.

A policy of delivery between 36 and 38 weeks of gestation for women with established diabetes is common in this country and is often applied to gestational diabetics. Figures shown in Table 10.7 reveal that the incidence of delivery by Caesarean section was as high as 58 per cent amongst mothers with established diabetes. Even amongst the gestational diabetic group, the incidence was 33 per cent. It seems likely that this is the result of a combination of failed induction of labour in many mothers in the presence of an unfavourable cervix and of elective Caesarean section for presumed fetal risk. Now that good diabetic control has considerably improved the prognosis for the baby it seems reasonable to review established delivery policies.

There is increasing evidence of the safety of allowing mothers to go into spontaneous labour, providing their diabetes is well controlled and the pregnancy is uncomplicated. Drury (1982) in Dublin has reported on a personally managed series of 113 pregnant women with established diabetes (*see* Table 10.7). His practice is to allow diabetic women to go into spontaneous labour with the safeguards already mentioned, and the results are in marked contrast with those of the UK Survey of Diabetic Pregnancy (1979–80). The incidence of preterm delivery is at least three times lower in Dublin and the direct result of the less interventionist policy is also a threefold reduction in Caesarean section rate. When perinatal mortality is considered the two studies are not strictly comparable because it is likely that diabetic control was considerably better overall in the Dublin series, due to the individual care provided by one physician. Nevertheless the important point that can still be made is that there was no obvious adverse fetal or neonatal outcome from less interventionist obstetric management.

These results underline one of the basic tenets of modern obstetric practice. 'Across the board' policies on such an important issue as the route of delivery are no longer acceptable—each case should be assessed on the available evidence of fetal wellbeing. If the baby is in good condition, the mother's pregnancy is uncomplicated, and her diabetes is well controlled, there is no obvious case against allowing the pregnancy to continue. Nor is there any obvious reason for a repeat Caesarean section if the

Table 10.7 Comparison of the incidence of Caesarean section, preterm labour and perinatal mortality among mothers with established diabetes from the National Maternity Hospital, Dublin (Drury 1982) and the United Kingdom Survey of Diabetic Pregnancy (Lowry and Beard 1982).

| | | Caesarean section rate | | Gestation | PNM |
	n	Elective	Intrapartum	< 38 weeks	(per 1000)
UK Survey	664	43%	15%	51%	61
NMH Dublin	113	16%	5%	15%	26

indications for the operation in a previous pregnancy are non-recurrent. However, elective Caesarean section may be indicated for a number of valid reasons, such as demonstrable fetal compromise or a baby which on clinical and ultrasound assessment is so large that traumatic vaginal delivery is a serious hazard. It needs to be stressed that while a much more liberal view about allowing vaginal delivery can be taken nowadays, this approach must be accompanied by careful antenatal assessment by an experienced obstetrician, good control of the blood glucose of the mother, and monitoring of the condition of the fetus throughout labour.

Intrapartum monitoring

The fetus of the diabetic mother should always be regarded as being at particular risk during labour, however well controlled the diabetes. Fetal asphyxia and disproportion are particular hazards of attempted vaginal delivery of the diabetic mother which require careful monitoring of the fetal condition and of the progress of labour. Established methods of monitoring the fetus by continuous fetal heart rate, and pH measurement if indicated, are satisfactory. There is no good evidence that the well recognised FHR abnormalities and acidosis—which are diagnostic of fetal asphyxia in the nondiabetic—are in any way different in the diabetic (Brudenell and Beard 1975).

Breast feeding

There is no contraindication to breast feeding unless the mother is being treated with oral hypoglycaemic agents. Many diabetic mothers, however, resort to artificial feeding because of the difficulty they experience of looking after themselves and the physical demands of breast feeding.

Contraception

Advice on contraception before and after pregnancy is an important part of the present day care of diabetic women during the reproductive years. The subject is a difficult one in diabetics because of the adverse effects of some methods of contraception on metabolic and circulatory systems. Equally, diabetes may interfere with the effectiveness of contraceptives. The reader is referred to papers by Oakley and Stanton (1982), Steel and Duncan (1980) and Adams and Oakley (1972) for a further account of the clinical and metabolic considerations of contraception for diabetic women.

ORAL CONTRACEPTIVES (OC)

There is well documented evidence that the combined OC interferes with the metabolism of women with subclinical diabetes (Beck 1975), although the explanations advanced so far remain speculative. Glucose tolerance declines and serum triglycerides rise. Interestingly, these changes are not nearly so predictable in women with insulin-requiring diabetes. Steel and Duncan (1980) observed an increase in insulin requirements in only 17 out of 88 diabetics who had started OC. The significance of these observations depends on their interpretation. If, as seems likely, deterioration of glucose tolerance in subclinical diabetes is the product of insulin resistance, then women who had transient diabetes during pregnancy (gestational diabetes) are more liable to remain diabetic if they are prescribed the OC after pregnancy.

An increased risk of thrombotic or thromboembolic lesions in diabetics on OC has long been postulated. The combination of proliferative intimal vascular lesions which are known to occur as a complication of diabetes, combined with an increase in platelet aggregation adhesiveness induced by oral contraceptives, sets the scene for thrombus formation. Steel and Duncan (1980) reported an alarming incidence of near fatal lesions in insulin-requiring diabetics aged less than 30 years on OCs compared with a similar group not on OCs. These ranged from cerebral ischaemia to myocardial infarction. These authors have argued that because it is the oestrogen component of the OC that induces the abnormal clotting, it is logical to use a 'progestogen-only' OC. The disadvantages of this method of contraception are an increased failure rate (6 per 100 woman years) and a 50 per cent rate of menstrual irregularity.

Table 10.8 (Oakley and Stanton 1982) shows the effect of diabetes and a combined OC (independently) on coronary artery risk factors. At present there is no information on whether the adverse effects of OC are additive to those of diabetes.

INTRAUTERINE CONTRACEPTIVE DEVICE (IUCD)

This should be an ideal method of contraception for women with diabetes. However, evidence suggests that copper-bearing devices are rendered ineffective more frequently in insulin-requiring diabetic women as compared with nondiabetic, by the tendency for the copper to become encrusted with sulphur and chloride, and to be eroded (Gosden *et al* 1982). In view of these findings it seems reasonable to recommend the use of plastic devices such as the Lippes loop for diabetic women.

Table 10.8   The effect of diabetes and a combined oral contraceptive, considered independently, on coronary artery risk factors (Oakley and Stanton 1982). + Increased effect, − decreased effect, 0 no effect.

	Fasting serum triglyceride	Fasting blood glucose	Glucose tolerance	Red cell flexibility	Platelet adhesiveness and aggregation	Intrinsic clotting system	Extrinsic clotting system	Antithrombin III	Individual clotting factors	Fibrinogen	Blood pressure
Diabetes	+/0	++	---	−	++	0	0	0	0	+/0	0
Combined OC	++	−/0	−/0	−	++	+	?+	−	+	+	+

OTHER METHODS

Mechanical methods (sheath and cap) are unfashionable but remain effective alternatives to the methods described.

STERILISATION

Sterilisation should only be performed after full consultation with the diabetic woman and her partner; it is particularly indicated when there is evidence of progressive vascular degeneration and/or nephropathy. All diabetic women should consider some limitation of their family. Laparoscopic sterilisation is the method of choice because it involves minimal disturbance of diabetic control and care of the baby.

Steel *et al* (1982) make the important point that pregnancy may have such disastrous consequences for the diabetic woman with severe nephropathy or progressive retinopathy that occasionally it is necessary to advise termination of pregnancy.

CONCLUSIONS

The ideal contraceptive which is fully effective, yet does not accelerate vascular complications of diabetes, is not available. However, it is possible to recommend the following working guidelines.

1   All young women with diabetes should be counselled about contraception and the effect of pregnancy on the disease well before they are at risk of becoming pregnant.
2   The combined oestrogen/progestogen-containing OC should not be prescribed to women with clinical or subclinical diabetes. The 'progestogen-only' pill is a suitable alternative, providing the woman is prepared to accept some menstrual irregularity.
3   The copper-containing IUCD should not be used in women with clinical diabetes because of the reported high failure rate, but as far as is known there is no contraindication to its use in women with subclinical diabetes or in those who have had gestational diabetes. Plastic devices such as the Lippes loop may be used in women with clinical or subclinical diabetes.
4   The use of 'barrier' methods of contraception should be encouraged in diabetic women who are prepared to persevere with them.
5   All diabetics should be prepared to accept some limitation of family size, although it is not possible to state precisely what this should be, because it will depend on the severity of the diabetes. Women with evidence of nephropathy or retinopathy are particularly at risk of accelerating the disease by becoming pregnant. Sterilisation is a matter for personal decision by the couple after the risks of pregnancy have been explained to them.

References

Adams P.W. & Oakley N.W. (1972) Oral contraceptives and carbohydrate metabolism. In Pike D.A. (ed.) *Diabetes and Related Disorders, Clinics in Endocrinology and Metabolism*, pp. 697–720. W.B. Saunders, Philadelphia.

Baker L., Egler J.M., Klein S.H. & Goldman A.S. (1981) Meticulous control of diabetes during organogenesis prevents congenital lumbo-sacral defects in rats. *Diabetes* **30,** 955–9.

Barnett A.H., Stubbs S.M. & Mander A.M. (1980) Management of premature labour in diabetic pregnancy. *Diabetologia* **18,** 365–8.

Beard R.W., Gillmer M.D.G., Oakley N.W. & Gunn P.J. (1980) Screening for gestational diabetes. *Diabetes Care* **3,** 468–71.

Beard R.W. & Hoet J.J. (1982) Is gestational diabetes a clinical entity? *Diabetologia* **23** 307–12.

Beard R.W. & Lowy C. (1982) The British Survey of Diabetic Pregnancies. Commentary. *British Journal of Obstetrics and Gynaecology* **89** 783–6.

Beard R.W. and Oakley N.W. (1976) The fetus of the diabetic. In Beard R.W. and Nathanielsz P.W. (eds), *Fetal Phytsiology and Medicine*, pp. 137–57. W.B. Saunders Co. Ltd., London, Philadelphia and Toronto.

Beck P. (1975) The effect of oral anticonceptual drugs on diabetes mellitus. In Camerini-Davalos R.A. and Cole H.S. (eds) *Early Diabetes in Early Life*, pp. 349–52. Proceedings of the 3rd International Symposium, Madeira, 1974. Academic Press, London.

Berendes H.W. (1975) Effect of maternal acetonuria on I.Q. of offspring. In Camerini-Davalos R.A. and Cole H.S. (eds) *Early Diabetes in Early Life*, p. 135. Proceedings of the 3rd International Symposium, Madeira. Academic Press, New York.

Borberg C., Gillmer M.D.G., Beard R.W. & Oakley N.W. (1978) Metabolic effects of beta-sympath-omimetic drugs and dexamethasone in normal and diabetic pregnancy. *British Journal of Obstetrics and Gynaecology* **85,** 184–9.

Brudenell M. & Beard R.W. (1975) Diabetes in pregnancy. In Pyke D.A. (ed.) *Diabetes and Related Disorders. Clinics in Endocrinology and Metabolism*, pp. 673–96, vol. 1, 3. W.B. Saunders Co., Ltd., London, Philadelphia and Toronto.

Burke J., Dixon G., Savage P.E., Owens C., Pennock C.A. & Sherriff R.J. (1981) Glycosylated haemoglobin in the assessment of diabetic control in pregnancy. *Journal of Obstetrics and Gynaecology* **1,** 153–6.

Cardell B.S. (1953) Hypertrophy and hyperplasia of the pancreatic islets in new born infants. *Journal of Pathology and Bacteriology* **66,** 335–8.

Cassar J., Gordon H., Dixon H.G., Cummins M. & Joplin G.F. (1978) Simplified management of pregnancy complicated by diabetes. *British Journal of Obstetrics and Gynaecology* **85,** 585–91.

Ciba Foundation Symposium, No. 63 (New Series) (1979) In Elliott K. and O'Conner M. (eds) *Pregnancy Metabolism Diabetes and the Fetus*. Excerpta Medica, Amsterdam, Oxford, New York.

Cunningham M.D., Desai N.S., Thompson S.A & Green J.M. (1978) Amniotic fluid phosphotidyl-glycerol in diabetic pregnancies. *American Journal of Obstetrics and Gynecology* **131,** 719–24.

Curet L.B. & Olson R.W. (1980) Oxytocin challenge tests and urinary oestriols in the management of high risk pregnancies. *Obstetrics and Gynecology* **55,** 296–300.

Deuchar E.M. (1979) Culture *in vitro* as a means of analysing the effect of maternal diabetes on embryonic development in rats. Elliott K. and O'Conner M. (eds) *Pregnancy, Metabolism, Diabetes and the Fetus*, pp. 181–97. Ciba Foundation Symposium, No. 63 (new series). Excerpta Medica, Amsterdam, Oxford, New York.

Dibble C.M., Kochenour N.K., Worley R.J., Tyler F.H. & Swartz M. (1982) Effect of pregnancy on diabetic retinopathy. *Obstetrics and Gynecology* **59,** 699–704.

Dorfman S.V. Dillaplain R.P. & Garnbrell R.D. (1979) Antepartum pituitary infection. *Obstetrics and Gynecology* (Suppl.) **53,** 21–4.

Drury M.I. (1982) Management of diabetes in the last trimester. Meeting on the Results of the United Kingdom Survey of Diabetic Pregnancy. Royal College of Obstetricians and Gynaecologists, April 1982.

Duraiswami P.K. (1952) Insulin induced skeletal abnormalities in developing chickens. *British Medical Journal* **2**, 384–390.

Essex N.L., Pyke D.A., Watkins P.J., Brudenell J.M. & Gamsu H.R. (1973) Diabetic pregnancy. *British Medical Journal* **4**, 89–93.

Freinkel N., Metzger B.E., Nitzan M., Hare J.W., Shambaugh G.E. III, Marshall R.T., Surmachyzka B.Z. & Natel T.C. (1972) Accelerated starvation and mechanisms for the conservation of maternal nitrogen during pregnancy. *Israeli Journal of Medical Science* **8**, 426–39.

Gentz J., Persson B. & Zetterström R. (1969) On the diagnosis of symptomatic neonatal hypoglycaemia. *Acta Paediatrica Scandinavica* **58**, 449–59.

Gillmer M.D.G. & Beard R.W. (1975) Fetal and placental function tests in diabetic pregnancy. In Sutherland H.W. and Stowers J.M. (eds) *Pregnancy and the Newborn*, pp. 168–98. Churchill-Livingstone, Edinburgh.

Gillmer M.D.G., Beard R.W., Brooke F.M. & Oakley N.W. (1975a) Carbohydrate metabolism in pregnancy. Part I. Diurnal plasma glucose profile in normal and diabetic women. *British Medical Journal* **3**, 399–402.

Gillmer M.D.G., Beard R.W., Brooke F.M. & Oakley N.W. (1975b) Carbohydrate metabolism in pregnancy. Part II. Relation between maternal glucose tolerance and glucose metabolism in the newborn. *British Medical Journal* **3**, 402–4.

Gillmer M.D.G., Oakley N.W. & Persson B. (1984) Diabetes mellitus and the fetus. In Beard R.W. and Nathanielsz P.W. (eds) *Fetal Medicine and Physiology*. Marcel-Dekker, New York (in press).

Gluck L. & Kulovich M.V. (1973) Lecithin-sphingomyelin ratios in amniotic fluid in normal and abnormal pregnancy. *American Journal of Obstetrics and Gynecology* **115**, 539–46.

Gosden C., Ross A., Steel J. & Springbett A. (1982) Intrauterine contraceptive devices in diabetic women. *Lancet* **i**, 530–5.

Gutgesell H.P., Mullins C.E., Gillette P.C., Speer M., Rudolph A.J. & McNamara D.G. (1976) Transient hypertrophic subaortic stenosis in infants of diabetic mothers. *Journal of Pediatrics* **89**, 120–5.

Guthberlet R.L. & Cornblath M. (1973) Infants born to diabetic women. In Gellis S.S. and Kagan B.M. (eds) *Current Pediatric Therapy*, pp. 327–9. W.B. Saunders, Philadelphia.

Guttorm E. (1975) Practical screening for diabetes mellitus in pregnant women. In Sutherland H.W. and Stowers J.M. (eds) *Carbohydrate Metabolism in Pregnancy and the Newborn*, pp. 142–52. Churchill-Livingstone, Edinburgh.

Halliday H.L. (1981) Hypertrophic cardiomyopathy in infants of poorly-controlled diabetic mothers. *Archives of Disease in Childhood* **56**, 258–63.

Hultquist G.T. & Olding L. (1975) Pancreatic islet fibrosis in young infants of diabetic mothers. *Lancet* **ii**, 1015–16.

Jervell J., Moe N., Skjaeraasen J., Blystad W. & Egge K. (1979) Diabetes mellitus and pregnancy—management and results at Riks Hospital et Oslo, 1970–1977. *Diabetologia* **16**, 151–5.

Jovanovic L., Druzin M. & Peterson C.M. (1981) Effect of euglycemia on the outcome of pregnancy in insulin-dependent diabetic women as compared with normal control subjects. *American Journal of Medicine* **71**, 921–7.

Kalhan S.C., Savin S.M. & Adam P.A.J. (1977) Attenuated glucose production rate in newborn infants of insulin-dependent diabetic mothers. *New England Journal of Medicine* **296**, 375–6.

Kalkoff R.K. & Kim H-J (1979) The influence of hormonal changes of pregnancy on maternal metabolism. In Elliott K. and O'Conner M. (eds) *Pregnancy Metabolism, Diabetes and the Fetus*, pp. 29–56. Ciba Foundation No. 63 (New Series). Excerpta Medica, Amsterdam.

Karlsson K. & Kjellmer I. (1972) The outcome of diabetic pregnancies in relation to the mother's blood sugar level. *American Journal of Obstetrics and Gynecology* **112**, 213–17.

Kitzmiller J.I., Cloherty J.P., Younger M.D., Tabatabah A., Rothchild S.B., Sosenko I., Epstein M.F., Singh S. & Neff R.K. (1978) Diabetic pregnancy and perinatal morbidity. *American Journal of Obstetrics and Gynecology* **131**, 560–80.

Larsson Y. & Ludvigsson J. (1974) Perinatal dödlighet vid diabetes-graviditet. *Läkartidningen* **71**, 155–7.

Leslie J., Shen S.C. & Strauss L. (1982) Hypertrophic cardiomyopathy in a midtrimester fetus born to a diabetic mother. *Journal of Pediatrics* **100**, 631–2.

Leslie R.D.G., Pyke D.A., John P.N. & White J.M. (1978) Haemoglobin A₁ in diabetic pregnancy. *Lancet* **ii**, 958–9.

Lowy C. & Beard R.W. (1982) *Report to the Meeting on the Results of the UK Survey of Diabetic Pregnancies.* Royal College of Obstetricians and Gynaecologists, London, April 1982.

Madsen H. & Ditzel J. (1982) Changes in red blood cell oxygen transport in diabetic pregnancy. *American Journal of Obstetrics and Gynecology* **143**, 421–4.

Malins J. (1979) Fetal anomalies related to carbohydrate metabolism. The epidemiological approach. In Sutherland H.W. and Stowers J.M. (eds) *Carbohydrate Metabolism in Pregnancy and the Newborn, 1978*, pp. 229–46. Springer-Verlag, Berlin.

Merkatz I.R., Duchon M.A., Yamashita T.S. & Houser H.B. (1980) A pilot community-based screening programme for gestational diabetes. *Diabetes Care* **3**, 453–7.

Metzger B.E., Phelps R.L., Freinkel N. & Navickas I.A. (1980) Effects of gestational diabetes on diurnal profiles of plasma glucose, lipids, and individual amino acids. *Diabetes Care* **3**, 402–9.

Miller E., Hare J.W., Cloherty J.P., Dunn P.J., Gleason R.E., Soeldner J.S. & Kitzmiller J.L. (1981) Elevated maternal haemoglobin A₁c in early pregnancy and major congenital anomalies in infants of diabetic mothers. *New England Journal of Medicine* **304**, 1331–4.

Milner R.D.G. & Hales C.N. (1965) Effect of intravenous glucose on concentration of insulin in maternal and umbilical cord plasma. *British Medical Journal* **1**, 284–6.

Molsted-Pedersen L. (1976) Perinatal mortality in diabetic pregnancy. In Rooth G. and Bratteby L-E (eds) *Perinatal Medicine, Proceedings of the 5th Congress, Uppsala, June 1976*, pp. 98–102. Almquist & Wiksell International, Stockholm, Sweden.

Molsted-Pedersen L. (1979) Preterm labour and perinatal mortality in diabetic pregnancy. Obstetric considerations. In Sutherland H.W. and Stowers J.M. (eds) *Metabolism in Pregnancy and the Newborn 1978*, pp. 392–406. Springer-Verlag, Berlin.

Murata Y. & Martin C.B. (1973) Growth of the biparietal diameter of the fetal head in diabetic pregnancy. *American Journal of Obstetrics and Gynecology* **115**, 252–6.

Naeye K.L. (1979) The outcome of diabetic pregnancies: a prospective study. In Elliott K. and O'Conner M. (eds) *Pregnancy, Metabolism, Diabetes and the Fetus*, pp. 227–38. Ciba Foundation Symposium No. 63 (new series), Excerpta Medica, Amsterdam, Oxford, New York.

Oakley N.W. (1976) The management of diabetes in pregnancy. In Rooth G. and Bratteby L-E (eds) *Perinatal Medicine. Proceedings of the 5th European Congress, Uppsala, June 1976*, pp. 92–7. Almquist & Wiksell International, Stockholm.

Oakley N.W., Beard R.W. & Turner R.C. (1972) Effect of sustained maternal hyperglycaemia on the fetus in normal and diabetic pregnancies. *British Medical Journal* **1**, 466–9.

Oakley N. & Stanton S.L. (1982) Contraception and diabetes. *British Journal of Family Planning* **8**, 55–8.

Oh W. (1982) Heading off problems in the diabetic's baby. *Contemporary Obstetrics and Gynecology* **19**, 91–3, 96.

O'Sullivan J.B., Charles D., Mahan C.M. & Dandrow R.V. (1973) Gestational diabetes and perinatal mortality rate. *American Journal of Obstetrics and Gynecology* **116**, 901–4.

O'Sullivan J.B. & Mahan C.M. (1964) Criteria for the oral glucose tolerance test in pregnancy. *Diabetes* **13**, 278–85.

O'Sullivan J.B. & Mahan C.M. (1980) Insulin treatment and high risk groups. *Diabetes Care* **3**, 482–5.

O'Sullivan J.B., Mahan C.M., Charles D. & Dandrow R.V. (1973) Screening criteria for high risk gestational diabetic patients. *American Journal of Obstetrics and Gynecology* **116**, 895–900.

Paisey R.B., Macfarlane D.G., Sherrif R.J., Hartog M., Slade R.R. & White D.A.J. (1980) The relationship between blood glycosylated haemoglobin and home capillary blood glucose levels in diabetics. *Diabetologia* **19**, 31–34.

Pedersen J. (1977) *The Pregnant Diabetic and Her newborn—Problems and Management.* Munksgaard, Copenhagen.

Pedersen J. (1979) Congenital malformations in newborn of diabetic mothers. In Sutherland H.W. and Stowers J.M. (eds) *Carbohydrate Metabolism in Pregnancy and the Newborn, 1978,* pp. 264–76. Springer-Verlag, Berlin.

Pedersen J. & Molsted-Pedersen L. (1965) Prognosis of the outcome of pregnancies in diabetics. A new classification. *Acta Endocrinologica (Kbh)* **50**, 70–4.

Pedersen J. & Molsted-Pedersen L. (1979a) Congenital malformations: the possible role of diabetes care outside pregnancy. In Elliott K. & O'Conner M. (eds) *Pregnancy, Metabolism, Diabetes and the Fetus (Ciba Symposium 63),* pp. 265–81. Excerpta Medica, Amsterdam.

Pedersen J.F. & Molsted-Pedersen L. (1979b) Early growth retardation in diabetic pregnancy. *British Medical Journal* **1**, 18–19.

Pedersen J.F. & Molsted-Pedersen L. (1981) Early fetal growth delay detected by ultrasound marks increased risk of congenital malformations in early pregnancy. *British Medical Journal* **283**, 269–71.

Persson B., Gentz J. & Lunell O. (1978) Diabetes in Pregnancy. In Scarpelli E.M. and Cosmi E.V. (eds) *Reviews in Perinatal Medicine* **2**, 1–55. Raven Press, New York.

Pettit D.J., Baird R., Aleck K.A., Bennett P.H. & Knowler W.C. (1983) Excessive obesity in offspring of Pima Indian women with diabetes during pregnancy. *New England Journal of Medicine* **308**, 242–5.

Roversi G.D., Gargiulo M., Nicolini U., Pedretti E. & Candiani G. (1977) Diabète de la mère et risque perinatal. *Revue Médicale de la Suisse Romande* **97**, 401–12.

Schneider J.M., Curet L.B., Olson R.W. & Stay G. (1980) Ambulatory care of the pregnant diabetic. *Obstetrics and Gynecology* **56**, 144–9.

Schwartz H.C., King K.C., Schwartz A.L., Edmunds D. & Schwartz R. (1976) Effects of pregnancy on haemoglobin A_{1c} in normal, gestational diabetic and diabetic women. *Diabetes* **25**, 1118–22.

Shelley H.J., Bassett J.M. & Milner R.D.G. (1975) Control of carbohydrate metabolism in the fetus and newborn. In Nathanielsz P.W. (ed.) *Perinatal Research. British Medical Bulletin* **31**, 37–43.

Sönksen P.H., Judd S.L. & Lowy C. (1978) Home monitoring of blood glucose. Method for improving diabetic control. *The Lancet* **i**, 729–32.

Steel J.M. & Duncan L.J.P. (1980) Contraception for the insulin-dependent diabetic woman: the view from one clinic. *Diabetes Care* **3**, 557–60.

Steel J.M., Johnstone F.D., Smith A.F. & Duncan L.J.P. (1982) Five years experience of a 'pre-pregnancy' clinic for insulin-dependent diabetics. *British Medical Journal* **285**, 353–6.

Steel J.M., Thomson P., Johnstone F. & Smith A.F. (1981) Glycosylated haemoglobin levels in mothers of large babies. *British Medical Journal* **282**, 1357–8.

Stowers J.M. & Beard R.W. (1982) Special features of diabetic pregnancies and their progeny. In Keen H. and Jarrett J. (eds) *Complications of Diabetes,* pp. 215–30. Edward Arnold, London.

Stubbs S.M., Leslie R.D.G. & John P.N. (1981) Fetal macrosomia and maternal diabetic control in pregnancy. *British Medical Journal* **282**, 439–40.

Stubbs W.A. & Stubbs S.M. (1978) Hyperinsulinism, diabetes mellitus and respiratory distress of the newborn: a common link? *Lancet* **i**, 308–9.

Sutherland H.W., Bewsher P.D., Cormack J.D., Hughes C.R.T., Reid A., Russell G. & Stowers J.M. (1974) The effect of moderate dosage of chlorpropamide in pregnancy on fetal outcome. *Archives of Diseases in Childhood* **49**, 283–91.

Sutherland H.W., Stowers J.M. & McKenzie C. (1970) Simplifying the clinical problem of glycosuria in pregnancy. *Lancet* **i**, 1069–71.

Szalay J., Kun L. & Somogyi J. (1975) Erfahrungen mit der kephalometric zur bestimung des entbindung-termins bei diabetischen schwangeren. *Zentralblatt für Gynaekologie* **97**, 871–4.

Thomson A.M., Billewicz W.Z. & Hytten F.E. (1968) The assessment of fetal growth. *Journal of Obstetrics and Gynaecology of the British Commonwealth* **75**, 903–16.

Titus R.S. (1937) Diabetes and pregnancy from the obstetric point of view. *American Journal of Obstetrics and Gynecology* **33**, 386–92.

Usher R.M., Allen A.C. & Maclean F.H. (1971) Risk of respiratory distress syndrome related to gestational age, route of delivery and maternal diabetes. *American Journal of Obstetrics and Gynecology* **111**, 826–9.

White P. (1965) Pregnancy and diabetes. Medical aspects. *Medical Clinics of North America* **49**, 1015–24.

Ylinen K., Raivio K. & Teramo K. (1981) Haemoglobin A_{1c} predicts the perinatal outcome in insulin-dependent diabetic pregnancies. *British Journal of Obstetrics and Gynecology* **88**, 961–7.

Yssing M. (1975) Long term prognosis of children born to mothers diabetic when pregnant. In Camerini-Davalos R.A. and Cole H.S. (eds) *Early Diabetes in Early Life* pp. 575–86. Proceedings of the 3rd International Symposium, Madeira. Academic Press, New York.

11 Thyroid Disease

Ian Ramsay

In most developed countries thyroid disease is relatively uncommon in pregnancy, only two per 1000 pregnancies being associated with hyperthyroidism and nine per 1000 being complicated by hypothyroidism (Niswander and Gordon 1972). In these countries the problems are that the obstetrician is usually unfamiliar with thyroid disease and the physician may be unaware of the ways in which the pregnant state may modify the clinical presentation of these diseases and may alter the results of thyroid function tests. However, in many parts of the Third World the major thyroid problem in pregnancy is that of iodine deficiency and endemic goitre. It is estimated that throughout the world up to 250 million people suffer from endemic goitre and that in some regions, such as Idjwi Island, Zaire, as many as 7.6 per cent of the children born may suffer from cretinism (Pharoah *et al* 1980). This terrible toll could be totally prevented by the prophylactic intramuscular injection of iodised oil every four or five years, at a cost of between three and four pence per head of the population each year. It is almost impossible to measure what effect this proportion of retarded and crippled beings has upon the productivity of people whose economic status is already very low.

No excuse, therefore, is made for including a section on the effect of endemic goitre in pregnancy but, before discussing thyroid disease, it is necessary to consider the normal physiology of the thyroid gland and the ways in which it is altered by pregnancy, the physiology of the fetal thyroid and the relationship between the thyroid status of mother and fetus.

Normal thyroid physiology

The thyroid gland produces two hormones thyroxine (T_4) and tri-iodothyronine (T_3). Although T_3 is secreted by the thyroid gland, a large proportion of it (70–80 per cent) is produced by the peripheral monodeiodination of T_4. It is thought that, functionally, T_3 is a more important hormone than T_4. In order to make T_4 and T_3 it is essential for the thyroid gland to have an adequate supply of iodine. Dietary iodide, absorbed from the gut into the blood stream is actively trapped by the follicular cells of the thyroid which can concentrate it 20 times more than in the perfusing blood. Between 100 and 200 μg of iodide are taken up by the thyroid each day.

The iodide in the thyroid is oxidised to iodine which then iodinates tyrosyl residues present in thyroglobulin to form monoiodotyrosine (MIT) and di-iodotyrosine (DIT). MIT and DIT molecules combine and form either thyroxine (tetra-iodothyronine) or tri-iodothyronine (Fig. 11.1).

Once the thyroid hormone has been formed it is stored, joined to thyroglobulin in the colloid of the follicle. In order for thyroid hormones to be released, colloid droplets are taken up by the apical border of the follicular cell. Lysosomes cause the release of T_4, T_3, MIT and DIT. MIT and DIT are deiodinated and the iodide is largely stored in the thyroid in order to be used again. Some of it passes into the blood. T_4 and T_3 are secreted in a ratio of 5:1. As noted before, 35–40 per cent of the T_4 is deiodinated peripherally to form T_3. An even greater proportion (50 per cent) is converted to an inactive hormone called reverse-tri-iodothyronine (rT_3) (Chopra 1976).

Thyroid hormones circulate in the blood almost entirely bound to plasma proteins. Eighty-five per cent of the bound hormone is attached to a specific protein called thyroxine-binding globulin (TBG). The rest is bound either to thyroxine-binding pre-albumin or to albumin itself (Woeber and Ingbar 1968). Only 0.05 per cent of T_4 is in the free, unbound, form. T_3 is bound to TBG to a lesser extent, so that 0.5 per cent of the hormone circulates in the free state. The half life of T_4 in the blood is about one week but that of T_3 is only $1-1\frac{1}{2}$ days.

The synthesis and secretion of thyroid hormones is controlled by thyroid stimulating hormone (TSH or thyrotrophin), synthesized in the pituitary, which binds to receptors on the thyroid follicular cell membrane. This binding to TSH receptors

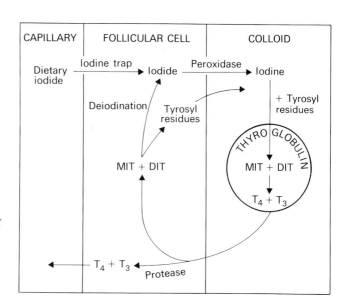

Fig. 11.1   The synthesis of thyroid hormones.
MIT mono-iodotyrosine,
DIT di-iodotyrosine,
T_4 thyroxine,
T_3 tri-iodothyronine.

activates adenyl cyclase which catalyses the formation of cyclic adenosine monophosphate (cyclic AMP) from adenosine triphosphate (ATP). TSH binding also seems to increase cytosol calcium and to cause increased synthesis of prostaglandins. All three mechanisms seem to play a part in thyroid hormone synthesis.

The amount of TSH stimulation of the thyroid depends upon how much is synthesised and released from the pituitary gland. This is controlled largely by the negative feedback of thyroid hormones on the pituitary, though the sensitivity of this feedback mechanism is modulated by a hypothalamic hormone called thyrotrophin-releasing hormone (TRH) which passes down the portal vessels of the pituitary stalk and renders the pituitary thyrotroph cells more sensitive to the feedback mechanism. Increased amounts of TSH are present in situations when thyroid hormone levels are low, as in hypothyroidism. Conversely, TSH is suppressed when thyroid hormone levels are high, as in hyperthyroidism. The net result in hypothyroidism is an enhanced basal release of TSH by the pituitary which can be increased even further by the administration of TRH (Ormston *et al* 1971). In hyperthyroidism the secretion of TSH is inhibited and cannot be increased by TRH (Hall *et al* 1973).

Thyroid hormones are important physiologically because of their major role in energy production. The hormones are bound to cell mitochondria which produce the high energy bonds of ATP. Small amounts of thyroid hormone encourage the formation of ATP but large amounts, as in hyperthyroidism, have a converse effect, causing a reduction in the amount of ATP and bringing about a waste of energy as heat. Two other important actions of thyroid hormones are their effect upon the stimulation of protein synthesis and upon growth in children.

EFFECT OF PREGNANCY ON THYROID PHYSIOLOGY

Before the twelfth week of pregnancy there is evidence of a reduction in the renal tubular absorption of iodide. As a result the urinary excretion of iodide doubles, the plasma level falls, and the thyroid gland is forced to triple its uptake of iodine from the blood (Aboul-Khair *et al* 1964). In situations where there is already at least a partial deficiency of iodine in the diet, the thyroid gland hypertrophies in order to be able to manufacture a sufficient amount of thyroid hormone. Thus, in Aberdeen, Crooks and his colleagues (1964) found that 70 per cent of pregnant women, when examined carefully, had a goitre. The same authors carried out a similar survey in Iceland, where the dietary intake of iodine is high, and found that there was no increase in the prevalence of goitre during pregnancy (Crooks *et al* 1967). Similarly in the United States, where domestic salt is almost always iodised, iodine balance was not found to be compromised during pregnancy (Dworkin *et al* 1966). Thus it seems that most cases of pregnancy goitre could be prevented by an adequate intake of iodine.

How the compensatory increase in thyroid size comes about is, at the moment, somewhat of a mystery. Theoretically the hypertrophy should be brought about by an increased secretion of TSH, but so far there is no general agreement that this occurs in pregnancy. Chorionic gonadotrophin has weak thyroid-stimulating properties but is unlikely to have an effect upon the thyroid in the quantities normally produced in pregnancy; amounts such as are found in hydatidiform mole, however, may stimulate the thyroid and even cause hyperthyroidism (Kenimer *et al* 1975; Nagataki *et al* 1976; Uchimura *et al* 1976). A chorionic thyrotrophin has been described by Hennen *et al* (1969), but its existence is doubted by others. Recently thyrotrophin-releasing hormone has been isolated from the placenta (Gibbons *et al* 1975). Any effect this might have on the thyroid would have to be mediated by TSH.

The second major effect of pregnancy upon thyroid economy is that of increased placental oestrogen secretion upon the synthesis of thyroxine-binding globulin (TBG) by the liver. By the twelfth week of pregnancy the serum concentrations of TBG have doubled (Man *et al* 1969; Mulaisho and Utiger 1977). The result is that increased amounts of both T_4 and T_3 are bound and this is reflected in increased concentrations of thyroid hormones in the blood. It is possible to measure the amount of binding of thyroid hormones to TBG by means of tests such as the T_3 resin uptake test, and from this and the total amount of hormone to calculate a free T_4 or free T_3 index. Unfortunately in situations such as pregnancy or oestrogen medication, the high TBG levels tend to make the estimation of free hormone a little erroneous (Burr *et al* 1979), the derived free hormone levels tending to be slightly higher than direct measurement of the free hormones actually shows. So far the latter techniques for measurement of free hormone (Ekins and Ellis 1976) are not available for general use in the management of thyroid disorders. When they are, they will greatly simplify the problems commonly dealt with.

Fig. 11.2 shows values of total T_4, T_3RU and FTI in normal pregnancy and also normal nonpregnant ranges. Free T_4 measured by equilibrium dialysis (Fig. 11.3) shows a close approximation to nonpregnant levels, though it is apparent that mean values are slightly less than in the normal nonpregnant female. Free T_3 (Fig. 11.3) concentrations are appreciably lower than the normal nonpregnant range.

THYROID FUNCTION IN THE FETUS

The fetal thyroid begins to secrete thyroxine by the twelfth week of intrauterine life and at the same time TSH is just detectable in fetal blood. Concentrations of both TSH and T_4 increase between 18 and 22 weeks of intrauterine life, after which TSH levels off, though the T_4 concentrations continue to rise until term. The fetal TSH at term is higher than that of the mother; the total T_4 is about the same or marginally greater (Fig. 11.2). Although fetal TBG is increased, owing to the effects of placental oestrogen (Dowling *et al* 1960), its concentration is not as high as in the mother. Consequently the fetal FTI at term is higher than in the mother (Robin *et al* 1970) (Fig. 11.2). Fetal free T_4 is also significantly higher in the term fetus than in the mother (Robin *et al* 1970) (Fig. 11.3). Fetal total T_3 is very much lower than in the mother, being about one-third of the value; free T_3 is also lower (Erenberg *et al* 1974) (Fig. 11.3). However the inactive hormone, reverse T_3, is increased in the fetus (Chopra *et al* 1975). It is possible that the low free T_3 levels are responsible for the slightly elevated amounts of TSH in fetal blood.

Within 30 minutes of birth, neonatal TSH levels rise sharply to a mean peak level of 86 μU/ml (Fisher and Odell 1969) and are followed within a few hours by rises in total

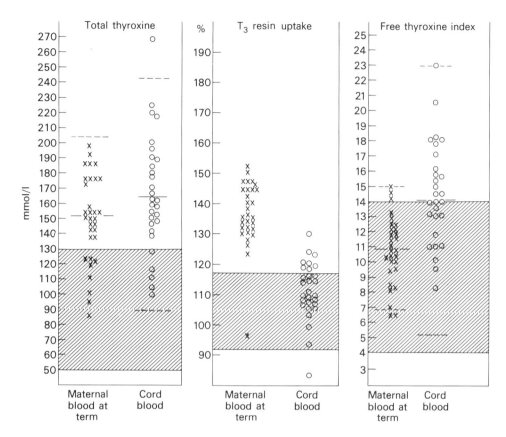

Fig. 11.2 Total thyroxine, T_3 resin uptake and free thyroxine index in maternal blood at term and in cord blood. The mean values are indicated by a solid line and 2 standard deviations from the mean by broken lines. The shaded areas indicate the normal adult nonpregnant ranges.

T_4 and T_3 (Abuid *et al* 1974; Erenberg *et al* 1974). Indeed, a state of physiological hyperthyroidism takes place, so that blood sampled a day or two after birth will be in the adult thyrotoxic range. It is possible that this surge of TSH and physiological hyperthyroidism is an adaptive phenomenon brought about by the immediate drop in ambient temperature consequent upon birth, or that it is due to more general 'stress' (Fisher and Odell 1969). After 72 hours (Fisher and Odell 1969) the TSH has returned virtually to normal. Total T_3 returns to normal values in the same length of time (Erenberg *et al* 1974), but T_4 takes about a week to return to normal. However, free hormone levels are raised for longer periods (Erenberg *et al* 1974). These factors must be borne in mind when testing thyroid function in the neonate.

For a fuller account of intrauterine and neonatal thyroid function, the reader is referred to the paper by Fisher and Klein (1981).

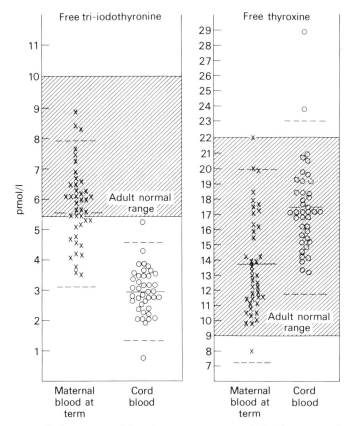

Fig. 11.3   Free tri-iodothyronine and free thyroxine in maternal blood at term and in cord blood. Mean values are indicated by solid lines and 2 standard deviations from the mean by broken lines. The shaded areas indicate the normal adult nonpregnant ranges.

RELATIONSHIP OF MATERNAL TO FETAL PITUITARY–THYROID AXIS

The control of the thyroid in mother and fetus is almost entirely separate. Although thyroid hormones do cross the placenta, they do so in only small amounts (Fisher *et al* 1964). However, it must be remembered that the fetal thyroid is totally dependent upon mother for supplies of iodine, and conversely, that pharmacological doses of iodine (Galina *et al* 1962) and the ingestion of antithyroid drugs or other goitrogens will cross the placenta and may cause both a goitre and hypothyroidism in the fetus. A full list of potential goitrogenic agents is shown in Table 11.1. It is important to avoid giving any of these substances to a pregnant woman and, if it is necessary (as in the treatment of maternal hyperthyroidism), the dose should be kept to the minimum necessary for the control of the disease. A difficult problem is self-medication, usually by iodine-containing cough preparations, of which the doctor may be unaware (Galina *et al* 1962).

Table 11.1 Potential goitrogens. Those which have been shown to produce fetal goitre are printed in italic type. The others do not normally cause goitre in the fetus but may possibly be goitrogenic in areas of endemic iodine deficiency (Fisher 1978; de Groot 1979; McLaren and Alexander 1979; Gaitan 1980).

Drugs used in the treatment of thyrotoxicosis
  Carbimazole
  Methimazole
  Propyl thiouracil
  Methyl thiouracil
  Potassium perchlorate
  Iodides in doses of more than 300 mg/day
  Radioactive iodine may cause fetal
  hypothyroidism but not goitre

Drugs used for other conditions
  Acetazolamide
  Aminoglutethimide
  Antihistamines
  Cobalt containing drugs
  Ethionamide
  Iodides in doses of more than 300 mg/day
  Lithium
  Methylxanthines
  Paraminobenzoic acid
  Phenylbutazone
  Resorcinol
  Sulphonamides
  Sulphonylureas
  Thiocyanate

Foodstuffs
  Cassava   ⎫ contain cyanogenic
  Maize   ⎪ glucosides which
  Sorghum   ⎬ may be converted
  Sweet potatoes ⎭ to thiocyanate
  Cabbage
  Cauliflower
  Brussels sprouts
  Piñon nuts
  Rutabagas
  Turnips

Other dietary factors
  Calcium
  E. coli in drinking water
  Fluoride
  Nitrate
  Rubidium
  Sulphurated hydrocarbons (from sedimentary
  rocks) in drinking water

Thyroid disease in pregnancy

ENDEMIC GOITRE

Up to 250 million people throughout the world are affected by endemic goitre due to iodine deficiency, though its prevalence may vary from area to area because of other factors, such as goitrogens in food and water, thyroiditis and genetic susceptibility. The areas most affected now are the Andes in South America, the Himalayan region, South-East Asia, Papua/New Guinea and Central Africa. In these areas up to 100 per cent of the female population may have a goitre (Kochupillai *et al* 1980), so clearly a goitre will frequently be present in a pregnant woman. In most patients with endemic goitre, frank hypothyrodism is not present because the fall in T_4 levels due to iodine deficiency leads to a compensatory rise in TSH. This stimulates the growth of the thyroid, leads to an increased uptake of iodine by the gland and causes the thyroid to secrete T_3 in preference to T_4. This is of advantage to the individual since each molecule of T_3 only requires three iodine atoms instead of the four necessary for T_4; T_3 is also the more important of the two hormones.

However, the presence of endemic goitre has a deleterious effect on the outcome of the pregnancy. In patients whose thyroid has not managed to compensate and who are hypothyroid, the fetal wastage will be about 30 per cent (McMichael *et al* 1980). Even in mothers who are euthyroid, the iodine deficiency during the first three months of pregnancy may lead to failure of proper development of the fetal central nervous system so that the baby is born with neurological cretinism. The baby is usually euthyroid, more often than not has a goitre, but is suffering from mental retardation, deafness and spasticity. This type of cretinism, which is due to iodine deficiency and not fetal hypothyroidism, is the type usually found in South America and Papua/New Guinea (Pharoah *et al* 1980). It does not respond to any form of treatment.

When iodine deficiency leads to fetal hypothyroidism in the second and third trimesters of pregnancy, the baby is born as a hypothyroid cretin. The baby is lethargic, has a large tongue, a hoarse cry, dry coarse skin, a pot belly and sometimes an umbilical hernia. Neonatal jaundice may be prolonged, the infant feeds badly, is constipated and has weak muscles. Goitre is rarely present. This type of cretinism responds to thyroid hormone replacement, the efficacy of which is directly related to how soon after birth it is started. The hypothyroid type of cretinism occurs commonly in Central Africa and affects up to 7.6 per cent of all babies born (Pharoah *et al* 1980). It is not known for certain why some areas of iodine deficiency have mainly cretins of the neurological variety while other areas have hypothyroid cretins. It is thought that, in the latter case, dietary ingestion of goitrogens, such as occur in cassava (a starchy root vegetable) may play some part.

Both forms of cretinism and the effects of maternal hypothyroidism on the outcome of pregnancy can be prevented by treatment with iodine before the pregnancy occurs. This can be done either by the use of iodised salt or by the intramuscular injection of 2–4 ml of iodised oil every 4 or 5 years (Hetzel *et al* 1980). Both forms of treatment are very cheap, the latter costing 3 or 4 pence per patient per year of protection. It is important for doctors practising in areas of endemic goitre to press for money to prevent this avoidable disease.

SPORADIC GOITRE

Most Western developed countries have got rid of endemic goitre by the use of iodised salt (e.g. Switzerland and the USA), but there nevertheless remains a residuum of patients who have a goitre. These patients are described as having 'sporadic goitre'. It is difficult to know in individual cases what factors are important in the aetiology of their particular goitre. Clearly relative iodine deficiency or ingested goitrogens may play a part, or there may be a partial defect in one of the enzymes necessary for the formation of thyroid hormones. Thyroiditis, as evidenced by the presence of significant titres of thyroid antibodies, is much more common than was thought previously (Gutteridge and Orell 1978), and probably accounts for two out of every three young girls presenting with what appears to be a 'simple goitre'. Recently a new class of thyroid antibody, a 'thyroid growth-stimulating immunoglobulin', has been described by Doniach and her colleagues (Drexhage *et al* 1980); the presence of this immunoglobulin may account for the growth of a goitre in those patients who have no other obvious cause.

During pregnancy pre-existing sporadic goitres tend to get bigger, because the effects of iodine deficiency in pregnancy are superimposed on whatever else was causing the goitre. In Aberdeen, 70 per cent of pregnant women were shown to have a goitre, whereas in Iceland—a country with a high iodine intake—there was no increase in the prevalence of goitre in pregnancy compared with the nonpregnant state (Crooks *et al* 1964, 1967).

It would seem sensible to promote an adequate iodine intake during pregnancy in a woman who has a simple goitre. This can be done simply by the use of iodised salt in cooking and at the table. One part of iodine per 40 000 of salt will give an average daily intake of 700 μg, which is adequate.

If there is evidence of thyroiditis (e.g. positive thyroid antibodies) or of a possible partial enzyme defect (elevated TSH level with or without normal thyroid hormone levels and no thyroid antibodies), it would seem reasonable either to monitor thyroid function on a monthly basis or to give the patient replacement thyroxine during pregnancy to obviate the possibility of subclinical hypothyroidism and further growth of the goitre. A useful guide to dosage is 2 μg of T_4 per kg bodyweight per day. An adequate amount has been given when the TSH has been suppressed into the normal range. Excessive dosage can be avoided by checking the FTI, but note that this may slightly overestimate the true level of free thyroxine in pregnancy (Burr *et al* 1979). Probably the best guide will be the measurement of free T_4 by the dialysis method, but at the moment this remains a research procedure.

HYPOTHYROIDISM

Hypothyroidism in pregnancy occurs in 9 per 1000 white women and in 3 per 1000 negroes (Niswander and Gordon 1972). The condition is usually mild, since severe hypothyroidism tends to cause infertility. However, it is important to diagnose hypothyroidism since the rate of fetal loss is twice that of normal women (Niswander and Gordon 1972), and it has been shown in a seven year folow-up study of the children of women who were hypothyroid during pregnancy, that their intelligence quotient was only 91.9 compared with 104.5 for children whose mothers received adequate amounts of thyroid hormone replacement during pregnancy (Man 1975).

The symptoms which should draw one's attention to the possible diagnosis of hypothyroidism are excessive weight gain despite a poor appetite, cold intolerance (a feature which is unusual in pregnancy), and a roughening of the skin. The pulse rate may be inappropriately slow for pregnancy and there may be delayed relaxation of the tendon reflexes ('hung-up jerks'). A goitre may be present in patients with thyroiditis or enzyme defects but will be absent in primary atrophic hypothyroidism.

A total thyroxine should be measured in any pregnant woman in whom there is the least suspicion of hypothyroidism. The T_4 will be inappropriately low for pregnancy, but note that it may be in the normal range for nonpregnant women (Fig. 11.4). This is because of the doubling of TBG concentration during pregnancy. A measurement of thyroid hormone binding, such as the T_3 resin uptake (T_3RU) test, will show a very large

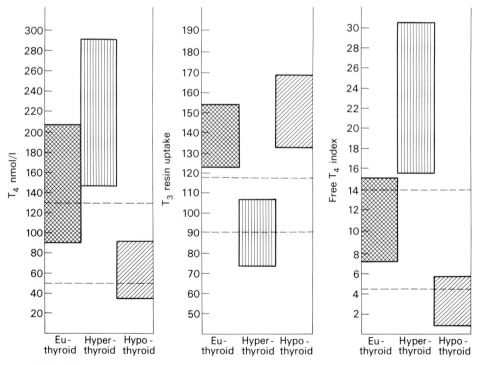

Fig. 11.4 Diagrammatic representation of the ranges of total thyroxine (T_4), T_3 resin uptake and free T_4 index which may be found in euthyroid, hyperthyroid and hypothyroid pregnant patients. The normal nonpregnant ranges are indicated by the broken lines. It should be emphasised that values will vary between laboratories.

number of vacant binding sites because of the high TBG and the low T_4. From the T_4 and the T_3RU the free thyroxine index (FTI) can be calculated and will be low, though it may still be in the normal nonpregnant range, since in situations where the TBG is high the FTI may overestimate the true value for free thyroxine (Souma *et al* 1973; Burr *et al* 1979). Again, actual measurement of free T_4 by dialysis methods (Ekins and Ellis 1976) should provide a much more accurate index of thyroid function in pregnancy. In patients with a low or low–normal FTI, a TSH level should be done. In primary hypothyroidism this will be elevated. However, it is important to be sure that the immunoassay used is specific for TSH, since in some assays the high hCG of pregnancy will crossreact and will give rise to falsely elevated 'TSH' concentrations.

Once hypothyroidism has been diagnosed, treatment should be instituted without delay. So long as the pregnant woman has no evidence of disease, replacement therapy can be instituted rapidly. Thyroxine can be given in an initial dose of 0.1 mg every morning for a week and then adjusted according to the patient's weight. A replacement dose of 2 μg/kg bodyweight provides a rough guide. After a month on this dosage, the FTI (or free T_4) and the TSH can be rechecked and the dosage altered if both results are not in the normal range. It is wise to continue to check the hormone levels monthly during the rest of pregnancy, because as the patient gains more weight, the dosage of T_4 may need to be increased.

Following childbirth, if the mother wishes to do so, there is no contraindication to breast feeding just because she is taking thyroxine. Usually the dose of thyroxine will need to be reduced postpartum because of the loss of weight.

It is wise to check the thyroid status of the neonate, because women with hypothyroidism due to Hashimoto's thyroiditis may have TSH–binding inhibitor immunoglobulins which pass across the placenta and cause intrauterine and temporary neonatal hypothyroidism (Matsuura *et al* 1980) (*see* thyroid stimulating antibodies, p. 399).

POSTPARTUM THYROIDITIS

In recent years it has become recognised that some women who complain of inability to lose weight, lethargy and cold intolerance after childbirth, may be suffering from postpartum thyroiditis (Amino *et al* 1977, 1982). It is thought that this condition, the prevalence of which is unknown, arises in a patient who is immunologically predisposed to thyroid antibody formation and who produces them in greater quantities, possibly as a rebound phenomenon after the immunosuppressive effect of pregnancy is removed (Amino *et al* 1978). The condition may be preceded by postpartum hyperthyroidism (Amino *et al* 1982). In addition to the signs of hypothyroidism a firm goitre is found. The patient should be treated with thyroxine, but it is important to stop this after 4–6 months, since about half of the patients will go into spontaneous remission. We do not know, however, how many of these patients will develop autoimmune thyroiditis and permanent hypothyroidism in later life. It is probably wise to advise the patients to have an annual check of thyroid function.

THYROTOXICOSIS

Thyrotoxicosis occurs in 2.2 per 1000 pregnant white women and in 1.7 per 1000 pregnant negroes (Niswander and Gordon 1972; Montgomery and Harley 1977). In the majority of instances the disease has been diagnosed before pregnancy and the patient is taking treatment; however, in a smaller number, the hyperthyroidism may start at about the same time as the patient became pregnant; in a few it may supervene later in pregnancy, though this is unusual. Severe, untreated thyrotoxicosis usually causes anovulatory infertility.

In a vast majority of cases the thyrotoxicosis is due to Graves' disease, but occasionally it may be due to a solitary toxic adenoma or to an autonomously functioning multinodular goitre. Rarely it occurs early on in de Quervain's thyroiditis (*see* p. 401).

The disease should be suspected in any pregnant patient who fails to gain weight satisfactorily despite a good appetite and who has either exophthalmos or lid lag. Many of the features of hyperthyroidism such as heat intolerance, palpitations, emotional lability, palmar erythema, goitre and thyroid bruit also occur in normal pregnancy and thus are not of much diagnostic help. However a family history of thyroid disease is found in about 50% of patients with Graves' disease and should act to increase one's diagnostic suspicion.

The T_4 will be inappropriately elevated even for normal pregnancy (Fig. 11.4), but the T_3RU will not be so 'hypothyroid' as normally occurs in pregnancy. The resultant FTI will be elevated, but remember that minor elevations of FTI may be found spuriously in pregnancy because of the high TBG levels (Souma *et al* 1973; Burr *et al* 1979). If it is possible, a direct measurement of free T_4 will determine whether or not the patient is hyperthyroid. If it is not available, a thyrotrophin-releasing hormone (TRH) test can be carried out (Ormston *et al* 1971). This is safe during pregnancy and consists of blood sampling at 0 minutes for TSH, the intravenous injection of 200 μg of TRH, and then further samples at 20 and 60 minutes. In a non-thyrotoxic subject, the initial TSH will be in the normal range (0–8 mU/l) and there will be a rise to more than 3.4 and less than 20 mU/l at 20 minutes, followed by a slight fall by 60 minutes. In a thyrotoxic patient, however, the pituitary will have been suppressed by the high thyroid hormone levels and will not contain TSH. It will therefore be unable to release TSH in response to TRH.

It is important to treat thyrotoxicosis during pregnancy since, without treatment, the fetal mortality may be as high as 48 per cent (Gardiner-Hill 1929).

Antithyroid drugs

The most convenient method of treatment is by means of antithyroid drugs, the commonly used ones being carbimazole and propyl-thiouracil. If thyrotoxicosis is newly diagnosed during pregnancy it should be controlled as quickly as possible. This can usually be achieved in four or five weeks by carbimazole in a dosage of 15 mg eight hourly or by propyl-thiouracil 150 mg eight hourly. The dose is then progressively lowered so that the maintenance dose of carbimazole is 15 mg per day or less and that of propyl-thiouracil 150 mg per day or less. The ability to use a fairly low maintenance dose is helped by a tendency for Graves' disease to ameliorate during the last trimester of pregnancy. It is necessary to use the lowest dose of antithyroid drug possible because these agents pass across the placenta very readily and may cause goitre and hypothyroidism in the fetus. The mother must be seen monthly during pregnancy, preferably by an endocrinologist, for a clinical evaluation and for measurements of T_4, FTI, free T_4 (if possible) and TSH. In this way the dose of antithyroid drugs can be adjusted more precisely. Some physicians try to stop antithyroid drugs completely during the last trimester of pregnancy because of a possible diminution in the activity of Graves' disease at this time. This manoeuvre has the advantage of avoiding the effects of the drug on the fetal thyroid, but necessitates very careful supervision of the mother in case she does become toxic again. This is most particularly likely to happen postpartum, when it may be overlooked, since weight loss and emotional disturbances are so common at that time.

Graves' disease, however, is a fluctuating condition (Wilkin *et al* 1979); these variations in disease activity are probably brought about by changes in the level of thyroid-stimulating antibodies (Mukhtar *et al* 1975). It is therefore possible for the dose of antithyroid drug, based on the results of thyroid function studies one month, to be inappropriately high or low by the time of the next month's clinical evaluation, so that the patient has become either hypothyroid or thyrotoxic. For this reason some authorities favour the additon of physiological replacement doses of thyroxine (*see* p. 393) to the antithyroid drug (Fraser and Wilkinson 1953; Selenkow *et al* 1973). In this way the fluctuations in maternal thyroid status are smoothed out and patient management becomes easier. Critics of this method of treatment object to it because of the need for slightly higher doses of antithyroid drugs than when these drugs are being used alone without supplementary thyroxine (Hamburger 1972). However, a comparison of the two methods of treatment shows that the combination of antithyroid drug with thyroxine produces less neonatal goitres and cretinism than are produced by the use of antithyroid drugs alone (Ramsay *et al* 1983). Moreover, in my own series (Ramsay *et al* 1983) of 20 babies whose mothers were treated with a combination of antithyroid drugs and thyroxine, all of them had normal total and free thyroid hormone concentrations in cord blood.

In a series of eleven mothers treated with propyl-thiouracil, seven of whom also received thyroid supplements (thyroxine and tri-iodothyronin), Cheron *et al* (1981) found a reduction of T_4 and FT_4I in the cord blood of their babies, compared with controls. They found no differences in the cord hormone levels of the four treated with propyl-thiouracil alone, compared with those receiving thyroid supplements. A larger study is needed finally to settle the issue. It is my feeling, however, that good results are likely to be achieved by either method. What matters is that the mother is closely observed during pregnancy and that the doses of drugs are adjusted according to the results of thyroid function tests.

At the time of delivery, cord blood should be taken for thyroid hormone and TSH concentrations and the paediatricians should be asked to examine the baby to make sure that it has not got a goitre, hypothyroidism or neonatal thyrotoxicosis (*see* p. 399).

Since antithyroid drugs are excreted in breast milk (Williams *et al* 1944), it has been the practice to recommend that mothers taking these drugs should not breast feed. Recent work (Low *et al* 1979; Kampmann *et al* 1980) has suggested that the amount of propyl-thiouracil present in breast milk is insufficient to materially affect neonatal thyroid function. The excretion of methimazole, the active metabolite of carbimazole, appears to be slightly greater than that of propyl-thiouracil (Low *et al* 1979). Until further evidence emerges it would seem wise to avoid breast feeding in women on antithyroid drugs (Tegler and Lindström 1980). If mothers do breast feed while taking anti-thyroid drugs thyroid function should be checked in the infant.

β-Adrenergic receptor blocking drugs

Over the last 15 years or so, there has been a vogue for the use of these drugs in the treatment of thyrotoxicosis, in order to ameliorate the sympathetically-mediated symptoms, such as tremor and tachycardia (Howitt and Rowlands 1966; Marsden *et al* 1968). Some people have advocated their use in the treatment of thyrotoxicosis in pregnancy (Langer *et al* 1974).

Beta blockers relieve mainly the symptoms of thyrotoxicosis, and not the metabolic derangement (Kaur *et al* 1981). Propranolol has been shown to decrease the peripheral conversion of T_4 to T_3 (Lottie *et al* 1977; Theilade *et al* 1977) and, since the drug crosses the placenta (Cottrill *et al* 1977), it would seem likely to have this effect on the fetus also, in a situation where circulating T_3 is already low (Fisher *et al* 1973). The other possible side-effects of $β$-adrenergic blockade—intrauterine growth retardation, acute fetal distress in labour, and hypoglycaemia in the neonate—are discussed on pp. 176–7. Although the incidence of side-effects is low, it would seem wise to continue to use the already well established antithyroid drugs as the mainstay of therapy and to only use $β$-adrenergic blockers, such as propranolol, in situations such as thyrotoxic crisis or in severe hyperthyroidism, where there is a very rapid heart rate.

Surgery

Some authors recommend surgery as the treatment of choice for thyrotoxicosis in pregnancy (Hawe and Francis 1962), preferably carried out during the middle trimester of pregnancy. However, the general consensus of opinion among endocrinologists is that it is unnecessary, since young women with mild-to-moderate thyrotoxicosis are the very group who are most likely to go into remission after a course of antithyroid drugs. Moreover, since up to 25 per cent of patients become temporarily hypothyroid during the first six months after partial thyroidectomy (Toft *et al* 1978), all women treated by surgery will have to be monitored as frequently during their pregnancy as if they were thyrotoxic, so that they can be treated with thyroxine as necessary.

There is no doubt, however, that surgery is indicated in certain pregnant women. If the goitre is very large and causing pressure symptoms, if there is any suspicion of malignancy or if the patient is uncooperative in the taking of antithyroid medication, then surgery would be justified. The latter group of patients, however, continue to be a problem because they frequently do not attend postoperative follow-up appointments and, if they need to be put on thyroxine, they often either do not take it or take it infrequently.

Radioactive iodine

Radioactive iodine should never be given in pregnancy. It is concentrated in the fetal thyroid from the twelfth week on, but ten times more avidly than in the mother's thyroid. The result will be fetal thyroid destruction and hypothyroidism. There are also risks of carcinoma of the thyroid and the worry of fetal gonadal irradiation.

FETAL AND NEONATAL THYROTOXICOSIS

The thyroid stimulating antibodies (TSAb's) which are the cause of Graves' disease (Volpé *et al* 1974; Mukhtar *et al* 1975)—being immunoglobulins—pass easily across the placenta and, if present in sufficient quantities, may stimulate the baby's thyroid to produce thyrotoxicosis. Although neonatal thyrotoxicosis is generally considered to be rare, the author has found it in 10 per cent of the babies of mothers with Graves' disease in pregnancy or with a previous history of it. Thyroid-stimulating antibodies should be measured as soon as possible in any pregnant woman who either has concurrent Graves' disease or who has a previous history of it. There are several different methods of measuring the TSAb's. If the long-acting thyroid stimulator–protector assay is used, then its presence in quantities of more than 20 units accurately predicts the subsequent development of neonatal thyrotoxicosis (Dirmikis and Munro 1975). Its level may decrease in pregnancy (Hardisty and Munro 1983).

If TSAb's are present in fetal blood, they may not cause intrauterine thyrotoxicosis if the mother is receiving antithyroid drugs, since these cross the placenta and may prevent fetal thyroid overactivity. However, in a woman who previously had Graves' disease and who may even have been rendered hypothyroid by partial thyroidectomy, appreciable concentrations of TSAb's may be present in the patient's blood. One such patient (Ramsay 1976) who was being treated with thyroxine for hypothyroidism following a partial thyroidectomy for Graves' disease at the age of 11, had one fetal death at the age of 21 at 28 weeks from intrauterine thyrotoxicosis and, at the age of 23, had a neonatal death due to thyrotoxicosis four days after birth. In her third pregnancy, in order to control fetal hyperthyroidism, she was treated with carbimazole 15 mg per day, together with her replacement dose of thyroxine. The fetal heart rate remained normal and the infant was clinically and biochemically euthyroid when born. Within 24 hours of birth the baby developed neonatal thyrotoxicosis which was successfully treated with carbimazole 0.75 mg t.d.s. The treatment usually needs to be given for only a few weeks, and in diminishing doses, since the thyroid-stimulating antibodies are broken down in the neonate. Occasionally, in severe cases, iodine may need to be used in addition to antithyroid drugs. Propranolol is useful if there are tachyarrhythmias, but should be used with caution if there is heart failure, when digoxin and diuretics will be needed.

Neonatal thyrotoxicosis may be diagnosed in the baby of a woman with a previous history of Graves' disease by measuring cord blood thyroid hormone levels. This procedure, however, will not necessarily be useful in a woman who has been receiving antithyroid drugs during pregnancy. If her baby is going to develop neonatal thyrotoxicosis it will generally do so during the first day or two of life, after the effect of the antithyroid drugs has worn off, though occasionally the disease may occur even later than this. What is important is to realise the possibility of its occurrence and to ask the paediatricians to keep a close watch on the baby. The physical features consist of a weight loss (which is greater than is usually found in a neonate), irritability, hyperactivity, avid (but sometimes poor) feeding, tachycardia, goitre, exophthalmos, splenomegaly and petechiae. It is important to make the diagnosis and to initiate treatment, since without therapy the mortality is 12 per cent (Samuel *et al* 1971), usually from cardiac failure.

THYROID NODULES

Solitary thyroid nodules appearing during pregnancy are always a worry because of the possibility of cancer. If there is a history of radiation in childhood to the neck or upper chest, the nodule should be assumed to be a carcinoma and should be removed, no matter what the stage of pregnancy. Likewise the presence of voice change, a hard fixed lump, lymph gland enlargement of Horner's syndrome demand immediate thyroid surgery.

Solitary thyroid nodules which have none of the above features may not require surgery. It is important to measure total thyroxine and tri-iodothyronine to exclude a toxic adenoma. An isotope scan to confirm this diagnosis (10 per cent of all solitary nodules) cannot be done in pregnancy because of the risk of fetal irradiation. For this reason it will be impossible to discover which nodules are hypofunctioning (70 per cent) and which are working normally (20 per cent). However, an alternative investigation, thyroid ultrasound examination, is safe and provides useful information (Thijs 1971; Blum *et al* 1972). It will indicate whether the lesion is solid, cystic or mixed solid/cystic. Generally speaking, cystic lesions are benign unless the cyst occurs in a nodule which is more than 4 cm in diameter (Miller *et al* 1974) or has an irregular lining, when there is a possibility of malignancy. These nodules should be removed; benign cysts can be aspirated.

Thyroid nodules which are solid or have a mixed pattern can be biopsied by the fine needle technique (Einhorn and Franzen 1962; Walfish *et al* 1976), which is being increasingly used in Continental Europe and North America, though hardly at all in Britain. If the technique is not available, these solid or mixed nodules should be removed, since about 15 per cent will turn out to be malignant.

It is important after thyroid surgery in pregnancy to give the patient replacement thyroxine in order to obviate the deleterious effects of even temporary hypothyroidism.

Larger doses should be given in cases where thyroid carcinoma has been diagnosed, in order to suppress TSH, since many tumours are TSH-dependent.

Other investigations which may modify one's diagnostic approach to the solitary thyroid nodule in pregnancy include the finding of an inappropriately low T_4, a raised TSH, and strongly positive thyroid antibodies—in which case the diagnosis is Hashimoto's thyroiditis. If the appearance of the nodule has been preceded by sore throat and systemic upset, and if the nodule is tender, a raised ESR may indicate subacute (de Quervain's, viral) thyroiditis. Thyroid function tests done early on may indicate mild thyrotoxicosis; later temporary hypothyroidism may occur, but ultimate recovery nearly always takes place.

References

Aboul-Khair S.A., Crooks J., Turnbull A.C. & Hytten F.E. (1964) The physiological changes in thyroid function during pregnancy. *Clinical Science* **27**, 195–207.

Abuid J., Klein A.H., Foley T.P. Jr & Larsen P.R. (1974) Total and free triiodothyronine and thyroxine in early infancy. *Journal of Clinical Endocrinology and Metabolism* **39**, 263–8.

Amino N., Miyai K., Kuro R., Tanizawa O., Azukizawa M., Takai S., Tanaka F., Nishi K., Kawashima M. & Kumahara Y. (1977) Transient postpartum hypothyroidism: fourteen cases with autoimmune thyroiditis. *Annals of Internal Medicine* **87**, 155–9.

Amino N., Kuro R., Tanizawa O., Tanaka F., Hayashi C., Kotani K., Kawashima M., Miyai K. & Kumahara Y. (1978) Changes of serum anti-thyroid antibodies during and after pregnancy in autoimmune thyroid diseases. *Clinical and Experimental Immunology* **31**, 30–7.

Amino N., Mori H., Iwatani Y., Tanizawa O., Kawashima M., Tsuge I., Ibaragi K., Kumahara Y. & Miyai K. (1982) High prevalence of transient post-partum thyrotoxicosis and hypothyroidism. *New England Journal of Medicine* **306**, 849–52.

Blum M., Goldman A.B., Herskovic A. & Hernberg J. (1972) Clinical applications of thyroid echography. *New England Journal of Medicine* **287**, 1164–9.

Burr W.A., Evans S.E., Lee J., Princé H.P. & Ramsden D.B. (1979) The ratio of thyroxine to thyroxine-binding globulin in the assessment of thyroid function. *Clinical Endocrinology* **11**, 333–42.

Cheron, R.G., Kaplan M.M., Larsen P.R., Selenkow H.A. & Crigler J.F. Jr (1981) Neonatal thyroid function after propylthiomail therapy for maternal Graves' disease. *New England Journal of Medicine* **304**, 525–8.

Chopra I.J., Sack J. & Fisher D.A. (1975) 3,3',5'-triiodothyronine (reverse T_3) and 3,3',5-triiodothyronine (T_3) in fetal and adult sheep: studies of metabolic clearance rates, production rates, serum binding, and thyroidal content relative to thyroxine. *Endocrinology* **97**, 1080–8.

Chopra I.J. (1976) An assessment of daily production and significance of thyroidal secretion of 3,3',5-triiodothyronine (reverse T_3) in man. *Journal of Clinical Investigation* **58**, 32–40.

Cottrill C.M., McAllister R.G. Jr., Gettes L. & Noonan J.A. (1977) Propranolol therapy during pregnancy, labor and delivery: evidence for transplacental drug transfer and impaired neonatal drug disposition. *Journal of Pediatrics* **91**, 812–4.

Crooks J., Aboul-Khair S.A., Turnbull A.C. & Hytten F.E. (1964) The incidence of goitre during pregnancy. *Lancet* **2**, 334–6.

Crooks J., Tulloch M.I., Turnbull A.C., Davidsson D., Skulason T. & Snaedal G. (1967) Comparative incidence of goitre in pregnancy in Iceland and Scotland. *Lancet* **2**, 625–7.

Dirmikis S.M. & Munro D.S. (1975) Placental transmission of thyroid-stimulating immunoglobulins. *British Medical Journal* 2, 665–6.

Dowling J.T., Freinkel N. & Ingbar S.H. (1960) The effect of oestrogens upon the peripheral metabolism of thyroxine. *Journal of Clinical Investigation* 39, 1119–30.

Drexhage H.A., Bottazzo G.F., Doniach D., Bitensky L. & Chayen J. (1980) Evidence for thyroid-growth-stimulating immunoglobulins in some goitrous thyroid diseases. *Lancet* 2, 287–92.

Dworkin H.J., Jacquez J.A. & Beierwaltes W.H. (1966) Relationship of iodine ingestion to iodine excretion in pregnancy. *Journal of Clinical Endocrinology and Metabolism* 26, 1329.

Einhorn J. & Franzen S. (1962) Thin-needle biopsy in the diagnosis of thyroid disease. *Acta Radiologica (Stockholm)* 58, 321–36.

Ekins R.P. & Ellis S.M. (1976) The radioimmunoassay of free thyroid hormones in serum. In Robbins J. and Braverman L.E. (eds) *Thyroid Research. Proceedings of the Seventh International Thyroid Conference, Boston, Massachusetts, June 9–13, 1975*, pp. 597–600. Excerpta Medica, Amsterdam.

Erenberg A., Phelps D.L., Lam R. & Fisher D.A. (1974) Total and free thyroid hormone concentrations in the neonatal period. *Pediatrics* 53, 211–16.

Fisher D.A., Lehman H. & Lackey C. (1964) Placental transport of thyroxine. *Journal of Clinical Endocrinology and Metabolism* 24, 393–400.

Fisher D.A. & Odell W.D. (1969) Acute release of thyrotropin in the newborn. *Journal of Clinical Investigation* 48, 1670–7.

Fisher D.A., Dussault J.H., Hobel C.J. & Lam R. (1973) Serum and gland triiodothyronine in the human fetus. *Journal of Clinical Endocrinology and Metabolism* 36, 397–400.

Fisher, D.A. (1978) In Werner S.C. and Ingbar S.H. (eds) *The Thyroid, a Fundamental and Clinical Text*, p. 955. Harper & Row, Hagerstown, Maryland.

Fisher, D.A. & Klein, A.H. (1981) Thyroid development and disorders of thyroid function in the newborn. *New England Journal of Medicine* 304, 702–11.

Fraser R. & Wilkinson M. (1953) Simplified method of drug treatment for thyrotoxicosis using a uniform dosage of methyl thiouracil and added thyroxine. *British Medical Journal* 1, 481–4.

Gaitan E. (1980) Goitrogens in the etiology of endemic goiter. In Stanbury J.B. and Hetzel B.S. (eds) *Endemic Goiter and Endemic Cretinism*, pp. 219–236. John Wiley & Sons, New York.

Galina M.P., Avnet N.L. & Einhorn A. (1962) Iodides during pregnancy. An apparent cause of neonatal death. *New England Journal of Medicine* 267, 1124–7.

Gardiner-Hill H. (1929) Pregnancy complicating simple goitre and Graves's disease. *Lancet* 1, 120–4.

Gibbons J.M., Mitnik M. & Chieffo V. (1975) *In-vitro* biosynthesis of TSH- and LH-releasing factors by the human placenta. *American Journal of Obstetrics and Gynecology* 121, 127.

de Groot L.J. (1979) Thyroid physiology: endocrine and neural relationships. In de Groot L.J. *et al* (eds) *Endocrinology*, Vol. 1, pp. 381–2. Grune & Stratton, New York.

Gutteridge D.H. & Crell S.R. (1978) Non-toxic goitre: diagnostic role of aspiration cytology, antibodies and serum thyrotrophin. *Clinical Endocrinology* 9, 505–14.

Hall R., Evered D.C. & Tunbridge W.M.G. (1973) The role of TSH and TRH in thyroid disease. In G. Walker (ed.) *9th Symposium on Advanced Medicine*, pp. 15–26. Pitman Medical, London.

Hamburger J.I. (1972) Management of the pregnant hyperthyroid. *Obstetrics and Gynecology* 40, 114–17.

Hardisty C.A. & Munro D.S. (1983) Serum long acting thyroid protector in pregnancy complicated by Graves' disease. *British Medical Journal* 283, 934–5.

Hawe, P. & Francis H.H. (1962) Pregnancy and thyrotoxicosis. *British Medical Journal* 2, 817–23.

Hennen G., Pierce J.G. & Freychet P. (1969) Human chorionic thyrotropin; further characterisation and study of its secretion during pregnancy. *Journal of Clinical Endocrinology and Metabolism* **29**, 581.

Hetzel B.S., Thilly C.H., Fierro-Benitez R., Pretell E.A., Buttfield I.H. & Stanbury J.B. (1980) Iodised oil in the prevention of endemic goiter and cretinism. In Stanbury J.B. and Hetzel B.S. (eds) *Endemic Goiter and Endemic Cretinism. Iodine Metabolism in Health and Disease*, pp. 513–32. John Wiley & Sons, New York.

Howitt G. & Rowlands D.J. (1966) Beta-sympathetic blockade in hyperthyroidism. *Lancet* **1**, 628–31.

Kampmann J.P., Johansen K., Hansen J.M. & Helweg J. (1980) Propyl thiouracil in human milk: revision of a dogma. *Lancet* **i**, 736–8.

Kaur S., Krassas G. & Ramsay I. (1981) Sotalol in hyperthyroidism. *Clinical Endocrinology* **15**, 627–34.

Kenimer J.G., Hershman J.M. & Higgins H.P. (1975) The thyrotropin in hydatidiform moles is human chorionic gonadotropin. *Journal of Clinical Endocrinology and Metabolism* **40**, 482.

Kochupillai N., Ramalingaswami V. & Stanbury J.B. (1980) South East Asia. In Stanbury J.B. and Hetzel B.S. (eds) *Endemic Goiter and Endemic Cretinism. Iodine Nutrition in Health and Disease*, pp. 101–21. John Wiley & Sons, New York.

Langer A., Hung C.T., McA'nulty J.A., Harrigan J.T. & Washington E. (1974) Adrenergic-blockade—a new approach to hyperthyroidism during pregnancy. *Obstetrics and Gynecology* **44**, 181–6.

Lotti G., Delitala G., Devilla L., Alagna S. & Masala A. (1977) Reduction of plasma triiodothyronine (T_3) induced by propranolol. *Clinical Endocrinology* **6**, 405–10.

Low L.C.K., Lang J. & Alexander W.D. (1979) Excretion of carbimazole and propylthiouracil in breast milk. *Lancet* **2**, 1011.

Man E.B. (1975) Maternal hypothyroxinaemia: development of 4 and 7 year old offspring. In Fisher D.A. and Burrow G.N. (eds) *Perinatal Thyroid Physiology and Disease*, p. 117. Raven Press, New York.

Man E.B., Reid W.A., Hellegers A.E. & Jones W.S. (1969) Thyroid function in human pregnancy. III. Serum thyroxine-binding prealbumin (TBPA) and thyroxine-binding globulin (TBG) of pregnant women aged 14 through to 43 years. *American Journal of Obstetrics and Gynecology* **103**, 338.

Marsden C.D., Gimlette T.M.D., McAllister R.G., Owen D.A.L. & Miller T.N. (1968) Effect of β-adrenergic blockade on finger tremor and Achilles reflex time in anxious and thyrotoxic patients. *Acta Endocrinologica (København)* **57**, 353–62.

Matsuura N., Yamada Y., Nohara Y., Konishi J., Kasagi K., Endo K., Kojima H. & Wataya K. (1980) Familial neonatal transient hypothyroidism due to maternal TSH-binding inhibitor immunoglobulins. *England Journal of Medicine* **303**, 738–41.

McLaren E.H. & Alexander W.D. (1979) Goitrogens. *Clinics in Endocrinology and Metabolism* **8**, 129–44.

McMichael A.J., Potter J.D. & Hetzel B.S. (1980) Iodine deficiency, thyroid function, and reproductive failure. In Stanbury J.B. and Hetzel B.S. (eds) *Endemic Goiter and Endemic Cretinism. Iodine Nutrition in Health and Disease*, pp. 445–460. John Wiley & Sons, New York.

Miller J.M., Zafar S.U. & Karo J.J. (1974) The cystic thyroid nodule: recognition and management. *Radiology*, **110**, 257–61.

Montgomery D.A.D. & Harley J.M.G. (1977) Endocrine disorders. *Clinics in Obstetrics and Gynaecology* **4**, 339–70.

Mukhtar E.D., Smith B.R., Pyle G.A., Hall R. & Vice P. (1975) Relation of thyroid-stimulating immunoglobulins to thyroid function and effects of surgery, radioiodine, and antithyroid drugs. *Lancet* **1**, 713–15.

Mulaisho C. & Utiger R.D. (1977) Serum thyroxine-binding globulin: determination by competitive ligand-binding assay in thyroid disease and pregnancy. *Acta Endocrinologica (København)* **85**, 314.

Nagataki S., Mizuno M., Sakamoto S., Irie M., Shizume K., Nakao K., Galton V.A., Arky R.A. & Ingbar S.H. (1976) Thyroid function in molar pregnancy. In Robbins J. and Braverman L.E. (eds) *Thyroid Research*, p. 535. Excerpta Medica, Amsterdam.

Niswander K.R. & Gordon M. (1972) *The Women and Their Pregnancies*, p. 246. W.B. Saunders, Philadelphia.

Ormston B.J., Garry R., Cryer R.J., Besser G.M. & Hall R. (1971) Thyrotrophin-releasing hormone as a thyroid-function test. *Lancet* **2**, 10–14.

Pharoah P., Delange F., Fierro-Benitez R. & Stanbury J.B. (1980) Endemic cretinism. In Stanbury J.B. and Hetzel B.S. (eds) *Endemic Goiter and Endemic Cretinism. Iodine Metabolism in Health and Disease*, pp. 395–421. John Wiley and Sons, New York.

Ramsay I. (1976) Attempted prevention of neonatal thyrotoxicosis. *British Medical Journal* **2**, 1110.

Ramsay I., Kaur S. & Krassas G. (1983) Thyrotoxicosis in pregnancy: results of treatment by antithyroid drugs combined with T₄. *Clinical Endocrinology* **18**, 75–85.

Robin N.I., Refetoff S., Gleason R.E. & Selenkow H.A. (1970) Thyroid hormone relationships between maternal and fetal circulations in human pregnancy at term; a study of patients with normal and abnormal thyroid function. *American Journal of Obstetrics and Gynecology* **108**, 1269–76.

Samuel S., Pildes R.S., Lewison M. & Rosenthal I.M. (1971) Neonatal hyperthyroidism in an infant born of an euthyroid mother. *American Journal of Diseases of Children* **121**, 440.

Selenkow H.A., Birnbaum M.D. & Hollander C.S. (1973) Thyroid function and dysfunction during pregnancy. *Clinical Obstetrics and Gynecology* **16**, 66–108.

Souma J.A., Niejadlik D.C., Cottrell S. & Rankel S. (1973) Comparison of thyroid function in each trimester of pregnancy with the use of triiodothyronine uptake, thyroxine iodine, free thyroxine, and free thyroxine index. *American Journal of Obstetrics and Gynecology* **116**, 905–910.

Tegler L. & Lindstrom B. (1980) Antithyroid drugs in milk. *Lancet* **2**, 591.

Theilade P., Hansen J.M., Skovsted L., Faber J., Kirkegård C., Friis T. & Siersbaek-Nielsen K. (1977) Propranolol influences serum T₃ and reverse T₃ in hyperthyroidism. *Lancet* **2**, 363.

Thijs L.J. (1971) Diagnostic ultrasound in clinical thyroid investigation. *Journal of Clinical Endocrinology and Metabolism* **32**, 709–16.

Toft A.D., Irvine W.J., Sinclair I., McIntosh D., Seth J. & Cameron E.H.D. (1978) Thyroid function after surgical treatment of thyrotoxicosis. *New England Journal of Medicine* **298**, 643–7.

Uchimura H., Nagataki S., Tabuchi T., Mizuno M. & Ito K. (1976) The thyroid stimulating activity of highly purified preparations of human chorionic gonadotrophin. In Robbins J. and Braverman L.E. (eds) *Thyroid Research*, p. 37. Excerpta Medica, Amsterdam.

Volpé R., Farid N.R., von Westarp C. & Row V.V. (1974) The pathogenesis of Graves' disease and Hashimoto's thyroiditis. *Clinical Endocrinology* **3**, 239–61.

Walfish P.G., Miskin M., Rosen I.B. & Strawbridge H.T.G. (1976) Application of special diagnostic techniques in the management of nodular goitre. *Canadian Medical Association Journal* **115**, 35–40.

Wilkin T.J., Swanson Beck J., Crooks J., Isles T.E. & Gunn A. (1979) Time and tides in Graves' disease; their implications in predicting outcome of treatment. *British Medical Journal* **1**, 88–89.

Williams R.H., Kay G.A. & Jandorf B.J. (1944) Thiouracil. Its absorption, distribution and excretion. *Journal of Clinical Investigation* **23**, 613–27.

Woeber K.A. & Ingbar S.H. (1968) The contribution of thyroxine-binding prealbumin to the binding of thyroxine in human serum, as assessed by immunoabsorption. *Journal of Clinical Investigation* **47**, 1710–21.

12 Diseases of the Pituitary and Adrenal Glands

Michael de Swiet

Pituitary gland

During pregnancy, diseases of the pituitary gland may manifest themselves either because of the associated endocrine disturbance, or because a tumour arising from the pituitary gland causes local pressure; effects which either specifically damage the optic nerve, or generally cause a rise in intracerebral pressure. Secretion of one or more of the gland hormones may be increased (usually as a result of a tumour) or decreased. Since underactivity may also be due to the local pressure of a pituitary tumour or its treatment, the presentation of patients with these tumours can be very varied. Nevertheless, there are specific clinical syndromes associated with pituitary disease.

PITUITARY TUMOURS

Pituitary tumours comprise 10 per cent of all cerebral tumours (Russell and Rubinstein 1977). They may secrete any or a mixture of the hormones of the anterior pituitary: prolactin, growth hormone, ACTH, FSH, LH or TSH. However, only tumours secreting the first three hormones are at all common clinically, and these will be considered in this chapter. In the past, these tumours have been classified on the basis of their reactions with haematoxylin and eosin stains. Prolactin and growth hormone-secreting tumours may be chromophobic or acidophilic; ACTH-secreting tumours are basophilic (Gemzell and Wang 1979).

Hyperprolactinaemia

The advent of widely available, specific assays for prolactin has shown that about 12 per cent of nonpregnant women with secondary amenorrhoea during their reproductive life have the pituitary prolactinoma syndrome (Jeffcoate 1978); this proportion rises to 50 per cent if galactorrhoea is also present (Scammell et al 1982). Hyperprolactinaemia may be due to drugs which interfere with dopamine function (e.g. reserpine, methyldopa, phenothiazines), renal or liver disease, hypothyroidism, or

405

disease of the pituitary gland itself. This may be a macroadenoma (greater than 10 mm in diameter) which can extend beyond the pituitary fossa, or a microadenoma (less than 10 mm in diameter) (Gemzell and Wang 1979). In the absence of any other cause of hyperprolactinaemia, it is usually considered that it is due to pituitary disease, even if the lesion cannot be demonstrated radiologically (Thorner *et al* 1979).

Until recently, the standard technique for the anatomical diagnosis of pituitary tumours has been tomography of the pituitary fossa, with air encephalography in suspicious cases, to demonstrate upward or lateral expansion of the tumour. Considerable expertise is needed to interpret the subtle changes that may be seen in tomographs (Thorner *et al* 1979; Doyle and Maclachlan 1977), and some doubt has been cast on their relevance since similar changes may be seen in the pituitary fossae of other patients, who have no clinical or laboratory evidence of pituitary tumour (Swanson and Du Boulay 1975).

The advent of computerised tomography, with or without contrast enhancement (McGregor *et al* 1979; Zervas and Martin 1980; Jung *et al* 1982), has markedly improved discrimination, but now that dopamine agonist therapy has become accepted, even for large tumours, localisation is less of a problem. An alternative approach in those with doubtful or negative pituitary tomography has been to consider the absolute level of prolactin. A normal level is up to 1000 mu/l (30 ng/ml) (Jeffcoate 1983). A basal level in excess of 1500 mu/l (45 ng/ml) is suggestive of pituitary tumour, though patients with tumours may have lower levels than this (Jacobs *et al* 1976). It is also believed that patients with adenomas are less likely to show a further rise in prolactin when challenged with thyrotropin-releasing hormone (TRH) or metoclopramide (Cowden *et al* 1979); however, the value and specificity of these tests has been questioned (*Lancet* 1980).

The effect of pregnancy on prolactin-secreting tumours

The pituitary prolactinoma syndrome can be treated in over 80 per cent of women by bromocriptine (Zervas and Martin 1980); thus these patients frequently become pregnant. They may also become pregnant spontaneously (Chang *et al* 1983). The main problem in their management in pregnancy is that, under the influence of oestrogen stimulation, the pituitary adenoma (if present) may enlarge—threatening vision or even life. (Episodes of visual loss in a patient with a prolactin-secreting adenoma, while taking an oestrogen-containing contraceptive, have also been reported (Mills *et al* 1979).) Before bromocriptine therapy and prolactin estimations were available, it was possible to achieve pregnancy in about 80 per cent of patients with amenorrhoea and galactorrhoea, using gonadotrophin, and Gemzell (1975) reported the outcome of pregnancy in 250 of 700 anovulatory women who became pregnant with pituitary stimulation. In the light of modern knowledge, it is likely that the 250 women who did succeed in becoming pregnant would have included a number with hyperprolactinaemia. In only four of these pregnancies (1.6 per cent) were there symptoms of tumour expansion in pregnancy, and only one patient required neurosurgery.

More recently, Thorner *et al* (1979) cited literature reports of 32 cases of visual field defects in patients with tumours around the pituitary fossa, and a number of unreported cases. Of the 32 cases, 29 had pituitary tumours, and the remainder had a craniopharyngioma or a meningioma. Some of these 32 cases have been reported to the manufacturers, who have given details of over 800 pregnancies achieved with the aid of bromocriptine (Griffith *et al* 1979). There was evidence of pituitary tumour in 116 completed pregnancies, and amongst these were nine tumour-related complications (7.8 per cent). Gemzell and Wang (1979) on the basis of a questionnaire sent to interested doctors, suggest that the risk of tumour-related complications in pregnant patients with previously untreated microadenomas is 5.5 per cent; however, in 56 pregnancies with previously untreated macroadenomas, they found an incidence of tumour-related complications of 37.5 per cent. These figures include four of 17 patients with tumour-related complications in pregnancy, reported by Bergh *et al* (1978), but they do not include the nine pregnancies of Lamberts *et al* (1979) in which there were three tumour-related complications. The data of Gemzell and Wang (1979) suggest that patients who have macroadenomas are much more likely to suffer from expansion of their tumours in pregnancy than those who have microadenomas, but Lamberts *et al* (1979) believe that it is not possible to predict which tumours will enlarge sufficiently in pregnancy to cause symptoms. This may possibly be related to the varied prolactin response that was found by White *et al* (1981) when they gave oestrogen (oestradiol benzoate) to women with prolactinomas. Nevertheless, the patients with the largest tumours studied by White *et al* (1981) did appear to increase their prolactin levels most when given oestrogen.

Other favourable studies of prolactin-secreting tumours in pregnancy with minimal or zero tumour-related complication rates are those of Zarate *et al* (1979), Jewelwicz and Van de Wiele (1980) and Hancock *et al* (1980). The response of women with prolactin-secreting tumours in successive pregnancies can be quite varied (Gemzell and Wang 1979), although Thorner *et al* (1979) found that, in women with visual field defects in one pregnancy, the defects increased in succeeding pregnancies.

If the risk of tumour-related complications in pregnancy is considered to be greater in those with macroadenomas than in those with microadenomas, the question arises whether they should be managed differently before they become pregnant?

First, all patients with hyperprolactinaemia who are treated with bromocriptine should be warned of the risks of tumour expansion if they become pregnant. As we have seen, these risks vary depending on whether or not there is a demonstrable tumour, and how large it is. In the past, a number of treatments have been used for the pituitary prolactinoma syndrome, including both external (Thorner *et al* 1979) and internal radiation with yttrium-90 (Child *et al* 1975), and surgery (Hardy *et al* 1978). It was particularly advocated that 'definitive' treatment be performed before pregnancy, because of the risk of tumour complications in pregnancy. However, more recently, the consensus of opinion is that the dopamine agonist bromocriptine can be used to decrease prolactin secretion and the size of the tumour in all patients with the pituitary prolactinoma syndrome (*Lancet* 1982). If tumour-related complications do develop in pregnancy, they can usually be treated with further bromocriptine (*see below*). Patients with macroadenomas should defer pregnancy until their tumours have been shrunk by bromocriptine, and the risk of tumour-related complications in pregnancy is lower. However, patients with macroadenomas usually do not get pregnant until after bromocriptine therapy.

Alternative forms of therapy, such as radiation, are unpleasant for the patient, and surgery is not always effective in treating the condition (Chang *et al* 1977; Franks *et al* 1977; Shearman and Fraser 1977) or in preventing complications in pregnancy (Lamberts *et al* 1979); it may also result in permanent hypopituitarism (Hardy *et al* 1978; Werder *et al* 1978; Franks *et al* 1977). External irradiation has been reported to cause sarcoma and damage to other intracerebral structures, i.e. loss of vision (Harries and Levene 1976) and bone necrosis. External irradiation may also be ineffective in preventing tumour complications in pregnancy, particularly if the tumour is large (Lamberts *et al* 1977).

The effect of prolactin-secreting tumours on pregnancy

The overall prevalence of the specific complications of prolactin-secreting tumours in pregnancy has been considered above. The most common and clearly documented complication is a visual field defect, typically a bitemporal hemianopia. Patients may also complain of headache, due presumably to raised intracerebral pressure. Very occasionally diabetes insipidus develops. All these complications are more likely after 30 weeks' gestation, but they have been reported in the first month of pregnancy (Thorner *et al* 1979). They almost invariably regress after delivery.

The incidence of spontaneous abortion is between 13 and 32 per cent of pregnancies that have been confirmed by elevated hCG levels (Thorner *et al* 1979; Bergh *et al* 1978; Gemzell and Wang 1979). This is rather higher than the 10 per cent suggested as normal by Llewelyn Jones (1969), possibly due to the inhibiting effect of prolactin on progesterone synthesis (McNeilly *et al* 1974) although this now seems rather unlikely. However, it must be remembered that the majority of these women will have been infertile before taking bromocriptine; pregnancy is more likely to be diagnosed early, and therefore there will be very few cases of abortion that are 'missed'. The incidence of abortion is also about 25 per cent in pregnancies following clomiphene or pergonal treatment.

Kelly *et al* (1979) found a high incidence of operative delivery in their series of patients with pituitary tumour, but the indications for intervention were varied, and they, and others, have not found any specific complication of pregnancy. Assuming that there is not a miscarriage, there are no specific fetal complications.

Management of pregnancy in patients with hyperprolactinaemia

All patients with previous hyperprolactinaemia should be followed carefully in pregnancy, since tumour expansion has occurred in some where there was no previous radiological abnormality (Kajtar and Tomkin 1971). The patients have usually conceived while taking bromocriptine. They should have been shown before pregnancy to have otherwise normal anterior pituitary function. Alternatively, the appropriate therapy with thyroxine and/or cortisone should have been started (*see* p. 416). When the pregnancy is confirmed, bromocriptine should be discontinued (Jewelewicz and Van de Wiele 1980) except in the unlikely event that a patient with a large pituitary tumour conceives without any prior therapy. Here, I believe, the risk of tumour-related complication is so high (*see above*) that bromocriptine should be continued throughout pregnancy. There is considerable experience in the use of bromocriptine in pregnancy, and no association with congenital abnormalities has been documented (Griffith *et al* 1979). At one time (Child *et al* 1975), bromocriptine was even continued for the first 12 weeks of pregnancy, because of the suggestion that prolactin depressed progesterone levels. In Child's series there was no excess teratogenicity, confirming the safety of bromocriptine in early pregnancy.

At least every month the visual fields should be plotted by an experienced observer. This objective documentation is helpful, although most patients know when their visual acuity or visual fields are deteriorating. Particular note should be taken of any headaches or thirst: these symptoms are an indication for further investigation, initially by conventional tomography of the pituitary fossa and, if necessary, by CT scanning. Some clinicians have followed serum prolactin levels in an attempt to monitor tumour activity during pregnancy (Dommerholt *et al* 1981). However, prolactin levels rise rather variably during pregnancy, and the within-patient hour-to-hour variability is also much greater in pregnancy than in the nonpregnant state (Whittaker *et al* 1982). Reported values for prolactin in normal pregnancy are shown in Table 12.1. The considerable variability is evident in the large standard deviations.

If there is evidence of tumour expansion during pregnancy, the patient should restart bromocriptine therapy (Bergh *et al* 1978). Additional treatment that may be indicated includes therapeutic abortion, early delivery, the use of dexamethasone (Jewelewicz *et al* 1977) or hydrocortisone (Lamberts *et al* 1979) and pituitary surgery (Lamberts *et al* 1979). Also, those centres that use ^{90}Y implants have successfully controlled tumour expansion in pregnancy in this way (Child *et al* 1975). Whether any of these additional measures is necessary depends on the severity of the condition, and which are used depends on the maturity of the fetus. Blindness in early pregnancy would be an indication for abortion, followed probably by surgery, although very severe visual field abnormalities have been treated successfully surgically without interruption of the pregnancy (Dommerholt *et al* 1981; Mills *et al* 1979). Deteriorating visual fields at 38 weeks' gestation could be managed by early delivery (Thorner *et al*

Table 12.1   Serum prolactin levels in normal pregnancy (mu/l$\pm$SD). Data of Whittaker *et al* (1982). $n=20$.

3 weeks	12 weeks	25 weeks	36 weeks
210$\pm$98	612$\pm$285	3185$\pm$1161	4426$\pm$1962

1975) since visual field defects regress after delivery (Bergh *et al* 1978). Diabetes insipidus has responded to intranasal synthetic vasopressin, but it usually regresses after delivery (Child *et al* 1975).

No special precautions are necessary in labour. Labour itself proceeds normally, despite the possible interruption of the pathways from the hypothalamus to the posterior pituitary (Kelly *et al* 1979), and possible interference with oxytocin release. Breast feeding is possible (Jewelwicz and Van de Wiele 1980; Kelly *et al* 1979), and there is no evidence that breast feeding causes pituitary tumours to enlarge. Presumably they are insensitive to the stimulae which, in normal women, cause a further rise in prolactin during the first few weeks of lactation. Certainly prolactin levels do not rise on suckling in these patients (Dommerholt *et al* 1981).

Contraception

Because of the remote risk of tumour expansion caused by the oestrogen component of oral contraceptive (Mills *et al* 1979), barrier methods are theoretically preferable. In practice, many patients have used oral contraceptives without any problems.

Acromegaly

In normal individuals, growth hormone secretion is inhibited by somatostatin, and stimulated by a peptide growth hormone-releasing factor. Acromegaly is caused by excess secretion of growth hormone from the anterior pituitary, most commonly because of the presence of an adenoma, but possibly because of loss of hypothalamic control (Lawrence *et al* 1970). Some mixed tumours may secrete both growth hormone and prolactin (Nabarro 1982).

Estimation of growth hormone in pregnancy is complicated by possible cross-reaction with human placental lactogen (Hytten and Lind 1973). However, Yen *et al* (1967), using a specific antiserum to human growth hormone, showed that growth hormone levels were no different in pregnancy compared to the nonpregnant state. The diagnosis of growth hormone excess is made by demonstration of elevating fasting levels, above 4 mu/l (2 ng/ml) (Zervas and Martin 1980) which are not suppressed by a glucose load of 1 g/kg bodyweight (Lawrence *et al* 1970). Before puberty and epiphyseal fusion hypersecretion of growth hormone causes gigantism; after puberty it causes coarsening of the features: acromegaly. Acromegaly may also be associated with diabetes mellitus and hypertension; patients frequently complain of headache. The pituitary tumour, like the prolactinoma, can cause hypopituitarism by compression of other pituitary cells, visual field defects and symptoms and signs of raised intracranial pressure.

The same forms of treatment are used as have been used in the treatment of prolactinomas: trans-sphenoidal microsurgery (Wilson and Dempsey 1978), internal and external irradiation (Eastman *et al* 1979) and bromocriptine (Wass *et al* 1977).

Patients with acromegaly whether treated or not rarely become pregnant (Fisch *et al* 1974). For example, in the series of Gemzell and Wang (1979) there were only three women with growth hormone or ACTH-secreting adenomas amongst 187 patients with pituitary adenoma. These three had each had their tumours treated before pregnancy, which was subsequently uncomplicated. Not only are growth hormone-secreting tumours rarer than prolactinomas, but ovulation is also suppressed, either because of pressure effects on other pituitary cells or because of concomitant hyperprolactinaemia. During pregnancy in treated patients, the tumour may expand or symptoms may recur, as in the case of O'Herlihy (1980). These complications should be managed in the same way as tumour expansion in prolactinomas, with the resumption of bromocriptine therapy, irradiation or surgery.

To ensure that the mother is not hyperglycaemic, it is advisable to perform a blood sugar series at 12 weeks' gestation or on presentation, and repeat these at 28 and 36 weeks' gestation. If the patient has more than one blood glucose in excess of 8 mmol/l, or two between 7.5 and 8 mmol/l, she should be managed as a diabetic (Chapter 10).

The infants may be growth retarded (O'Herlihy 1980) or macrosomic (Fisch *et al* 1974), possibly because of maternal hyperglycaemia. Growth hormone does not cross the placenta (King *et al* 1971). However, pregnancy is usually normal, producing an appropriately grown infant.

The infants are appropriately grown even in the absence of growth hormone, either in the mother or in the fetus (Rimoin *et al* 1968) possibly due to the presence of hPL, the 'growth hormone of pregnancy'. These patients with isolated growth hormone deficiency (sexual ateliosis) also lactate normally.

Cushing's syndrome

Cushing's syndrome has been included in the pituitary rather than the adrenal section of this chapter, because of the finding that in 80 per cent of cases the primary pathology is in the pituitary gland or, possibly, the hypothalamus (Cushing's disease) (Zervas and Martin 1980). A pituitary adenoma secretes excess ACTH which inappropriately stimulates the adrenal glands to produce glucocorticoids. However, a benign or malignant tumour in the adrenal cortex can cause a similar clinical picture. Primary pathology in the adrenal gland is relatively more common in Cushing's syndrome in pregnancy than in the nonpregnant state, although adrenal hyperplasia (presumably pituitary in origin) was still slightly more common (55 per cent) than adrenal tumour in a survey of 23 patients with Cushing's syndrome in pregnancy (Anderson and Walters 1976). Nevertheless, Cushing's syndrome is exceedingly rare in pregnancy. Even amongst 187 patients with microadenomas of the pituitary in pregnancy, there were at most three ACTH-producing tumours (Gemzell and Wang 1979).

Cushing's syndrome has been reported to appear in pregnancy, and then remit after delivery (Kreines *et al* 1964; Calodney *et al* 1973); it is not clear to what extent pregnancy is a specific risk factor in the development of Cushing's syndrome.

Occasionally, neoplasms arising outside the hypothalamo–pituitary–adrenal axis may also cause Cushing's syndrome, but this has not been reported in pregnancy. Treatment with corticosteroid drugs can also reproduce the clinical features of Cushing's syndrome. These are well known and need not be described further.

Although most female patients with the condition have irregular periods or amenor-rhoea, the precise mechanism of infertility has not been determined. However, because of the associated infertility, patients do not usually present with Cushing's syndrome *de novo* in pregnancy. More commonly the condition has been diagnosed before pregnancy and only partially treated, or a relapse has occurred during pregnancy.

The treatments that have been employed depend to some extent on the primary cause of the condition. Bilateral adrenalectomy entails lifelong corticosteroid therapy. Also, because there is considerable morbidity associated with the procedure, and because of the subsequent possible development of ACTH-secreting pituitary adenomas (Nelson's syndrome), it is becoming less popular (Zervas and Martin 1980). Because irradiation of the pituitary fossa is not always successful (Zervas and Martin 1980), some authors have used the serotonin antagonist cyproheptadine to decrease ACTH activity (Krieger *et al* 1975). Pituitary microsurgery may be the optimal treatment for those with pituitary-dependent Cushing's syndrome where an adenoma can be demonstrated (Tyrell *et al* 1978), although the results vary from centre to centre (Burch 1983).

The clinical features of Cushing's syndrome in women include bruising, myopathy, hypertension, plethora, oedema, hirsuitism, red striae, menstrual irregularity, truncal obesity, headaches, acne, generalised obesity and impaired glucose tolerance. The presence of these does not necessarily indicate that the patient has Cushing's syndrome: the first three are the most powerful discriminators (Ross and Linch 1982).

In addition, the diagnosis of Cushing's syndrome in pregnancy will depend on finding elevated cortisol levels in plasma with a lack of diurnal variation, and a failure to suppress with exogenous steroids (dexamethasone suppression test). Estimation of ACTH in the plasma may be helpful, although it is difficult. All these parameters are changed in pregnancy (Galvão-Teles and Burke 1973; Rees and Lowry 1978); the normal pregnant woman has total cortisol levels similar to those seen in Cushing's syndrome; this is partly due to the oestrogen-mediated increase in cortisol binding globulin (Doe *et al* 1964), but there is also an increase in plasma free cortisol. Normal values for total and free plasma cortisols, free urinary cortisol and ACTH in pregnancy and the nonpregnant state are given in Table 12.2. Note the higher levels at 9.00 a.m. and those at midnight. Table 12.2 also shows the normal range for 24-hour urinary free cortisol in pregnancy. This is an estimate of the daily cortisol production rate. If, as is likely, there are not the facilities for estimation of plasma free cortisol, urinary cortisol estimation should be performed, particularly in pregnancy, because of varying levels of cortisol binding globulin.

Elevated ACTH levels indicate a pituitary or ectopic cause for the condition, although the placenta may secrete some ACTH-like material (Rees *et al* 1975) and the neurointermediate lobe of the pituitary secretes peptides in pregnancy which may cross-react with ACTH (Rees 1977).

Anderson and Walters (1976) gave dexamethasone 1 mg to four normal pregnant women (Table 12.3) to compare the result with that in a patient with Cushing's syndrome. Cortisol levels may be nonspecifically elevated because of obesity or anxiety. In nonpregnant patients, Cushing's syndrome has been confirmed by the failure of

Table 12.2 Morning and evening plasma cortisol, urinary free cortisol and plasma ACTH in pregnancy and the nonpregnant state.*

		Nonpregnant	2nd trimester	3rd trimester
Total cortisol† nmol/l	9.00 a.m. midnight	324 ± 100 103 ± 76		1029 ± 200 470 ± 124
Free cortisol† nmol/l	9.00 a.m. midnight	18 ± 9 6 ± 4		38 ± 12 17 ± 5
Urinary free cortisol† nmol/day		103 (13–256)		348 (229–680)
ACTH ng/ml		(15–70)‡	30 (20–70)§	50 (20–120)§

* Values are means ± SD or (range)
† Galvão-Teles and Burke (1973)
‡ Ratcliffe and Edwards (1971)
§ Rees and Lowry (1978).

cortisol levels to fall after small quantities (2 mg per day) of dexamethasone. Preservation of diurnal rhythm and subsequent suppression by dexamethasone 8 mg per day suggest a pituitary cause. Failure of suppression by dexamethasone 8 mg per day usually indicates an adrenal cause—adenoma or carcinoma. However, there is not sufficient experience to know if these criteria apply to patients who are pregnant. The data of Anderson and Walters (1976), shown in Table 12.3, would suggest that even normal patients do not suppress cortisol secretion so well in pregnancy with dexamethasone, but these authors understandably only used the lower dose dexamethasone suppression test giving 1 mg at midnight, since they were giving the medication to healthy controls.

A skull X-ray should be taken and visual fields checked because of the possibility of upward expansion of the pituitary tumour.

Table 12.3 Plasma cortisol—diurnal variation and response to dexamethasone, 1 mg in late pregnancy. Data of Anderson and Walters (1976).

	Control		After dexamethasone 1 mg at midnight
Normal pregnant nmol/l	8.00 a.m. 830 (560–1070)	5.00 p.m. 520 (360–600)	8.00 a.m. 450 (320–560)
Nonpregnant nmol/l	(200–770)		(100–400)

Values given are means with range in parentheses.

There have been about 30 cases reported of the association of Cushing's syndrome and pregnancy (*see* Anderson and Walters 1976 for details). A more recent case report is by Kasperlik-Zaluska *et al* (1980) who reported two pregnancies in a patient after treatment with cyproheptadine. Griffith and Ross (1981) have also reported a successful case following cyproheptadine therapy. However, it is noteworthy that one of the infants born following this therapy *in pregnancy* died three months later from gastroenteritis (Kasperlik-Zaluska *et al* 1980); this raises the possibility that this form of treatment may suppress the fetal hypothalamo–pituitary–adrenal axis, as suggested in one of the cases of Kreines and Devaux (1971). These authors (Kreines *et al* 1964) also reported marked hypoplasia of the fetal zone of the adrenal cortex in two stillborn babies born to mothers with Cushing's syndrome. Although neonatal adrenal insufficiency appears to be a risk in these circumstances, it is exceptionally rare in the neonates of patients taking therapeutic steroids in pregnancy, occurring in only 1 of 260 cases studied by Bongiovanni and MacPadden (1960) (*see* Chapter 1). Since the elevated levels of cortisol binding globulin which are present in pregnancy limit placental transfer of cortisol, the mechanism of suppression of the fetal hypothalamo–pituitary adrenal axis may be other than simple transference of glucocorticoids across the placenta. Indeed, the fetal outcome is not good in Cushing's syndrome, with a fetal loss of 10 in 25 cases (400 per 1000), where pregnancy was not interrupted (Anderson and Walters 1976). The reason for this high fetal loss rate is not known but, since there were 4 stillbirths, maternal hyperglycaemia may also be a factor (Check *et al* 1979). Certainly the fetus may be macrosomic, as in non-Cushing's diabetic pregnancy (Anderson and Walters 1976).

If Cushing's syndrome is newly diagnosed during pregnancy, particular care should be taken to exclude an adrenal cause (low ACTH levels, high cortisol not suppressed by dexamethasone). If the condition is pituitary dependent, radiotherapy (Anderson and Walters 1976) or pituitary microsurgery are the treatments of choice. Management of possible adrenal adenoma or carcinoma is very difficult in pregnancy. CT scanning of the adrenal glands for localisation and proof of the tumour cannot be used, unless it has been decided to terminate the pregnancy before viability. Ultrasound examination may be helpful. Nevertheless, if it is believed that there is an adrenal tumour, exploration should be performed whatever the gestation, because of the difficulty in distinguishing adenoma from carcinoma (Ramsey 1976).

If pregnancy does continue in the presence of Cushing's syndrome, treated or not, patients should be checked for hyperglycaemia, as in acromegaly (*see above*) and hypertension. If there is any possibility of a pituitary tumour, the visual fields should be checked regularly. The newborn infant should be carefully watched for adrenal failure.

Lactation has been discouraged (Kaperlik-Zaluska *et al* 1980) because of the possibility of permanent galactorrhoea (Anderson and Walters 1976), because of the justifiable concern that drugs such as cyproheptadine may be secreted in breast milk, and possibly because of the unjustified concern that lactation will maintain the 'Cushingoid state of pregnancy'.

HYPOPITUITARISM

The classical studies of Sheehan have shown that the pituitary gland is very vulnerable during pregnancy and the puerperium and that severe postpartum haemorrhage can cause permanent hypopituitarism by avascular necrosis (Sheehan 1937, 1939; Sheehan and Murdoch 1938). The vulnerability of the anterior pituitary during pregnancy is presumably related to its two- to threefold increase in size at this time. Several hundred cases of Sheehan's syndrome have been reported, with 39 subsequent pregnancies in 19 well documented cases reviewed by Grimes and Brooks (1980). Almost invariably it is the anterior pituitary that is affected by postpartum haemorrhage, possibly because its blood supply is via the superior hypophyseal artery, whereas the posterior pituitary and hypothalamus are supplied by the inferior hypophyseal artery and the circle of Willis (Bayliss *et al* 1980). Only two cases of diabetes insipidus following postpartum haemorrhage have been reported (Bayliss *et al* 1980; Collins *et al* 1979). Other rare causes of hypopituitarism in pregnancy are the pressure effect of pituitary tumours—either adenoma (*see above*) or craniopharyngioma (Van der Wilt *et al* 1980)—and eosinophilic granuloma, histiocytosis X or Hand–Schüller–Christian disease (Ogburn *et al* 1981). Occasionally no cause can be found (Gossain *et al* 1980). Antepartum pituitary infarction has been described in eight cases but only in insulin-dependent diabetics (Dorfman *et al* 1979). The patient develops a severe headache, usually in the third trimester, and her insulin requirements decrease markedly. She is then very liable to hypoglycaemic episodes. After delivery, she does not lactate, and has other features of hypopituitarism, most frequently lack of growth hormone and gonadotrophins.

In those cases of Sheehan's syndrome presenting during the puerperium, there is usually a history of severe postpartum haemorrhage and hypotension, followed by lack of lactation. The patients rapidly become apathetic and are often thought to be depressed in the puerperium. Subsequently, there is persistant amenorrhoea, with loss of axillary and pubic hair, and the symptoms and signs of hyperthyroidism and adrenocortical insufficiency. The diagnosis is rarely made during the puerperium, but any patient with a history of severe postpartum haemorrhage and impaired lactation should be followed for at least one year with this complication in mind. The diagnosis is confirmed by demonstrating impaired secretion by the pituitary target organs (low thyroxine and plasma cortisol, etc.) with low levels of the pituitary hormones (TSH, ACTH, FSH, LH and growth hormone) that do not rise on provocative stimulation.

The provocative tests that have been used include administration of LH- and TSH-releasing hormones. The ability of the hypothalamo–pituitary axis to secrete ACTH, growth hormone and prolactin is tested by insulin-induced hypoglycaemia. The dose of insulin is 0.1 units/kg bodyweight, or 0.05 units/kg if hypopituitarism is strongly suspected. Insulin hypoglycaemia is not without risk, since patients who are deficient in glucocorticoids, either because of adrenal or pituitary failure, can have very severe hypoglycaemic reactions. The test should not be performed unless an intravenous infusion has already been set up for the subsequent emergency administration of glucose and hydrocortisone. Occasionally metyrapone, which is a metabolic inhibitor of cortisol synthesis, may be used to test ACTH secretion by the hypothalamo–pituitary axis.

Diabetes insipidus is diagnosed by demonstrating a high urine volume with low osmolality, which is maintained as the plasma osmolality increases with water deprivation. Pituitary-dependent diabetes insipidus is reversed by giving a synthetic analogue of vasopressin, DDAVP; nephrogenic diabetes insipidus is not (*see* p. 418).

Since patients may have a wide spectrum of disease, with only one or all pituitary hormones affected, each aspect of pituitary function should be studied as far as possible. Any patient who is considered to have hypopituitarism should have an assessment of visual fields, standard tomography of the pituitary fossa and, ideally, computer-assisted tomography to exclude pituitary tumour.

Most patients with hypopituitarism become pregnant with the diagnosis already made; pregnancy without treatment is unusual. However, the condition can present in pregnancy for the first time even if, in retrospect, it is clear that the patient had some evidence of prior hypopituitarism (Grimes and Brooks 1980); this is particularly likely if the syndrome is incomplete (Satterfield and Williamson 1976; Smallridge *et al* 1980).

Most indices of pituitary function have now been tested in pregnancy in patients with hypopituitarism. Grimes and Brooks (1980) demonstrated levels of TSH that were not elevated despite subnormal thyroxine values. It is said that the pituitary is more sensitive to TRH in pregnancy than in the nonpregnant state (Burrows 1975). Low ACTH levels (Bowers and Jubiz 1974), which did not rise above 20 pg/ml (normal range 10–70 pg/ml) during antepartum haemorrhage, have also been reported (Grimes and Brooks 1980)—the assumption being that the hypothalamo–pituitary axis was unable to react to the stress of hypotension. It has been suggested that the response to metyrapone is blunted in pregnancy (Beck *et al* 1968). However, the outcome of the test was judged by a relative lack of increase in urinary steroids rather than the direct assay of ACTH. In early pregnancy, the cortisol and ACTH response to insulin hypoglycaemia (0.1 unit per kg) is similar to that in nonpregnant individuals (Kauppila *et al* 1976).

In patients with hypopituitarism diagnosed and treated before pregnancy, the outcome of pregnancy is good (Table 12.4). Where treatment is absent or inadequate the mother is at risk, and three fatalities have been reported (Israel and Conston 1952; Smallridge *et al* 1980). Apart from glucocorticoid deficiency (hypopituitarism, Addison's disease) the differential diagnosis of hypoglycaemia in pregnancy includes hypothyroidism, insulinoma (Serrano-Rios *et al* 1976), and self-administration of insulin; thyroxine and insulin levels should be measured to exclude these conditions. Other causes of hypoglycaemia such as liver failure (acute fatty liver of pregnancy, p. 308) are usually obvious. Overwhelming infection with falciparum malaria is a recently described cause of hypoglycaemia in pregnancy (White *et al* 1983).

For patients with anterior pituitary deficiency replacement therapy with hydrocortisone up to 30 mg per day, and thyroxine up to 300 μg per day should be sufficient. It may be necessary to start this therapy, particularly hydrocortisone, before a precise diagnosis is made. It is unlikely to cause any harm, and may be life-saving (Smallridge *et al* 1980). In contrast to patients with Addison's disease, these patients usually secrete

Table 12.4 Outcome of pregnancy in patients with Sheehan's syndrome.* Data from Grimes and Brooks (1980).

	Without therapy		With therapy	
Pregnancies	24		15	
Live births	13	(54%)	13	(87%)
Spontaneous abortion	10	(42%)	2	(13%)
Stillbirth	1	(4%)	0	
Maternal death	3	(12%)	0	

* The figures in parenthesis are the proportions (%) of
the total number of pregnancies in each case.

sufficient mineralocorticoid not to need fludrocortisone. Additional parenteral hydro-cortisone 100 mg 6 hourly should be given to cover the acute stress of labour and intercurrent illness. However, parenteral treatment may be necessary in more chronic conditions, such as hyperemesis. Exogenous gonadotrophin may be necessary before pregnancy to stimulate ovulation, but once the patient is pregnant, replacement gonadotrophin, oestrogen and progesterone will not be necessary because of their production by the fetoplacental unit.

Abortion is the major fetal risk in untreated hypopituitarism (Table 12.4). Stillbirth has also been reported (Schneeberg *et al* 1960). Lactation may also be impaired because of prolactin deficiency (Grimes and Brooks 1980).

DIABETES INSIPIDUS

Diabetes insipidus may also present in pregnancy when it can be a sign of tumour expansion—either pituitary adenoma (*see above*) or craniopharyngioma (Van der Wilt *et al* 1980). It may also be caused by skull trauma which has occurred in pregnancy (Phelan *et al* 1978) or be idiopathic (Hime and Richardson 1978). These latter authors have reviewed the subject and commented on 67 cases of diabetes insipidus in pregnancy in the world literature. Patients with pre-existing, isolated diabetes insipidus have no impairment in fertility and the incidence of the disease in pregnancy is about the same as in the general population: 1 in 15 000 (Hendricks 1954). Hime and Richardson (1978) found that, in 67 cases, 58% deteriorated in pregnancy, 20 per cent improved, and 15 per cent remained the same. There were inadequate data to assess the remaining 7 per cent. A number of reasons have been put forward why diabetes insipidus should deteriorate in pregnancy; the increase in glomerular filtration rate (Chapter 7) appears to be the most convincing.

Diabetes insipidus presents with excessive thirst and polyuria. After exclusion of diabetes mellitus diagnosis is made as above. However, to achieve maximum urine concentration, fluid deprivation is necessary for 22 hours (Miles *et al* 1954) which is very distressing for the patient. The synthetic analogue of vasopressin DDAVP is therefore frequently used for the primary diagnosis (Hutchon *et al* 1982). The latter group have compared the responses to DDAVP (20 μg intranasally) and 15 hour fluid deprivation. Although 15 hours' fluid deprivation was a greater stimulus to urine concentration in the nonpregnant state, DDAVP was an equally effective stimulus in pregnancy, and these authors conclude that this should be the method of choice for diagnosis of diabetes insipidus in pregnancy. The maximum urine concentration achieved in normals was about 1000 mosmol/kg. Any value over 700 mosmol/kg in the 11 hours after instillation of DDAVP should be considered normal (Huchon *et al* 1982).

A possible risk of using DDAVP late in pregnancy for the diagnosis of diabetes insipidus is premature labour, even though it has minimal oxytocic action (*see below*). Van der Wilt *et al* (1980) infused 1 μg in one patient at 36 weeks' gestation, and noted a marked increase in uterine contractility. The patient went into labour three days later.

Treatment of diabetes insipidus in pregnancy should be with DDAVP (Sack *et al* 1980; Oravec and Lichardus 1972). The drug is given as intranasal drops 10–20 μg, 2–3 times daily. Its particular advantage in pregnancy is that it has 75 times less oxytocic action than preparations of arginine vasopressin (Vavra *et al* 1968). However, Van der Wilt *et al* (1980) did find that DDAVP caused some uterine contraction when given at 36 weeks' gestation (*see above*). DDAVP is also less likely to cause abdominal pain than vasopressin which, in turn, can cause rhinitis and allergic pulmonary lesions (*BMJ* 1977). Patients with some residual pituitary function, and those with nephrogenic diabetes insipidus, have been treated with chlorpropamide (Arduino *et al* 1966). This drug increases the renal responsiveness to endogenous vasopressin, but it should not be used in pregnancy because of the risk of fetal hypoglycaemia (Chapter 10). Carbamazepine acts in a similar way (Meinders *et al* 1974), and is reasonably safe in pregnancy (Chapter 14).

Labour proceeds normally in patients with diabetes insipidus; breast feeding is usually successful (Van der Wilt *et al* 1980; Sack *et al* 1980; Ogburn *et al* 1981).

The adrenal gland

ADDISON'S DISEASE

Addison's disease is characterised by atrophy of the adrenal cortex and subsequent lack of glucocorticoid and mineralocorticoid activity. The clinical picture—of vomiting, hypotension and weakness with hyperpigmentation due to excess ACTH secretion—is well known, although less florid cases are often not diagnosed. At one time, the commonest cause was tuberculosis, with autoimmune destruction of the adrenal gland accounting for a minority of cases. The situation is now reversed.

The most comprehensive historical account of the interaction between Addison's disease and pregnancy was given by Davis and Plotz (1956). Before hormone therapy was possible, there were 18 cases reported with a maternal mortality of 77 per cent; when extracts of the adrenal cortex became available, there were 17 cases with a maternal mortality of 30 per cent. Once desoxycorticosterone could be used, the mortality dropped to 11 per cent in 34 cases. Now that we have experience of the use of full steroid replacement therapy, pregnancy should not be any risk in cases with previously diagnosed Addison's disease, and there should be no excess maternal mortality (Khunda 1972). Patients are at risk from the nausea and vomiting of early pregnancy, from labour (when they will not be able to increase their output of steroids from the adrenal glands), and during the puerperium when the physiological diuresis may cause profound hypotension. All of these complications can be treated with extra parenteral hydrocortisone, and with intravenous saline if there is any question of hypovolaemia. Labour should be managed with hydrocortisone 100 mg i.m. 6 hourly; because of the risk of hypovolaemia in the puerperium, this dose should be reduced only slowly in the first six days following delivery.

The only consistently recorded fetal complication is intrauterine growth retardation (Osler 1962). Baum and Chantler (1968) reported one case of fetal hyperinsulinism which they thought was due to fetal hypoglycaemia secondary to a temporary Addisonian state, caused by transplacental passage of maternal antibodies.

The diagnosis of Addison's disease in pregnancy is difficult, because so many of the features of Addison's disease may be associated with normal pregnancy (vomiting, syncope, weakness, hyperpigmentation). However, persistence of nausea and vomiting after 20 weeks' gestation and weight loss should be considered abnormal. The diagnosis will be made on the basis of high levels of endogenous ACTH and low plasma cortisol levels which do not rise 30 minutes after the patient is given synacthen 0.25 mg i.m. Fortunately, most patients with undiagnosed Addison's disease usually tolerate pregnancy well. The diagnosis is often made when they suffer Addisonian collapse after delivery (Brent, 1950).

Patients who are being treated with corticosteroids for other reasons such as bronchial asthma (Chapter 1) or systemic lupus erythematosus (Chapter 8) should be managed during labour or in other crises in the same way as patients with Addison's disease. They do not require increased steroid medication for the same period after delivery; 24 hours is usually sufficient.

ACUTE ADRENAL FAILURE

This is a rare complication, not necessarily associated with Addison's disease, which is said to result from thrombosis or haemorrhage in the adrenal glands. It normally follows some obstetric catastrophe, such as eclampsia or postpartum haemorrhage. The patient presents with rigors, abdominal pain, circulatory collapse and vomiting. It is almost invariably fatal. The largest review is that of Macgillivray (1951) which describes nine patients who died, all with haemorrhage in the adrenal glands. It may well be that acute adrenal failure is not a specific entity, but another manifestation of disseminated intravascular coagulation (Chapter 3).

CONGENITAL ADRENAL HYPERPLASIA

This term covers a group of inborn errors of metabolism affecting glucocorticoid and mineralocorticoid synthesis. Due to the absence or reduced levels of these hormones, the pituitary gland produces large quantities of ACTH which stimulates the adrenal gland to produce excessive quantities of alternative steroid hormones; these have virilising and hypertensive actions. For management and diagnostic purposes, the level of 17-hydroxyprogesterone is usually monitored. In 90 per cent of cases there is a deficiency of 21-hydroxylase; other causes are 11-hydroxylase, 3 beta-hydroxysteroid dehydrogenase and 17-hydroxylase deficiencies (Kaplan 1979). The condition is inherited as an autosomal recessive. If a woman has had one child with congenital adrenal hyperplasia, she has a 1 in 4 chance that subsequent pregnancies will be affected. If she, herself, has the condition and her husband is a carrier (risk 1 in 200 to 1 in 400), there is a 1 in 2 chance that her children will be affected (Burrow 1975). The condition may be diagnosed antenatally by estimation of the steroid pattern in amniotic fluid (Barson 1981) although most would not consider congenital adrenal hyperplasia an indication for termination of pregnancy.

The diagnosis is usually made in infancy, either because of the presence of ambiguous genitalia in a female child, or because the child becomes acutely ill due to hyponatraemia. Treatment is with glucocorticoid and sometimes mineralocorticoid replacement with sodium supplementation as indicated. This reduces pituitary secretion of ACTH and the subsequent formation of alternative steroid hormones. In addition, reconstructive plastic surgery may be necessary for the ambiguous female genitalia.

Effect on pregnancy

In two series (Grant *et al* 1983; Kligensmith *et al* 1978) menarche was delayed by about two years compared to normal girls. Although the incidence of regular menstruation is related to the degree with which the condition is controlled by hormone replacement therapy, this rule is not invariable, since some patients do not menstruate, despite adequate biochemical control (Grant *et al* 1983). The fertility of these patients is therefore reduced. Kligensmith *et al* (1978) found that of 14 patients who wished to become pregnant, six were unable to do so. Grant *et al* (1983) reported on 53 female patients amongst whom at least four, who wished to become pregnant, were unable to do so. However, the necessity for plastic surgery is not a bar to pregnancy. For example, Andersen *et al* (1983) studied one individual who was originally named as a boy and then, after hormone therapy and construction of an artificial vagina, had a successful pregnancy.

The outcome of pregnancy, where it has been reported, is shown in Table 12.5. Since there has only been a total of 22 pregnancies reported, it is difficult to be certain about the likely outcome of pregnancy in patients with congenital adrenal hyperplasia. However, it does not appear that these pregnancies are particularly at risk. There is no reason to believe that the steroid replacement therapy with prednisone, hydrocortisone or fludrocortisone is teratogenic (*see* Chapter 1).

Table 12.5   Outcome of pregnancy in 22 patients with congenital adrenal hyperplasia.

Normal pregnancy	Abortion	Termination	Complications	Total
8	3	2	1 premature and spastic 1 multiple congenital abnormalities	15
4		1	1 eclampsia	6
1				1
Total 13	3	3	3	22

1 Kligensmith *et al* (1978); 2 Grant *et al* (1983); 3 Andersen *et al* (1983).

Management of pregnancy

In patients who are not pregnant, the dose of steroid replacement therapy is usually based on clinical judgement, and assay of serum 17-hydroxyprogesterone; the aim being to achieve a level of 17-hydroxyprogesterone less than 10 nmol/l, without the patient becoming Cushingoid; however, if this cannot be achieved, levels of 20–40 nmol/l are probably acceptable. During pregnancy, the level of 17-hydroxyprogesterone is unreliable as an estimate of adrenal suppression, but Kligensmith *et al* (1978) did not find it necessary to change the dose of steroid replacement, and this has also been our experience (Porter & de Swiet 1983).

Some of these patients may be hypertensive, and can require antihypertensive therapy. Despite this, one of our patients developed postpartum eclampsia, but her lack of cooperation may also have contributed (Porter & de Swiet 1983).

Labour should be covered by increased and parenteral steroid medication. Our usual practice in these and all patients who may have depression of the hypothalamo–pituitary axis is to give hydrocortisone 100 mg intramuscularly 6 hourly, while the patient is in labour. This will also contain sufficient mineralocorticoid activity if the patient is also taking fludrocortisone.

There is controversy concerning the need for Caesarean section in these patients. Kligensmith *et al* (1978) reported nine Caesarean sections for disproportion, possibly due to the presence of an android pelvis caused by masculinising influence of abnormal hormone secretion. Grant *et al* (1983) reported only one Caesarean section and that for severe pre-eclampsia, but they only studied six pregnancies in four women. This is clearly an issue that requires further study.

Cushing's syndrome

This condition, which may have an adrenal cause (adenoma or carcinoma) has been considered earlier in the chapter, amongst the diseases of the pituitary gland.

References

Anderson K.J. & Walters W.A.W. (1976) Cushing's syndrome and pregnancy. *Australian and New Zealand Journal of Obstetrics and Gynaecology* **16**, 225–30.

Andersen M., Andreasen E., Jest P. & Larsen S. (1983) Successful pregnancy in a woman with severe gongenital 21-hydroxylase deficiency of the salt-loosing type. *Pediatric & Adolescent Gynecology* **1**, 47–52.

Archer D.F., Lattanzi D.R., Moore E.E., Harger J.H. & Herbert D.L. (1982) Bromocryptine treatment of women with suspected pituitary prolactin-secreting microadenomas. *American Journal of Obstetrics and Gynecology* **143**, 620–5.

Arduino F., Ferrar F.P.J. & Rodrigues J. (1966) Antidiuretic action of chlorpropromide in idiopathic diabetes insipidus. *Journal of Clinical Endocrinology and Metabolism* **26**, 1325–8.

Bayliss P.H., Milles J.J., London D.R. & Butt W.R. (1980) Post partum cranial diabetes insipidus. *British Medical Journal* **1**, 20.

Beck P., Eaton C.J., Young K. & Upperman H.S. (1968) Metyrapone response in pregnancy. *American Journal of Obstetrics and Gynecology* **100**, 327–30.

Bergh T., Nillius S.J. & Wide L. (1978) Clinical course and outcome of pregnancies in amenorrhoeic women with hyperprolactinaemia and pituitary tumours. *British Medical Journal* **1**, 875–80.

Biswas S. & Rodeck C.H. (1976) Plasma prolactin levels in pregnancy. *British Journal of Obstetrics and Gynaecology* **83**, 683–7.

Bongiovanni A.M. & McPadden A.J. (1960) Steroids during pregnancy and possible fetal consequences. *Fertility and Sterility* **11**, 181–6.

Bowers J.H. & Jubiz W. (1974) Pregnancy in a patient with hormone deficiency. *Archives of Internal Medicine* **133**, 312–14.

British Medical Journal (1977) (Editorial) Diabetes insipidus—turning off the tap. *British Medical Journal* **1**, 1050.

Burch W. (1983) A survey of results with transsphenoidal surgery in Cushing's disease. *New England Journal of Medicine* **308**, (2), 103–4.

Burrow G.N. (1975) Adrenal, pituitary and parathyroid disorders. In Burrow G.N. and Ferris T.F. (eds) *Medical Complications During Pregnancy*, p. 259. W.B. Saunders & Co., Philadelphia.

Calodney L., Eaton R.P., Black W. & Cohn F. (1973) Exacerbation of Cushing's disease during pregnancy. Report of a case. *Journal of Clinical Endocrinology and Metabolism* **36**, 81–6.

Chang R.J., Keye W.R., Young J.R., Wilson C.B. & Jaffe R.B. (1977) Detection, evaluation and treatment of pituitary microadenomas in patients with galactorrhea and amenhorrhea. *American Journal of Obstetrics and Gynecology* **128**, 356–63.

Check J.H., Caro J.F., Kendall B., Peris L.A. & Wellenbach B.L. (1979) Cushing's syndrome in pregnancy: Effect of associated diabetes on fetal and neonatal complications. *American Journal of Obstetrics and Gynecology* **133**, 846.

Child D.F., Gordon H., Mashiter K. & Joplin G.F. (1975) Pregnancy, prolactin and pituitary tumours. *British Medical Journal* **2**, 87–9.

Ch'ng J.L., Rosenstock J., Mashiter K. & Joplin G.F. (1983) Pregnancy in untreated hyperprolactinaemic women. *Journal of Obstetrics and Gynaecology* **3**, 258–61.

Collins M.L., O'Brien P. & Cline A. (1979) Diabetes insipidus following obstetric shock. *Obstetrics and Gynaecology* (Suppl.) **53**, 16–17S.

Costello R.T. (1936) Subclinical adenoma of the pituitary gland. *American Journal of Pathology* **12**, 205–15.

Cowden E.A. & Thomson J.A. (1979) Resolution of hyperprolactinaemia after bromocriptine-induced pregnancy. *Lancet* **1**, 613.

Cowden E.A., Thomson J.A., Doyle D., Ratcliffe J.G., MacPherson P. & Teasdale G. (1979) Tests of prolactin secretion in diagnosis of prolactinomas. *Lancet* **1**, 1156–8.

Doe R.P., Fernandez R. & Seal U.S. (1964) Measurement of corticosteroid-binding globulin in man. *Journal of Clinical Endocrinology and Metabolism* **24**, 1029–39.

Dommerholt H.B.R. & Assies J. Van Der Werf (1981) Growth of a prolactinoma during pregnancy. Case report and review. *British Journal of Obstetrics and Gynaecology* **88**, 62–70.

Dorfman S.G., Dillaplain R.P. & Gambrell R.D. (1979) Ante partum pituitary infarction. *Obstetrics and Gynaecology* (Suppl.) **53**, 21–4S.

Doyle F. & McLachlan M. (1977) Radiological aspects of pituitary-hypothalamic disease. *Clinics in Endocrinology and Metabolism* **6**, 53–81.

Eastman R.C., Gorden P. & Roth J. (1979) Conventional supervoltage irradiation is an effective treatment for acromegaly. *Journal of Clinical Endocrinology & Metabolism* **48**, 931–40.

Lancet editorial (1980) Hyperprolactinaemia: Pituitary tumour or not? *Lancet* **1**, 517–19.

Fisch R.O., Prem K.A., Feinberg S.B. & Gehrz R.C. (1974) Acromegaly in a gravida and her infant. *Obstetrics and Gynecology* **43**, 861–5.

Franks S., Jacobs H.S., Hull M.G.R., Steele S.J. & Nabarro J.D.N. (1977) Management of hyperprolactinaemic amenorrhoea. *British Journal of Obstetrics and Gynaecology* **84**, 241–53.

Franks S., Jacobs H.S. & Nabarro J.D.N. (1975a) Studies of prolactin in pituitary disease. *Journal of Endocrinology* **67**, 55P.

Franks S., Murray M.A.F., Jequier A.M., Steele S.J., Nabarro J.O.N. & Jacobs H.S. (1975b) Incidence and significance of hyper-prolactinaemia in women with amenorrhoea. *Clinical Endocrinology* **4**, 597–607.

Galvão-Teles A. & Burke C.W. (1973) Cortisol levels in toxaemic and normal pregnancy. *Lancet* **1**, 737–40.

Gemzell C. (1975) Induction of ovulation in infertile women with pituitary adenoma. *American Journal of Obstetrics and Gynecology* **121**, 311–15.

Gemzell C. & Wang C.F. (1979) Outcome of pregnancy in women with pituitary adenoma. *Fertility and Sterility* **31**, 363–72.

Gomez F., Reyes F.I. & Faiman C. (1977) Nonpuerperal galactorrhea and hyperprolactinemia. Clinical findings, endocrine features and therapeutic responses in 56 cases. *American Journal of Medicine* **62**, 648–60.

Gordon G. & Bradford W.P. (1970) Pregnancy in patient with diabetes insipidus following induction of ovulation with clomiphene. *Journal of Obstetrics and Gynaecology of the British Commonwealth* **77**, 467–9.

Gossain V.V., Rhodes C.E. & Rovner D.R. (1980) Pregnancy in hypothalamic hypopituitarism. *Obstetrics and Gynecology* **56**, 762–6.

Grant D., Muram D. & Dewhurst C. J. (1983) Menstrual and fertility patterns in patients with congenital adrenal hyperplasia. *Pediatric & Adolescent Gynecology* **1**, 97–103.

Griffith D.N. & Ross E.J. (1981) Pregnancy after cyproheptadine treatment for Cushing's disease. *New England Journal of Medicine* **305**, 893–4.

Griffith R.A., Turkalj I. & Braun P. (1979) Pituitary tumours during pregnancy in mothers treated with bromocriptine. *British Journal of Clinical Pharmacology* **7**, 393–6.

Grimes H.G. & Brooks M.H. (1980) Pregnancy in Sheehan's Syndrome. Report of a case and review. *Obstetrical and Gynaecological Survey* **35**, 481–8.

Hancock K.W., Scott J.S., Lamb J.T., Myles Gibson R. & Chapman C. (1980) Conservative management of pituitary prolactinomas: evidence of bromocriptine-induced regression. *British Journal of Obstetrics and Gynaecology* **87**, 523–9.

Hardy J., Beauregard H. & Robert F. (1978) Prolactin-secreting pituitary adenomas: transphenoidal microsurgical treatment. In Rolyn C. and Harter M. (eds) *Progress in Prolactin Physiology and Pathology*, pp. 361–70. Amsterdam: Elsevier/North-Holland Biomedical Press.

Harris J.R. & Levene M.B. (1976) Visual complications following irradiation for pituitary adenomas and craniopharyngiomas. *Radiology* **120**, 167–71.

Hendricks C.H. (1954) The neurohypophysis in pregnancy. *Obstetrical and Gynecological Surgery* **9**, 323–41.

Hime M.C. & Richardson J.A. (1978) Diabetes insipidus and pregnancy. A case report, incidence and review of literature. *Obstetric and Gynecological Survey* **33**, 375–9.

Hutchon D.J.R., Van Zijl J.A.W.M., Campbell-Brown B.M. & McFadyen I.R. (1982) Desmopressin as a test of urinary concentrating ability in pregnancy. *Journal of Obstetrics and Gynaecology* **2**, 206–9.

Hytten F.E. & Lind T. (1973) *Diagnostic Indices in Pregnancy.* Documenta Geigy, Basle.

Israel S.L. & Conston A.S. (1952) Unrecognised pituitary necrosis (Sheehan's Syndrome). A cause of sudden death. *Journal of the American Medical Association* **148**, 189–93.

Jacobs H.S., Franks S., Murray M.A.F., Hull M.G.R., Steele S.J. & Nabarro J.O.N. (1976) Clinical and endocrine features of hyperprolactinaemic amenorrhoea. *Clinical Endocrinology* **5**, 439–54.

Jacobs H.S. (1980) Hypothalamus and pituitary gland. In Hytten F. and Chamberlain G.V.P. (eds) *Clinical Physiology in Obstetrics.* Blackwell Scientific Publications, Oxford.

Jeffcoate S.L. (1978) Diagnosis of hyperprolactinaemia. *Lancet* **2**, 1245–7.

Jewelwicz R. & Van de Wiele R.L. (1980) Clinical course and outcome of pregnancy in twenty-five patients with pituitary microadenomas. *American Journal of Obstetrics and Gynecology* **136**, 339–43.

Jewelewicz R., Zimmerman E.A. & Carmel P.W. (1977) Conservative management of a pituitary tumour during pregnancy following induction of ovulation with gonadotrophins. *Fertility and Sterility* **28**, 35–40.

Jung R.T., White M.C., Bowley N.B., Bydder G., Mashiter K. & Joplin G.F. (1982) CT abnormalities of the pituitary in hyperprolactinaemic women with normal or equivocal sellae radiologically. *British Medical Journal* **285**, 1078–81.

Kajtar T. & Tomkin G.H. (1971) Emergency hypophysectomy in pregnancy after induction of ovulation. *British Medical Journal* **4**, 88–90.

Kaplan S.A. (1979) Diseases of the adrenal cortex. *Pediatric Clinics of North America* **26**, 77.

Kasperlik-Załuska A., Migdalska B., Hartwig W., Wilczyńska J., Marianowski L., Stopińska-Gluszak U. & Łozińska D. (1980) Two pregnancies in a woman with Cushing's Syndrome treated with cyproheptadine. Case report. *British Journal of Obstetrics and Gynaecology* **87**, 1171–3.

Kauppila A., Ylikorkalma O., Järvinen P.A. & Haapalahti J. (1976) The function of the anterior pituitary-adrenal cortex axis in hyperemesis gravidarum. *British Journal of Obstetrics and Gynaecology* **83**, 11–16.

Kelly W.F., Doyle F.H., Mashiter K., Banks L.M., Gordon H. & Joplin G.F. (1979) Pregnancies in women with hyperprolactinaemia: clinical course and obstetric complications of 41 pregnancies in 27 women. *British Journal of Obstetrics and Gynaecology* **86**, 698–705.

Kelly W. & Joplin G.F. (1978) Hyperprolactinaemia and pituitary tumours. *British Medical Journal* **1**, 1050–1.

Kelly W.F., Mashiter K., Doyle F.H., Banks L.M. & Joplin G.F. (1978) Treatment of prolactin secreting pituitary tumours in young women by needle implantation of radioactive yittrium. *Quarterly Journal of Medicine* **47**, 473–93.

King K.C., Adam P.A.J., Schwartz R. & Teramo K. (1971) Human placental transfer of human growth hormone I-125. *Pediatrics* **48**, 534–9.

Kleinberg D.L., Noel G.L. & Frantz A.G. (1977) Galactorrhea: a study of 235 cases including 48 with pituitary tumours. *New England Journal of Medicine* **296**, 589–600.

Klingensmith G.J., Jones H.W. & Blizzard R.M. (1977) Glucocorticoid treatment of girls with congenital adrenal hyperplasia. Effects on height, sexual maturation and fertility. *Journal of Pediatrics* **90**, 996.

Kreiger D.T., Amorosa L. & Linick F. (1975) Cyproheptadine-induced remission of Cushing's disease. *New England Journal of Medicine* **293**, 893–6.

Kreines K. & Devaux W.D. (1971) Neonatal adrenal insufficiency associated with maternal Cushing's syndrome. *Pediatrics* **47**, 516–19.

Kreines K., Perin E. & Salzer R. (1964) Pregnancy in Cushing's Syndrome. *Journal of Clinical Endocrinology and Metabolism* **24**, 75.

Lamberts S.W.J., Klijen J.G.M., de Lange S.A., Singh R., Stefanilo S.Z. & Birkenhäger J.C. (1979) The incidence of complications during pregnancy after treatment of hyperprolactinaemia with bromocriptine in patients with radiologically evident pituitary tumours. *Fertility & Sterility* **31**, 614–9.

Lamberts S.W.J., Seldenlath H.J., Kwa H.G. & Birkenhäger J.C. (1977) Transient bitemporal hemianopia during pregnancy after treatment of galactorrhea-amenhorrhea syndrome with bromocriptine. *Journal of Clinical Endocrinology and Metabolism* **44**, 180–4.

Lawrence A.M., Goldfine I.D. & Kirsteins L. (1970) Growth hormone dynamics in acromegaly. *Journal of Clinical Endocrinology and Metabolism* **31**, 239–47.

Llewellyn-Jones D. (1969) *Fundamentals of Obstetrics and Gynaecology*, p. 157. Faber & Faber Ltd., London.

Lloyd G.M., Meares J.D. & Jacob J. (1975) Effects of oestrogen and bromocriptine on in vivo secretion and mitosis in prolactin cells. *Nature* **255**, 497 8.

McGregor A.M., Scanlon M.F., Hall R. & Hall K. (1979) Effects of bromocriptine on pituitary tumor size. *British Medical Journal* **2**, 700–3.

McNeilly A.S. (1974) Prolactin and human reproduction. *British Journal of Hospital Medicine* **12**, 57–62.

Meinders A.E., Cejka V. & Robertson G.L. (1974) The antidiuretic action of carbamazepine in man. *Clinical Science* **47**, 289–99.

Miles B.E., Paton A. & de Wardener H.E. (1954) Maximum urine concentration. *British Medical Journal* **2**, 901–4.

Mills R.P., Harris A.B., Heinrichs L. & Burry K.A. (1979) Pituitary tumor made symptomatic during hormone therapy and induced pregnancy. *Annals of Opthalmalogy* **11**, 1672–6.

Ogburn P.L., Cefalo R.C., Nagel T. & Okagaki T. (1981) Histiocytosis X and pregnancy. *Obstetrics and Gynecology* **58**, 513–51.

O'Herlihy C. (1980) Pregnancy in an acromegalic after bromocriptine therapy. *Irish Journal of Medical Science* **149**, 281–2.

Oravec D. & Lichardus B. (1972) Management of diabetes insipidus in pregnancy. *British Medical Journal* **4**, 114–15.

Phelan J.P., Guay A.T. & Newman C. (1978) Diabetes insipidus in pregnancy. *American Journal of Obstetrics and Gynecology* **130**, 365–6.

Polishuk W.Z., Palti Z., Rabau E., Lunenfeld B. & David A. (1965) Pregnancy in a case of Sheehan's Syndrome following treatment with human gonadotropins. *Journal of Obstetrics and Gynaecology of the British Commonwealth* **72**, 778–80.

Porter R.J. & de Swiet M. (1983) Pregnancy in a patient with congenital adrenal hyperplasia. *Pediatric & Adolescent Gynecology* **1**, 39–45.

Ramsay I. (1976) Thyroid and adrenal disease in pregnancy. *British Journal of Hospital Medicine* **15**, 373–80.

Rees L.H., Burke C.W., Chard T., Evans S.W. & Letchworth A.T. (1975) Possible placental origin of ACTH in normal pregnancy. *Nature* **254**, 620–2.

Rees L.H. & Lowry P.J. (1978) ACTH and related peptides. In James V.H.T., Serio M., Guisli G. and

Martini L. (eds) *Endocrine Function of the Human Adrenal Cortex*, p. 33. Academic Press, London.

Rigg L.A., Lein A. & Yen S.S.C. (1977) Pattern of increase in circulating prolactin levels during human gestation. *American Journal of Obstetrics and Gynecology* **129**, 454–6.

Rimoin D.L., Holzman G.B. Merimee T.J., Rabinowitz D., Barnes A.C., Tyson J.E.A. & McKusick V.A. (1968) Lactation in the absence of human growth hormone. *Journal of Clinical Endocrinology and Metabolism* **28**, 1183–8.

Ross E.J. & Linch D.C. (1983) Cushing's Syndrome—killing disease: discriminatory value of signs and symptoms during early diagnosis. *Lancet* **2**, 646–9.

Sack J., Friedman E., Katznelson D. & Frenkel Y. (1980) Long-term treatment of diabetes insipidus with a synthetic analog of vasopressin during pregnancy. *Israel Journal of Medical Science* **16**, 406–7.

Satterfield R.G. & Williamson H.O. (1976) Isolated ACTH deficiency and pregnancy. *Obstetrics and Gynecology* **48**, 693–6.

Schneeberg N.G., Perloff W.H. & Israel S.L. (1960) Incidence of unsuspected Sheehan's Syndrome. Hypopituitarism after post partum haemorrhage and/or shock—Clinical and laboratory study. *Journal of American Medical Association* **172**, 20–7.

Serrano-Rios M., Cifuentes I., Prieto J.C., De Oya M., Navarro V. & Makin G. (1976) Insulinoma in a pregnant woman. *Obstetrics and Gynecology* **47**, 361–4.

Shearman R.P. & Fraser K. (1977) Impact of the new diagnostic methods on the differential diagnosis and treatment of secondary amenorrhoea. *Lancet* **1**, 1195–7.

Sheehan H.L. (1937) Postpartum necrosis of the anterior pituitary. *Journal of Pathology and Bacteriology* **45**, 189–214.

Sheehan H.L. (1939) Simmond's disease due to post partum necrosis of anterior pituitary. *Quarterly Journal of Medicine* **8**, 277–309.

Sheehan H.L. & Murdoch R. (1938a) Postpartum necrosis of the anterior pituitary; pathological and clinical aspects. *Journal of Obstetrics and Gynaecology of the British Empire* **45**, 456–89.

Sheehan H.L. & Murdoch R. (1938b) Postpartum necrosis of the anterior pituitary. Effect of subsequent pregnancy. *Lancet* **2**, 123–5.

Smallridge R.C., Corrigan D.F., Thomason A.M. & Blue P.W. (1980) Hypoglycemia in Pregnancy. *Archives of Internal Medicine* **140**, 564–5.

Swanson H.A. & Du Boulay G. (1975) Borderline variations of the normal pituitary fossa. *British Journal of Radiology* **48**, 366–9.

Thorner M.O., Besser G.M., Jones A., Dacie J. & Jones A.E. (1975) Bromocriptine treatment of female infertility: report of 13 pregnancies. *British Medical Journal* **4**, 694–7.

Thorner M.O., Edwards C.R.W., Charlesworth M., Dacie J.E., Moult P.J.A., Rees L.H., Jones A.E. & Besser G.M. (1979) Pregnancy in patients presenting with hyperprolactinaemia. *British Medical Journal* **2**, 771–4.

Tyrell J.B., Brooks R.M., Fitzgerald P.A., Cofoid P.B., Forsham P.H. & Wilson P.B. (1978) Cushing's disease: selective trans-sphenoidal resection of pituitary microadenomas. *New England Journal of Medicine* **298**, 753–8.

Tyson J.E., Hwang P., Guyda H. & Friesen H.G. (1972) Studies of prolactin secretion in human pregnancy. *American Journal of Obstetrics and Gynecology* **113**, 14–20.

Van der Wilt B., Drayer J.I.M. & Eskes T.A.B. (1980) Diabetes insipidus in pregnancy as a first sign of a craniopharyngioma. *European Journal of Obstetrics, Gynecology and Reproductive Biology*. **10**, 269–74.

Vávra I., Machová A., Holeček V., Cort J.H., Zaoral M. & Šorm F. (1968) Effects of a synthetic analogue of vasopressin in animals and in patients with diabetes insipidus. *Lancet* **1**, 948–52.

Wass J.A.H., Moult P.J.A., Thorner M.O., Dacie J.E., Charlesworth M., Jones A.E. & Besser G.

(1979) Reduction of pituitary-tumour size in patients with prolactinomas and acromegaly treated with bromocriptine with or without radiotherapy. *Lancet* **2**, 66–9.

Wass J.A.H., Thorner M.O., Morris D.V., Rees L.H., Mason A.S., Jones A.E. & Besser G.M. (1977) Long term treatment of acromegaly with bromocriptine. *British Medical Journal* **1**, 875–8.

Werder K.V., Fahlbusch R., Landgraf R., Pickardt C.G., Rjosk H.K. & Scriba P.C. (1978) Treatment of patients with prolactinomas. *Endocrinological Investigation* **1**, 47–58.

White M.C., Anapliotu M., Rosenstock J., Mashiter K. & Joplin G.F. (1981) Heterogenity of prolactin responses to oestradiol benzoate in women with prolactinomas. *Lancet* **1**, 1394–6.

White N.J., Warrell D.A., Pornthep Chanthavanich M.D. *et al* (1983) Severe hypoglycaemia and hyperinsulinemia in falciparum malaria. *New England Journal of Medicine* **309**, 61–6.

Whittaker P.G., Wilcox T. & Lind T. (1982) The effect of stress upon serum prolactin concentrations in pregnant and non-pregnant women. *Journal of Obstetrics and Gynaecology* **2**, 149–52.

Wilson C.B. & Dempsey L.C. (1978) Transsphenoidal removal of 250 pituitary adenomas. *Journal of Neurosurgery* **48**, 13–22.

Yen S.S.C., Samaan N. & Pearson H. (1967) Growth hormone levels in pregnancy. *Journal of Clinical Endocrinology and Metabolism* **27**, 1341–47.

Zarate A., Canales E.S., Alger M. & Forsbach G. (1979) The effect of pregnancy and lactation on pituitary prolactin-secreting tumours. *Acta Endocrinalogica* **92**, 407–12.

Zervas N.T. & Martin J.B. (1980) Management of Hormone-secreting pituitary adenomas. *New England Journal of Medicine* **302**, 210–14.

13 Bone Disease, Disease of the Parathyroid Glands and some other Metabolic Disorders

Barry Walters*

The association of pregnancy with bone disease is by no means common in the Western world. Nevertheless, there are very real changes in bone physiology and calcium and phosphate homeostasis in pregnancy. An understanding of these changes and their derangements is necessary for a full appreciation of the problems that occur from time to time in pregnancy. This chapter is devoted firstly to a consideration of normal physiology in the nongravid state, secondly to the changes seen in pregnancy, and thirdly to the relevant clinical problems that may be seen.

Bone structure and function

The skeletal framework of the body is in a state of constant metabolic activity. Simultaneous processes of new bone formation and dissolution of older osteons achieve remodelling of individual bones in response to the changing needs of the organism. Further, bone acts as the major repository for calcium and phosphate in the body. Regulation of these ions is effected largely through changes in bone mediated by certain hormones.

Bone as a tissue is composed of cells, organic matrix and mineral. Osteoblasts synthesise and mineralise bone. Osteocytes are osteoblasts incorporated into the bony

* The author is the recipient of the P. F. Sobotka Postgraduate Scholarship of the University of Western Australia.

matrix they have secreted. The osteoclast, probably of macrophage origin, appears as a multinucleate cell responsible for bone resorption.

After epiphyseal closure, the cellular activities of the skeleton are confined to repair and remodelling. Remodelling begins when osteoblasts and osteoclasts appear at a focus on the bone's surface. The osteoclasts dissolve bone, leaving a bay (Howship's lacuna), into which the osteoblasts nestle and deposit new bone matrix, which later undergoes mineralisation. This organic matrix (osteoid) is 90–95 per cent collagen, but also contains mucopolysaccharides and lipids. Mineralisation seems to be part of the function of the osteoblast. It involves the deposition of calcium and phosphorous as amorphous salts. Over days, these assume a more crystalline structure resembling hydroxyapatite, $Ca_{10}(PO_4)_6(OH)_2$, the dominant mineral found in mature bone. The majority of the mineral phase is accomodated in spaces interspersed throughout the collagen fibrils.

Osteoblasts are rich in alkaline phosphatase. Its serum level rises when their activity increases as in conditions of rapid bone turnover. It is possible that alkaline phosphatase locally inactivates inhibitors of precipitation (such as inorganic pyrophosphate) resulting in formation of crystals.

Calcium and phosphate

The total body calcium content is 25–30 moles (1000–1500 g) and 99 per cent of this is incorporated in bone crystals. This pool is in equilibrium with the extracellular fluid calcium. Total exchange of the ions of extracellular fluid occurs several times daily. Bone deposition and resorption, which also contribute to calcium economy, proceed much more slowly.

The daily dietary intake of calcium averages 25 mmol (1 g) and faecal excretion accounts for the unabsorbed moiety of this (19 mmol). Absorption occurs in the proximal small intestine by active transport. Further modification of circulating calcium levels is effected in the kidney by adjustments in tubular reabsorption and, under normal circumstances, 98 per cent of filtered calcium is reabsorbed proximally.

Total serum calcium includes protein bound (45 per cent) and free ionised fractions. A small amount is present as diffusible complexes. Binding is largely to albumin and variations in its concentration will lead to misinterpretation of effective calcium concentration unless corrective calculations are performed, since the biological activity of calcium relates to its free ionised concentration.

The normal total serum calcium in the nonpregnant state, after correction for albumin concentration, is 2.25–2.65 mmol/l. The normal ionised calcium is 1.1–1.4 mmol/l. Many clinical laboratories can now measure ionised calcium directly. If ionised calcium cannot be measured directly, it can be derived from the total serum calcium, albumin and globulin concentrations by the following formula:

% protein bound $= 0.8 \times$ albumin (g/l) $+ 0.2 \times$ globulin (g/l) $+ 3$
% ionised $= 100 - \%$ protein bound

Of the total body phosphorous, 85 per cent is in the skeleton and the remainder is found inside cells throughout the body. One-third of the plasma phosphorus is present as inorganic phosphate (0.8–1.4 mmol/litre) whilst two-thirds is in phospholipid form. In contrast to calcium, about 88 per cent of inorganic phosphate is free and not protein bound. Phosphate concentration is very labile and alters from hour to hour. After eating, plasma phosphate falls because phosphate enters the cells with glucose. For these reasons, samples for phosphate estimation should be taken with the patient fasting in the early morning.

Phosphate is abundant in normal foods. Its absorption is very efficient. For this reason, dietary privation, short of actual starvation, does not lead to deficiency. However, non-absorbable antacids, if taken in large amounts, can interfere with phosphate absorption by binding it in the gut lumen. Under normal circumstances, the normal daily requirement of 40 mmol is easily satisfied by gastrointestinal absorption.

The kidney is the major regulator of phosphate balance. After glomerular filtration, 80–90 per cent of phosphate is reabsorbed in the proximal convoluted tubule. A rise in plasma phosphate is countered by increased renal excretion. Parathyroid hormone (PTH) achieves this by inhibiting tubular phosphate reabsorption. Bone uptake and release of phosphate also contribute to homeostasis, but the renal mechanism predominates.

Hormonal regulation of calcium, phosphate and bone

The functions of bone, kidney and gut in calcium and phosphate homeostasis are regulated by hormones. These are chiefly PTH and vitamin D although thyroid and adrenal hormones, as well as glucagon, growth hormone and the sex steroids also have influence. The place of calcitonin in this system has not been fully characterised.

VITAMIN D

The healing effect of ultraviolet light on rachitic bone lesions was recognised in 1919. Soon after, it was demonstrated that sunlight activates a sterol in the skin to become the antirachitic agent. This is the photochemical conversion of 7-dehydrocholesterol to cholecalciferol or vitamin D3 (Fig. 13.1). To a lesser extent, the diet contributes to the body stores of vitamin D but about 90 per cent of circulating vitamin D is skin-derived (Arnaud *et al* 1977a). Natural dietary sources include fish oils, eggs, butter and liver and these yield both vitamin D3 and vitamin D2 (ergocalciferol). Absorption from the proximal small intestine is aided by bile salts as for the other fat soluble vitamins. Vitamin D is transported bound to a plasma globulin to the liver. Its first metabolic activation step yields 25-hydroxycholecalciferol (25 OHD)—the dominant circulating form of the vitamin. The same transport protein conveys 25 OHD to the kidney, the only known site of the 1-alpha hydroxylase enzyme (though there may be extrarenal sites in pregnancy (Gray *et al* 1979; Weissman *et al* 1979). Hydroxylation at either the C_1 or C_{24} position takes place in cells of the proximal convoluted tubule producing 1-alpha 25-dihydroxycholecalciferol and 24,25-dihydroxycholecalciferol (1,25 OHD and 24,25 OHD).

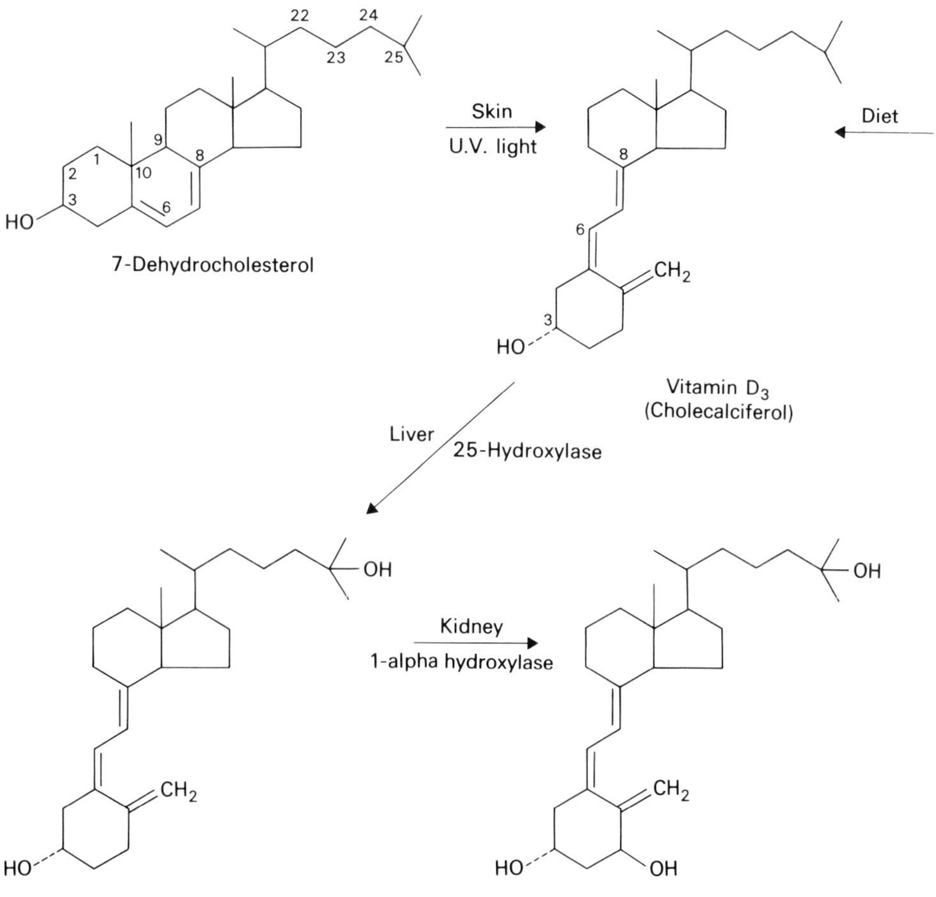

Fig. 13.1 Metabolic activation of vitamin D to 1,25-OHD. In addition the kidney also synthesizes 24,25-OHD, but its function is uncertain.

The biological importance of 24,25 OHD is not settled. It may have a role in bone mineralisation (Goodwin *et al* 1978) as its synthesis is favoured by hypercalcaemia, which inhibits 1,25 OHD formation. The reverse situation pertains when serum calcium is low (Boyle *et al* 1971). However, 1,25 OHD clearly has a very significant role and is the most potent vitamin D metabolite. Its serum concentration (30–40 pg/ml) is a thousand times less than that of 25 OHD (20–30 ng/ml) but, in its absence, the complete syndrome of vitamin D deficiency develops. As it is synthesised in the kidney yet exerts its chief effects elsewhere after circulation in the blood stream, it can correctly be regarded as a hormone. There are several other vitamin D metabolites of weaker activity which will not be considered here.

The prime function of 1,25 OHD is to sustain plasma levels of calcium and phosphate. This permits normal mineralisation of newly forming bone. It acts on at least three target organs: gut, bone and kidney (Fig. 13.2). In the small intestine it induces synthesis of brush border proteins which bind calcium and phosphate, promoting their active transport from lumen to blood stream. In the absence of vitamin D, gut absorption of these ions virtually ceases.

Its action in the kidney is of uncertain nature and significance. By a direct action on the proximal convoluted tubule, calcium and phosphate reabsorption are probably enhanced. However, even in the absence of vitamin D, 99 per cent of all calcium filtered at the glomerulus can still be reabsorbed. In X-linked familial hypophosphataemia, where the tubule does not respond to vitamin D, phosphate is lost in the urine and rickets results.

Although vitamin D clearly has major effects on the skeleton, its action is complex. The various metabolites have disparate effects and no explanation is yet available to integrate them all. 1,25 OHD is a potent direct stimulator of bone resorption (Holtrop *et al* 1981; Raisz *et al* 1972), but the physiological effect of this is not established. Vitamin D also is essential for normal growth and mineralisation of the skeleton. Whether it has a direct growth-promoting action or acts only indirectly by providing the optimum milieu for bone growth is not certain.

Hypocalcaemia, by stimulating PTH secretion, activates renal 1-alpha-hydroxylase. This increases production of 1,25 OHD resulting in enhanced gut calcium absorption. Hypophosphataemia also stimulates 1,25 OHD synthesis (but without the

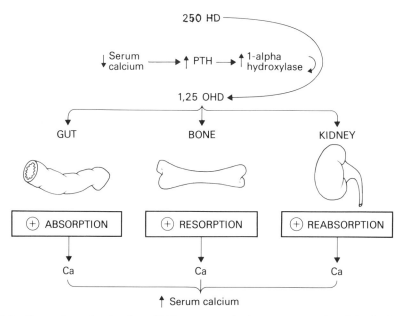

Fig. 13.2 Hypocalcaemia stimulates PTH secretion which activates renal 1-alpha-hydroxylase. Increased production of 1,25-OHD raises serum calcium by effects on gut, bone and kidney. + Stimulant effect.

mediation of PTH). This causes a fall in phosphate excretion. It appears that the gonadal steroids, growth hormone, human placental lactogen and prolactin as well as PTH and phosphate deficiency have the capacity to stimulate 1-alpha-hydroxylase (Spanos *et al* 1976; Brown *et al* 1980).

PARATHYROID HORMONE

PTH is the second major hormone influencing calcium balance and bone. Its effects are mediated by intracellular cyclic AMP and its physiological function is to sustain, within narrow limits, extracellular fluid calcium concentration. Any fall in ionised calcium is countered by secretion of PTH. The fall in calcium is checked by the direct effects of PTH on bone and kidney, and its indirect stimulation of calcium absorption by gut mediated by 1,25 OHD.

In bone, PTH stimulates the activity of osteoclasts and osteoblasts causing bone resorption with calcium and phosphate mobilisation. As it stimulates secretion of osteoclast collagenases and similar lytic enzymes, it acts to accomplish metabolic destruction of the bony matrix. This is reflected in increased urinary and plasma hydroxyproline. In general, remodelling activity is stimulated, but osteoclast function predominates. However, the action of PTH on bone is more complex than this and not yet fully elucidated.

In the kidney, PTH acts firstly to inhibit phosphate reabsorption by the proximal tubule. Phosphate released from bone is thereby rapidly excreted with resulting hypophosphataemia and hyperphosphaturia in states of PTH excess. By a different mechanism, probably operating distally in the tubule, PTH tends to increase calcium reabsorption. Nevertheless, the flood of calcium from bone exceeds the capacity for calcium reabsorption so that hypercalciuria ensues. PTH also inhibits proximal tubular reabsorption of bicarbonate so that states of PTH excess are often accompanied by a mild metabolic acidosis.

CALCITONIN

In the absence of thyroid and parathyroid glands, the response to a calcium load is blunted and the return to normocalcaemia delayed. This observation led to a search for a hypocalcaemic factor, the hormone calcitonin, secreted by the parafollicular C cells of the thyroid. Its output is stimulated by a rise in ionised calcium concentration but also by the gut hormones gastrin and cholecystokinin. Hypocalcaemia has the opposite effect. The effect of calcitonin in lowering serum calcium is accompanied by a fall in serum phosphate and both probably result from a direct inhibition of bone breakdown. Also calcitonin inhibits the bone resorption produced by a number of substances, including PTH and vitamin D metabolites. The place of calcitonin in the complex system of calcium balance is not yet certain. In medullary carcinoma of the thyroid, where there is hypersecretion of this hormone, there are no overt bony changes and no disturbance of calcium or phosphate levels. An intriguing observation has been that of osteopetrosis in the newborn babies of women with medullary carcinoma, but this may represent genetic linkage of two disorders rather than causation (Verdy *et al* 1971).

Changes in bone, calcium and phosphate homeostasis during pregnancy

Pregnancy is a time of increased demand on maternal calcium stores. The fetus is known to accumulate nearly 30 g of calcium and half as much phosphorus in its own tissues (Hytten and Leitch 1971) and all of this must be maternally derived. Seventy per cent of the calcium accumulation occurs in the third trimester when fetal skeletal growth is maximal. Without an anticipatory rise in calcium absorption, the necessary calcium would be drawn from the maternal skeleton. Furthermore, lactation continues the calcium demand. Human milk contains 6–9 mmol/l of calcium (2–3 times the maternal serum level) and the intake of a normal 3 kg infant is 1–1.5 l/week, increasing with age. In addition, as well as protection of the maternal skeleton from resorption, there may even be a need for increased bone deposition. This would provide the added structural support made necessary by the increased bodyweight of pregnancy. What then are the physiological changes which have evolved in pregnancy and how are they achieved?

Early in pregnancy gut absorption of calcium increases. It has doubled by the beginning of the third trimester and remains elevated in the puerperium during lactation (Heaney and Skillman 1971; Shenolikar 1970). Calcium is progressively retained throughout the course of pregnancy and maternal bone accretion accounts for that proportion not absorbed by the fetus. Urinary loss of calcium rises early and then falls to normal levels near term but the net effect is of permanent incorporation of calcium into mother and fetus.

The explanation for the enhanced calcium absorption may lie in the steady rise in plasma 1,25 OHD that occurs throughout pregnancy (Kumar *et al* 1979; Whitehead *et al* 1981) (Fig. 13.3). After delivery in the lactating mother, the level falls, but remains higher than in nongravid women (Kumar *et al* 1979; Lund and Selnes 1979). The newborn infant is born with a low 1,25 OHD concentration which, by 24 hours of age,

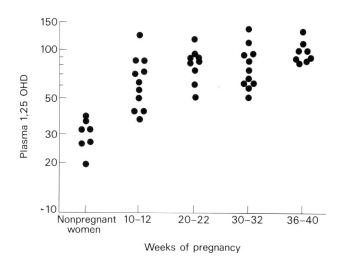

Fig. 13.3 Plasma 1,25 dihydroxyvitamin D concentrations in control women and during pregnancy. (After Whitehead *et al* 1981.) Units are ng/l.

equals normal adult levels (Steichen *et al* 1980). This can be seen as an adaptive response by the baby to the new need to absorb calcium across the gut lumen.

What accounts for the stimulation of maternal 1-alpha hydroxylase activity? It is tempting to postulate that the initial stimulus is a slight fall in ionised calcium which causes PTH release, thus stimulating the enzyme. But PTH is an unlikely candidate. Whether it rises in pregnancy (Cushard *et al* 1972; Pitkin *et al* 1979) or is unchanged (Whitehead *et al* 1981), is disputed. Moreover, the timing of the demonstrated rise in PTH does not coincide with the onset of enhanced calcium absorption. After delivery, 1,25-OHD falls rapidly whilst PTH levels decline slowly to normal levels (Lund and Selnes 1979).

Whether PTH levels rise or not, there is no need to invoke PTH as the sole cause of enhanced calcium absorption, because there are several other stimulators of renal 1-alpha hydroxylase activity (*see* above). Oestrogens are known to do this, at least in postmenopausal osteoporotic women (Gallagher *et al* 1978; Nordin *et al* 1980) and egg-laying birds (Castillo *et al* 1979). The stimulatory effect in the bird is fortified by the presence of progesterone (Tanaka *et al* 1978). Both these hormones, of course, are high in pregnancy, but fall promptly after delivery. Prolactin or hPL may be involved, or even growth hormone (Brown *et al* 1980) which bears structural similarities to hPL. Another potent stimulator of the enzyme is lowered plasma phosphate content (*see below*).

In summary, the enhanced calcium absorption of pregnancy is probably due to activation of renal 1-alpha hydroxylase. This results in rising concentrations of 1,25 OHD. The initiating stimulus has not been identified.

Total serum calcium and phosphorus fall in pregnancy (Fig. 13.4). The fall in calcium continues from soon after conception until mid third trimester when there is a slight rise (Pitkin *et al* 1979). Phosphate falls until about 30 weeks and then rises to normal levels at term (Newman 1957). It is likely that the fall in serum proteins accounts for the decline in serum calcium and the closely parallel patterns for calcium and albumin support this. Futhermore, it has been demonstrated in longitudinal studies that the fall must be due to the protein-bound fraction, as ionised calcium either rises very slightly (Andersen and Larsen 1981) or remains constant (Pitkin *et al* 1979).

Early in gestation the fetal serum calcium is lower than maternal (Westin *et al* 1959). At term, however, fetal levels exceed maternal (Delivoria-Papandopoulos *et al* 1967) and the existence of a placental active transport mechanism seems likely. Experimental data lend support to this idea (Whitsett and Tsang 1980). Further, circumstantial evidence lies in the observation that serum calcium levels fall promptly in the newborn after abrupt separation from placental supply (Steichen *et al* 1980; Tsang *et al* 1979). It is possible that maternal 1,25 OHD stimulates a carrier protein to accomplish transplacental passage in the same way that it stimulates transmucosal importation of calcium from the gut lumen.

The state of vitamin D nutrition is most conveniently assessed by the plasma level of 25 OHD. This is no different in pregnancy from the nonpregnant range, at least in Caucasian women (Whitehead *et al* 1981; Dent and Gupta 1975; MacLennan *et al* 1980). Also, a seasonal fluctuation in plasma levels is apparent (Cockburn *et al* 1980).

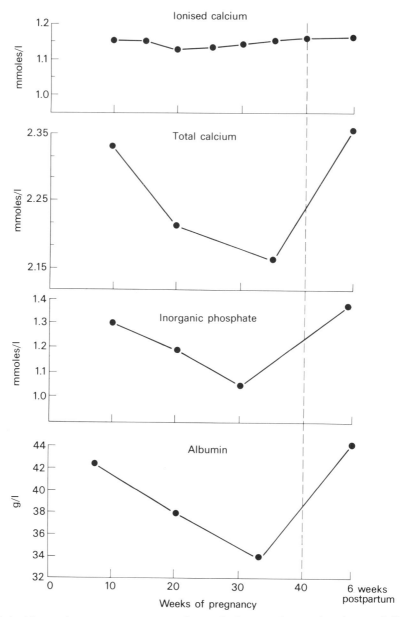

Fig. 13.4 Maternal serum concentrations of ionised calcium, calcium, phosphate and albumin during and after pregnancy. (After Pitkin *et al* 1979.)

Moreover, a careful longitudinal study (MacLennan *et al* 1980) (Fig. 13.5) demonstrated a fall during the third trimester where it occurred in the winter months (January to March). The implication was that, in normal Caucasian women, vitamin D levels withstand the challenge of pregnancy except when the period of greatest demand (the third trimester) coincides with the time of least supply (winter). Further, it was shown

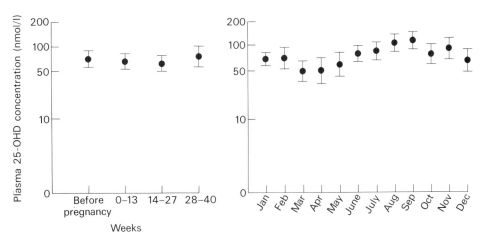

Fig. 13.5 (*Left*) Plasma 25-OHD concentrations before and during pregnancy in 26 women (mean ± 1.96 SD). (*Right*) Seasonal variation (northern hemisphere) of plasma 25-OHD concentration before or during pregnancy in 26 women (mean ± 1.96 SD). After Maclennan *et al* 1980.)

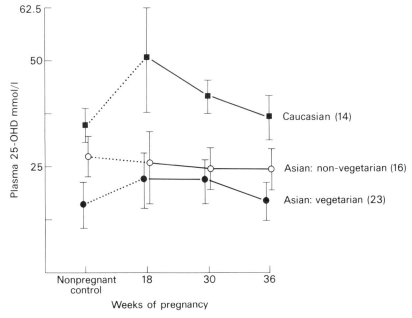

Fig. 13.6 Plasma 25-OHD concentrations in nonpregnant women and during pregnancy. (After Dent and Gupta 1975.)

in another study (Watney *et al* 1971) that there is a seasonal variation of serum calcium in newborn Asian babies, the lowest levels occurring when late gestation coincides with the period of least sunlight (January to March).

The linear relationship between maternal and cord blood concentrations of 25 OHD suggests direct transfer across the placenta (Hillman and Haddad 1974; MacLennan *et al* 1980; Brooke *et al* 1980). On the other hand, 1,25 OHD is significantly lower in the newborn baby than in maternal blood at delivery and bears no relationship to it (Steichen *et al* 1980). This certainly implies that it does not cross the placenta.

A definite rise in calcitonin secretion can be detected during pregnancy and lactation (Whitehead *et al* 1981; Stevenson *et al* 1979). Bearing in mind the considerable ability of calcitonin to inhibit bone resorption, including that caused by PTH and vitamin D, it is possible that it has a role in protecting the maternal skeleton from demineralisation. The newborn baby also has high calcitonin levels (Samaan *et al* 1975; Kovarik *et al* 1980).

The net effect of pregnancy and lactation on skeletal mineral content is not finally established. A retrospective study of Bantu and Caucasian women showed no radiological evidence of bone loss after multiple pregnancies and long lactations in either group (Walker *et al* 1972). There was also no difference in bone density. In other studies, bone mass tended to increase with parity (Goldsmith *et al* 1975; Nilsson 1969). Contrasting results came from photon scanning of the femur in ten lactating women which suggested mineral losses of 2.2 per cent over 100 days (Atkinson and West 1970). Furthermore, there is evidence that some adolescent mothers demonstrate bone demineralisation after 16 weeks of lactation, perhaps because of low dietary intake of calcium and phosphorus (Chan *et al* 1982).

X-ray spectrophotometry was used in a prospective investigation in 1977 (Lamke *et al*) and showed a small but significant loss of mineral from trabecular but not cortical bone during normal pregnancy. Part of this diversity in findings can be attributed to the lack of a standardised method for the assessment of bone mineral content. Nevertheless, in normal pregnancy there is probably no great change in maternal bone content. Perhaps this is what one would expect as the calcium content of a term infant is less than 5 per cent of that of its mother and maternal absorption of calcium spread over a 40 week period is more than adequate to provide for this under normal circumstances. During lactation, however, adequate dietary intake of calcium and phosphorus is important to prevent bone loss.

Table 13.1 summarises the changes in normal pregnancy discussed above. There is the possibility that there are changes in end organ responsiveness to these hormones in pregnancy, but this had not been taken into account. If this were so, there could be changes in metabolism without quantifiable changes in serum levels of the hormones.

Metabolic bone disease

Metabolic bone diseases are those that affect the whole skeleton, though often the involvement is not uniform. We will discuss here a number of disorders which are important in pregnancy and which can be understood on the basis of aberrations in the

Table 13.1   Mineral metabolism, changes in serum concentrations in normal pregnancy. Values are representative means from the literature. Individual studies show wide variation.

	Nonpregnant	3rd Trimester
Total calcium (mmol/l)	2.48[1]	2.34[1,2]
Ionized calcium (mmol/l)	1.18[3]	1.22[3]
Total phosphate (mmol/l)	1.24[1]	1.05[1,2]
Albumin (g/l)	42.0[1]	32.0[1]
25 OHD (nmol/l)	35[4]	38[4]
1,25 OHD (ng/l)	29.5[5]	100[5]

[1] Turton *et al* 1977; [2] Cockburn *et al* 1980; [3] Fogh-Andersen and Schultz-Larsen 1981; [4] Dent and Gupta 1975; [5] Whitehead *et al* 1981.

normal functions considered above. Complete descriptions of each clinical entity in the nonpregnant state can be found elsewhere.

The diseases of rickets and osteomalacia have been classified by Harrison (1979) into two types. Type I is secondary to deficiency of 1,25 OHD and an important feature is secondary hyperparathyroidism. Type II rickets and osteomalacia is the result of hypophosphataemia, most commonly due to impaired renal tubular phosphate reabsorption. Secondary hyperparathyroidism is not a prominent feature. The pathological disorders within each type are listed in Table 13.2. Most of them will be discussed here.

NUTRITIONAL OSTEOMALACIA

Delay in or failure of bone mineralisation is the hallmark of osteomalacia. If it occurs in childhood before closure of the epiphyses, it results in the characteristic disorder of

Table 13.2   Classification of rickets and osteomalacia (after Harrison 1979).

Type I	Type II
Vitamin D deficiency	Fanconi syndrome
sunlight deficiency	Renal tubular acidosis
dietary deficiency	cystinosis
Vitamin D malabsorption	tyrosinosis
Liver disease	idiopathic
Drug-induced	Familial primary hypophosphataemia
anticonvulsants	Acquired primary hypophosphataemia
corticosteroids	
heparin	
Renal insufficiency	

rickets. The rachitic epiphysis, with widened growth plate and distorted architecture, demonstrates hyperosteoidosis, i.e. the presence of excess (unmineralised) osteoid. The same histopathological features are seen in adults with osteomalacia, but in different sites. The epiphyses having closed, the changes can be seen throughout the skeleton wherever remodelling occurs.

Many disorders cause the syndrome of osteomalacia, but all exert their pathological effects through abnormalities in vitamin D metabolism or through hypophosphataemia (Table 13.2). The biochemical triad of low serum calcium and phosphate combined with high alkaline phosphatase (heat labile or bone component to be distinguished in pregnancy) is generally seen with osteomalacia. Urinary hydroxyproline is almost always raised. The diagnosis of nutritional osteomalacia, however, should also include low plasma 25 OHD and high PTH concentrations (reflecting secondary hyperparathyroidism). X-ray features will not be discussed here. In pregnant Asians in Britain, nutritional osteomalacia seems to be common, though often unrecognised. The first manifestation of vitamin D lack may be the birth of a baby with rickets (Ford 1973; Moncrieff 1974) or hypocalcaemia in the first week of life (Heckmatt *et al* 1979). Enamel defects may develop in the teeth later on in life (Purvis *et al* 1973; Cockburn *et al* 1980).

In an investigation of maternal factors relevant to neonatal hypocalcaemia, Watney *et al* (1971) demonstrated lower total calcium levels (serum) in Asian women than in Caucasian. The difference was significant at booking, 36 weeks and 6 weeks after delivery, and the Asian babies had lower serum calcium levels on the sixth day of life. West Indian babies had the highest mean serum calcium. Elsewhere it was shown prospectively that 25 OHD levels in Asians were lower than in Caucasians at every occasion when they were sampled throughout late pregnancy (Dent and Gupta 1975) (Fig. 13.6). Brooke *et al* (1981a) showed that vegetarian Asians had significantly lower levels on each occasion studied and 70 per cent of them had undetectable 25 OHD levels in the puerperium (compared with 12 per cent of non-vegetarians). Nearly half of the babies of vegetarian women had hypocalcaemia whilst none of the other babies developed this problem. These studies supported the findings of a number of previous investigations into the vitamin D and calcium status of pregnant Asian women in Britain (Heckmatt *et al* 1979; Brooke *et al* 1980; Dent and Gupta 1975; Polanska *et al* 1976). Studies from Pakistan (Rab and Baseer 1976) and India (Rizvi and Vaishnava 1977) have shown a high prevalence of subclinical and even overt osteomalacia in pregnant women.

In a recent study, cord 25-OHD levels of a group of Asian babies were less than half those of Asian babies whose mothers had received 1000 units of vitamin D daily in the third trimester and one-fifth the level found in white babies. Despite this, there was no difference between the three groups in bone mineral content of the forearms as assessed by photon absorptiometry (Congdon *et al* 1983). The conclusion was that fetal skeletal mineralisation is not impaired by maternal vitamin D deficiency. Unfortunately, as neither maternal 1,25 OHD nor 25 OHD were measured this conclusion may not be justifiable. Others have also disputed that pregnancy leads to an increased requirement for vitamin D. Dent and Gupta (1975) showed that 25 OHD levels were low in a group of

Asian women and remained so throughout pregnancy without further fall. They argued that this suggested there was no increased need for vitamin D in pregnancy.

Nevertheless the association between pregnancy and osteomalacia, at least in Asians (Wilson 1931; Maxwell 1934) is undeniable. It may be that pregnancy brings a vitamin D-deficient woman to medical attention for the first time and that pregnancy is coincident with the D deficiency rather than causative. What is unknown at present is whether these women with very low vitamin D levels can furnish the normal pregnancy rise in 1,25 OHD concentration. If there is a tendency for pregnancy to unmask latent osteomalacia, it may be explicable on this basis.

It is well established that low maternal 25 OHD levels are associated with neonatal morbidity (Watney *et al* 1971; Cockburn *et al* 1980; Heckmatt *et al* 1979) and impaired first year growth in some groups (Brooke *et al* 1981b). This is sufficient reason to support the recommendation that vitamin D supplements be made available in the UK to all Pakistani women and vegetarian Asians in pregnancy and lactation. The basis for their deficiency seems to lie in dietary inadequacy (even in the non-vegetarian, the diet usually contains little vitamin D) and equally, if not more so, in lack of skin exposure to sunlight (related to the Pakistani custom of covering the body extensively). Of course indoor dwelling, northern latitudes, and the winter season all tend to aggravate the problem. The World Health Organisation (1965) and National Academy of Sciences (*Recommended Dietary Allowances*, 1979) recommend 400 IU (10 μg) of vitamin D daily during pregnancy and lactation. In the absence of widespread supplementation of milk with vitamin D as practised in the USA, prescription of vitamin D by doctors is necessary. In a controlled trial (Cockburn *et al* 1980) 400 IU of ergocalciferol seemed as effective in preventing neonatal problems as 1000 IU had been (Brooke *et al* 1980). The preferred dose would, therefore, seem to be 400 IU. The added loss of calcium in milk in the puerperium makes the consumption of either 1–2 pints of cows' milk per day or of some cheese advisable in all lactating women.

Rickets

Childhood rickets results in stunting of bone growth so that the pelvis does not attain normal size and structure. This often results in reduction of the pelvic diameters. In particular, the anteroposterior diameter of the brim is reduced (Fig. 13.7). Whilst the bone structure cannot be improved in the short-term, it remains essential that these women receive vitamin D during pregnancy as the fetus is at risk of bone disease.

GASTROINTESTINAL AND HEPATIC OSTEOMALACIA

Osteomalacia due to vitamin D and calcium deficiency may complicate any disorder where intestinal absorptive function is compromised. Patients with inflammatory bowel disease, particularly Crohn's disease after intestinal resection, are at high risk. Seventy per cent of patients in an American series had subnormal 25 OHD levels complicating their Crohn's disease (Genant *et al* 1976). Moreover, these patients may need very high doses of vitamin D (2000–20 000 IU) to reverse the bone disease

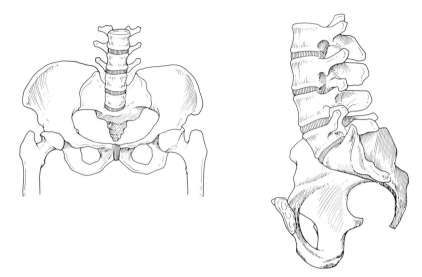

Fig. 13.7 (*Left*) Rachitic flat pelvis. (*Right*) Sagittal section of rachitic flat pelvis with false promontory and reduced AP diameter of pelvic inlet.

(Driscoll *et al* 1977), probably because little of the administered dose is absorbed. They may also have osteoporosis related to corticosteroid therapy and complex metabolic disturbances, as well as osteomalacia.

Despite all these potential problems, neither bony nor calcium complications in mother or baby have been noticed in pregnancies complicated by Crohn's disease (Mogadam *et al* 1981). Nevertheless, it is advisable to monitor calcium and phosphate levels of women who have had bowel resection. Vitamin D should be administered in the usual recommended dose and in a dose of 2000 IU per day if the mother has ever had evidence of vitamin D deficiency. Also the infant should be closely monitored for hypocalcaemia. One study of Asian mothers who did not have inflammatory bowel disease (Watney *et al* 1971) has indicated that elevated maternal heat-labile alkaline phosphatase and lowered serum phosphate are predictors of neonatal hypocalcaemia. These findings would still be relevant to the pregnant patient with Crohn's disease.

Depression of serum 25 OHD, possibly temporary, has been seen in 33–60 per cent of patients after jejunoileal bypass for morbid obesity, in spite of supplementation with 800 IU of vitamin D per day (Schoen *et al* 1978; Teitelbaum *et al* 1977) and bone loss also occurs in these patients (Parfitt *et al* 1978). More of these women are now becoming pregnant (Olow 1976; Ayromlooi & Parsa 1977) and supplementation is warranted, as well as monitoring of mother and baby as detailed above.

Gluten-sensitive enteropathy (coeliac disease) also affects vitamin D absorption (Arnaud *et al* 1977a) and osteomalacia may result. There is a suggestion that 25 OHD may be better absorbed than vitamin D itself in this condition but the first prerequisite of care must be the obsessional adherence to a gluten-free diet. Such dietary treatment can reverse infertility and normal pregnancies have been reported (Morris *et al* 1970) (*see* Chapter 9).

Modern treatment of cystic fibrosis of the pancreas allows increasing numbers of women to successfully conceive and complete pregnancy (Cohen *et al* 1980; *see* Chapter 1). Whilst bone disease is far from their most serious problem, it can exist and low 25 OHD levels with decreased bone mass have been detected, even in the face of dietary vitamin D supplementation (Hahn *et al* 1979). Exocrine pancreatic enzyme replacement must also be continued throughout the pregnancy.

Since the liver is the site of synthesis of 25 OHD, it is not surprising that liver diseases are associated with low serum 25 OHD concentrations. However, osteomalacia is seen more frequently with cholestatic liver disorders than with hepatocellular disease. This probably reflects the paucity of bile salts in the intestinal lumen rendering vitamin D absorption inadequate. Even so, malabsorption is not the only problem since, even if vitamin D is given parenterally, large doses (100 000 IU/month) are required to raise 25 OHD levels in patients with primary biliary cirrhosis (Skinner *et al* 1977).

The only cholestatic disease seen with any frequency in pregnancy is idiopathic cholestasis of pregnancy (Chapter 9). Although a temporary deficit of 25 OHD might be expected in this condition, it has not been reported.

RENAL BONE DISEASE

Bone lesions are common in kidney disease. In general they are seen in two different clinical settings. Firstly osteomalacia and retardation of growth in children result from conditions causing renal tubular acidosis. There may also be renal calculi and nephrocalcinosis. The bone lesions probably result from loss of calcium and phosphate in the urine, but may also be related to the acidosis itself, causing osteolysis and liberation of calcium from bone.

Secondly in the presence of chronic renal failure, the pathogenesis of osteomalacia is related to deficiency of 1,25 OHD. Also, there is phosphate retention and hypocalcaemia causing secondary hyperparathyroidism. Treatment involves administration of vitamin D and calcium and lowering of phosphate absorption from the gut with nonabsorbable antacids. The more potent forms of vitamin D seem more effective.

Pregnancy is occasionally encountered in women with chronic renal failure. Congenital rickets has been reported as a complication in their babies (Savdie *et al* 1982). Certainly, vitamin D should be administered (and the 1-alpha preparation should be used), but the exact dose is not yet established.

DRUG-INDUCED OSTEOPENIA

Drugs that affect bone which are likely to be used in pregnancy are the anticonvulsants, heparin and corticosteroids. Steroids will not be discussed here, since steroid-induced bone disease is rarely a problem in pregnancy; heparin-induced osteopenia is considered in Chapter 4.

Anticonvulsants

Anticonvulsant osteomalacia results from drug-induced disturbance of vitamin D metabolism, and disordered mineral ion transport in bone and intestine. Most of the currently used anticonvulsants have been implicated and the changes are dose dependent.

Most anticonvulsants stimulate activity of the hepatic microsomal oxidase enzymes, bringing about conversion of vitamin D and 25 OHD to inactive metabolites (Hahn *et al* 1972a). Furthermore, phenytoin may also inhibit transintestinal calcium transport (Hahn and Halstead 1979). Phenytoin and phenobarbitone can inhibit bone resorption caused by PTH and 25 OHD (Jenkins *et al* 1974). These observations would only be of theoretical significance if it were not for the known occurrence of osteomalacia with these drugs. The usual manifestations of this problem are a slightly low serum calcium and a distinctly low serum 25 OHD level, often with elevated alkaline phosphatase (Hahn *et al* 1972b). Bone loss can be detected by radiology, by photon-absorption, and, of course, by bone biopsy. Only in the most severe cases will the complete picture of osteomalacia (or rickets in children) develop.

Christiansen *et al* (1981) found that the bone content of epileptic gravidas was 86 per cent of that of age-matched controls at 18 weeks. This same differential persisted at eight days and six months postpartum. The babies' bone content was no different from a control group. It is noteworthy that all epileptics and controls received vitamin D supplementation throughout. Fleischman *et al* (1978) reported reduced 25 OHD levels in epileptic mothers and their babies, and hypocalcaemia in one infant. At present there does not seem to be adequate evidence to advise vitamin D supplementation in these patients, but monitoring of serum calcium and phosphate and surveillance of the baby is prudent.

PARATHYROID DISEASE

Primary hyperparathyroidism

The use of multichannel analysers has led to a great increase in the detection of patients with asymptomatic hypercalcaemia. Many of them have primary hyperpara-thyroidism, but the diagnosis depends on exclusion of other causes. In pregnancy, hypercalcaemia will be overlooked unless the total serum calcium is corrected for hypoalbuminaemia.

Hyperparathyroidism in pregnancy is a serious condition associated with a high rate of fetal loss and increased perinatal morbidity and mortality. In a review of the world literature, Shangold *et al* (1982) found 63 women with the problem. Of 159 pregnancies, 84 ended with delivery of normal full-term babies and 35 with neonatal tetany. There were four neonatal deaths, 11 intrauterine deaths and 13 spontaneous abortions. The neonatal deaths all followed tetany. Wagner *et al* (1964) found the presence of maternal bone disease (osteitis fibrosa or bone cysts) to be a worrying feature as all perinatal deaths came from this group. Conversely, pregnancy outcome was not correlated with renal involvement.

The neonatal hypocalcaemia is a result of parathyroid suppression by high ambient calcium levels during intrauterine life. Recovery of normal parathyroid gland function appears to take a considerable time in these infants and hypocalcaemia may continue for many weeks if untreated (Better *et al* 1973). The intrauterine deaths probably relate to severe fetal hypercalcaemia, as fetal calcium levels exceed maternal (Steichen *et al* 1980) because of active transplacental transfer.

Most women with hyperparathyroidism tolerate pregnancy well. It is possible that pregnancy offers some protection against hypercalcaemia because of the low serum albumin and loss of calcium to the fetus. Even so, there are several reports of hypercalcaemic crisis in pregnancy (Thomason *et al* 1981; Clark *et al* 1981; Whalley 1963). What might seem more likely is postpartum crisis, but this has only been reported twice (Salem and Taylor 1979; Schenker and Kallner 1965).

There is no doubt that the definitive treatment of hyperparathyroidism involves surgery. Moreover, neck exploration seems to be a relatively safe procedure in pregnancy. In 16 of the cases reported by Shangold, operation was performed during pregnancy and in only one was the baby lost (stillborn at six months after neck exploration; Whalley 1963). The remaining 27 of the 28 fetal losses described occurred in the absence of surgical treatment, as did all of the 35 cases of neonatal tetany. For the fetus, therefore, operation at diagnosis seems to be the best course of action. If, for any reason, neck exploration cannot be performed, medical treatment with a low calcium diet, high fluid intake and oral phosphate should be commenced. Montoro *et al* (1980) reported success with oral phosphate therapy in pregnancy.

Hypoparathyroidism

In young women this is usually subsequent to thyroid surgery. Rarely, it is part of an autoimmune disorder where antibodies are directed against adrenal, thyroid, gastric and ovarian tissue as well. Treatment is intended to maintain serum calcium within normal limits and utilises vitamin D and oral calcium supplements. In pregnancy the requirement for vtamin D has been seen to increase 2–3 fold, as its behaviour in normal pregnancy might suggest (Sadeghi-Nejad *et al* 1980; Salle *et al* 1981).

For the fetus, the consequences of untreated maternal hypoparathyrodisim are serious. Intrauterine parathyroid overactivity has been reported (Landing and Kamoshita 1970; Sann *et al* 1976) and fatal rickets may occur (Gradus *et al* 1981). All of these cases occurred when the maternal condition had either been undiagnosed or inadequately treated. In these cases chronic maternal hypocalcaemia leads to fetal hypocalcaemia and parathyroid hyperplasia, which has been demostrated at autopsy.

Therapy with oral vitamin D and calcium prevents deleterious effects in the fetus (Graham *et al* 1964). Recently the successful use of oral 1,25 OHD has been reported, but this must be applied carefully as one baby showed increased density of skull and long bones consistent with excessive mineralisation (Salle *et al* 1981). Frequent monitoring of maternal calcium and phosphate is necessary. As we have seen, it will usually be necessary to increase the dosage to maintain adequate serum calcium as pregnancy progresses. However, there is also the danger of provoking hypercalcaemia, particularly if using the potent synthetic analogue of vitamin D, dihydrotachysterol (Jensen *et al* 1980).

OSTEOPOROSIS AND NECROSIS OF THE FEMORAL HEAD

A number of patients present with severe idiopathic osteoporosis during pregnancy. A group of these were studied in their first pregnancy and no exacerbation during subsequent pregnancies was found (Dent and Friedman 1965). These authors concluded there was no definite relationship between pregnancy and osteoporosis.

The neck of the femur seems to be particularly susceptible in pregnancy to osteoporosis and avascular necrosis. Some women complain of pain in the hip during pregnancy, but X-ray is seldom performed. Some of these patients may have osteoporosis as described by Longstreth *et al* (1973). Many other cases have been reported and the disorder seems to be limited to the duration of the pregnancy. The progression to femoral head necrosis is very uncommon and usually seen in women with predisposing causes such as steroid ingestion. However, there are some cases occurring in pregnancy where no cause is apparent (Kay *et al* 1972; Zolla-Pazner *et al* 1980). These patients will complain of increasingly severe pain in the hip which may be of very sudden onset.

Other inherited metabolic disorders

MARFAN SYNDROME

This generalised disorder of connective tissue displays autosomal dominant inheritance. The underlying biochemical abnormality is unknown, but its chief defects are manifested in the skeletal, ocular and cardiovascular systems. Weakness in the media of the aorta predisposes all these patients to progressive dilatation and aneurysmal widening of the ascending aorta (Brown *et al* 1975). This often leads to aortic regurgitation. Also, mitral valve prolapse can be revealed in most patients using echocardiography. There is an increase in length of the tubular bones and weak yielding ligaments leading to joint laxity and kyphoscoliosis. These abnormalities usually cause no problem in pregnancy; neither is there any severe structural problem with the pelvis.

Women with the Marfan syndrome have an increased risk of spontaneous abortion and low birthweight babies (Pyeritz 1981). The gravest risk to these patients in pregnancy is that of aortic dissection, and maternal deaths due to this complication have been reported (Pyeritz 1981). The cardiovascular aspects of this syndrome have been discussed in Chapter 5. Spontaneous uterine inversion in association with Marfan syndrome has been reported (Quinn and Mukerjee 1982).

OSTEOGENESIS IMPERFECTA

This is another generalised disorder of connective tissue. The most common variety (tarda) has autosomal dominant inheritance. The basic defect is not known but the fully developed syndrome involves blue sclerae, deafness from otosclerosis, multiple fractures and joint laxity. The bones are porotic and fragile and repeated fractures leave the sufferer with skeletal deformity. The pelvis is often misshapen with subsequent cephalopelvic disproportion. Of 17 cases reported, nine delivered vaginally including one who sustained a pelvic fracture and another who died of haemorrhage from uterine laceration. Most of these cases are reviewed by Key and Horger (1978).

If the decision is made to deliver by Caesarean section, the vulnerability of the skeleton under general anaesthesia should be remembered and care taken in positioning the patient. There is a suggestion that these patients may develop hyperthermia if succinyl choline is used as a muscle relaxant, and it is therefore best avoided (Solomons and Myers 1971). Lumbar epidural anaesthesia is not contraindicated, although accurate needle placement may be difficult.

Scoliosis is the most common deformity. If severe it is accompanied by diminished lung volume, as in the case of Sengupta *et al* (1977). Despite the fact that respiratory difficulties have not been prominent in the reported cases, pulmonary function should be monitored. Ultrasound or radiography of the fetus should be performed before delivery. If the baby is affected, it is best to minimise birth trauma and this usually means delivery by Caesarean section.

No therapy is of proven benefit in this disorder. Even so, all patients should be given calcium supplements as a propensity for hypocalcaemia in pregnancy has been demontrated (Freda *et al* 1961).

ACHONDROPLASIA

Inheritance is autosomal dominant, but many cases represent new mutations. Women with this bony disorder tend to have early menarche and early menopause. They have an increased incidence of uterine fibroids.

During pregnancy, cardiorespiratory compromise is a risk as the fetus grows larger. All women with achondroplasia require Caesarean section because of pelvic contraction. Moreover, general anaesthesia should be used because spinal stenosis is usual in these patients making epidural anaesthesia technically difficult. Furthermore, particular care must be taken in manipulating the neck during tracheal intubation because of cervical spinal stenosis (Hall 1981)

Other inherited disorders of bone

There are a number of very rare bone dysplasias. They will not be discussed here but details can be found in the article by Hall (1981).

PHENYLKETONURIA

Classical phenylketonuria is an inborn error of metabolism, inherited as an autosomal recessive, whereby phenylalanine is not metabolised to tyrosine, because of the absence of phenylalanine hydroxylase. Its metabolic precursor, phenylpyruvic acid, is then excreted in the urine. It is usually diagnosed in the newborn by the Guthrie test, which detects the excess of phenylalanine in the blood; the diagnosis is confirmed by quantifying the high levels of phenylalanine and low levels of tyrosine. If left untreated, the condition is associated with severe mental retardation in the growing child.

Since phenylalanine is present in nearly all proteins, dietary treatment consists of virtual elimination of natural proteins, and substitution of a hydrolysate of aminoacid with very low phenylalanine content. Children can often continue this diet for the first years of life and, if they do, their subsequent development is nearly normal. However, when they return to a normal diet, at between four and eight years of age, blood levels of phenylalanine rise again. Many such girls previously treated in childhood, are now reaching reproductive age and, in addition, some individuals with milder forms of previously undiagnosed hyperphenylalaninaemia are also being detected in screening programmes (Hyanek *et al* 1979). The importance of these observations is that maternal hyperphenylalaninaemia greater than 1.2 mmol/l is associated with a very high incidence of abortion, intrauterine growth retardation, fetal congenital abnormalities, almost exclusively congenital heart disease (Lenke and Levy 1980), and also microcephaly and mental retardation (Hyanek *et al* 1979; Mabry *et al* 1966; Yu and O'Halloran 1970). The risk of microcephaly and mental retardation appears to be 75 per cent in the infants of women with phenylalanine levels between 0.96 and 1.2 mmol/l (Lenke and Levy 1980). Some 95 per cent of mothers with blood phenylalanine levels greater than 1.2 mmol/l will have at least one abnormal child (Lenke and Levy 1980). The association is not complete. Some normal infants have been born to mothers with documented hyperphenylalaninaemia in pregnancy (Woolf *et al* 1961) but the chance of producing a normal infant in these circumstances is very low.

The reintroduction of dietary therapies certainly improves the fetal prognosis (Davidson *et al* 1981; Arthur and Hulme 1970) even if started in the second trimester (Zaleski *et al* 1979). However, abnormal fetuses have been born to women taking adequate dietary therapy (Smith 1970; Scott *et al* 1980), including one case of congenital heart disease in a woman who started a diet at six weeks' gestation (Bouvierre-Lapierre *et al* 1974). Although the precise relationship between the risk of fetal impairment and maternal serum phenylalanine level has not been established (Farquhar 1980), it would appear that control of maternal phenylalanine levels (like the control of maternal glucose levels in diabetes) should be optimal before conception (Scott *et al* 1980).

The target of dietary therapy should be a phenylalanine level of less than 0.6 mmol/l. The precise level is not clear since Hyanek *et al* (1979) have shown a mild degree of retardation in the offspring of women with serum phenylalanine concentrations greater than 0.24 mmol/l: such patients do not have phenylketonuria. It is even possible that abnormal, low maternal levels of phenylalanine are also harmful to the fetus. Since there is some suggestion that low maternal tyrosine levels may also harm the fetus (Bessman *et al* 1978), dietary tyrosine supplementation has also been used (Davidson *et al* 1981). The diet will also require supplementation with glucose, vitamins and minerals (Davidson *et al* 1981). Since the reintroduction of a low phenylalanine diet is unpleasant, and, since conception may be unexpected, girls should be encouraged to continue the diet from the time of first diagnosis, until after they stop having children (Murphy & Troy 1979).

Some children with phenylketonuria may be lost to follow-up and, because of the evidence that moderate elevations of phenylalanine in the blood do not cause phenylketonuria, but are still harmful to the fetus (Hyanek 1979), there is a case for a routine screening test in pregnancy. Ideally, the test should be for hyperphenyla-laninaemia (Hyanek *et al* 1979). The Guthrie test has also been used (Scott *et al* 1980) as have urine screening tests (Arthur and Hulme 1970). Since the maximum gain appears to be from treatment instituted before conception, such a screen should really be part of a prepregnancy or premarital screening service (Scott *et al* 1980). Nevertheless, the yield of such screening tests is low: 1 in 10 000 Guthrie tests performed in pregnancy in Glasgow (Scott *et al* 1980). Screening may be more worthwhile in populations where the risk of phenylketonuria is greater. Hyanek *et al* (1979) found nine cases of abnormal aminoacid metabolism in 15 000 women screened by blood paper chromatography in Czechoslovakia.

There are no specific pregnancy complications in maternal phenylketonuria, apart from a slight excess of intrauterine growth retardation. Furthermore, the emotional strain put on the mother, both by worrying about the fetal outcome and by having to follow an unpleasant diet, may be considerable. Breast feeding can be allowed, since the increased dietary load of phenylalanine in breast milk will not cause hyperphenyla-laninaemia in the newborn (Davidson *et al* 1981).

HYPERXANTHINURIA, HYPERGLYCINAEMIA, HYPERTYROSINAEMIA

In the few cases of hyperxanthinuria reported in pregnancy there has been no evidence of excess fetal abnormalities (McKeran 1977; Curiel and Bandinelli 1979). Neverthe-less, one patient lost two out of three pregnancies, both associated with prematurity (Curiel and Bandinelli 1979). The mothers are at risk from the formation of xanthine urinary stones. Maternal uric acid levels—which are helpful in the management of hypertensive disease in pregnancy (*see* Chapter 6)—cannot be relied upon because of the impairment of uric acid formation which is part of the metabolic block (Curiel and Bandinelli 1979).

Hyanek *et al* (1979) report that one of two cases of maternal hyperglycinaemia was associated with mental retardation in the newborn. Two children from a woman with hypertyrosinaemia were normal.

References

Aarskog D., Aksnes L. & Lehmann V. (1980) Low 1,25-dihydroxyvitamin D in heparin-induced osteopenia. *Lancet* **ii**, 650.

Arnaud S.B., Matthusen M. *et al* (1977a) Components of 25-hydroxyvitamin D in serum of young children in upper midwestern United States. *American Journal of Clinical Nutrition* **30**, 1082.

Arnaud S.B., Newcomer A.D. *et al* (1977b) Serum 25-OHD and the pathogenesis of osteomalacia in patients with non-tropical sprue. *Gastroenterology* **72**, 1025.

Arthur L.J.H. & Hulme S.R.D. (1970) Intelligent, small-for-dates baby born to oligophrenic phenylketonuric mother after low phenylalanine diet during pregnancy. *Pediatrics* **46**, 235–9.

Atkinson P.J. & West R.R. (1970) Loss of skeletal calcium in lactating women. *Journal of Obstetrics and Gynaecology of the British Commonwealth* **77**, 555.

Ayromlooi J. & Parsa H. (1977) Pregnancy following jejunoileal bypass for obesity. *American Journal of Obstetrics and Gynecology* **129**, 921.

Bessman S.P., Williamson M.L. & Koch R. (1978) Diet, genetics and mental retardation interaction between phenylketonuric heterozygous mother and fetus to produce non-specific diminution of IQ: evidence in support of the justification hypothesis. *Proceedings of the National Academy of Sciences USA* **75**, 1562–6.

Better O., Levi J. *et al* (1973) Prolonged neonatal parathyroid suppression: A sequel to asymptomatic maternal hyperparathyroidism. *Archives of Surgery* **106**, 722.

Bouvierre-Lapierre M., Saint-Dizier C., Freycon F., David M., Dorche C. & Jeune M. (1974) Deux enfants nés de mère phénylcetonurique. Échec d'un régime pauvre en phénylalanine institue pendant la deuxième grossesse. *Pediatrie* **29**, 51–72.

Boyle I.T., Gray R.W. & DeLuca H.F. (1971) Regulation by calcium of in vivo synthesis of 1,25 dihydroxycholecalciferol and 24,25 dihydroxycholecalciferol. *Proceedings of the National Academy of Sciences USA* **68**, 2131.

Brooke O.G., Brown I.R.F. *et al* (1980) Vitamin D supplements in pregnant Asian women: effects on calcium status and fetal growth. *British Medical Journal* **1**, 751.

Brooke O.G., Brown I.R.F. & Cleeve H.J.W. (1981a) Observations on the vitamin D state of pregnant Asian women in London. *British Journal of Obstetrics and Gynecology* **88**, 18.

Brooke O.G., Butters F. & Wood C. (1981b) Intrauterine vitamin D nutrition and postnatal growth in Asian infants. *British Medical Journal* **283**, 1024.

Brown D.J., Spanos E. & MacIntyre I. (1980) Role of pituitary hormones in regulating renal vitamin D metabolism in man. *British Medical Journal* **1**, 277.

Brown O.R., DeMots H., Kloster F.E. *et al* (1975) Aortic root dilatation and mitral valve prolapse in Marfan's syndrome. *Circulation* **52**, 651.

Castillo L., Tanaka Y. *et al* (1979) Production of 1,25-dihydroxyvitamin D_3 and formation of medullary bone in the egg-laying hen. *Endocrinology* **104**, 1598.

Chan G.M., Slater P., Ronald N. *et al* (1982) Bone mineral status of lactating mothers of different ages. *American Journal of Obstetrics and Gynecology* **144**, 438.

Christiansen C., Brandt N.J. *et al* (1981) Bone mineral content during pregnancy in epileptics on anticonvulsant drugs and in their newborns. *Acta Obstetrica et Gynecologica Scandinavica* **60**, 501.

Clark D., Seeds J.W. & Cefalo R.C. (1981) Hyperparathyroid crisis and pregnancy. *American Journal of Obstetrics and Gynecology* **140**, 840.

Cockburn F., Belton N.R. *et al* (1980) Maternal vitamin D intake and mineral metabolism in mothers and their newborn infants. *British Medical Journal* **281**, 11.

Cohen L.F., di Sant'Agnese P.A. & Friedlander J. (1980) Cystic fibrosis and pregnancy. *Lancet* **ii**, 842.

Congdon P., Horsman A., Kirby P.A. *et al* (1983) Mineral content of the forearms of babies born to Asian and white mothers. *British Medical Journal* **286**, 1233–5.

Curiel P. & Bandinelli R. (1979) Pregnancy in a woman with xanthinuria: study of amniotic fluid uric acid. *American Journal of Obstetrics and Gynecology* **134**, 721–2.

Cushard W.G., Creditor S., Canterbury J.M. & Reiss E. (1972) Calcium, magnesium, phosphorus, and parathyroid hormone interrelationships in pregnancy and newborn infants. *Journal of Clinical Endocrinology and Metabolism* **34**, 767.

Davidson D.C., Isherwood D.M., Ireland J.T. & Rae P.G. (1981) Outcome of pregnancy in a phenylketonuric mother after low phenylalanine diet introduced from the ninth week of pregnancy. *European Journal of Pediatrics* **137**, 45–8.

Delivoria-Papandopoulos M., Battaglia F.C., Bruns P.D. & Meschia G. (1967) Total, protein-bound, and ultrafilterable calcium in maternal and fetal plasmas. *American Journal of Physiology* **213**, 363.

Dent C.E. & Friedman M. (1965) Pregnancy and idiopathic osteoporosis. *Quarterly Journal of Medicine* **34**, 341.

Dent C.E. & Gupta M.M. (1975) Plasma 25-hydroxyvitamin D levels during pregnancy in Caucasians and in vegetarian and non-vegetarian Asians. *Lancet* **ii**, 1057–60.

Driscoll R.H., Meredith S. *et al* (1977) Bone histology and vitamin D status in Crohn's disease: assessment of vitamin D therapy. *Gastoenterology* **72**, 1051.

Farquhar J.W. (1980) Commentary. *Archives of Disease in Childhood* **55**, 636–7.

Fleischman A.R., Rosen J.F. & Nathenson G. (1978) 25-hydroxyvitamin D. Serum levels and oral administration of calcifediol in neonates. *Archives of Internal Medicine* **138**, 869.

Fogh-Andersen N.F. & Schultz-Larsen P.S. (1981) Free calcium ion concentration in pregnancy. *Acta Obstetrica et Gynecologica Scandinavica* **60**, 309.

Ford J.A., Davidson D.C. *et al* (1973) Neonatal rickets in Asian immigrant population. *British Medical Journal* **3**, 211.

Freda V.J., Vosburgh G.J. & Diliberti C. (1961) Osteogenesis imperfecta congenita. *Obstetrics and Gynecology* **18**, 535.

Gallagher J.C., Riggs B.L. *et al* (1978) Effect of estrogen therapy on calcium absorption and vitamin D metabolism in postmenopausal osteoporosis. *Clinical Research* **26**, 415A.

Genant H.K., Mall J.C. *et al* (1976) Skeletal demineralisation and growth retardation in inflammatory bowel disease. *Investigative Radiology* **11**, 541.

Goldsmith N.F. & Johnston J.O. (1975) Bone mineral: Effects of oral contraceptives, pregnancy and lactation. *Journal of Bone and Joint Surgery* **57A**, 657.

Goodwin D., Noff D. & Edelstein S. (1978) 24,25 Dihydroxyvitamin D is a metabolite of vitamin D essential for bone formation. *Nature* **276**, 517.

Gradus D., Le Roith D. *et al* (1981) Congenital hyperparathyroidism and rickets secondary to maternal hypoparathyroidism and vitamin D deficiency. *Israel Journal of Medical Sciences* **17**, 705.

Graham III W.P., Gordon G.S. *et al* (1964) Effect of pregnancy and of the menstrual cycle on hypoparathyroidism. *Journal of Clinical Endocrinology and Metabolism* **24**, 512.

Gray T.K., Lester G.E. & Lorenc R.S. (1979) Evidence for extrarenal 1-hydroxylation of 25-hydroxyvitamin D_3 in pregnancy. *Science* **204**, 1311.

Hahn T.J. & Halstead L.R. (1979) Anticonvulsant drug-induced osteomalacia: alterations in mineral metabolism and response to vitamin D_3 administration. *Calcified Tissue International* **27**, 13.

Hahn T.J., Birge S.J. *et al* (1972a) Phenobarbital-induced alterations in vitamin D metabolism. *Journal of Clinical Investigation* **51**, 741.

Hahn T.J., Hendin B.A. *et al* (1972b) Effect of chronic anticonvulsant therapy on serum 25-hydroxycalciferol levels in adults. *New England Journal of Medicine* **287**, 900.

Hahn T.J., Squires A.E. *et al.* (1979) Reduced serum 25-hydroxyvitamin D concentration and disordered mineral metabolism in patients with cystic fibrosis. *Journal of Pediatrics* **94**, 38.

Hall J.G. (1981) Disorders of connective tissue and skeletal dysplasia. In Schulman J.D. and Simpson J.L. (eds) *Genetic Diseases in Pregnancy*, p. 79. Academic Press, New York.

Harrison H.E., (1979) Vitamin D, the parathyroid and the kidney. *Johns Hopkins Medical Journal* **144**, 80.

Heaney R.P. & Skillman T.G. (1971) Calcium metabolism in normal human pregnancy. *Journal of Clinical Endocrinology and Metabolism* **33**, 661.

Heckmatt J.Z., Peacock M. *et al* (1979) Plasma 25-hydroxyvitamin D in pregnant Asian women and their babies. *Lancet* **2**, 546.

Hillman L.S. & Haddad J.G. (1974) Human perinatal vitamin D metabolism. I. 25-hydroxyvitamin D in maternal and cord blood. *Journal of Pediatrics* **84**, 742.

Holtrop M.E., Cox K.A. *et al* (1981) 1,25 Dihydroxycholecalciferol stimulates osteoclasts in rat bones in the absence of parathyroid hormone. *Endocrinology* **108**, 2293.

Hyánek J., Homolka J., Trnka J., Seemanóva E., Cervenka J., Třesoh Lavá Z., Kapras J., Doležal A., Sraček J., Vácha V., Hoza J., Losān F., Nevšímalová S., Malá M. & Viletová H. (1979) Results of screening for phenylalanine and other amino acid disturbances among pregnant women. *Journal of Inherited and Metabolic Diseases* **2**, 59–63.

Hytten F.E. & Leitch I. (1971) *The Physiology of Human Pregnancy*, 2nd edn, p. 383. Blackwell Scientific Publications, Oxford.

Jenkins M.V., Harris M. & Wills M.R. (1974) The effect of phenytoin on parathyroid extract and 25-hydroxycholecalciferol-induced bone resorption. *Calcified Tissue Research* **16**, 163.

Jensen L.P., Ras G. & Boes E.G.M. (1980) Hypercalcaemia in pregnancy. A case report. *South African Medical Journal* **57**, 712.

Kay N.R.M., Park W.M. & Bark M. (1972) The relationship between pregnancy and femoral head necrosis. *British Journal of Radiology* **45**, 828.

Key T.C. & Horger E.O. (1978) Osteogenesis imperfecta as a complication of pregnancy. *Obstetrics and Gynecology* **51**, 67.

Kovarik J., Woloszczuk W. *et al* (1980) Calcitonin in pregnacy. *Lancet* **i**, 199.

Kumar R., Cohen W.R., Silva P. & Epstein F.H. (1979) Elevated 1,25 Dihydroxyvitamin D plasma levels in normal human pregnancy and lactation. *Journal of Clinical Investigation* **63**, 342.

Lamke B., Brundin J. & Moberg P. (1977) Changes of bone mineral content during pregnancy and lactation. *Acta Obstetrica et Gynecologica Scandinavica* **56**, 217.

Landing B.H. & Kamoshita S. (1970) Congenital hyperparathyroidism secondary to maternal hypoparathyroidism. *Journal of Pediatrics* **77**, 842.

Lenke R.R. & Levy H.L. (1980) Maternal phenylketonuria and hyperphenylalaninemia. An international survey of the outcome of untreated and treated pregnancies. *New England Journal of Medicine* **303**, 1202–8.

Longstreth P.L., Malinak L.R. & Hill C.S. (1973) Transient osteoporosis of the hip in pregnancy. *Obstetrics and Gynecology* **41**, 563.

Lund B. & Selnes A. (1979) Plasma 1,25 dihydroxyvitamin D levels in pregnancy and lactation. *Acta Endocrinologica* **92**, 330.

Mabry C.C., Denniston J.C. & Coldwell J.G. (1966) Mental retardation in children of phenylketonuric mothers. *New England Journal of Medicine* **275**, 1331–6.

McKeran R.O. (1977) Xanthinuria and Pregnancy. *Lancet* **ii**, 86–7.

MacLennan W.J., Hamilton J.C. & Darmady J.M. (1980) The effects of season and stage of pregnancy on plasma 25-hydroxyvitamin D concentrations in pregnant women. *Postgraduate Medical Journal* **56**, 75.

Maxwell J.P. (1934) Further studies of adult rickets (osteomalacia) and foetal rickets. *Proceedings of the Royal Society of Medicine* **28**, 265.

Mogadam M., Dobbins W.O. *et al* (1981) Pregnancy in inflammatory bowel disease: Effect of sulfasalazine and corticosteroids on fetal outcome. *Gastroenterology* **80**, 72.

Moncrieff M.W. & Fadahunsi T.O. (1974) Congenital rickets due to maternal vitamin D deficiency. *Archives of Disease in Childhood* **49**, 810.

Montoro M.N., Collea J.V. & Mestman J.H. (1980) Management of hyperparathyroidism in pregnancy with oral phosphate therapy. *Obstetrics and Gynecology* **65**, 431.

Morris J.S., Adjukiewicz A.B. & Read A.E. (1970) Coeliac infertility: an indication for dietary gluten restriction. *Lancet* **i**, 213.

Murphy D. & Troy E.M. (1979) Maternal phenylketonuria. *Irish Journal of Medical Science* **48**, 310–13.

Newman R.L. (1957) Serum electrolytes in pregnancy, parturition and the puerperium. *Obstetrics and Gynecology* **10**, 51.

Nilsson B.E. (1969) Parity and osteoporosis. *Surgery, Gynecology and Obstetrics* **129**, 27.

Nordin B.E.C., Heyburn P.J. *et al* (1980) Osteoporosis and osteomalacia. *Clinical Endocrinology and Metabolism* **9**, 177.

Olow B., Akesson B.A. *et al.* (1976) Pregnancy after jejuno-ileostomy because of obesity. *Acta Chirurgica Scandinavica* **142**, 82.

Parfitt A.M., Miller M.J. *et al* (1978) Metabolic complications after intestinal bypass for treatment of obesity. *Annals of Internal Medicine* **89**, 193.

Pitkin R.M., Reynolds W.A. *et al* (1979) Calcium metabolism in normal pregnancy: A longitudinal study. *American Journal of Obstetrics and Gynecology* **133**, 781.

Polanska N., Dale R.A. & Wills M.R. (1976) Plasma calcium levels in pregnant Asian women. *Annals of Clinical Biochemistry* **13**, 339.

Purvis R.J., Barrie W.J.M. *et al* (1973) Enamel hypoplasia of the teeth associated with neonatal tetany: a manifestation of maternal vitamin D deficiency. *Lancet* **ii**, 811.

Pyeritz R.E. (1981) Maternal and fetal complications of pregnancy in the Marfan syndrome. *American Journal of Medicine* **71**, 784.

Quinn R.J. & Mukerjee B. (1982) Spontaneous uterine inversion in association with Marfan's syndrome. *Australian & New Zealand Journal of Obstetrics & Gynaecology* **22**, 163.

Rab S.M. & Baseer A. (1976) Occult osteomalacia amongst healthy and pregnant women in Pakistan. *Lancet* **ii**, 1211.

Raisz L.G., Trummel C.L. *et al* (1972) 1,25 Dihydroxycholecalciferol: a potent stimulator of bone resorption in tissue culture. *Science* **175**, 768.

Recommended Dietary Allowances, 9th edn. (1979) Food and Nutrition Board. Washington D.C. National Research Council-National Academy of Sciences.

Rizvi S.N.A. & Vaishnava H. (1977) Occult osteomalacia in pregnant women in India. *Lancet* **i**, 1102.

Sadeghi-Nejad A., Wolfsdorf J.I. & Senior B. (1980) Hypoparathyroidism and pregnancy: treatment with calcitriol. *Journal of the American Medical Association* **243**, 254.

Salem R. & Taylor S. (1979) Hyperparathyroidism in pregnancy. *British Journal of Surgery* **66**, 648.

Salle B.L., Berthezene F. *et al* (1981) Hypoparathyroidism during pregnancy: treatment with calcitriol. *Journal of Clinical Endocrinology and Metabolism* **52**, 810.

Samaan N.A., Anderson G.D. & Adam-Mayns M.E. (1975) Immunoreactive calcitonin in the mother, neonate, child and adult. *American Journal of Obstetrics and Gynecology* **121**, 622.

Sann L., David L. *et al* (1976) Congenital hyperparathyroidism and vitamin D deficiency secondary to maternal hypoparathyroidism. *Acta Paediatrica Scandinavica* **65**, 381.

Savdie E., Caterson R.J. *et al* (1982) Successful pregnancies in women treated by haemodialysis. *Medical Journal of Australia* **2**, 9.

Schenker J. & Kallner B. (1965) Fatal postpartum hyperparathyroid crisis. *Obstetrics and Gynecology* **25**, 705.

Schoen M.S., Lindenbaum J. *et al* (1978) Significance of 25-hydroxycholecalciferol level in gastrointestinal disease. *Digestive Diseases* **23** (2), 137.

Scott T.M., Morton Fyfe W. & McKay Hart D. (1980) Maternal phenylketonuria: abnormal baby despite low phenylalanine diet during pregnancy. *Archives of Disease in Childhood* **55**, 634–9.

Sengupta B.S., Sivapragasam S. *et al* (1977) Osteogenesis imperfecta: Its physiopathology in pregnancy. *Journal of the Royal College of Surgeons of Edinburgh* **22**, 358.

Shangold M.M., Dor N. *et al* (1982) Hyperparathyroidism and pregnancy: A review. *Obstetrics and Gynecology Survey* **37**, 217.

Shenolikar I.S. (1970) Absorption of dietary calcium in pregnancy. *American Journal of Clinical Nutrition* **23**, 63.

Skinner R.K., Long R.G. *et al* (1977) 25-hydroxylation of vitamin D in primary biliary cirrhosis. *Lancet* **i**, 720.

Smith J., Macartney F.J., Erdohazim M., Pincott J.R., Wolff O.H., Brenton D.P., Biddle S.A., Fairweather D.V.I. & Dobbing J. (1979) Fetal damage despite low-phenylalanine diet after conception in a pheylketonuric woman. *Lancet* **i**, 17–19.

Solomons C.C. & Myers D.N. (1971) Hyperthermia of osteogenesis imperfecta and its relationship to malignant hyperthermia. In Gordon R.A., Gritt B.A., Kalow W. (eds) *International Symposium on Malignant Hyperthermia*, pp. 319–31. Thomas, Springfield, Illinois.

Spanos E., Pike J.W., Haussler M.R. *et al* (1976) Circulating 1 alpha, 25 dihydroxyvitamin D in the chicken: enhancement by injection of prolactin and during egg laying. *Life Sciences* **19**, 1751.

Steichen J.J., Tsang R.C., Gratton T.L. *et al* (1980) Vitamin D homeostasis in the perinatal period. *New England Journal of Medicine* **302**, 315.

Stevenson J.C., Hillyard C.J. *et al* (1979) A physiological role for calcitonin: Protection of the maternal skeleton. *Lancet* **ii**, 769–70.

Tanaka Y., Castillo L. *et al* (1978) Synergistic effect of progesterone, testosterone, and estradiol in the stimulation of chick renal 25-hydroxyvitamin D-1 alpha-hydroxylase. *Endocrinology* **103**, 2035.

Teitelbaum S.L., Halverson J.D. *et al* (1977) Abnormalities of circulating 25-OH vitamin D after jejunoileal bypass for obesity and evidence of an adaptive response. *Annals of Internal Medicine* **86**, 289.

Thomason J.L., Sampson M.B. *et al* (1981) Pregnancy complicated by concurrent primary hyperparathyroidism and pancreatitis. *Obstetrics and Gynecology* **57**, 345.

Tsang R., Abrams L. *et al* (1979) Ionised calcium in neonates in relation to gestational age. *Journal of Pediatrics* **94**, 126.

Turton C.W.G., Stanley P. *et al.* (1978) Altered vitamin D metabolism in pregnancy. *Lancet* **i**, 222–5.

Verdy M., Beaulieu R., Demers L. *et al* (1971) Plasma calcitonin activity in a patient with thyroid medullary carcinoma and her children with osteopetrosis. *Journal of Clinical Endocrinology* **32**, 216.

Wagner G., Transbol I. & Melchior J. (1964) Hyperparathyroidism and pregnancy. *Acta Endocrinologica* **47**, 549.

Walker A.R.P., Richardson B. & Walker F. (1972) The influence of numerous pregnancies and lactations on bone dimensions in South African Bantu and Caucasian mothers. *Clinical Science* **42**, 189.

Watney P.J., Chance G.W. *et al* (1971) Maternal factors in neonatal hypocalcemia: a study in three ethnic groups. *British Medical Journal* **2**, 432–6.

Weissman A., Harell A. *et al* (1979) 1,25-dihydroxyvitamin D and 24,25 dihydroxyvitamin D in vitro synthesis by human placenta and decidua. *Nature* **280**, 317.

Westin B., Kaiser I.H. *et al* (1959) Some constituents of umbilical venous blood of previable human fetuses. *Acta Paediatrica Scandinavica* **48**, 609.

Whalley P. (1963) Hyperparathyroidism and pregnancy. *American Journal of Obstetrics and Gynecology* **86**, 517.

Whitehead M., Lane G. & Young O. (1981) Interrelations of calcium regulating hormones during normal pregnancy. *British Medical Journal* **283**, 10.

Whitsett J.A. & Tsang R.C. (1980) Calcium uptake and binding by membrane fractions of human placenta: ATP-dependent calcium accumulation. *Pediatric Research* **14**, 769.

Wilson D.C. (1931) The incidence of osteomalacia and late rickets in Northern India. *Lancet* **ii**, 10.

Wise P.H. & Hall A.J. (1980) Heparin-induced osteopenia in pregnancy. *British Medical Journal* **iii**, 110.

Woolf L.I., Ounsted C., Lee D., Humphrey M., Cheshire N.M. & Steed G.R. (1961) Atypical phenylketonuria in sisters with normal offspring. *Lancet* **ii**, 464–5.

WHO (1965) Nutrition in Pregnancy and Lactation. Report of a WHO expert Committee. *World Health Organisation Technical Report Series Number* **302**, p. 37.

Yu J.S. & O'Halloran M.T. (1970) Children of mothers with phenylketonuria. *Lancet* **i**, 210–12.

Zaleski A. Casey R.E. & Zaleski W. (1979) Maternal phenylketonuria: dietary treatment during pregnancy. *Canadian Medical Association Journal* **121**, 1591–4.

Zolla-Pazner S., Pazner S.S. *et al* (1980) Osteonecrosis of the femoral head during pregnancy. *Journal of the American Medical Association* **244**, 689.

14 Neurological Disorders

Anthony Hopkins

Neurological disease is uncommon in youth and middle life. It is unlikely that any single obstetrician or neurologist will have an extensive experience in the management of pregnancy and labour in any of the disorders discussed in this chapter. The incidence of epilepsy, for example, is only about 50 per 100 000 per year in the third and fourth decades. The incidence of multiple sclerosis—generally considered amongst neurologists to be a common neurological disease in the USA and northern Europe, is only about one-tenth of this—about 5 per 100 000 per year. However, because the duration of many neurological diseases is long, the prevalence rates are much higher. Whereas an obstetrician is unlikely to see the onset of a neurological illness, such as multiple sclerosis in pregnancy, he is quite likely to be called upon to manage the pregnancy and labour of a woman who already has one of these illnesses. A further general point is that an obstetrician has a crucial role to play in the prevention of neurological disorders.

Antenatal screening

Awareness of the possibility of neural tube defects may allow selective abortion based on elevated maternal serum alpha fetoprotein, elevated alpha fetoprotein in the amniotic fluid, and ultrasound examination of the fetus. Useful reviews are those of Golbus *et al* (1979), Milunsky (1976), and the Working Party of the Medical Research Council (1978). Amniocentesis may also reveal markers of genetically transmitted diseases, such as Tay–Sachs disease. Alternatively, fetal sex may be identified, and allow a selective termination of pregnancy of male fetuses, for example, in the case of Duchenne muscular dystrophy. Table 14.1 lists those commoner neurological conditions in which antenatal diagnosis has proved to be possible and useful. New advances are continually being made. For example, Mahoney *et al* (1977) suggest the estimation of phosphocreatine kinase in fetal blood as a marker of Duchenne dystrophy. The advent of human gene probes should further increase our ability to detect genetic abnormalities.

There may be occasions when termination of pregnancy is justified for genetic disease, even if the sex is unimportant or there is no recognised marker of the disease. For example, 50 per cent of the children of a mother who is already showing the chorea of Huntington's disease will carry the gene. More often, of course, the probabilities are not so clear cut as this. For example, a daughter whose father has Huntington's disease may be pregnant before he has reached the age at which it is clear whether he has the gene or not. The fetus has a risk of carrying the gene of rather less than 0.25—the extent to which it is less than 0.25 being based upon the age that her father has reached without yet showing overt symptoms.

Unfortunately some malformations of the fetal nervous system result from relatively banal infections in pregnancy. For example, mumps virus may cause aqueduct stenosis and hydrocephalus in suckling mice, and possibly also in children (Johnson 1972) (*see also* Chapter 15).

Epilepsy

In September 1980, a Workshop on epilepsy, pregnancy and the child was held in West Berlin, and the proceedings have been published in abstract form (Workshop 1981) and in monograph form (Janz *et al* 1983). This Workshop covers many of the main points which need to be considered in the management of a mother with epilepsy. Other useful reviews are those of Montouris *et al* (1979) and So and Penry (1981).

INHERITANCE OF EPILEPSY

An epileptic mother may first consult her obstetrician about the probabilities of bearing a child with epilepsy. Until about thirty years ago it was believed that the genetic endowment was a major factor in the causation of epilepsy. Belief in the 'epileptic constitution' led, in the case of some states of America and in Scandinavian countries, to the promulgation of laws banning the marriage of those with epilepsy.

There undoubtedly is a genetic component, but it is very difficult to prove. Calculations by Metrakos and Metrakos (1974) have shown that quite modest assumptions about the genetic basis of epilepsy—for example that epilepsy was entirely due to three denes, one dominant and two recessive—could nearly fully account for the

Table 14.1 Prenatal diagnosis of neurological disorders.

Category of disorder	Method of diagnosis
Malformations*	
with dilated lateral ventricles or an abnormality of ventricular system such as absent corpus callosum (e.g. X-linked hydrocephalus) spina bifida,	Ultrasound
anencephaly, iniencephaly, encephalocoele, microcephaly†	Maternal serum and amniotic α-fetoprotein; ultrasound Serial head and body measurements by ultrasound
if associated with anopthalmia, micropthalmia, limb defect, renal agenesis or polycystic disease of kidneys	Ultrasound
Autosomal recessive or X-linked recessive disorder	
with an established metabolic error‡ (e.g. Tay–Sachs disease, Lesch–Nyhan syndrome)	Usually by amniotic cell culture; occasionally using amniotic fluid
with a consistent abnormality of cultured cells (e.g. xeroderma pigmentosum, Cockayne's syndrome, Menkes disease)	Amniotic cell culture
Autosomal dominant disorders	
by linkage to markers in amniotic fluid or fetal blood§ (e.g. myotonic dystrophy Charcot–Marie– Tooth disease, type 1)	Secretor genotype of amniotic fluid
because of consistently associated abnormalities, such as of skin, eye, limbs, kidneys	Duffy blood group in fetal blood Ultrasound
X-linked mental retardation associated with fragile X-chromosome	Fetal blood
X-linked disorders without a specific metabolic or chromosomal defect (e.g. Duchenne muscular dystrophy; other forms of X-linked mental retardation)	Fetal sexing only, using amniotic cells

* *See* Hobbins *et al* (1979) for a recent review.
† Note that some varieties of genetic microcephaly do not develop until after 30 weeks' gestation.
‡ *See* Prenatal Diagnosis Group Newsletter for a recent list of metabolic disorders recognisable prenatally (available from Departments of Clinical Genetics, or from South West Regional Cytogenetic Centre, Southmead Hospital, Bristol).
§ Not all families will be informative for linkage studies.
This table has been prepared with the kind cooperation of Dr Sarah Bundey, Department of Clinical Genetics, Infant Development Unit, Queen Elizabeth Medical Centre, Edgbaston, Birmingham, England.

known prevalence of one in 200. However, we know that, taking a sample of people with epilepsy in the community, the risk of an epileptic adult having a child with epilepsy is only about one chance in 30 (*see below*).

There is one type of epilepsy in which the situation is more clear cut. Metrakos and Metrakos (1974) have published a number of studies about the siblings and parents of those with primary generalised ('constitutional') epilepsy—epilepsy with generalised symmetrical three cycle per second spike, slow wave discharges of which petit-mal attacks are the archetype, and without any structural cause. The studies show that these individuals also have a high probability of having similar electroencephalo-graphic discharges, and a lesser probability of overt seizures. If an allowance is made for the decline of the expression of the gene with age, it appears that the transmission is through an autosomal dominant gene.

Some idea of the overall risk of an epileptic mother bearing an epileptic child in other types of epilepsy can be found in the data from the Workshop (1981). Janz and his colleagues reported on a retrospective study of 768 children of 414 families in which one parent had epilepsy, and the other neither epilepsy nor febrile convulsions. Epilepsy occurred in 3.4 per cent of all children—a risk about five times that of the general population. The risks were higher when the parent had epilepsy of unknown origin, when it was the mother rather than the father who was epileptic, and when the children themselves had already shown febrile convulsions. This risk, and the increased likelihood of the affected parent being a woman was also found in another study reported in the same Workshop, although no clear reason has been advanced for this.

From these studies, it follows that correct counselling of a prospective parent with epilepsy depends upon the sex of the parent affected, and an accurate clinical and electroencephalographic classification of the seizure type of the parent. The risks will be highest if there is clear evidence of primary generalised epilepsy in the family, but will still be greater than for the general population, even if the epilepsy results from a clear cut structural cause, such as a depressed skull fracture, because of the presumed polygenic inheritance of a seizure 'threshold'.

A related question is the probability of the child of an epileptic parent having febrile convulsions. Another study from Berlin (Workshop 1981) showed that the cumulative incidence rate of such convulsions was 4.7 per cent by the age of five years, which is not significantly different from that experienced in the general population. Factors relatively increasing the risk of febrile convulsions are a family history of febrile convulsions, epilepsy with generalised seizures, and a history of perinatal complica-tions. Furthermore, as noted above, if a child of an epileptic parent does have febrile convulsions, then the child's chances of having epilepsy are increased.

MAY PREGNANCY START EPILEPSY?

It must be remembered that the age-specific annual incidence rate for epilepsy is roughly constant at about 50 per 100 000 throughout the childbearing period. Pregnancy and the onset of noneclamptic seizures will therefore coincide by chance alone in a number of women. Although there are some women whose first (of many) seizures occur in pregnancy, there is no study which provides statistical evidence that pregnancy is likely to start epilepsy.

A rather different problem is noneclamptic nonfebrile seizures which occur for the first time in pregnancy, remit in the puerperium, and then return only in subsequent pregnancies. Knight and Rhind (1975) found only two such patients amongst their 59 epileptic mothers studied through 153 pregnancies. Furthermore, it is rare, in a case of pre-existing epilepsy, for seizures to recur during pregnancy after a prolonged seizure-free period. The apparent rarity of these phenomena suggests that pregnancy *per se* is not a particularly potent epileptogenic agent.

GENERALISED SEIZURES OCCURRING IN THE PUERPERIUM

Our clinical impression is that patients are more at risk from seizures during labour and the puerperium. Perhaps this is because the patients are more likely to be under medical supervision at this time, or the emotional strain, fatigue and hyperventilation of labour may account for the increase. One major problem is the differential diagnosis between epilepsy and eclampsia. Eclamptic fits very rarely commence more than three days after delivery; neither do they occur in the absence of hypertension (diastolic blood pressure greater than 90 mmHg) or albuminuria. The patient who is a known epileptic might require intravenous anticonvulsant therapy if her labour is at all prolonged, since the absorption of all drugs is impaired at this time. (Some intramuscular preparations are poorly absorbed and acidic.) The patient who has her first epileptic fit during labour or the puerperium should be treated briefly with anticonvulsant drugs because of the apparent increased risk of further seizures occurring at this time. If she has only one seizure, it would be reasonable to limit therapy to two weeks; repeated seizures will necessitate longer treatment. Phenytoin is probably the drug that is most frequently used, given in a loading dose of 10 mg/kg bodyweight followed by 5 mg/kg/24 hours, monitored, if possible, by estimation of serum levels. Patients who develop generalised seizures for the first time in pregnancy or the puerperium should be investigated in the same way as those developing epilepsy unassociated with pregnancy. A particularly likely cause during pregnancy is expansion of an arteriovenous malformation or meningioma. In the puerperium, a seizure may be the first evidence of cortical venous thrombosis (p. 467).

DOES PREGNANCY MAKE EPILEPSY WORSE?

The effect of pregnancy on the course of epilepsy has been extensively reviewed in recent years. Ramsay *et al* (1978) list seven studies between 1938 and 1976 which show an enormous variation in the frequency of seizures during pregnancy. In one study, 61 per cent of patients had more seizures and 6 per cent fewer; in another study 33 per cent had more seizures and 52 per cent fewer! The average experience from all studies on a total of 155 reported patients was an increase in frequency in 45 per cent of women, a decrease in 12 per cent of women, the frequency remaining unchanged in 43 per cent (Ramsey *et al* 1978). These figures are close to those found in the most recent

British study by Knight and Rhind (1975). They found that whether the epilepsy was idiopathic or symptomatic did not make much difference to these figures, but it should be noted that this study contained an excessively large number of mothers with so-called 'idiopathic' epilepsy, suggesting that classification of seizures was not accurate. Those who had very frequent seizures (monthly or more frequently) were four times more likely to have an increased frequency of seizures during pregnancy than those with occasional seizures (less than one in three months). Knight and Rhind also found that mothers carrying a male fetus were twice as likely to deteriorate than those carrying a female fetus. This rather surprising tendency has been found in two other studies quoted by these authors.

The studies reviewed by Ramsey *et al* (1978) and by So and Penry (1981) will—or indeed already have—become out of date as control of seizures becomes better guided by frequent estimates of serum anticonvulsant levels during pregnancy. For example, one report from the Workshop in Berlin (1981) showed that, in a prospective study of 32 women with epilepsy, seizure frequency did not change in 87 per cent of 38 pregnancies. Improvement in seizure frequency followed the attainment of adequate anticonvulsant drug levels, or replacement of one drug by a more effective one during pregnancy. A larger study from Janz's group, published since this chapter was prepared (Schmidt *et al* 1983), supports these views and places particular stress upon the problems of non-compliance and inadequate supervision of anticonvulsant therapy. These authors also suggest that sleep deprivation during pregnancy may precipitate seizures.

Good compliance and adequate levels of anticonvulsant drugs are not easily attained. First of all, the pregnant epileptic woman is probably increasingly aware of the teratogenic effects of anticonvulsant drugs, which are discussed below. Therefore, either she or another physician, may reduce or stop anticonvulsant drugs in an attempt to reduce the possibility of bearing an abnormal baby. Secondly, pregnancy has multiple effects upon anticonvulsant drug levels.

THE EFFECT OF PREGNANCY UPON ANTICONVULSANT DRUGS

This is reviewed by Lander *et al* (1977) in the Berlin Workshop (1981) and by Janz *et al* (1982). The effects include the following (*see* Fig. 14.1).

1 Fluid retention and the volume of fetal tissues and placenta increase the volume of distribution of the anticonvulsant drugs given orally. This in itself will tend to lower the serum level, if the oral dose is left unchanged.

2 The plasma protein binding of some drugs may be reduced. Ruprah *et al* (1980) have reported in detail upon the binding of phenytoin to serum proteins in the last three months of pregnancy. They have shown that the level of binding is considerably reduced, this reduction largely being accounted for by the concomitant fall in serum albumen. In the presence of such reduced binding, any previous relation between serum phenytoin concentration and therapeutic effect will no longer hold, since a greater proportion of the total drug concentration will be pharmacologically active. These authors point out that in such circumstances the clinical value of measuring

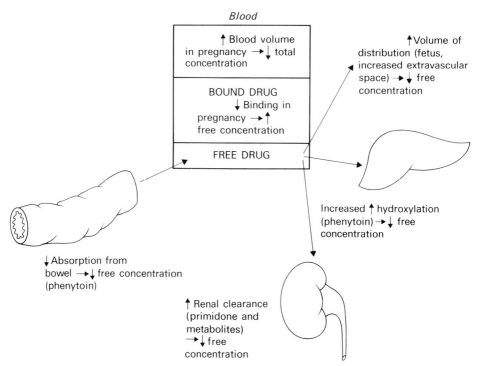

Blood

↑ Blood volume in pregnancy → ↓ total concentration

↑ Volume of distribution (fetus, increased extravascular space) → ↓ free concentration

BOUND DRUG
↓ Binding in pregnancy → ↑ free concentration

FREE DRUG

Increased ↑ hydroxylation (phenytoin) → ↓ free concentration

↓ Absorption from bowel → ↓ free concentration (phenytoin)

↑ Renal clearance (primidone and metabolites) → ↓ free concentration

Fig. 14.1   Anticonvulsant metabolism in pregnancy.

phenytoin levels in whole serum is greatly reduced unless serum binding capacity is measured, or at least some account taken of the fall in serum albumen.

3   The maternal liver may develop an increased capacity for hydroxylation from some anticonvulsant drugs, such as phenytoin (Mygind *et al* 1976).

4   Renal clearance may increase during pregnancy; this has been shown for primidone and its metabolites (Workshop 1981).

5   The absorption of anticonvulsants from the bowel may be reduced. Ramsey *et al* (1978) report a pregnant woman with seizures who had extremely low serum levels of phenytoin, complicated by the occurrence of status epilepticus until the oral dose of phenytoin was increased to 1200 mg per day. Metabolic studies showed that, whereas the proportion of unmetabolised phenytoin in the urine remained unchanged, a very large proportion (56 per cent, normal range 5–15 per cent) was excreted in the stool, this proportion falling to 23 per cent in the postpartum period. The malabsorption was not specific for phenytoin, affecting also d-xylose and dietary fat.

6   Interaction with other drugs occurs. For example, benzodiazepines, which may be given to pregnant women, also lower the serum concentration of phenytoin.

The relationship between folic acid and anticonvulsants deserves special mention. Folic acid, often given during pregnancy, is known to cause a reduction in the level of at least one anticonvulsant drug, phenytoin, and may itself have an epileptogenic effect

(Strauss and Bernstein 1974). However, patients taking anticonvulsants may become folate deficient in pregnancy with deleterious consequences (*see* p. 49). Hiilesmaa *et al* (1983) showed that, although there was an inverse correlation between serum folate and phenytoin or phenobarbitone levels, the number of epileptic seizures during pregnancy showed no relation to serum folate levels. They suggest that a low dose of 100 or 1000 μg of folate is sufficient supplement for pregnant women on these drugs.

Although most of the work has been done on phenytoin, there is little doubt that the metabolisms of carbamazepine, primidone and phenobarbitone are also changed during and after pregnancy.

If the oral dose of an anticonvulsant drug has been increased during pregnancy, as is sometimes indicated, then it is essential that appropriate adjustments are made after delivery, in order that intoxication is avoided.

THE EFFECTS OF EPILEPSY AND ITS THERAPY ON THE FETUS

The Berlin Workshop (1981) reported a number of brief reviews on the outcome of pregnancy in women with epilepsy. Birthweights tend to be lower, and head circumference at birth also lower than in children with mothers without epilepsy and the still-birth rate is increased. These findings were confirmed in the much larger Collaborative Perinatal Project of the National Institute of Neurological and Communicative Disorders and Stroke (Nelson and Ellenberg 1982). The Berlin Workshop also noted an increased rate of surgical intervention, which the authors thought might be explained by '. . . the insecurity on the part of obstetricians in handling epileptic women'.

It is now well recognised that there is an increased chance of fetal abnormality occurring in the pregnancies of epileptic mothers. A large proportion of this increased risk is apparently due to medication, to be discussed below, but some studies have shown that untreated epileptic mothers still have a slightly increased risk of bearing an abnormal child than control mothers. This subject is reviewed by Nakane *et al* (1980). In the 14 studies quoted by them, 4.5 per cent of 825 infants of untreated epileptic mothers were malformed. These authors also examined 18 reports of the outcome of pregnancies of treated epileptic mothers, when the incidence of malformation was 7.1 per cent. Nakane and his colleagues do point out that '. . . although there is considerable discrepancy among previous authors (reviewed) as to the definitions of and criteria for malformation, and it would be difficult to draw specific conclusions about these results as a whole, they do serve to point out the general trend.'

Another way of distinguishing between the contribution of epilepsy *per se*, and its treatment is to compare the children of men with epilepsy, and the children of women with epilepsy. Two such studies were reported at the Workshop (1981). Anneggers and Hauser found that the children of men with epilepsy did not have increased rates of congenital malformations of specific types. However, studies from Janz's department in Berlin found that facial clefts were found with a higher incidence than expected in children of epileptic fathers.

Another approach has been to study the incidence of epilepsy among parents with children with facial clefts—the commonest abnormality found in the children of epileptic mothers (Friis 1979). Friis found that the point prevalence of epilepsy amongst the parents of facial cleft probands was 2.3 per cent, about three times the expected value ($P<0.05$). A teratogenic effect of anticonvulsant medication would be reflected in a higher number of female than male epileptic parents. However, there was no significant difference between the sex of the parents in the study. Friis *et al* (1981) have furthermore shown that the incidence of facial clefts among those with epilepsy is twice that expected from the general population. The studies by Friis, by Janz and by Nakane all suggest that epilepsy *per se* is a factor in the genesis of facial clefts. It could be that there is a specific genetic linkage between epilepsy and fetal abnormality; or it could be argued that women with epilepsy are limited in their choice of husband who may be less biologically 'fit'.

These studies do not exclude the possibility that, in other epileptic mothers, anticonvulsant drugs are still teratogenic. Indeed, the review by Nakane *et al* (1980) showed that in all published studies the incidence of malformation for treated epileptics was 7.1 per cent, compared to 4.5 per cent for untreated epileptic mothers. The figure of 7.1 per cent from their review of the literature was close to their own figure of 8.7 per cent of 657 treated epileptic patients. It is generally accepted that the malformations which are most increased by the effect of anticonvulsant medication and epilepsy are hare lip and cleft palate, but cardiac lesions and hypoplasia of nails and digits are also more frequent. Hypoplasia of the optic nerve has also recently been reported (Hoyt and Billson 1978). Of course, in any large retrospective survey some abnormal children will be found in which the abnormality is coincident to the epilepsy and anticonvulsant treatment.

Until recently, many people with epilepsy have been taking more than one drug, so it is difficult to ascribe blame to any particular drug; however, analysis of all the reports incriminate hydantoins and barbiturates in particular. The large survey by Nakane and colleagues shows clearly that the malformation rate increased dramatically when drugs are used in combination. When four anticonvulsant drugs were used in 69 patients, the malformation rate rose to approximately 25 per cent.

Paulson and Paulson (1981) and Janz (1982) have recently reviewed again the whole problem of the teratogenic effects of anticonvulsants. They, and a number of earlier workers quoted by them, call attention to the fetal hydantoin syndrome, the defects of which include small digits, midline fusion failures, reduced mental abilities, and possibly congenital heart disease, trigonocephaly, microcephaly and hypertelorism. Other patients have abnormal ears, a short neck, and other skeletal abnormalities.

It is not known why anticonvulsants particularly affect the closure of the facial cleft. Proliferation of mesenchymal cells is active in the fetus at the tips of the palatal shelves. Phenytoin, which in adults causes fibroblastic proliferation in lips and gums, may interfere with such cell proliferation at the edge of the facial cleft. It is also important to remember that genetic factors and phenytoin may interact. It has been shown that the incidence of malformations induced by phenytoin in mice varies with the strain of mouse as well as with the dose used.

When talking to patients along these lines, it is reassuring to remind them that the incidence of facial clefting is still low even in patients taking anticonvulsants. The random incidence in the population is of the order of 1 per 1000: even if the risk is increased tenfold, 990 babies will still have normal faces and palates.

Paulson and Paulson (1981) review various animal studies carried out on anticonvulsants. They point out that many such studies have been performed with doses of medications tenfold or more than the usual dose, but that malformations also occur at doses more comparable with human therapeutic levels. In general, carbamazepine seems less teratogenic in mice than phenytoin. There is a particular interest in sodium valproate at present, as it is a very effective anticoagulant drug and, in those not pregnant, the drug of choice for primary generalized epilepsy. It is relatively free from unwanted effects. Paulson and Paulson review the teratogenic effects of sodium valproate on mice. At doses between 15 and 25 times the human therapeutic range, up to 31 per cent of the fetuses are resorbed or dead, and 6 per cent show exencephaly. Other studies suggest that the risk of spina bifida in the infants of mothers taking valproate may be even higher. For example up to 30 per cent of all malformations in the infants of mothers taking valproate may be cases of spina bifida and it has been estimated that valproate may increase the risk of this condition by 15-fold (Leck 1983). Bailey *et al* (1983) reviewed the literature concerning valproate teratogenicity, and reported two cases of multiple congenital abnormalities associated with its use in pregnancy. Clearly valproate should be avoided in early pregnancy, as the manufacturers have always stated. After appropriate counselling, those women who do inadvertently take valproate in the first few months of pregnancy should be offered amniocentesis for alpha-fetoprotein estimation.

Troxidone should not be used now in pregnancy. Feldman *et al* (1977) review the fetal trimethadime syndrome previously recognised.

The obstetrician and neurologist have to balance two conflicting interests in managing a pregnant woman with epilepsy. On the one hand, she may be advised to continue to take anticonvulsant drugs during pregnancy, probably in increased oral dosage so that adequate serum levels can be maintained, in order to avoid the risks of seizures and in particular of status epilepticus occurring during pregnancy (Goodwin and Lawson 1947). On the other hand, reducing or stopping anticonvulsant drugs may be suggested in order to reduce the chances of a congenital malformation. A careful review of all the relevant factors is necessary before a decision can be reached, but it must be remembered that more harm than good may result if a woman has an increased number of major seizures due to reduction or arrest of anticonvulsant medication.

In these litigious days, it is probably wise to advise the mother taking anticonvulsant drugs of the broad outlines of the problems reviewed above.

THE PERINATAL PERIOD

Even if a baby is born without significant malformation to an epileptic mother, its problems are not necessarily over. Immediately after delivery, the level of anticonvulsants, which have freely crossed the placenta, begin to decline in the baby. The rate of clearance from the new-born has been described in the Berlin Workshop (1981) and elsewhere (Koup *et al* 1978). The half life for ethosuximide is 41 hours, for sodium valproate 40–45 hours, for primidone 23 hours, and for phenobarbitone 113 hours.

Desmond *et al* (1972) described the effects of barbiturate withdrawal in the neonate. The clinical signs are hyperexcitability, occasional seizures, tremulousness and impaired suckling. Kaneko and his colleagues have recently studied 42 infants and 32 epileptic mothers for harmful side-effects of anticonvulsant therapy (Berlin Workshop 1981). They compared these infants with 50 infants of normal mothers and found less efficient suckling and slower gains in weight in the infants of epileptic mothers. Expectant supervision of such children is usually adequate, but if tremulousness or, in particular, if seizures occur, small doses of phenobarbitone (3–5 mg/kg/day) may be given.

Some infants have bled as a result of drug-induced depression of vitamin K-dependent clotting factors, such as prothrombin and Factors V and VII (Solomon *et al* 1973). Vitamin K 20 mg/day should be routinely administered for the last two weeks of pregnancy to the mother treated with anticonvulsants and also given intramuscularly to her new-born infant (p. 49).

BREAST FEEDING

Mothers will wish to know whether it is safe to breast feed their children, wondering whether the anticonvulsant drug passes into the milk. Coradello (1973) studied this point for the older drugs, and the Berlin Workshop reports on sodium valproate. With the exception of phenobarbitone, negligible quantities of drugs pass into the milk; there is, however, significant transmission of phenobarbitone and if the mother desires to breast feed it would be preferable to change the medication before or during pregnancy.

Cerebrovascular disease

Much of the published work in this field is confusing. For example, Amias (1970a) records a series of cases of intracranial haemorrhage in pregnancy, but it is only with difficulty that the cases of primary intracerebral haemorrhage are disentangled from those with primary subarachnoid haemorrhage—two types of intracranial bleeding in which the pathology and prognosis is very different. Similarly, hemiplegia in pregnancy and the puerperium has been attributed to cerebral venous thrombosis in reports published before the more or less routine investigative use of carotid arteriography; these must be regarded with suspicion. Cross *et al* (1968) and Amias (1970b) have subsequently shown the high incidence of arterial occlusive disease in pregnancy. It is necessary to consider arterial occlusive disease, venous occlusive disease, intracerebral haemorrhage and subarachnoid haemorrhage quite separately.

ARTERIAL OCCLUSIVE DISEASE

It is not generally realised that occlusions of major arteries occur with some frequency in both sexes of the age group 15–45. Jennett and Cross (1967) found that about 12 per cent of all their proved occlusions of all ages in the years 1956–65 were in women in this age group. Glasgow, the centre from which they write, then acted as virtually the only specialised centre capable of undertaking arteriography in a population of about three million. Jennett and Cross (1967) and Cross *et al* (1968) analysed the relationship of pregnancy and the puerperium to arterial occlusive disease. Of the 65 women aged 15–45 with proven arterial occlusion, 23 (35 per cent) were pregnant—a pregnancy rate more than three times the general population pregnancy rate. The incidence of an arterial occlusion in pregnancy and the puerperium was assessed at 1 per 20 000 live births. The mortality rate was more than twice that of males of the same age group and three times that of nonpregnant females of the same age group. Middle artery occlusion is the commonest finding in pregnancy, and internal carotid artery occlusion in the puerperium.

The pathological basis of occlusion of major arteries is uncertain. As oral contraceptive therapy also increases the incidence of arterial occlusion some 3–4 times (Collaborative Group for the Study of Strokes in Young Women 1973), hormonal factors are probably important. References to the changes in levels of clotting factors and lipids that occur during pregnancy are available in the paper of Bansal *et al* (1974) (*see also* p. 73), but there is no evidence linking these changed levels to the occurrence of the occlusion.

Once an occlusion of a major cerebral artery has occurred, there is no really effective treatment. Some studies suggest that it is worth giving glycerol or dexamethasone in order to reduce oedema, or low-molecular-weight dextran to prevent further sludging, but controlled trials have failed to show a consistent effect.

CEREBRAL VENOUS THROMBOSIS

As noted above, this entity is probably overdiagnosed. Cross *et al* (1968) did not encounter a single case during the ten years in which 23 pregnant and puerperal women presented with arterial occlusion. At the other extreme Abraham *et al* (1970), writing from India, record that 25 per cent of all strokes in women under 40 were due to puerperal phlebothrombosis or thrombophlebitis. Such an enormous difference is presumably accounted for by national differences in the incidence of postpartum haemorrhage and sepsis. Faced with such extremes, it is advisable to confine one's attention to those few cases adequately investigated by arteriography (e.g. Kalbag and Woolf 1967; Krayenbühl 1967; Estanol *et al* 1979).

The chief symptoms are headache, drowsiness and vomiting, associated with a hemiplegia taking several hours or so to develop. Partial motor or generalised convulsions are frequent. Both paresis and seizures may spread to the other hemisphere, indicating involvement of the tributaries of the superior sagittal sinus in the contralateral hemisphere.

Confirmation of the diagnosis of cerebral venous thrombosis may be obtained by cerebral arteriography with special emphasis taken on films taken in the later phases after injection—up to twelve seconds. Oblique and subtraction films are often desirable, and sometimes essential, to show abnormalities of filling in cortical venous drainage.

It is not clear why women in the postpartum period or indeed women on the oral contraceptive pill should be specially predisposed to cerebral venous thrombosis. Bansal *et al* (1974) compared the serum lipid and the blood fibrinolytic activity in 17 patients of clinically diagnosed puerperal cerebral venous thrombosis, with normal puerperal controls. A significant rise in serum triglycerides, phospholipids, free fatty acids, and a fall in blood fibrinolytic activity was found in the cases of thrombosis. Estanol *et al* (1979) found some evidence of a hypercoagulable state in ten out of 14 young women with intracranial thrombosis, some of whom were pregnant. Occasionally, cerebral venous thrombosis is found in association with thrombosis in the venous system elsewhere. Such a case is reported by Lavin *et al* (1978). This lends some credence to the view that in pregnancy there is a hypercoagulable state. In Lavin's case, quite exceptionally, the thrombosis occurred in the first trimester. Apart from changes in the coagulability of the blood, other suggestions have been advanced. It has been suggested that there may be embolism of pelvic thrombi via the paravertebral venous plexus to the cerebral vein (Batson 1940).

An interesting clinical variant of cortical venous thrombosis has recently been reported by Beal and Chapman (1980). They call attention to the occurrence of visual field defects, and even cortical blindness as a result of bilateral cortical venous infarction. It is recognised that bizarre behaviour, even denial of apparent blindness, may be seen in those with occipital lobe infarction (Anton's syndrome). Singh *et al* (1980) report a similar case.

As soon as the diagnosis of cortical venous thrombosis is made, anxiety will naturally follow about the best method of treatment. Although anticoagulation may seem the obvious choice, the frequent presence of red blood cells in the spinal fluid (Carroll *et al* 1966) is a worry. Some workers (Castaigne *et al* 1977) have reported very worthwhile improvement after heparin infusions, even in patients who have had large numbers of red cells in the spinal fluid. A reasonable compromise, suggested by Beal and Chapman (1980), is to do a cranial CT scan and, if there is no visible intracranial haemorrhage and the patient's condition is rapidly deteriorating, a trial of heparin might be justified. Another suggestion, made by Kalbag and Woolf (1967), is the use of low-molecular-weight dextran. In addition to these measures, designed to prevent further thrombosis, the use of steroids to reduce cerebral oedema and intracranial pressure is advisable. A suitable dose would be dexamethasone 20 mg/24 hours. Furthermore, anticonvulsants should be given even if the subject has not had a seizure, as the risk of seizures is so high. An intravenous infusion of phenytoin 10 mg/kg bodyweight will rapidly produce therapeutic serum anticonvulsant levels, which should thereafter be monitored by daily measurements, the oral dose of approximately 5 mg/kg bodyweight/24 hours meanwhile being continued.

Estanol *et al* (1979) treated a small number of patients with thrombosis of the superior sagittal sinus by surgical thrombectomy, passing a Fogarty catheter in each direction down the sinus through a midline incision. One of their four patients died, and Estanol suggests that the operation is indicated only if there is rapidly deteriorating vision and medical treatment to control life-threatening intracranial pressure has failed.

SUBARACHNOID HAEMORRHAGE

This has been the subject of many reviews and case reports. Reviews in the neurosurgical literature include those of Robinson *et al* (1972, 1974) and, in the obstetric literature, of Amias (1970a). Although it is generally considered that pregnancy does not greatly increase the chances of an *aneurysm* bleeding, a recent paper by Garcia *et al* (1979) suggested that a more active process may occur in pregnancy. Histology of their patient's ruptured spinal aneurysm showed a frayed and disintegrated lamina elastica and muscularis, with dilatation, focal haemorrhagic dissection, necrosis and polymorphonuclear inflammatory reaction—rather like the histology of a mycotic aneurysm, though no organisms were found.

There is no clear relationship to parity, and bleeding may occur at any time, though it is more likely later in pregnancy. Haemorrhage during labour is exceptional. Aneurysms are at the typical sites: on the circle of Willis or on proximal or major branches from the circle. The neurosurgical management of a bleed is, ideally, as if the woman were not pregnant—early arteriography and early definitive neurosurgical occlusion of the aneurysm if possible. The obstetric management is assisted delivery with epidural anaesthesia because of the remote risk of rupture. Patients who are deeply comatose from subarachnoid haemorrhage, or even those who have clinical brain death, may still have a normal labour (Friedman *et al* 1983).

Arteriovenous malformations, however, are clearly more likely to bleed during pregnancy (Robinson *et al* 1974), and they seem more prone to rupture during labour. Whereas they are an uncommon cause of subarachnoid bleeding in nonpregnant patients in Europe and North America, they do account for about half the cases of subarachnoid haemorrhage in pregnancy. It has been suggested that circulating steroid hormones in pregnancy cause the smooth muscle wall of angiomas to dilate. If angiography shows that the angioma is accessible to neurosurgery, then definitive operation should be undertaken as soon as possible, since Robinson *et al* (1974) show that untreated arteriovenous malformations carry a 33 per cent mortality rate in pregnancy. If neurosurgical management is not practical, then it would be wise to deliver the baby by Caesarean section.

INTRACEREBRAL HAEMORRHAGE

Apart from haemorrhage occurring during eclampsia, primary intracerebral haemorrhage in pregnancy is rare. When it occurs, it is almost always due to a leak from a buried arteriovenous malformation. Amias (1970b), for example, reported 52 cases of intracranial haemorrhage in pregnancy and the puerperium, of which aneurysms accounted for 21 and angiomas for 19. The cause was undetermined in twelve but in only four of these was the site of bleeding primarily intracerebral, and only one of these was at a site at which it commonly occurs in older people—the midbrain. These and other papers make it clear that there is little possibility of an intracranial bleed from a Charcot–Bouchard aneurysm of the type common in the elderly hypertensive.

Cerebral and spinal tumours

PITUITARY TUMOUR (*see* Chapter 12)

MENINGIOMA

Bickerstaff *et al* (1958) describe two cases and review others in which meningiomas in the parasellar region or on the medial sphenoid wing caused cranial nerve palsies or deterioration of vision in pregnancy, with subsequent remission of symptoms on delivery. Relapse of symptoms may take place during subsequent pregnancies. Spinal meningiomas may expand rapidly in pregnancy to cause a paraparesis.

ASTROCYTOMA

It is generally believed that pregnancy accelerates the course of astrocytomas, but the behaviour of these tumours is so variable that the point has not been firmly established. Certainly, the literature contains no study demonstrating remission of symptoms following delivery or termination.

ANGIOMA

Pregnancy certainly provokes subarachnoid haemorrhage from intracranial angiomas, as discussed earlier. Aminoff and Logue (1974) also record the episodic presence of spinal symptoms in each of three pregnancies, in a woman with a spinal angioma, and give references to similar case reports.

NEUROFIBROMA

Swapp and Main (1973) describe ten pregnant patients with cutaneous neurofibromatosis. In five of the patients, lesions appeared for the first time during pregnancy and in the others the lesions increased in size and number only to regress after delivery. All ten patients were hypertensive, but there was no evidence of increased excretion of catecholamines. A similar study has been reported by Edwards *et al* (1983). Jarvis and Crompton (1978) could not confirm this high incidence of hypertension in their series.

Acoustic neuromas have also been shown to expand sharply during pregnancy. Allen *et al* (1974) described acoustic neuromas in five women who noted the onset of symptoms during the second half of pregnancy, and a further woman whose earlier symptoms became substantially worse.

Benign intracranial hypertension

The course of benign intracranial hypertension in pregnancy has been reviewed by Greer (1963), by Powell (1972) and by Shekleton *et al* (1980). The cases reported presented between the second and fifth month of pregnancy. Greer comments that this is the time in pregnancy that oestrogen levels rise and urinary corticoid excretion falls. Occasionally the problem recurs in subsequent pregnancies (Nickerson and Kirk 1965).

The disease is self-limiting and of shorter duration in pregnant than in nonpregnant women. Nevertheless, if papilloedema is severe and vision threatened, treatment must be undertaken urgently. In nonpregnant women operative subtemporal decompression is now virtually never required, diuretic therapy with chlorthalidone being successful in reducing papilloedema and the area of the blind spot (Jefferson and Clark 1976). It is probable that this would be sufficient in pregnant women.

The traditional treatment of draining the subarachnoid space by repeated lumbar punctures has now fallen into disuse as continuous records of intracranial pressure, measured by extradural transducer, have shown that it 'bounces back' within an hour or so of lumbar puncture.

In nonpregnant women, large doses of oral steroids may be successful in controlling the intracranial pressure, but this treatment has not been used in pregnancy.

Powell (1972) points out that, in those cases reported in the literature, spontaneous resolution of papilloedema usually followed delivery or termination—suggesting that in rare cases termination might be justified if vision were threatened—probably more justified than subtemporal decompression.

Multiple sclerosis and pregnancy

The question of whether the course of multiple sclerosis is affected by pregnancy is reviewed at length in the monograph of McAlpine *et al* (1972). It is necessary to compare the relapse rate per woman year for those pregnant and those not pregnant, bearing in mind the fact that, as the course of the disease is so variable, the series must contain sufficient numbers of patients matched closely for age of onset and clinical state on entering the study.

The relapse rate for single and married women is about 0.1/woman/year. The relapse rate per pregnant woman year is about 0.25—the pregnancy year including three months after delivery. At least as many relapses occur during these three months as in the nine months of pregnancy.

If a woman asks about the risks of deterioration as a result of pregnancy she should therefore be warned to take as much rest as possible in the puerperium. But there is another factor to be remembered. If the mother is already much affected when she becomes pregnant, she may be so disabled within a year or so of birth that the burden of child-rearing will fall on other members of the family.

Multiple sclerosis itself has no effect upon the course of pregnancy or labour (Sweeney 1958). If the disease has caused paraplegia, then the same principles apply as are discussed below.

Chorea gravidarum

At the time of Willson and Preece's exhaustive account (1932), this disease was relatively uncommon, yet the authors could collect accounts of 104 choreic pregnancies, and study a further 846 reported in the literature. Chorea gravidarum is now exceptionally rare, and the obstetrician or gynaecologist is more likely to see chorea as a complication arising between about two and six months after he has prescribed an oral contraceptive. Numerous reports of 'contraceptive chorea' have appeared in recent years (Riddoch *et al* 1972; Pulsinelli and Hamill 1978). Chorea may arise because oestrogen affects catecholamine turnover within the brain, but the exact mechanism is uncertain.

Chorea gravidarum is most likely to begin in the first trimester, but may begin at any stage of pregnancy. A previous history of Sydenham's chorea is found in about half the cases. Beresford and Graham (1950) also showed that about 4 per cent of those with a history of Sydenham's chorea developed chorea gravidarum. Once chorea has occurred in one pregnancy, subsequent pregnancies are also likely to be complicated by chorea. The mechanism of reactivation of chorea is totally obscure, but the association of chorea with contraceptives does suggest that humoral factors are important. Bird *et al* (1976) have shown that minimal persistent signs after Sydenham's chorea are much more frequent than was previously recognised.

Not only has chorea gravidarum become much less frequent in recent years, it has also become much milder. Maternal mortality dropped from 13 per cent in Willson and Preece's series (1932) to 2 per cent in Beresford and Graham's series (1950). The principal 'complications'—or really manifestations of the same process—are cardiac lesions (35 per cent in 1950) and psychosis (3 per cent in 1950). Ichikawa *et al* (1980) have recently reported neuropathological observations on a fatal case of chorea gravidarum, the first extensive autopsy reported since 1936. This unfortunate patient was a primigravida whose pregnancy had been uneventful until approximately the 36th week when she began to notice increasing anxiety and restlessness. In the 39th week of her pregnancy, she was noted to be suffering from choreiform movements, and these worsened within a few days to the point where she could only with great difficulty eat, drink or sleep. She developed a high fever, and this was accompanied by a severe generalised rhabdomyolysis. The principal findings were sharply circumscribed foci of acute tissue necrosis in the cerebral cortex, caudate nucleus and thalamus, sometimes in close proximity to capillaries occluded by fibrin thrombi. There was also a mild-to-moderate loss of nerve cells in the caudate nucleus and putamen, with a striking proliferation of mildly hypertrophied astrocytes.

These authors justifiably point out that chorea in pregnancy should not necessarily be assumed to be of rheumatic origin. For example, the choreiform movements of Huntington's disease may also make their initial appearance during pregnancy. Furthermore certain sedative drugs of the phenothiazine group, particularly fluphenazine, may cause dystonic reactions resembling chorea. Therefore the previous drug history of those with chorea should be reviewed to see if these drugs have been administered. Chorea is also a rare complication of SLE in pregnancy (p. 260).

Successful management of the pregnancy and labour complicated by rheumatic chorea depends largely on any associated cardiac lesion. Adequate rest, quiet and reassurance will help the chorea, but sedation by a benzodiazepine or chlorpromazine may be required. Termination of pregnancy is now unlikely to be required.

Migraine

Two series of interviews on large numbers of pregnant women have been carried out in Ireland and Australia, to determine the effect of pregnancy on migraine (Callaghan 1968; Somerville 1972). By and large, the studies confirm the old belief that pre-existing migraine is strikingly improved during pregnancy in about 80 per cent of women. Somerville investigated the possibility that alterations in plasma progesterone levels might be associated with this improvement, but he found no evidence for this view, insofar as the mean levels in those whose symptoms were better during pregnancy were no different from those whose symptoms did not change or deteriorate. It is still possible, however, that the generally raised level of progesterone does inhibit cranial vasomotor responses. Any hypothesis linking improvement to pregnancy also has to take into account the fact that most studies contain numbers of patients who begin migraine for the first time during pregnancy. It is possible that investigation of social factors (e.g. whether the mother was pleased to be pregnant) may be more meaningful.

Attacks of migraine occurring during pregnancy are best treated by soluble aspirin, in association with metoclopramide. If attacks are frequent, attention should be paid to the dietary factors which precipitate migraine in some women—alcohol (and, in particular, red wine), strong cheeses and chocolate. Regular small meals may be advised, as relative hypoglycaemia may trigger an episode.

Those interested in menstrual migraine can consult two other papers by Somerville (1975a, 1975b), in which he finds no support for the previously expressed view that the rapidly declining progesterone levels just before menstruation are responsible for the precipitation of migraine at that time.

Neuropathies

MONONEUROPATHIES

The carpal tunnel syndrome

The median nerve passes from forearm to hand behind the flexor retinaculum, in company with the flexor tendons and their sheaths. The weight gain of pregnancy is sometimes sufficient to limit further the already small space available for this nerve, and tingling in the lateral three or four digits results. This tingling is classically nocturnal and extremely painful. Progression to weakness of abductor pollicis brevis is not common but may occur. The association of this now well recognised syndrome with pregnancy was first reported by Wallace and Cook (1957). Computed scanning of the wrists has shown a range of cross-sectional areas of the carpal tunnel. It is probable that those with congenitally narrow tunnels are those most likely to have symptoms.

If the pregnancy is near term, it would be reasonable to tide the mother over with splints which dorsiflex the hand at night, or with an injection of hydrocortisone into the carpal tunnel, as the symptoms commonly remit after delivery. However, operative decompression is so simple that it should not be long delayed in the face of persistent symptoms. It should certainly be recommended if weakness occurs.

Meralgia paraesthetica

The lateral cutaneous nerve of the thigh passes through the inguinal ligament. The weight gain of pregnancy, and the tension on the connective tissue of the abdominal wall, may lead to compression of the nerve. Pearson (1957) amongst others, has recorded the onset of symptoms of paraesthesia and numbness in the anterolateral aspect of the thigh occurring in pregnancy, and slowly remitting after delivery. Operative decompression is often disappointing.

Bell's palsy

The facial nerve passes through a long bony canal as it leaves the skull, and oedema may again be responsible for the greatly increased incidence of Bell's palsy in pregnancy. Hilsinger *et al* (1975) have shown that the risk of idiopathic facial paralysis in pregnant women is 45 per 100 000 births—3.3 times the risk to nonpregnant women in the same age group.

The palsy is most likely to occur in the third trimester. The outcome is just as favourable as in the nonpregnant woman; there is no evidence that prednisone is beneficial unless given within 24 hours of the onset. Other relative contraindications to steroid therapy, apart from delay after the onset of symptoms, include diabetes and hypertension. If steroids are used, a reasonable regime would be prednisone 60 mg per day in divided doses for three days, reducing the dose to zero over a period of about ten days. Operative decompression of the facial nerve is no longer performed, as the results have proved poor.

Pressure palsies in the pelvis and lumbar disc protrusions

Common peroneal nerve palsies are sometimes seen if the supports which maintain the thighs in the lithotomy position have been incorrectly adjusted. But sometimes after labour a foot drop is seen without any obvious trauma to a peripheral nerve. Brown and MacDougall (1957) hold that the fetal head can compress the fourth and fifth lumbar roots as they form a cord to pass into the pelvis.

Foot drop is also more common after instrumental vaginal delivery, particularly those deliveries involving rotation with Kielland's forceps. Exceptionally, fibroids which are rapidly increasing in size during pregnancy may have the same effect (Hefferman *et al* 1980). O'Connell (1944) wrote that the majority of cases of sciatic pain and foot drop are due to lumbar disc protrusions occurring late in pregnancy or in labour. Although distressing to the patient, foot drop occurring in labour usually remits spontaneously, even though it may take several months to achieve complete recovery. Physiotherapy helps the patient's morale.

POLYNEUROPATHIES

In developing countries it is probable that some cases of polyneuropathy in pregnancy are caused by thiamine deficiency. In Western countries, acute infective polyneuro-pathy (Guillain–Barré syndrome) occasionally occurs in pregnancy, but not more often than would be expected by chance. The management has been reviewed by Sudo and Weingold (1975). They believe that termination of pregnancy is not necessary. A review of their paper suggests that if tracheostomy and intermittent positive pressure ventilation is needed because of respiratory paralysis, the prognosis is grave. Three out of the four patients in this group died. It appears that Caesarean section might have improved this mortality.

In milder cases, there is no reason why the pregnancy should not go to term. The children are not affected.

Calderon-Gonzales and his colleagues (1970) described a patient with a relapsing polyneuropathy that occurred three times in three pregnancies, and once while taking oral contraceptives. Conductive velocity was very slow, so the neuropathy was probably of the demyelinating type.

Neuromuscular diseases

DYSTROPHIA MYOTONICA

Dystrophia myotonica is a dominantly inherited dystrophic disorder characterised by muscular weakness, myotonia (repetitive contractions of muscle fibres in response to a single neural discharge, resulting in delayed relaxation of muscles), frontal alopecia, lenticular opacities and testicular atrophy in males. Those affected are usually of below-average IQ.

There have been a number of case reports and reviews of the effects of pregnancy on this condition (Hopkins and Wray 1967; Shore and MacLachlan 1972; Sarnat *et al* 1976). Although fertility in affected women may be decreased, pregnancy is not uncommon. The degree of muscular weakness and myotonia suffered by the mother may increase, usually by about the 28th week of pregnancy. Improvement may occur after delivery. Some mothers do not deteriorate. Hopkins and Wray (1967) suggested that deterioration might be related to the effect of progesterone on the intracellular/extracellular potassium concentration ratio.

There is a high rate of fetal loss due to spontaneous abortion, premature delivery, and neonatal death from congenital myotonic dystrophy. Premature labour may be related to uterine myotonia or to polyhydramnios, which is frequently associated.

Abnormalities of all three stages of labour have been described—either inert (responsive to oxytocin) or precipitate. The second stage may be prolonged due to maternal weakness; postpartum haemorrhage then may occur.

Children with the genotype may not develop overt evidence of the disease until late in life; in others, there is congenital myotonic dystrophy, characterised by facial diplegia, talipes and arthrogryposis multiplex. Clinical myotonia is seldom seen in the affected infants, but electromyography reveals it. Severely affected children can be born to mildly affected mothers, and vice versa.

Affected mothers should be offered termination of pregnancy, as 50 per cent of the fetuses will carry the gene. Medication (with procainamide) has little effect on either myotonia or weakness. Delivery should certainly take place in hospital.

MYOTONIA CONGENITA (THOMSEN'S DISEASE)

As in dystrophia myotonica, weakness may become more pronounced during the second half of pregnancy (Hakim and Thomlinson 1969).

MYASTHENIA GRAVIS

The prevalence of myasthenia is about 1 per 20 000 of the general population. The disease is commoner in females than in males, and the peak decades of incidence are in the years of childbearing. Weakness and easy fatiguability of muscles affects particularly the external ocular, facial and bulbar muscles, and the proximal muscles of the limbs. In severely affected cases, ventilation is impaired. There is increasing evidence that the disorder is caused by circulating antibody to acetylcholine receptor protein (Pinching *et al* 1976). Approximately 60 per cent of cases have thymic enlargement and 8 per cent a malignant thymoma. Thymectomy relieves symptoms in about 40 per cent of cases, but treatment with anticholinesterase compounds such as prostigmine is often necessary.

The obstetric management of myasthenia gravis has been reviewed in a number of series (Frazer and Turner 1953; Plauche 1964; Chambers *et al* 1967). Some patients continue unchanged throughout pregnancy, some few remit, and some deteriorate in the second trimester; however, by far the most likely time for deterioration to occur is in the postpartum period. Plauche, in his review, shows that there are no factors which will allow an accurate prediction of the outcome in any one case.

Vaginal delivery is usually uneventful in the mildly affected case, but the obstetrician must be prepared to shorten the second stage with a low forceps delivery if ventilation or voluntary muscular assistance to the unaffected uterine musculature shows signs of fatigue. It must be remembered that muscular relaxants are extremely poorly tolerated in myasthenic patients, and should be avoided if general anaesthesia is necessary. It is also important, for all concerned in the management of the myasthenic patient, to know of the possibility of deterioration in muscle strength due to overdosage with anticholinesterase compounds. Skilled neurological assessment is often necessary. However, it may be remembered that meiotic pupils usually indicate overdosage. The response to a 1 mg dose of edrophonium (Tensilon) will also help—if brisk transient deterioration occurs, then the crisis is cholinergic (overdosage) rather than myasthenic. Perry *et al* (1975) state that anticholinesterase medication does not enter breast milk, so that the infant can be breast fed.

About 10 per cent of all children born to myasthenic mothers will have transient neonatal myasthenia (Teng and Osserman 1956). Symptoms are present at birth or a day or two afterwards. The principal signs are of limpness and hypotonia, with an absent or impaired Moro reflex, inability to suck, and poor cry. In contrast to adults, the external ocular muscles are seldom affected. The infants improve spontaneously over a few days, but if there is difficulty in breathing, small doses of anticholinesterase compounds may be given (e.g. 0.05 mg of prostigmine by injection). Exceeding care should be taken before larger doses are given (Namba *et al* 1970).

Finally, the very limited experience of malignant thymoma in pregnancy (Goldman 1974), suggests that pregnancy precipitates the extrathoracic spread of tumour and termination would be justifiable.

CARNITINE DEFICIENCY

Cornelio *et al* (1978) and Angelini *et al* (1978) have both described patients with carnitine deficiency whose muscles have become profoundly weak during pregnancy or in the immediate postpartum period. Carnitine is apparently essential in the transport of longchain fatty acids into mitochondria. If deficient, excessive lipid accumulates in muscle fibres and is easily visible on muscle biopsy. The metabolic defect, probably inherited through a recessive gene, is of great interest, as oral supplement of the diet with carnitine can reverse the process.

Pregnancy and labour in paraplegia

Robertson (1972) has reviewed the experience of Guttmann's pioneering unit at Stoke Mandeville in England. During the years 1952–72 26 paraplegic women had 39 babies. The principal complication of pregnancy to be feared is renal tract infection and, if renal function is already impaired as a consequence of recurrent infections, it would be wise to advise against pregnancy. If the spinal cord is completely divided above the 10th thoracic segment, labour is painless and because of this the onset may be difficult to diagnose, and premature labour in unfavourable circumstances may result. Robertson gives the following example, 'A patient . . . in the 34th week of pregnancy gave birth, unaware labour had started. She rang her bell at 4.00 a.m. and told the nurse that she could hear a baby crying. When the nurse pulled back the bed-clothes, there was no doubt which baby was crying.' Normal polarised uterine contractions do occur, but forceps delivery is often necessary, due to the paralysis of muscles assisting the expulsive efforts. Caesarean section is very rarely needed but was in the case described by Nath (1979), in whom hypertensive crises (autonomic hyperreflexia), in association with labour, complicated a high spinal lesion. In less severe cases, β-adrenergic blockade might well prove sufficient.

Other neurological disorders

ENCEPHALITIS

Encephalitis is occasionally associated with pregnancy, by chance. One case report is that of Jewett (1975).

WERNICKE'S ENCEPHALOPATHY

Wernicke's encephalopathy, due to thiamine deficiency, may result from profound hyperemesis gravidarum (Berkwitz and Lufkin 1932; Victor *et al* 1971; Wood *et al* 1983). Very early recognition of the diagnosis, based on some clouding of consciousness, nystagmus, diplopia and ataxia, is essential, and immediate treatment by intravenous thiamine should be given on suspicion, without waiting for biochemical confirmation.

References

Abraham J., Rao P.S.S., Inbaraj S.G., Shetty G. & Jose C.J. (1970) An epidemiological study of hemiplegia due to stroke in South India. *Stroke* **1**, 477–82.

Allen J., Eldridge R. & Koerber T. (1974) Acoustic neuroma in the last months of pregnancy. *American Journal of Obstetrics and Gynecology*, **119**, 516–20.

Amias A.G. (1970a) Cerebral vascular disease in pregnancy. 1. Haemorrhage. *Journal of Obstetrics and Gynaecology of the British Commonwealth* **77**, 100–20.

Amias A.G. (1970b) Cerebral vascular disease in pregnancy. 2. Occlusion. *Journal of Obstetrics and Gynaecology of the British Commonwealth* **77**, 312–25.

Aminoff M.J. & Logue V. (1974) Clinical features of spinal vascular malformations. *Brain* **97**, 197–210.

Angelini C., Govoni E., Bragaglia M. & Vergani L. (1978) Carnitine deficiency: acute post-partum crisis. *Annals of Neurology* **4**, 558–61.

Bailey C.J., Pool R.W., Foskitt E.M.E. & Harris F. (1983) Valproic acid and fetal abnormality. *British Medical Journal* **286**, 190 (1 page only).

Bansal B.C., Prakash C., Gupta R.R. & Brahmanandam K.R.V. (1974) Study of serum lipid and blood fibrinolytic activity in cases of cerebral venous/venous sinus thrombosis during the puerperium. *American Journal of Obstetrics and Gynecology* **119**, 1079–82.

Batson D.V. (1940) Function of the vertebral veins. *Annals of Surgery* **112**, 138–49.

Beal M.F. & Chapman P.H. (1980) Cortical blindness and homonymous hemianopia in the post-partum period. *Journal of the American Medical Association* **244**, 2085–7.

Beresford O.D. & Graham A.M. (1950) Chorea gravidarum. *Journal of Obstetrics and Gynaecology of the British Empire* **57**, 616–25.

Berkwitz N.J. & Lufkin N.H. (1932) Toxic neuronitis of pregnancy; a clinicopathological report. *Surgery, Gynecology and Obstetrics* **54**, 743–57.

Bickerstaff E.R., Small J.M. & Guest I.A. (1958) The relapsing course of certain meningiomas in relation to pregnancy and menstruation. *Journal of Neurology, Neurosurgery and Psychiatry* **21**, 89–94.

Bird M.T., Palkes H. & Prensky A.L. (1976) A follow up study of Sydenham's chorea. *Neurology (Minneapolis)*, **26**, 601–6.

Brown J.T. & McDougall A. (1957) Traumatic maternal birth palsy. *Journal of Obstetrics and Gynaecology of the British Empire* **64**, 431–5.

Calderon-Gonzalez R., Gonzalez-Canta N. & Rizzi-Hernandez H. (1970) Recurrent polyneuropathy with pregnancy and oral contraceptives. *New England Journal of Medicine* **282**, 1307–8.

Callaghan N. (1968) The migraine syndrome in pregnancy. *Neurology (Minneapolis)* **18**, 197–201.

Carroll T.D., Leak O. & Lee H.A. (1966) Cerebral thrombophlebitis in pregnancy and the puerperium. *Quarterly Journal of Medicine* **35**, 347–68.

Castaigne P., Laplane D. & Rousser M.G. (1977) Superior sagittal sinus thrombosis. *Archives of Neurology* **34**, 788–9.

Chambers D.C., Hall H.E. & Boyce J. (1967) Myasthenia gravis and pregnancy. *Obstetrics and Gynecology* **29**, 597–603.

Collaborative Group for the Study of Strokes in Young Women (1973) Oral contraception and increased risk of cerebral ischaemia or thrombosis. *New England Journal of Medicine* **288**, 871–8.

Coradello H. (1973) Über die Ausscheidung von Antiepiliptika in die Muttermilch. *Weiner Klinische Wochenschrift* **85**, 695–7.

Cornelio F., di Donato S., Peluchetti D., Bizzi A., Bertagnolio A., d'Angelo A. & Wiesmann U. (1977) Fatal cases of lipid storage myopathy with carnitine deficiency. *Journal of Neurology, Neurosurgery and Psychiatry* **40**, 170–8.

Cross J.N., Castro P.O. & Jennett W.B. (1968) Cerebral strokes associated with pregnancy and the puerperium. *British Medical Journal* **3**, 214–17.

Davis L.E. (1979) Normal laboratory values of c.s.f. during pregnancy. *Archives of Neurology* **36**, 443.

Desmond M.M., Schwanecke R.P., Wilson G.S., Yasunaga S. & Burgdorff R.N. (1972) Maternal barbiturate utilisation and neonatal symptomatology. *Journal of Pediatrics* **90**, 190–7.

Donaldson J.O. (1978) *Neurology of Pregnancy*, pp. 271. W.B. Saunders Co., Philadelphia, London & Toronto.

Edwards J.N.T., Fooks M. & Davey D.A. (1983) Neurofibromatosis and severe hypertension in pregnancy. *British Journal of Obstetrics and Gynecology* **90**, 528–30.

Estanol B., Rodriguez A., Conte G., Aleman J.M., Loyo M. & Pizzuto J. (1979) Intracranial venous thrombosis in young women. *Stroke* **10**, 680–4.

Falconer M.A. & Stafford-Bell M.A. (1975) Visual failure from pituitary and parasellar tumours occurring with favourable outcome in pregnant women. *Journal of Neurology, Neurosurgery and Psychiatry* **38**, 919–30.

Feldman G.L., Weaver D.D. & Lourie E.W. (1977) The fetal trimethadione syndrome. *American Journal of Diseases of Childhood* **131**, 1389–92.

Frazer D. & Turner J.W.A. (1953) Myasthenia gravis and pregnancy. *Lancet* **2**, 417–20.

Friedman M., Zimmer E.L., Peretz B.A., Borowich B., Zaarur M. & Paldi E. (1983) Spontaneous delivery in a woman with clinical brain death. *Journal of Obstetrics and Gynaecology* **3**, 323 (1 page only).

Friis M.L. (1979) Epilepsy among parents of children with facial clefts. *Epilepsia* **20**, 69–76.

Friis M.L., Boveng-Nielsen B., Sindrup E.J., Lund M., Fogh-Andersen P. & Hauge M. (1981) Facial clefts among epileptic patients. *Archives of Neurology* **38**, 227–9.

Garcia C.A., Dulcey S. & Dulcey J. (1979) Ruptured aneurysm of the spinal artery of Adamkiewicz during pregnancy. *Neurology* **29**, 394–8.

Golbus M.S., Longhman W.D., Epstein C.J., Halbaoch G., Stephens J.D. & Hall B.D. (1979) Prenatal genetic diagnosis in 3000 amniocenteses. *New England Journal of Medicine* **300**, 157–63.

Goldman K.P. (1974) Malignant thymoma in pregnancy. *British Journal of Diseases of the Chest* **68**, 279–83.

Goodwin J.F. & Lawson C.W. (1947) Status epilepticus complicating pregnancy. *British Medical Journal* **2**, 332–3.

Greer M. (1963) Benign intracranial hypertension in pregnancy. *Neurology (Minneapolis)* **13**, 670–2.

Hakim C.A. & Thomlinson J. (1969) Myotonia congenita in pregnancy. *Journal of Obstetrics and Gynaecology of the British Commonwealth* **76**, 561–2.

Hefferman L.P.M., Fraser R.C. & Purdy R.A. (1980) L5 radiculopathy secondary to a uterine leiomyoma in a primigravid patient. *American Journal of Obstetrics and Gynecology* **138**, 460–1.

Hiilesmaa V.K., Teramo K., Granström M.-L. & Bardy A.H. (1983) Serum folate concentrations in women with epilepsy: relation to antiepileptic drug concentrations, number of seizures and fetal outcome. *British Medical Journal* **287**, 577–9.

Hilsinger R.L., Adour K.K. & Doty H.E. (1975) Idiopathic facial paralysis, pregnancy and the menstrual cycle. *Annals of Otology, Rhinology and Laryngology* **84**, 433–42.

Hobbins J.C., Grannum P.A.T., Berkowitz R.l., Silverman R. & Mahoney M.J. (1979) Ultrasound in the diagnosis of congenital anomalies. *American Journal of Obstetrics and Gynecology* **134**, 331–45.

Hopkins A.P. & Wray S. (1967) The effect of pregnancy on dystrophia myotonica. *Neurology (Minneapolis)* **17**, 166–8.

Hoyt C.S. & Billson F.A. (1978) Maternal anticonvulsants and optic nerve hypoplasia. *British Journal of Ophthalmology* **62**, 3–6.

Hunter D.J.S. (1971) Acute intermittent porphyria and pregnancy. *Journal of Obstetrics and Gynaecology of the British Commonwealth* **78**, 746–50.

Ichikawa K., Kim R.C., Givelber H. & Collins G.H. (1980) Chorea Gravidarum. Report of a fatal case with neuropathological observations. *Archives of Neurology* **37**, 429–32.

Janz D. (1982) Anti-epileptic drugs and pregnancy: altered utilisation patterns and teratogenesis. *Epilipsia* **23** (suppl.), 353–63.

Janz D., Bossi L., Dam M., Helge H., Richens A. & Schmidt D. (1982) *Epilepsy, Pregnancy and the Child.* Raven Press, New York.

Jarvis, G.J. & Crompton, A.C. (1978) Neurofibromatosis and pregnancy. *British Journal of Obstetrics and Gynaecology* **85**, 844–6.

Jefferson A. & Clark J. (1976) Treatment of benign intracranial hypertension by dehydrating agents. *Journal of Neurology, Neurosurgery and Psychiatry* **39**, 627–39.

Jennett W.B. & Cross J.N. (1967) Influence of pregnancy and oral contraception on the incidence of strokes in women of child-bearing age. *Lancet* **1**, 1019–23.

Jewett J.F. (1975) Committee on maternal welfare. Herpes simplex encephalitis. *New England Journal of Medicine* **292**, 530.

Johnson R.T. (1972) Effects of viral infections on the developing nervous system. *New England Journal of Medicine* **287**, 599–604.

Kalbag R.M. & Woolf A.L. (1967) *Cerebral Venous Thrombosis*, pp. 280. Oxford University Press.

Knight A.H. & Rhind E.G. (1975) Epilepsy and pregnancy: a study of 153 pregnancies in 59 patients. *Epilepsia*, **16**, 99–110.

Koup J.R., Rose J.Q. & Cohen M.E. (1978) Ethosuximide pharmokinetics in a pregnant patient and her new-born. *Epilepsia* **19**, 535–9.

Krayenbühl H.A. (1967) Cerebral venous and sinus thrombosis. *Clinical Neurosurgery* **14**, 1–24.

Lander C.M., Edwards V.E., Eadie M.J. & Tyrer J.H. (1977) Plasma anticonvulsant concentrations during pregnancy. *Neurology* **27**, 128–31.

Lavin P.J.M., Bone I., Lamb J.T. & Swinburne L.M. (1978) Intracranial venous thrombosis in the first trimester of pregnancy. *Journal of Neurology, Neurosurgery and Psychiatry* **41**, 726–9.

Leck I. (1983) Spina bifida and anencephaly: fewer patients, more problems. *British Medical Journal* **286**, 1679–80.

Mahoney M.J., Haseltine F.P., Hobbins S.C., Banker B.Q., Caskey T. & Golbus M.S. (1977) Prenatal diagnosis of Duchenne's muscular dystrophy. *New England Journal of Medicine* **297**, 968–73.

Marecek Z. & Graf M. (1976) Pregnancy in penicillamine treated patients and Wilson's disease. *New England Journal of Medicine* **295**, 841–2.

McAlpine D., Lumsden C.E. & Acheson E.D. (1972) *Multiple Sclerosis: a Reappraisal*, 2nd ed., pp. 653. Churchill Livingstone, London.

Metrakos K. & Metrakos J.D. (1974) Genetics of epilepsy. In Vinken P.J. and Bruyn G.W. (eds) *Handbook of Clinical Neurology*. Elsevier, Amsterdam.

Milunsky A. (1976) Current concepts in genetics. Prenatal diagnosis of genetic disorders. *New England Journal of Medicine* **295**, 377–80.

Montouris G.D., Fenichal G.M. & McLain, W. (1979) The pregnant epileptic. A review and recommendations. *Archives of Neurology* **36**, 601–3.

Mygind K.I., Dam M. & Christiansen J. (1976) Phenytoin and phenobarbitone plasma clearance during pregnancy. *Acta Neurologica Scandinavica* **54**, 160–6.

Nakane Y., Okuma T., Takahishi R. *et al* (1980) Multi-institutional study on the teratogenicity and foetal toxicity of anti-epileptic drugs: a report of a collaborative study group in Japan. *Epilepsia* **21**, 663–80.

Namba T., Brown S.B. & Grob D. (1970) Neonatal myasthenia gravis. *Pediatrics* **45**, 488–504.

Nath M., Vivian J.M. & Cherny W.B. (1979) Autonomic hyperreflexia in pregnancy and labor. *American Journal of Obstetrics and Gynecology* **134**, 390–2.

Nelson K.B. & Ellenberg J.H. (1982) Maternal seizure disorder, outcome of pregnancy, and neurologic abnormalities in the children. *Neurology* **32**, 1247–54.

Nickerson C.W. & Kirk R.F. (1965) Recurrent pseudotumor cerebri in pregnancy. *Obstetrics and Gynaecology* **25**, 811–13.

O'Connell J.E.A. (1944) Maternal obstetrical paralysis. *Surgery, Gynecology and Obstetrics* **79**, 374–82.

Paulson R.B., Paulson G.W. & Jreissaty M.S. (1979) Phenytoin and carbamazepine in production of cleft palates in mice. *Archives of Neurology* **36**, 832–9.

Paulson G.W. & Paulson R.B. (1981) Teratogenic effects of anticonvulsants. *Archives of Neurology* **38**, 140–3.

Pearson M.G. (1957) Meralgia paraesthetica, with reference to its occurrence in pregnancy. *Journal of Obstetrics and Gynaecology of the British Empire* **64**, 427–30.

Perry C.P., Hilliard G.D., Gilstrap L.C. & Harris R.E. (1975) Myasthenia gravis in pregnancy. *American Journal of Medical Sciences* **12**, 219–21.

Pinching A.J., Peters D.K. & Newsom-Davis J. (1976) Remission of myasthenia gravis following plasma exchange. *Lancet* **2**, 1373.

Plauche W. (1964) Myasthenia gravis in pregnancy. *American Journal of Obstetrics and Gynecology* **88**, 404–17.

Powell J.L. (1972) Pseudo tumour cerebri and pregnancy. *Obstetrics and Gynecology* **40**, 713–18.

Pulsinelli W.A. & Hamill R.W. (1978) Chorea complicating oral contraceptive therapy. *American Journal of Medicine* **65**, 557–9.

Ramsay R.E., Strauss R.G., Wilder J. & Willmore L.J. (1978) Status epilepticus in pregnancy: effect of phenytoin malabsorption on seizure control. *Neurology* **28**, 85–9.

Riddoch D., Jefferson M. & Bickerstaff E.R. (1971) Chorea and the oral contraceptives. *British Medical Journal* **4**, 217–19.

Robertson D.N.S. (1972) Pregnancy and labour in the paraplegic. *Paraplegia* **10**, 209–12.

Robinson J.L., Hall C.J. & Sedzimir C.B. (1972) Subarachnoid haemorrhage in pregnancy. *Journal of Neurosurgery* **36**, 27–33.

Robinson J.L., Hall C.H. & Sedzimir C.B. (1974) Arteriovenous malformations, aneurysms and pregnancy. *Journal of Neurosurgery* **41**, 63–70.

Ruprah M., Perucca E. & Richens A. (1980) Decreased serum protein binding of phenytoin in late pregnancy. *Lancet* **2**, 316–17.

Sarnat H.B., O'Connor T. & Byrne P.A. (1976) Clinical effects of myotonic dystrophy on pregnancy and the neonate. *Archives of Neurology* **33**, 459–65.

Scheinberg I.H. & Sternlieb I. (1975) Pregnancy in penicillamine treated patients with Wilson's disease. *New England Journal of Medicine* **293**, 1300–2.

Shekleton, P., Fidler, J. & Grimwade, J. (1980) A case of benign intracranial hypertension in pregnancy. *British Journal of Obstetrics and Gynaecology* **87**, 345–7.

Shore R.N. & MacLachlan T.B. (1971) Pregnancy with myotonic dystrophy. *Obstetrics and Gynecology* **38**, 448–54.

Singh B.M., Morris L.J. & Strobos R.J. (1980) Cortical blindness in puerperium. *Journal of the American Medical Association* **243**, 1134.

So E.L. & Penry J.K. (1981) Epilepsy in adults. *Annals of Neurology* **9**, 3–16.

Solomon G.E., Hillgartner M.W. & Kutt H. (1973) Coagulation defects caused by phenobarbitol and primidone. *Neurology (Minneapolis)* **23**, 445–51.

Somerville B.W. (1972) A study of migraine in pregnancy. *Neurology (Minneapolis)* **22**, 824–8.

Somerville B.W. (1975a) Estrogen—withdrawal migraine. I. *Neurology (Minneapolis)* **25**, 239–44.

Somerville B.W. (1975b) Estrogen—withdrawal migraine. II. *Neurology (Minneapolis)* **25**, 245–50.

Strauss R.G. & Bernstein R. (1974) Folic acid and Dilantin antagonism in pregnancy. *Obstetrics and Gynecology* **44**, 345–8.

Sudo N. & Weingold A.B. (1975) Obstetric aspects of the Guillain–Barré syndrome. *Obstetrics and Gynecology* **45**, 39–43.

Swapp G.H. & Main R.A. (1973) Neurofibromatosis in pregnancy. *British Journal of Dermatology* **80**, 431–5.

Sweeney W.J. (1958) Pregnancy and multiple sclerosis. *Clinical Obstetrics and Gynecology* **1**, 137–45.

Teng P. & Osserman K.E. (1956) Studies in myasthenia gravis—neonatal and juvenile types. *Journal of Mount Sinai Hospital* **23**, 711–40.

Thorner M.O., Besser G.M. & Jones A.M. (1975) Bromocriptine treatment of female infertility. *British Medical Journal* **4**, 694–7.

Victor M., Adams R.D. & Collins G.H. (1971) *The Wernicke–Korsakoff Syndrome.* Davis, Philadelphia.

Wallace J.T. & Cook A.W. (1957) Carpal tunnel syndrome in pregnancy. *American Journal of Obstetrics and Gynecology* **73**, 1333–6.

Willson P. & Preece A.A. (1932) Chorea gravidarum. *Archives of Internal Medicine* **49**, 471–533 and 671–97.

Wood P., Murray A., Sinha B., Godley M. & Goldsmith H.J. (1983) Wernicke's encephalopathy induced by hyperemesis gravidarum. *British Journal of Obstetrics and Gynaecology.* In press.

Working Party of the Medical Research Council (1978) An assessment of the hazards of amniocentesis. *British Journal of Obstetrics and Gynaecology* (Suppl. 2), 1–41.

Workshop (1981) Workshop on Epilepsy, Pregnancy and the Child. *Epilepsia* **22**, 365–75.

15 Fever and Infectious Diseases

Rosalinde Hurley

Pathophysiology

Persistent elevation of the body temperature above those levels that are normal in an individual is defined as fever. Regardless of race or climatic environment, the body temperature usually lies between 37.0°C and 37.5°C with diurnal variations so that evening temperatures are 0.5–1.0°C higher than those of the morning. Oral and axillary temperatures are 0.4°C and 1.0°C lower than that of the blood, but both are more reliable recordings than that taken per rectum.

Several explanations have been offered to explain disturbance of temperature regulation in disease. Shifts in body water may interfere with heat production and heat loss, and inadequate hydration causes temperature elevation in the newborn, although *per se* it does not seem to have this effect in adults. Metabolic rate affects body temperature, which is raised in thyrotoxicosis and lowered in myxoedema. Abnormalities of etiocholanolone metabolism occur in some patients with 'periodic fever' and administration of this substance, or of progesterone and some of its congeners, results in fever in man. Following intravenous injection of purified bacterial endotoxin or killed bacteria such as typhoid vaccine, the body temperature rises after about an hour. The patient feels cold, shivers, and has a rigor lasting some 10–20 minutes. The skin is pale and cold. As the rigor subsides, the patient feels warmer and complains of feeling feverish as the skin flushes. Profuse sweating begins, and the body temperature starts to fall toward normal. The underlying pathophysiological sequence of events seems to be the rapid removal of endotoxin from the blood stream by the fixed phagocytes of the reticuloendothelial system followed by margination of polymorphonuclear leucocytes along the walls of vessels. These and the fixed phagocytes are activated to release endogenous pyrogen (Bennett and Beeson 1950), which exists in the cells in inactive form, into the circulation. The pyrogen is a protein of low molecular weight produced in response to toxic, immunological, or infectious stimuli. Its production is induced through the release of lymphocytic lymphokines arising in response to antigenic recognition, and it acts on the hypothalamic thermoregulatory centre, transmitting information to the vasomotor centre, possibly through local production of prostaglan-

483

din. Heat generation is increased, heat loss is prevented and the body temperature rises. The release of endogenous pyrogen by phagocytic cells appears to be the common factor in the pathogenesis of fever, irrespective of its cause (Table 15.1). More detailed accounts of fever are given by Weinstein and Swartz (1979) and Dinarello and Wolff (1978).

The pattern of the febrile response, be it intermittent (falling to normal each day), remittent (falling each day, but still remaining elevated above the baseline), sustained (without significant diurnal variation), or relapsing (alternating with periods of one or several days of normal temperatures) is not particularly helpful clinically, although relapsing fever characterises malaria, relapsing fever itself, rat-bite fever, obstructive infection of the biliary or ureteric tracts, and some cases of Hodgkin's disease ('Pel–Ebstein fever'). Though not strictly a relapsing fever, listeriosis during pregnancy characteristically presents as two or more febrile episodes, the first usually being diagnosed as urinary tract infection (*see below*).

The perception of fever in individuals varies markedly, some patients, notably those with tuberculosis, being unaware of body temperatures as high as 39°C. Repeated rigors, though typical of septicaemia with pyogenic bacteria, may occur in non-infectious diseases, such as lymphoma but are rare in viral infections. Antipyretic drugs themselves may evoke or perpetuate a rigor. Some fevers, especially in pneumococcal and streptococcal infections, malaria, or meningococcal septicaemia are heralded or accompanied by cold sores. Prostration, malaise, backache and headache often accompany infectious fevers, and delirium may occur in bacterial fevers.

Fever is likely to be infectious in origin, its likely cause depending on the clinical circumstances and variations in locally endemic disease, although drug or serum fever, fever associated with malignant or thromboembolic disease, haemolytic disease or metabolic disorder may have to be considered in its differential diagnosis. Acute febrile illnesses of less than two weeks' duration are amongst the most frequent occurrences in medical practice; many are self-limiting, perhaps viral in origin, and definitive aetiological diagnosis is seldom made. However, prolonged febrile illnesses, in which the diagnosis remains obscure for weeks or months, do occur, and in some patients fever is the dominant sign or symptom. Before diagnosis is established, this condition is called pyrexia (or fever) of unknown (or uncertain) origin (FUO, PUO (Tables 15.2 and

Table 15.1   Pathogenesis of fever.

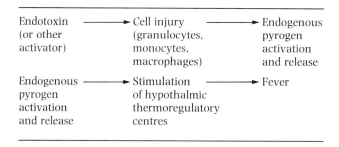

Table 15.2   Infectious diseases associated with prolonged fever (Europe and the United States).

Tuberculosis (Chapter 1)
Systemic mycoses
Cholecystitis, cholangitis and empyema of the gall bladder (Chapter 9)
Subphrenic hepatic and other intra-abdominal abscess
Appendicitis and diverticulitis
Pelvic inflammatory disease
Some types of urinary tract infection, e.g. ureteric obstruction (Chapter 7)
Retroperitoneal infection
Septicaemias—meningococcal, gonococcal, listeric, vibriosis, brucellosis
Infective endocarditis (Chapter 5)
Epstein–Barr, cytomegalovirus and coxsackie B virus disease
Q-fever and psittacosis
Parasitic infestations—malaria, amoebiasis, trichinosis
Leptospirosis and relapsing fever

15.3)), although the term should be reserved for those patients who have had episodes of fever in excess of 38°C for a period of at least three weeks, and who have been investigated for at least one week (Petersdorf and Beeson 1961).

Any of the acute or chronic specific infectious diseases may be contracted during the course of pregnancy or the puerperium, and conception may occur in women already subject to infection. In labour and in the early part of the puerperium, parturient women are peculiarly susceptible to serious infections of the genital tract, and child-bed fever has always been one of the most important causes of maternal death. Urinary tract infections are common in women, and are frequent during pregnancy and the puerperium (Brumfitt and Condie 1977). Wound infections, postoperative pneumonia,

Table 15.3   Non-infectious disease associated with prolonged fever.

Neoplasms
Metastatic carcinoma
Melanoma
Lymphomas—Hodgkin's disease
Leukaemias (Chapter 2)
Retroperitoneal sarcoma
Tumours of lung, kidney, pancreas, liver, heart

Connective tissue disease
Rheumatic fever (Chapter 5)
Systemic lupus erythematosus (Chapter 8)
Rheumatoid arthritis (Chapter 8)

Miscellaneous
Drug fever
Embolic disease
Sarcoidosis
Haemolytic disease

---

mastitis and breast abscess and thrombophlebitis may all occur in the puerperium. Most of the conditions enumerated above give rise to fever, and those that are most likely to occur in temperate climates are listed in Tables 15.4 and 15.5. Charles (1980) and Monif (1982) give good accounts of these diseases.

Casual or chance infections occurring during pregnancy range from mild illnesses to the major microbial diseases. In the Far East and in other parts of Asia, Africa and South America, pregnant women may be exposed to epidemic disease such as cholera, plague, the dysenteries (amoebic and bacillary), and enteric fevers. Pandemic influenza may also occur. In parts of Africa and in the Americas, systemic fungal infections (Table 15.6) such as coccidioidomycosis, histoplasmosis, and North and South American blastomycosis occur, and fever characterises certain parasitic infestations (Table 15.7).

Although serious microbial disease is well controlled in the UK and the USA, mothers of young children, particularly of those at school, are exposed to the specific infectious diseases of childhood and in addition to the common upper respiratory tract infections; in this way they may contract mumps, chickenpox, measles, rubella, scarlet

Table 15.4 Non-specific bacterial infections with fever complicating pregnancy or the puerperium.

Urinary tract infection (Chapter 7)
acute lower urinary tract infection
acute pyelonephritis
chronic pyelonephritis
Puerperal or post-abortal sepsis
endometritis
peritonitis
pelvic abscess
thrombophlebitis (Chapter 4)
intraperitoneal abscess
Septicaemia
Mastitis and breast abscess
Wound infection
Infective endocarditis (Chapter 5)

Table 15.5 Specific bacterial infections with fever complicating pregnancy or the puerperium.

Gonococcal septicaemia
Gonococcal salpingitis (acute, purulent)
Secondary syphilis (fever is unusual and low-grade)
Acute bacterial tonsillitis (streptococcal), rheumatic fever (Chapter 5)
Streptococcal septicaemia
Staphylococcal septicaemia
Other septicaemia (Gram-negative rods)
Listeriosis
Tuberculosis (Chapter 1)
Gas gangrene
Tetanus

Table 15.6 Fungal diseases with fever.

Disease	Geographical distribution	Remarks
Systemic candidosis	Worldwide	Rare during pregnancy, opportunistic infection
Cryptococcosis	Worldwide	Fever usually absent
North American blastomycosis	Southern, south eastern mid-western USA	Fever often low-grade
Paracoccidioidomycosis	South America	Fever often low-grade
Coccidioidomycosis (Chapter 1)	South western USA and Argentina	Half the infections are asymptomatic and afebrile—placental involvement is common in disseminated disease but congenital infection is not documented
Histoplasmosis	Americas, Africa, parts of Asia	Fever prolonged in severe cases
Phycomycosis	Worldwide	Opportunistic infection, rare
Aspergillosis	Worldwide	Fever lasts weeks or months in disseminated disease

Table 15.7 Parasitic diseases with fever.

Disease	Geographical distribution	Fever	Hazards to pregnancy
Fulminating amoebic dysentery	Worldwide	High	Pregnancy precipitates attack
Malaria	South and Central America, Africa, Asia	High relapsing	Anaemia, debility, cachexia of chronic or repeated infection more severe in pregnant women. Congenital disease Adventitious bacterial infection likely, and tuberculosis likely to extend and disseminate
Visceral leishmaniasis	Middle and Far East, Mediterranean, South and Central America	High irregular	
Trypanosomiasis	Mid, west and east Africa, Central and South America	High continuous or recurrent	
Toxoplasmosis	Worldwide	Usually absent	Risk of congenital transmission and congenital disease

fever or acute bacterial tonsillitis, whooping cough, dysentery or viral or other bacterial diarrhoea. As young adults, they may contract poliomyelitis, or toxoplasmosis, and hepatitis A, B, or non-A non-B may also occur (Hurley 1983). Enterovirus and echovirus infections, together with those ascribable to herpes viruses, in particular, to

Table 15.8 Viral infections during pregnancy implicated in fetal or neonatal disease (from Hurley 1982b).

Virus	Potential effect on mother	Potential effect on fetus or newborn
Coxsackie A	Herpangina, hand-foot-and-mouth disease; myocardiopathy	?Congenital defect
Coxsackie B	Often unnoticeable; aseptic meningitis; Bornholm disease	Myocarditis/meningoencephalitis ?Congenital heart disease ?Urogenital anomalies
Cytomegalovirus	Usually asymptomatic, but sometimes moderate to high fever in primary infection	Chronic infection; ?Congenital malformation; Mental retardation
Echoviruses	Rubella-like illness, fever, aseptic meningitis	Fatal disseminated viral infection (hepatic necrosis)
Hepatitis A and Hepatitis B (Chapter 9)	Flu-like illness; chills and high fever, constitutional symptoms and jaundice, increased severity during pregnancy	Prematurity, fetal death, neonatal hepatitis; vertical transmission of HBsAg
Herpes virus hominis	Oral or genital infection probably more severe in pregnancy	?Abortion ?Prematurity fatal disseminated infection
Influenza	Increased mortality in pandemics	?Increased fetal mortality ?Congenital defects ?Increase in childhood leukaemia and other malignant disease
Lymphocytic choriomeningitis	Meningitis/Meningoencephalitis	Congenital disease
Measles (Rubeola)	No special effect	Probably increased fetal mortality
Mumps	No special effect	?Endocardial fibroelastosis ?Fetal or neonatal growth aberrations
Poliomyelitis	Increased susceptibility, severity and mortality during pregnancy	Fetal death, neonatal poliomyelitis
Polyoma viruses	Asymptomatic	?Increased risk of jaundice
Rubella	Often asymptomatic, or very mild illness	Fetal death; chronic persisting infection; congenital malformations
Varicella-zoster	Often more severe; maternal death	Neonatal varicella; probable specific defect
Vaccinia and variola	Increased severity and mortality	Fetal death; intrauterine neonatal smallpox or vaccinia
Venezuelan and western equine encephalomyelitides	Meningoencephalitis	Neonatal encephalitis

cytomegalovirus and herpes virus hominis types 1 and 2, are not uncommon, although few give rise to systemic disturbance. The common virus infections of pregnancy are shown in Table 15.8. Fever may be marked in some of these infections, for example, in hepatitis, primary herpes or cytomegalovirus infections, influenza, mumps, measles and the meningoencephalitides, but is often low grade and transitory. Their diagnosis is, however, important because of their known or reported deleterious effects on the fetus. Accounts of the clinical manifestations of the viral diseases commonly occurring during pregnancy are given by Hurley (1977, 1982b), Hanshaw and Dudgeon (1978), and Charles (1980).

Most fevers presenting during pregnancy do not give rise to diagnostic difficulties, related as they are to disorders of the urinary or reproductive tracts, or to intercurrent infections that are common and frequent in the community. However, as in the nonpregnant, prolonged fever poses problems of investigation and diagnosis. With so many possible causes, it is not feasible to outline a scheme of investigation that is pertinent to every cause of fever. Clinical acumen, based on careful history-taking and accurate recording of the chronology of symptoms and signs, together with thorough clinical examination provide important leads. The place of residence, visits abroad, occupation and hobbies, keeping of pets, contact with known cases of infectious disease, localising symptoms, skin rashes, heart murmurs, presence of masses, enlargement of spleen or liver, all give clues to the differential diagnosis.

Useful laboratory tests, particularly in prolonged fever, include the following: cultures of blood or bone marrow (endocarditis, septicaemia, brucellosis, salmonellosis, listeriosis); serum enzymes (hepatocellular disease); blood counts and smears (blood dyscrasias, typhoid fever, parasitic infestation, lupus erythematosis, glandular fever, acute pyogenic infections); tests for specific antibody (viral diseases, enteric fever, toxoplasmosis, venereal diseases); immunological tests (connective tissue diseases); and cold agglutinins (mycoplasma infections). During pregnancy, the urine should always be examined microbiologically, and physical examination may indicate that throat or vaginal swabs should be cultured. If specific lesions (e.g. herpetic vesicles) are present or there is reason to suspect viral infection, viriculture or electronmicroscopy is indicated, although diagnosis is usually established serologically. In the puerperium, specimens from throat, genital and urinary tracts, and a blood culture should always be examined. If there is any indication of breast pathology, expressed breast milk should also be examined. The erythrocyte sedimentation rate, haemoglobin concentration, haemoglobin electrophoresis, blood smears and blood counts should be performed if the cause of fever remains obscure.

Infections associated with pregnancy and the puerperium

ASSOCIATED INFECTIONS

These are all acute infections, though recrudescence of chronic infection may occur. None is peculiar to pregnancy, but their incidence is increased in pregnant as compared with nonpregnant women.

URINARY TRACT INFECTIONS (*see also* Chapter 7)

These are fully described by Brumfitt and Condie (1977) and by Charles (1980). Infections of the urinary tract afflict some 6–7 per cent of pregnant women, occurring also with increased frequency during the puerperium. Much emphasis is placed on their early diagnosis and treatment. Any part of the renal tract may be involved and, with modern bacteriological techniques, infection by significant numbers of organisms can be detected before the onset of symptoms. The infections may be acute and primary, or recrudescences of chronic infection; they range from urethritis to acute pyelonephritis, which, in former days, was sometimes accompanied by blood stream infection ('catheter fever'). The usual causes during pregnancy are members of the *Enterobacteriaceae* and other Gram-negative rods, as well as the pathogenic Gram-positive cocci. The relationship of the less flagrant forms of urinary tract sepsis to abortion, prematurity, low birthweight and stillbirth is not established with certainty.

Three major clinical syndromes are distinguishable: acute lower urinary tract infection, acute pyelonephritis, and chronic pyelonephritis. Infections of the lower urinary tract can be followed by acute pyelonephritis, but in adult women without obstruction, it is rare for the acute infection to become chronic. In any case, chronic pyelonephritis probably has several causes, of which infection is but one. The presenting symptoms include frequency of micturition, dysuria, strangury and suprapubic discomfort (urethral syndrome, cystitis), often with no fever or one of low grade. Although the infection may settle spontaneously within a few days, there is some danger of recurrence, and urinary reflux may result in ascending infection with acute pyelonephritis. About 5 per cent of pregnant women have significant bacteriuria (more than 100 000 organisms per ml) and some 40 per cent of these will develop overt urinary tract disease as pregnancy advances. Dilatation of the ureters, and urinary stasis contribute to this outcome. Those with asymptomatic bacteriuria are usually given a week's course of antibiotic therapy (sulphonamide, ampicillin or other).

The onset of acute pyelonephritis is usually sudden, with fever, shivering and rigors, malaise, pain in the loins, frequency and dysuria and tenderness in the renal angle. Pus appears in the urine and there is a leucocytosis. Bedrest is important, and the fluid intake should be at least three litres a day. If the urine is acid, as it is with *Escherichia coli* infection, an alkaline mixture should be given. The results of bacteriological examination help in the choice of antibiotic to which the infecting microbe is sensitive. Nevertheless, treatment is usually started 'blind' with ampicillin or cephalosporin before the sensitivities are known. The urine should be cultured again, after apparent cure, to ensure that bacteriuria has not persisted.

Chronic pyelonephritis may present as chronic renal failure, sometimes preceded by symptomless proteinuria, or as a febrile illness, similar in presentation to the acute form. Eradication of infection, if demonstrated, may take many months of therapy, and antibiotics may have to be used in reduced dosage. The urine must be cultured at regular intervals.

Pyelonephritis, or 'pyelitis of pregnancy' was once the most frequent and important of the medical complications of pregnancy, with an incidence of just over 1 per cent and a maternal mortality of 3–4 per cent at the beginning of the antibiotic era. Fetal loss, from prematurity was 16–30 per cent. The complete clinical picture of frank pyelonephritis is seen far less frequently nowadays, almost certainly owing to early diagnosis and the prompt administration of antibiotics. Characteristically, the onset of the acute disease is about the fifth or sixth month of pregnancy or in the first week of the puerperium.

Most studies have shown that 4–7 per cent of women examined during pregnancy have significant bacteriuria, figures not unlike those recorded for the adult female population in general. Pregnancy itself need not cause any increase in prevalence of bacteriuria, though few would dispute the relationship of asymptomatic bacteriuria during early pregnancy to the subsequent development of symptoms referable to urinary tract infection. Acute pyelonephritis is particularly liable to develop in bacteriuric women, early treatment substantially reducing its incidence. For this reason, many antenatal clinics send urine to be screened for bacteriuria by quantitative methods. The term 'significant bacteriuria' implies that bacteria are multiplying in the bladder urine and, therefore, that infection as opposed to microbial contamination is present. Under the circumstances, the bacterial population, usually of known urinary pathogens, will ordinarily exceed 100 000 per ml of urine. The specimen must be taken correctly and either processed promptly or stored at 4°C for examination later on the same day.

The principal route of infection is probably an ascending one, and the risk of introducing infection by catheterisation has long been recognised. Much hospital-acquired infection, following catheterisation or operations on the bladder, is associated with organisms that are being disseminated in the wards. Another route of infection is the lymphatic system, for the right kidney has a direct connection, via the lymphatics, with the ascending colon, to which it is directly related. Infection may be blood-borne and blood cultures are often positive in pyelonephritis. Experimentally, the intravenous injection of some urinary pathogens into laboratory animals causes localised disease of the kidney, but in the case of *Escherichia coli*, the ureter must have been ligated or the kidney previously damaged, suggesting that local anatomical anomaly or malfunction is important in its genesis.

In the female, the proximity of the urethral orifice to the rectum, and the moist environment of the perineum, favour growth of microbes, including pathogens of the urinary tract. The distal 4 cm of the urethra is colonised by bacteria. Local minor trauma such as that occasioned by sexual intercourse may favour bacterial multiplication and, during pregnancy, increased concentrations of aminoacids and lactose are believed to encourage growth of *E. coli* in the urine.

Mechanical factors, especially those that obstruct urinary flow, are important in promoting bacterial infection, and the immediate predisposing cause of urinary tract infections during pregnancy is stasis. Progesterone causes dilation of the ureters and oestrogens cause muscular hypertrophy at a time when changing anatomical relationships in the pelvis lead to a compression of the right ureter. Complete bladder emptying is important, for present evidence suggests that bacteria coming into contact with the mucosa are killed. Interference with normal micturition, such as may occur during delivery or in operations to repair the pelvic floor, promotes infection. Ureteric valve incompetence leading to reflux during pregnancy has been postulated but not demonstrated.

Most of the infections that occur sporadically in the population are caused by *E. coli* which is also most frequently isolated in obstetric and gynaecological practice. Organisms less frequently isolated include *Proteus* spp., *Str. faecalis*, *Klebsiella* spp., staphylococci and *Ps. aeruginosa*, *Micrococcus* spp. and *Staph. epidermidis* as well as *Enterobacteriaceae* carried in the introitus which are associated with the 'frequency–dysuria' or 'urethral' syndrome, in which patients have symptoms suggestive of cystitis.

The bacteriological diagnosis of urinary tract infection depends on quantitative examination of freshly voided urine. Care must be taken in collection of specimens from women, and catheterisation should be avoided. If the results of culture are equivocal or if there is persistent contamination, the urine may be sampled directly by suprapubic aspiration, which is quite safe in pregnant women. The presence of 100 000 organisms per ml is generally accepted as the criterion of infection within the urinary tract and special methods, including serotyping, may serve to distinguish relapse from reinfection.

Sulphonamides, ampicillin, cephalexin and other cephalosporins, and nitrofurantoin are all used in treatment. Cotrimoxazole is also effective, though not generally recommended because of its potential toxicity.

With early diagnosis and prompt and successful treatment, the long-term prognosis in terms of chronic infection and renal damage is good. However, it is prudent to follow the outcome in those who have responded slowly or only partially to treatment, and further urine examinations and intravenous pyelography—the latter carried out not less than three months postpartum—may be required.

Puerperal sepsis and wound infections

Puerperal sepsis includes a series of febrile disorders of the lying-in period that share the common aetiology of being wound infections of the genital tract. It may occur after delivery or abortion and is occasioned by several genera of pathogenic bacteria, of which the most notorious and dangerous are *Clostridium* and *Streptococcus*. In the great majority of fatal cases, the microbes are introduced from without, and such infections are preventable. In general, endogenous microbes, harboured in the vagina, such as *Enterobacteriaceae* and *Staphylococcus* cause less severe forms of sepsis.

Since the establishment of rigid schedules of asepsis and antisepsis in maternity units over the last century and since the introduction of chemotherapeutic agents and antibiotics, the aetiological pattern of serious puerperal sepsis has altered. Formerly, exogenous microbes accounted for the majority of fatal cases, being mainly Lancefield Group-A β haemolytic streptococci originating from the attendants, the patient's own body outside the genital tract, and from visitors; they spread to the parturient patient by droplet infection, infected dust, infected hands and contaminated fomites, such as instruments and dressings. Nowadays, aerobic non-haemolytic streptococci, anaerobic streptococci, members of the *Enterobacteriaceae*, occasionally staphylococci, *Cl. welchi*, *Str. faecalis* (Lancefield Group D) or haemolytic streptococci of other groups are encountered. As well as having extrinsic origins, all can be isolated from the vagina regularly. *Bacteroides*, *Mycoplasma* and other genera may be implicated in puerperal sepsis, as in other infections of the genital tract, but their causal relationship to disease therein and their relative frequency has been less thoroughly studied.

Puerperal sepsis is a wound infection which may involve any part of the parturient genital tract from infected episiotomies, perineal or cervical lacerations, metritis and endometritis, to involvement of the uterine appendages, with local or generalised peritonitis and invasion of the blood stream. Disease localised to the genital tract proper does not run a fatal course, but the prognosis is poor if peritonitis or blood stream infection supervenes as it is very likely to do if the causative agent is an unchecked streptococcus. The factors predisposing to infection include premature rupture of the membranes, repeated examination of the vagina, instrumentation and internal monitoring of labour, lacerations of the birth canal, episiotomy, manual rotation, and forceps delivery. An increased rate of postpartum endometritis follows Caesarean section. Factors tending to lower general resistance, such as malnutrition, intercurrent disease, anaemia, haemorrhage and maternal exhaustion also promote infection. The retention of blood clot, or of fragments of membrane or placenta encourages infection by providing a nidus in which bacteria may multiply. The basis of prevention is scrupulous hygiene, with a short labour and few vaginal examinations, followed by an uncomplicated vaginal delivery.

Fever is the cardinal sign of puerperal sepsis, and may arise before, during or after labour. Puerperal pyrexia occurring in the 48 hours succeeding delivery or abortion may also be caused by urinary tract infection, administration of contaminated intravenous infusions, aspiration pneumonia, or retained products of conception. Septic thrombophlebitis, 'third day fever', infection of an abdominal wound, breast engorgement with or without incipient mastitis or breast abscess, drug fevers, surgical misadventure with swabs or other foreign bodies, and fortuitous infection in sites remote from the genitourinary tract should all be considered, especially when fever arises later in the puerperium. Patients with streptococcal endometritis appear acutely ill, with temperatures up to 39.5°C (104°F). The induration and purulent uterine discharge associated with less severe and more localised disease are usually absent, being replaced by diffuse slight pelvic tenderness and clear cervical discharge, in which Gram-positive cocci can be seen on staining. Treatment must be instituted without awaiting laboratory reports (*see below*). Low grade endometritis is characterised by diminution in the lochial flow before the onset of fever, uterine tenderness and a foul-smelling discharge from the endocervical canal.

The diagnosis of puerperal sepsis is made on clinical grounds, and the identity of the infecting microbes is established by the laboratory. Direct Gram-stained smears of exudate from the cervix or from within the uterus, are examined and the specimen is cultured. The nature and the sensitivity of the pathogen to antibiotics is usually established in less than 48 hours. The patient is treated with appropriate antibiotics, penicillin with an aminoglycoside being used for incipient severe infection, and safe, broad spectrum antibiotics being used for low grade infections if the aetiological diagnosis is completely open. Surgical measures are used as indicated, and supportive therapy is given, including bedrest, fluids, and oral hygiene.

Septic abortion and shock

The availability of contraceptive techniques and the legalisation of abortion has led to diminution in the number of women with septic abortion, but the diagnosis should be suspected in every febrile woman who is bleeding in the first trimester of pregnancy. In the majority of cases the cervical os is open, and there is evidence of the passage of the products of conception. High, spiking fevers and the presence of hypotension are bad prognostic signs. Pelvic examination, with assessment of uterine size is important, for most serious infections follow attempts to terminate pregnancy in women beyond the twelfth week of gestation. As in puerperal sepsis following delivery, extension of the infection beyond the uterus is attended by correspondingly grave risk for the patient. Plain X-rays of the abdomen with the patient both in the supine and the upright positions may demonstrate the presence of intraperitoneal or myometrial gas. Exploratory laparotomy may be required. Myometrial gas suggests *Cl. welchi* (perfringens) infection, and operative intervention may be required. Foreign bodies such as an intrauterine contraceptive device, may require removal. Many patients respond successfully to curettage and antibiotic therapy or even antibiotic therapy alone (*see* p. 244). Many antibiotics have been used, but the most favoured regimen is a combination of intravenous penicillin and metronidazole with intramuscular aminoglycoside in high dosage. The blood pressure and urinary output should be measured at regular intervals, and antibiotic concentrations should be assayed.

The microbes causing septic abortion are similar to those causing postdelivery sepsis, but nonsporing anaerobes, such as *Bacteroides fragilis*, may be implicated more frequently and with Gram-negative aerobes, such as *E. coli* and *Klebsiella* spp. are related to endotoxic shock. The onset of bacteraemia is accompanied by fever, rigors, nausea, vomiting, diarrhoea and prostration. Tachycardia, tachypnoea, hypotension, usually with cool, pale extremities and often with peripheral cyanosis, oliguria and mental confusion are added to the development of septic shock.

The haematological manifestations of severe shock are considered in Chapter 3 and the renal problems in Chapter 7.

Listeriosis

There is probably only one common diagnostic pitfall in the investigation of fever during pregnancy and the puerperium. Though there are many forms of listeriosis, including superficial disease, characteristically in pregnant women, listeriosis is associated with two or more febrile episodes (Hurley 1982a). The first, recognised only in retrospect as listeriosis, is associated with malaise, headache, fever, backache and abdominal or loin pain. Pharyngitis, conjunctivitis and diarrhoea are present in some cases. The condition is usually diagnosed as pyelonephritis, for the kidneys are involved in the listeric process, and often there seems to be a concomitant urinary tract infection with *E. coli* or other coliform. The patient is usually treated with antibiotics to which *L. monocytogenes* is susceptible and fever resolves only to return in 2–3 weeks, usually within 1–20 days of premature delivery of an infected child. The true nature of these episodes of fever will be recognised if the often slowly growing *Listeria* is actively sought in cultures of blood and other sites, such as the genital tract and urine and, after delivery, in the placenta and various sites in the sick newborn. If the child is born dead, postmortem cultures of heart blood, cerebrospinal fluid and viscera should be made. In about 40 per cent of cases of maternal listeriosis, fever is not marked and the patient presents with an influenza-like illness. Maternal and perinatal infections may require prolonged therapy (Table 15.9). Ampicillin should be given in high doses—at least 8 g/day in adults and 150 mg/kg/day in infants. Impairment of renal function reduces the rate of excretion of ampicillin and the dose can be reduced accordingly. Very high serum concentrations may be associated with cerebral irritation. Less common than listerosis as a diagnostic problem, but equally important, is the occurrence of infective endocarditis, particularly when it occurs after prophylaxis with appropriate antibiotic (Hurley 1977). The diagnosis is established by blood culture.

Toxoplasmosis

Toxoplasmosis is probably unique amongst the parasitic diseases of man in that its congenital form was recognised before that of postnatally acquired infection. The reported incidence of the congenital disease in the UK, though not so high as in France, exceeds that of congenital syphilis. There is little difference in the prevalence rates between sexes although, clearly, the disease is more important and more frequently diagnosed in women of childbearing age. There are few data from which to derive morbidity, mortality or case fatality rates.

Although placental transmission has been demonstrated in chronically infected mice, in humans congenital infection is believed to follow primary infection and the prognosis for subsequent pregnancies is good. The risk to the fetus appears to be related to the gestational age at which primary maternal infection occurs, transmission being less likely in the first trimester, but resulting in more severe disease should it occur. Infection leading to stillbirth or neonatal death, or to survival with ocular and cerebral

Table 15.9   Listeriosis.

Treatment
Ampicillin and gentamicin
High doses parenterally (*see* above)
e.g. ampicillin 200 mg/kg BW/day, gentamicin 5–6 mg/kg/day
Continue for one week after fever subsides
Erythromycin or tetracycline for superficial disease

involvement occurs only in the offspring of mothers who acquire infection in the first or second trimester.

Although transmission rates as high as 33 per cent have been reported following primary maternal infection, 72 per cent of the infected newborn were spared overt clinical infection. Such asymptomatic infants may suffer no serious consequences or they may later develop chorioretinitis, blindness, strabismus, hydrocephaly or microcephaly, cerebral calcification, psychomotor or mental retardation, epilepsy, or deafness. Children known to have had congenital toxoplasmosis must, therefore, be kept under observation for months or years. The available data are insufficient to support or to refute the hypothesis that *T. gondii* causes malformations during the period of organogenesis. The infected infant should be treated with spiramycin, or pyrimethamine/sulphonamide and folinic acid. There is some evidence that treatment of the mother who has an acute attack in pregnancy with spiramycin decreases the fetal risk.

Viral infections

Nearly a fifth of all perinatal deaths are ascribed to congenital malformations, especially those of the central nervous system. Although the majority of maternal viral infections cause little harm, some may result in severe damage to the fetus. Very careful prospective studies performed on large cohort populations and other studies have failed to establish, unequivocally, teratogenic potential in viruses other than rubella virus and cytomegalovirus, although a strong case can be advanced linking varicella-zoster infection with specific defect. There are many reports, retrospective analyses and partly controlled epidemiological studies attempting to link congenital malformations with maternal infection with mumps, influenza, varicella-zoster, hepatitis virus, EB virus, herpes virus hominis, coxsackie A4 viruses and measles. There is also considerable evidence linking the cardiotropic coxsackie B3 and B4 viruses with fetal myocarditis, but the relationship to congenital heart disease cannot, as yet, be regarded as proven.

Leaving aside teratogenic effects (i.e. malformations consequent on infections blighting the fetus during the period of organogenesis), there is evidence of increased rates of abortion and stillbirth in intrauterine rubella and in cytomegalovirus infection, and fetal and perinatal death has been reported in the course of maternal herpes virus hominis infections, varicella-zoster, hepatitis, mumps, poliomyelitis, or vaccinia, measles and influenza. Fetal wastage is not necessarily caused by viral invasion, but may be the result of maternal exhaustion and toxaemia.

Neonatal illness and congenital infection may result following infection with rubella, cytomegalovirus, herpes virus hominis, varicella-zoster, variola or vaccinia, poliovirus, coxsackie B virus, the myxoviruses, and the hepatitis viruses. In general, neonatal infection is more likely to follow maternal infection at or about the time of delivery.

Diagnosis of congenital virus infection is based on serological tests that indicate primary infection in the mother, and active infection in the newborn. Viriculture is helpful.

Congenital infections are often grouped together under the apt, if unlovely, name of TORCH, or as some would have it, STORCH. The initials denote syphilis, toxoplasmosis, other viruses, rubella, cytomegalovirus and herpes virus hominis. A diagnostic laboratory, warned of the clinical possibility of congenital infection, will institute appropriate serological tests for these agents.

References

Bennett I.L. & Beeson P.B. (1950) The properties and biological effects of bacterial pyrogens. *Medicine* **29**, 365.

Brumfitt W. & Condie A.P. (1977) Urinary infection. In E.E. Philipp, Josephine Barnes and M. Newton (eds) *Scientific Foundations of Obstetrics and Gynaecology*, pp. 754–67. Heinemann Medical, London.

Charles D. (1980) *Infections in Obstetrics and Gynaecology*, pp. 103–82. W.B. Saunders, Philadelphia.

Dinarello C.A. & Wolff S.M. (1978) Pathogenesis of fever in man. *New England Journal of Medicine* **298**, 607–712.

Hanshaw J.B. & Dudgeon J.A. (1978) *Viral Diseases of the Fetus and Newborn*. W.B. Saunders, Philadelphia.

Hurley R. (1977) Viral diseases in pregnancy. In G.V.P. Chamberlain (ed.) *Contemporary Obstetrics and Gynaecology*, pp. 68–82. Northwood Publications, London.

Hurley R. (1977) Heart disease, parturition and antibiotic prophylaxis. In P.J. Lewis (ed.) *Therapeutic Problems During Pregnancy*, pp. 69–79. MTP Press, Lancaster.

Hurley R. (1982a) Listeriosis. In *Oxford Textbook of Medicine*. Oxford University Press, London.

Hurley R. (1982b) Virus infections in pregnancy and the puerperium. In A.P. Waterson (ed.) *Recent Advances in Clinical Virology—3*. Churchill Livingstone, Edinburgh.

Hurley R. (1982c) Infection in pregnancy. In *Oxford Textbook of Medicine*. Oxford University Press, London.

Hurley R. (ed.) (1983) *Viral Hepatitis: a Problem in Hospital Practice*. S.O.G. Srl, Padua.

Monif G.R.G. (ed.) (1982) *Infectious Diseases in Obstetrics and Gynaecology*, 2nd edn. Harper and Row, Philadelphia.

Petersdorf R.G. & Beeson P.B. (1961) Fever of unexplained origin: report on 100 cases. *Medicine (Baltimore)* **40**, 1.

Weinstein L. & Swartz M.N. (1979) Host responses to infection. In W.A. Sodeman and T.M. Sodeman (eds) *Pathology Physiology*, 6th edn., pp. 545–9. W.B. Saunders, Philadelphia.

16 Drug Dependence

Michael de Swiet

The increase in the numbers of young people who abuse or are addicted to drugs has brought a corresponding increase in the number of women who abuse drugs during pregnancy. This is more of a problem in the USA from where most of the large series concerning drug addiction in pregnancy have been published; however, we still see drug addicts in hospitals in the UK, particularly those catering for the patients from the centres of large towns. Most of the following comments concern opiate addiction, but since drug addicts usually abuse several different sorts of drugs, it is difficult to be certain that the effects ascribed to opiate addiction are not due to some of the other drugs taken in addition. Also, illicit drugs are so expensive that the drug addict is forced to adopt a very poor standard of living, often also indulging in prostitution (with its associated risk of sexually transmitted diseases) to pay for her drugs. These nutritional and social factors must also affect the outcome of pregnancy in drug addicts. For comprehensive reviews of the problem of drug addiction in pregnancy in America see Finnegan (1978, 1979, 1980).

Effect of opiate addiction on pregnancy and its outcome

Finnegan (1979) quotes a number of obstetric complications including abortion, abruption, breech presentation, previous Caesarean section, etc., but she has not controlled for the social deprivation that we have already mentioned. From this point of view, a better series is that of Ostrea and Chaver (1979) who studied 830 opiate-dependent mothers delivered in one hospital in Michigan, and compared them with 400 controls matched for social class and race (86 per cent black). The relative risks of meconium-stained amniotic fluid, anaemia, premature rupture of membranes, haemorrhage, multiple pregnancy and intrauterine growth retardation are shown in Table 16.1. It can be seen that the risk of these complications for the drug addict ranges between 1.5 and 5.5 times the risk in the control population. The perinatal mortality was 2.5 times that of the control group. In addition, once born the infants had greater risks of jaundice, aspiration pneumonia (particularly meconium aspiration), transient tachypnoea and congenital abnormalities. The question of neonatal withdrawal is considered below. In contrast to earlier studies (Glass *et al* 1971) the incidence of

498

Table 16.1 Antenatal problems and condition of infants at birth in opiate addicts compared to controls* (from Ostrea and Chavez 1979).

	Addict ($n=830$) %	Control ($n=400$)	Relative risk (addict/control)
Meconium staining	21.2	13.8	1.5
Anaemia†	13.4	8.2	1.6
Premature rupture of membranes	12.2	7.8	1.6
Haemorrhage (abruption and placenta praevia)	3.0	1.2	2.5
Multiple pregnancy	3.4	1.2	2.8
Premature delivery (<38 weeks)	18.5	9.8	1.9
Small for gestational age‡	16.5	3.0	5.5
Apgar <6 at 1 minute	19.9	10.0	2.0
Perinatal mortality	2.7	1.0	2.7

*All differences were statistically significant $p<0.05$.
† Haemoglobin $\leqslant 10$ gm/dl.
‡ Less than tenth percentile for weight in the Lubchenco curve.

hyaline membrane disease in the premature drug-addicted group was the same as in the premature deliveries from the control group.

The congenital abnormalities found were varied; an excess risk has not been found in other studies (Finnegan 1979). At present, this should be considered a chance finding, but something to watch carefully.

It has been suggested that the frequent occurrence of meconium staining of the liquor, and hence of meconium aspiration, is part of the fetal response to maternal drug withdrawal. Liu *et al* (1976) cite reports from mothers that increased fetal movements occur before the mothers' subjective symptoms of withdrawal. Cardiotocographic findings, and falling maternal oestriol levels, also suggest fetal stress at the time of maternal withdrawal (Liu *et al* 1976). In addition, fetal asphyxia may be precipitated by the increased oxygen consumption caused by excessive movement in an already compromised fetus (Zuspan *et al* 1975).

The excess rate of multiple pregnancy has also been noted by Rementeria *et al* (1975) who found an overall multiple pregnancy incidence of one in 32 pregnancies— about three times their usual rate. The excess was contributed by dizygotic twins. Perhaps opiates stimulate the ovary to release an extra follicle, either directly or via the hypothalamus and gonadotrophin release.

Neonatal withdrawal syndrome

This will occur in 60–90 per cent of infants born to drug-dependent mothers (Hill and Desmond 1963; Zelson *et al* 1971), at between four hours and two weeks of age. The timing is related to the rate of metabolism of the opiate drugs. Heroin and morphia are metabolised rapidly, and infants will develop signs between four and 24 hours after delivery. Methadone is metabolised much more slowly, and signs do not occur until one day or even one week (Challis and Scopes 1977) or two weeks (Finnegan 1979) after delivery.

The neonatal withdrawal syndrome is characterised by signs of central nervous hyperirritability (increased reflexes and tremor) with gastrointestinal dysfunction (continual finger sucking, with regurgitation of feeds and diarrhoea) and respiratory distress (Finnegan 1979). Paediatricians are undecided as to whether treatment should be with dilute opium solutions such as paregoric (Finnegan 1978) or barbiturates (Finnegan 1979). In addition, chlorpromazine (Challis and Scopes 1977) and diazepam have also been used, but the latter causes a marked impairment in suckling (Finnegan 1978).

Neonatal abstinence syndrome has also been reported with other non-narcotic drugs of addiction, such as barbiturates, pentazocine, ethyl alcohol and amphetamines (Finnegan 1979).

Infants born to opiate-dependent mothers have an increased risk of dying unexpectedly from sudden infant death syndrome. This risk varies from 1.6 per cent (Harper *et al* 1973) to 21.4 per cent (Pierson *et al* 1972) compared to the overall population risk of 0.3 per cent (Southall *et al* 1982). Although there must be social factors accounting, in part, for this increased incidence, it is of great theoretical importance, because of the possible interference by opiates with the normal development of cardiorespiratory control in the newborn infant, either directly or through maternal hypoventilation (Metcalfe *et al* 1980).

It is encouraging that Sardemann *et al* (1976) who studied 19 infants for two years after delivery from drug-addicted mothers in Denmark, did not find any evidence of behavioural disturbance, impaired intelligence, or growth retardation. However, most of the children had spent long periods in institutional care.

Other drugs of addiction

The fetal effects of other drugs of dependence are even harder to define than those of opiates, because their abusers do not form such a clear cut group. However, it is indisputable that alcohol, if taken in sufficient quantities, will produce a specific fetal alcohol syndrome, first described by Jones and Smith (1973). The newborn child is growth retarded, with a characteristic facies, narrow palpebral fissure, epicanthal folds, short nose and long philtrum. In addition, the children are often mentally retarded, and may have other major congenital abnormalities. Although the condition had been considered to be very uncommon in the UK, Beattie *et al* (1983) have reported 40 cases from the West of Scotland, an area with a notoriously high incidence of alcoholism.

Overlap between the fetal alcohol syndrome and the DiGeorge syndrome, where immunodeficiency is a major feature, has also been postulated (Ammann *et al* 1982).

It is not clear what is the minimum daily alcohol intake that will affect the fetus, or the maximum daily intake that is safe. The majority of affected fetuses with the full fetal alcohol syndrome have been born to mothers taking large quantities of alcohol: on average, 174 ml per day—the equivalent of at least 17 drinks (Ouellette *et al* 1977). However, growth retardation has been reported in patients taking much smaller quantities of alcohol, more than 100–140 ml per week (Wright *et al* 1983; Davis *et al* 1982). Even though growth retardation will not inevitably occur in women taking one or two drinks per day, the zero option of no alcohol intake at all during pregnancy—as advised by the United States Surgeon General (1981)—is the only safe recommendation.

It is very unlikely that the fetal alcohol syndrome is due to intercurrent consumption of other drugs, because the syndrome is specific to alcoholics, and those taking this quantity of alcohol do not, as a group, consistently abuse any other one drug.

Lysergic acid diethylamide (LSD) and cannabis may be teratogenic. There are several isolated reports of phocomelia (Hecht *et al* 1968) and other typical amniotic band lesions (Carakushansky *et al* 1969; Assemany *et al* 1970) which have been discussed by Blanc *et al* (1971). It remains controversial whether these agents cause chromosomal damage in man (Hecht *et al* 1968).

The possible teratogenic effects of barbiturates are considered in Chapter 14.

Management of pregnancy in the drug-dependent woman

The majority of problems which can occur in drug-dependent women during pregnancy are not specific to drug dependency and could, and do, occur in others of low social class and poor health and nutrition. The specific problems relate to the choice of which opiate should be used, and interactions between opiates and other drugs during pregnancy. One further practical problem is that drug addicts usually have very few patent, superficial veins. Indeed they may be the only people that can successfully perform venepuncture on themselves.

In 1973, Zelson *et al* published a study from New York which purported to show that heroin-exposed infants had a much better neonatal outcome than methadone-exposed infants, with less severe withdrawal symptoms and no cases of hyaline membrane disease despite their prematurity. For these reasons, they suggested that mothers should not be taken off a 'street' supply of heroin by changing them to a methadone maintenance programme. This bold suggestion made quite an impact at the time, but it was challenged, largely because the groups of methadone- and heroin-treated addicts were not necessarily comparable (O'Brien 1974). The general view now is that patients and their offspring are much better managed in a methadone maintenance programme, than trying to obtain heroin or other more rapidly-acting opiates illegally. Such a programme will put the addict in contact with medical and social services, and this alone should improve her standard of living sufficiently to benefit her and her infant's health (Rosner *et al* 1982). The reason for using methadone is that it is metabolised much more slowly than heroin; its half life is 18–97 hours, and withdrawal symptoms do not occur until 72–96 hours after the last dose. The half life of heroin is 4–10 hours, and withdrawal symptoms may occur within 24 hours after the last dose. Patients may be maintained on an oral methadone regime and they and their fetuses are much less likely to have withdrawal symptoms than when they are taking heroin. In addition, most countries have narcotics' regulations which forbid the supply of heroin to addicts, but will legalise specific individuals to give methadone in cases of addiction. Unfortunately, patients may not like to change from heroin to methadone, because the latter does not produce the same feelings of pleasure. Nevertheless, for the reasons outlined above, all opiate addicts should be transferred to a methadone maintenance programme during pregnancy. The only exceptions are those that present in late pregnancy or during labour. Because drug addicts habitually lie, and because all 'street' heroin is diluted to a varying extent with fillers such as lactose, it is difficult to know exactly how much heroin the addict has in fact been taking. Therefore, transfer to an adequate methadone regime takes time, because of the need to find the right dose and the longer duration of methadone action. There is therefore a risk of precipitating a withdrawal state during transfer and, as indicated above, this may be particularly dangerous for the fetus. Indeed Liu *et al* (1976) have observed fetal distress in labour not due to recognised causes, which was relieved by administration of pethidine. For these reasons, it is best not to transfer to methadone the addict who presents late in pregnancy as an outpatient. Such patients should ideally be admitted and transferred to methadone with judicious use of short-acting narcotics, to render them symptom free, and to prevent fetal distress and premature labour (Fultz and Senay 1975). This is not an easy thing to do because of the manipulating, demanding characteristics of drug addicts, which cause considerable disruption in hospital routine, particularly in maternity hospitals, where the staff may not be experienced in managing such problems.

Analgesia during labour is best given by an epidural anaesthetic. If this is not possible, opiates such as pethidine can be given, but they will be less effective in an opiate addict. Because this effect is rather variable, it is better to give a standard dose, such as pethidine 100 mg intramuscularly more frequently, rather than a large (and possibly too large) dose at standard time intervals.

Pentazocine should not be used because it is a narcotic antagonist, and can precipitate a withdrawal reaction in an opiate addict (Fultz and Senay 1975). Overdose of opiate should be treated with the specific antagonist naloxone which is given in an initial dose of 200 μg, followed by 100 μg every two minutes according to response. The dose given to the neonate is 5–10 μg/kg. Nalorphine should not be used because it causes respiratory depression, even though it is an opiate antagonist. All opiate antagonists may cause very severe withdrawal symptoms in the mother or her child. If necessary, these can be treated with further doses of opiate.

Narcotics interact dangerously with other drugs causing CNS depression such as barbiturates, hypnotics, sedatives, general anaesthetics, and tranquillizers. These drugs should be given with great care, if at all, to drug addicts. In addition, muscle relaxants, such as D-tubocurarine can interact with opiates to cause severe respiratory depression.

Methadone is secreted in breast milk. The average concentration found by Blinick *et al* (1975) in a group of women taking an average of 52 mg per day was 0.27 μg/ml. This would be equivalent to a daily dose of 0.12 mg in an infant taking 450 ml of milk per day, or 0.04 mg/kg in a 3 kg infant. This is about one twentieth of the maternal dose of 0.74 mg/kg for a 70 kg mother, and is clearly very little. Since there have been no reports of adverse effects of breast feeding by drug-dependent mothers, it would seem sensible to encourage breast feeding in these patients, particularly since it may be difficult for them to bond to their children.

References

Ammann A.J., Wara D.W., Cowan M.J., Barrett D.J. & Stiehm E.R. (1982) The Di George Syndrome and the fetal alcohol syndrome. *American Journal of Diseases of Children* **136**, 906–8.

Assemany S.R., Neu R.L. & Gardner L.I. (1970) Deformities in a child whose mother took LSD. *Lancet* **1**, 1290.

Beattie J.O., Day R.E., Cockburn F. & Garg R.A. (1983) Alcohol and the fetus in the West of Scotland. *British Medical Journal* **287**, 17–20.

Blanc W.A., Mattison D.R., Kane R. & Chauhan P. (1971) L.S.D., intrauterine amputations and amniotic-band syndrome. *Lancet* **2**, 158–9.

Blinick G., Inturissi C.E., Jerez E. & Wallach R.C. (1975) Methadone assays in pregnant-women and progeny. *American Journal of Obstetrics and Gynecology* **121**, 617–21.

Carakushansky G., Neu K.L. & Gardner L.I. (1969) Lysergide and cannabis as possible teratogens in man. *Lancet* **1**, 150–1.

Challis R.E. & Scopes J.W. (1977) Late withdrawal symptoms in babies born to methadone addicts. *Lancet* **2**, 1230.

Davis P.J.M., Partridge J.W. & Storrs C.N. (1982) Alcohol consumption in pregnancy. How much is safe? *Archives of Disease in Childhood* **57**, 940–3.

Finnegan L.P. (1978) Management of pregnant drug-dependent women. *Annals of the New York Academy of Sciences* **311**, 135–46.

Finnegan L.P. (1979) Pathophysiological and behavioural effects of the transplacental transfer of narcotic drugs to the foetuses and neonates of narcotic-dependent mothers. *Bulletin on Narcotics* **31**, 1–59.

Finnegan L.P. (ed) (1980) *Drug Dependence in Pregnancy. Clinical Management of Mother and Child.* Castle House Publications.

Fultz J.M. & Senay E.C. (1975) Guidelines for the management of hospitalized narcotic addicts. *Annals of Internal Medicine* **82**, 815–18.

Glass L., Rajegowda B.K. & Evans H.E. (1971) Absence of respiratory distress syndrome in premature infants of heroin-addicted mothers. *Lancet* **2**, 685–6.

Harper G., Concepcion G.S. & Blenman S. (1973) Observations on the sudden death of infants born to addicted mothers. In *Proceedings Fifth National Conference on Methadone Treatment*, p. 1122. National Association for the Prevention of Addiction to Narcotics, New York.

Hecht F., Beals R.K., Lees M.H., Jolly H. & Romberts P. (1968) Lysergic-acid-diethylamide and cannabis as possible teratogens in man. *Lancet* **2**, 1087.

Hill R.M. & Desmond M.M. (1963) Management of the narcotic withdrawal syndrome in the neonate. *Pediatric Clinics of North America* **10**, 67–86.

Jones K.L. & Smith D.W. (1973) Recognition of the fetal alcohol syndrome in early infancy. *Lancet* **2**, 999–1001.

Liu D.T.Y., Tylden E. & Tukel S.H. (1976) Fetal response to drug withdrawal. *Lancet* **2**, 588.

Metcalfe J., Dunham M.J., Olsen G.D. & Krall M.A. (1980) Respiratory and haemodynamic effects of methadone in pregnant women. *Respiration Physiology* **42**, 383–393.

O'Brien C.P. (1974) Narcotic abuse during pregnancy. *New England Journal of Medicine* **291**, 311.

Ostrea E.M. & Chaver C.J. (1979) Perinatal problems (excluding neonatal withdrawal) in maternal drug addiction: A study of 830 cases. *Journal of Pediatrics* **94**, 292–5.

Ouellette E.M., Rosett H.L., Rosman P. & Weiner L. (1977) Adverse effects on offspring of maternal alcohol abuse during pregnancy. *New England Journal of Medicine* **297**, 528–30.

Pierson P.S., Howard P. & Kleber H.D. (1972) Sudden deaths in infants born to methadone-maintained addicts. *Journal of American Medical Association* **220**, 1733–4.

Rementeria J.L., Janakammal S. & Hollander M. (1975) Multiple births in drug-addicted women. *American Journal of Obstetrics and Gynecology* **122**, 958–60.

Rosner M.A., Keith L. & Chasnoff I. (1982) The North Western University Drug Dependence Program: The impact of intensive prenatal care on labor and delivery outcomes. *American Journal of Obstetrics & Gynecology* **144**, 23–7.

Sardemann H., Madsen K.S. & Friis-Hansen B. (1976) Follow-up of children of drug-addicted mothers. *Archives of Disease in Childhood* **51**, 131–4.

Southall D.P., Richards J.M., Shinebourne E.A., Franks C.I. & Wilson A.J. (1982) Prospective population-based studies into heart rate and breathing patterns in newborn infants; prediction of infants at risk of SIDS. *International Conference into SIDS*, Baltimore, 1982.

U.S. Surgeon General (1981) Surgeon General's Advisory on alcohol and pregnancy. *FDA Drug Bulletin* **11**, 9–10.

Wright J.T., Waterson E.J., Barrison I.G., Toplis P.J., Lewis I.G., Gordon M.G., MacRae K.D., Morris N.F. & Murray-Lyon I.M. (1983) Alcohol consumption, pregnancy and low birth weight. *Lancet* **i**, 663–5.

Zelson C., Rubio E. & Wasserman E. (1971) Neonatal narcotic addiction: 10 year observation. *Pediatrics* **48**, 178–89.

Zelson C., Lee S.J. & Casalino M. (1973) Neonatal narcotic addiction. Comparative effects of maternal intake of heroin and methadone. *New England Journal of Medicine* **289**, 1216–20.

Zuspan F.P., Gumpel J.A., Mejia-Zelaya A., Madden J. & Davis R. (1975) Fetal stress from methadone withdrawal. *American Journal of Obstetrics and Gynecology* **122**, 43–6.

Index

References to figures and tables are indicated by the prefix f or t.